2000

MCAT

THE SCIENCE OF REVIEW™

Complete Preparation for the
Medical College Admission Test

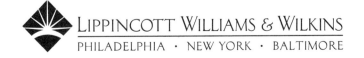
LIPPINCOTT WILLIAMS & WILKINS
PHILADELPHIA · NEW YORK · BALTIMORE

Acquisitions Editor: Elizabeth A. Nieginski
Marketing Manager: Jennifer Conrad
Compositor: Maryland Composition
Printer: Mack Printing Group

9 8 7 6 5 4 3 2 1

Library of Congress Cataloging-in-Publication Data

2000 MCAT : complete preparation for the Medical College Admission
Test.
        p.   cm.
    ''... the 2000 edition of Complete preparation for the MCAT ...''—Pref.
    Includes bibliographical references.
    ISBN 0-683-30779-7
    1. Medical colleges—United States—Entrance examinations—Study
guides.   2. Medicine—Examinations, questions, etc.   I. Title:
Complete preparation for the Medical College Admission Test.
    R838.5.C65   1999
    610'.76—dc21   98-55494
                                                             CIP

Test Dates

April 17, 1999	August 21, 1999

Selected Resources for Pre-Medical Information

Williams & Wilkins
Science of Review Hotline
1-800-634-4365
E-mail: mcatprep@wwilkins.com

Association of American
Medical Colleges
2450 N Street, NW
Washington, D.C. 20037
(202) 828-0416

MCAT Program Office
P.O. Box 4056
Iowa City, IA 52243
(319) 337-1357

Afrinatino, Inc.
1000 Ewing Road
Coraopolis, PA 15108
http://iweb4u.com/afrinatino

Student National Medical
Association, Inc.
National Office
1012 Tenth Street, NW
Washington, DC 20001
(800) 636-SMNA
E-mail: SMNA@SMART.NET

Columbia Review-Intensive
MCAT Preparation-Courses
220 Madison Avenue
San Francisco, CA 94134
(800) 300-PREP or (415) 337-2009

The Journal of Pre-Med Studies
P.O. Box 3029
Garden City, NY 11531
(516) 873-0626
E-mail: JMSFJEFF4@aol.com

Selected Internet Sites

Williams & Wilkins Homepage
http://www.wwilkins.com

AAMC Newsletter
http://www.aamc.org/events/aamcstat/
aamcnews.htm

Welcome to Premedical.com
http://www.premedical.com

American Medical
Student Association
http://www.amsa.org/

The Pre-Med and
Medical Information
http://www.efn.org/~brideb/Deb/medstuff/
Medstuff.html

World Wide Web for Premeds
http://www.washcoll.edu/WC.HTML/
academics/resources/premed.html

Pre Med Internet Resources
http://www.sc.edu/library/sciences/
premed/html

The Pre Med Major
http://ww2.globalvision.net/admissions/
pops/premed.html

UCI Chemistry/Instruction/
Online Resources/ Pre-Med
http://chem.ps.uci.edu/instructions/
premed.html

Finding Pre-Med Information
http://www.fas.harvard.edu/~cabref/
premed.html

MCAT Mania
http://mail.utep.edu/~lfloyd/hmome.html

Applying to Med School
http://www.geocities.com/Athens/7103/
apply.html

The Pre-Med Zone
http://www.netside.net/~hochstim/
index.html

Premed.Edu Hunter Pre-Med
http://www.spacelab.net/~premed/

Medical Servers
http://www.columbia.edu/cu/gspremed/
med.html

Premed@jhu
http://jhunix.hcf.jhu.edu/~scheel/aed/
v__two/v2for2top.html

Brad's Premed Resource Center
http://rio.atlantic.net/~xyz/premed.html

Alpha Epsilon Delta
http://www.utexas.edu/students/aed/

Students who have recently taken the MCAT had these comments:

I took the MCAT in April of 1996 as a senior undergraduate student at Brown University. I was fortunate in that I only had to take the exam once. I believe the most important thing to remember about taking the MCAT is that this exam is not necessarily about one's ability to retain tons of scientific information, it is about one's ability to solve problems logically. This does not mean you don't have to study if you are a good problem solver, it means memorizing facts and formulas should only be the beginning of your studying; spend enormous amounts of time taking the exams again and again. Try taking the exam in a crowded place to see if you can concentrate. Most importantly, remember it is only an exam. If you do not do well the first time, you can try again. Yes this is one of the more important exams you will have to take in your life, but keep everything in perspective. Good Luck!!!

Stephanie Davis

I needed to quickly relearn and synthesize the information. I felt overwhelmed about the amount of material I had to know. It frightened me and made me feel inadequate at times. However, I had a goal and I was going to accomplish that goal. Rather than getting stuck on a small point, I would try to understand major concepts, theories, and rules. It is important to understand the big picture. Also, I found it beneficial to take practice tests. I wish I had more time to take these tests and do an actual simulation. I would recommend that everyone take at least one full blown simulation and several other practice tests (including the writing sections). If I could go back and do it all over, I definitely would take more practice tests.

After taking the MCAT, I remember feeling relieved and accomplished. I had just completed something that I had invested lots of time, energy, and money into. However, I also had a great feeling of anxiety: did I do a certain problem correctly, did I write concise, to the point, and legibly, what are my scores going to be, and will my scores be good enough to get me into school? Though the MCAT tests some basic core science, I find it to be more of a test of endurance, dedication, and test taking strategies. The day my scores came, I didn't want to open the envelope. I was so relieved when I saw I did well enough to get into school. Preparation for the MCAT helped me fine tune my study habits and taught me ways to learn, memorize, and enhance test taking skills. As a medical student, I currently use many of these techniques. Overall, the MCAT helped me to prepare to be an efficient student.

Craig Flinders

The MCAT is not a true measure of intelligence. In fact, I believe everyone who meets the prerequisites for medical school has been exposed to the necessary concepts to do well on the test. Perhaps a more accurate description of the MCAT would include an element of desire. The desire and commitment to become a doctor. Like medical school, the MCAT requires time, repetition, and sacrifice. Think of the MCAT as a measure of your own personal commitment to the profession. The MCAT serves as a device to test your desire.

David Skolnick

I consider the MCAT to be a "catch 22" situation for most students. To answer all the questions, one needs to read very quickly. But if one reads very quickly, one is unlikely to answer the questions correctly. I found this to be a very difficult balance to achieve. The test day itself was stressful (since so much was at stake) and a great deal longer than I had expected since the test preparation manuals that I used did not account for breaks when indicating how long the test day was to be. The day was so long that one of the proctors fell asleep and actually snored. I found this to be immensely distracting. The room itself was comfortable and otherwise facilitated test-taking. I underestimated how much material was to be covered on the MCAT. I started to study for the test only four weeks beforehand and was, I felt, not thoroughly prepared. I consider the need to memorize a sizable number of physics formulas for the MCAT to be an unnecessary waste of time. Application, I believe, is more important than memorization and the physical sciences portion of the test should efficiently reflect this but does not. After taking the MCAT I felt as if I had spent 4 years in undergraduate school without learning a single thing. While taking the test I became very frustrated during the Physical Sciences and the Biological Sciences sections, the two I felt were most important. It seemed as if there were so many things on the test that I didn't know or couldn't remember. I was especially discouraged by the Physical Sciences section; so discouraged that I considered having my scores deleted after the lunch period. I thought that I had done horrible and I was concerned about admissions committees seeing a bad score. After finishing the test, I went home feeling very discouraged and disappointed. I felt that I had known so many more things when I took the practice tests and studied from the MCAT preparation books that I had purchased. I didn't feel any better about the test until my test scores came back. They turned out a lot better than I thought they would. It wasn't until then that I realized that I knew a lot of the things on the MCAT. It only seemed like I didn't because I was focusing only on the questions that I wasn't comfortable with and forgetting about the ones that I knew.

Brian Pollock

I hated taking the MCAT. Preparation for it was exhausting and drained my self-confidence. I felt as if the undergraduate science courses I had taken were inadequate in preparing me for this experience. I do not know how anyone could perform well on the rest without having taken some kind of preparatory course. The anxiety alone, associated with one's performance can be crippling on the day of the examination. I felt I would never take a more important test, or one that would have such an impact on the path I prayed my life would follow. The only positive thing I can now say, is that I'm here and all the hard work, tears and self-doubt were worth it to get here.

Ilysa Diamond

Contents

Writing Sample

Test-Taking Skills for the MCAT

Applied Math Concepts Required for Physical and Biological Sciences

Problem Solving in the Physical Sciences

Problem Solving in the Biological Sciences

Full-Length Practice MCAT

Preface to the 2000 Edition

The goal of the 2000 edition of *Complete Preparation for the MCAT: The Betz Guide* is to help busy students and practitioners prepare for all types of examinations in the health sciences, particularly the MCAT. Now in its seventeenth year of publication, the 2000 edition of this book is a culmination of our efforts in producing a self-managed MCAT study program. This edition includes advanced concepts from medical and premedical curricula. Problem-solving practice using passage-based problems is a special feature of this edition.

Information passages in this book, such as the paragraphs within each subsection, present material similar to that found in college textbooks. Review questions that follow each math and science section are organized at an increasing level of difficulty: straightforward review questions are followed by questions requiring problem-solving skills. The review questions demand a knowledge of the concepts presented, whereas the problem-solving questions, which are now more prevalent on the MCAT, require a greater ability to analyze, synthesize, and make judgments based on information presented or on knowledge acquired elsewhere.

Applied Concepts is a special feature of this edition. In each science topic of Chapters 7 and 8, current medical research, medical instrumentation, and experimental sciences are discussed. This feature also covers procedures and scientific models not covered in typical college courses. Familiarity with these concepts will provide you with current information about medical experimentation and scientific instruments used in medicine.

SCHEMATIC LAYOUT OF THIS BOOK

This layout provides a quick overview of the 2000 edition of *Complete Preparation for the MCAT*. The chapters are connected with arrows to emphasize the integration of knowledge and skills required by the Medical College Admission Test (MCAT).

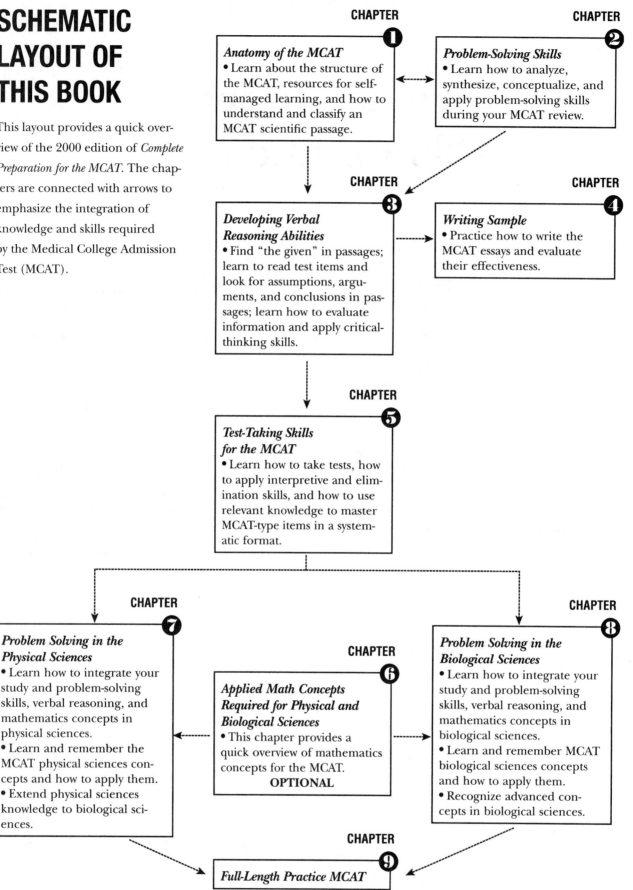

CHAPTER 1

Anatomy of the MCAT
• Learn about the structure of the MCAT, resources for self-managed learning, and how to understand and classify an MCAT scientific passage.

CHAPTER 2

Problem-Solving Skills
• Learn how to analyze, synthesize, conceptualize, and apply problem-solving skills during your MCAT review.

CHAPTER 3

Developing Verbal Reasoning Abilities
• Find "the given" in passages; learn to read test items and look for assumptions, arguments, and conclusions in passages; learn how to evaluate information and apply critical-thinking skills.

CHAPTER 4

Writing Sample
• Practice how to write the MCAT essays and evaluate their effectiveness.

CHAPTER 5

Test-Taking Skills for the MCAT
• Learn how to take tests, how to apply interpretive and elimination skills, and how to use relevant knowledge to master MCAT-type items in a systematic format.

CHAPTER 7

Problem Solving in the Physical Sciences
• Learn how to integrate your study and problem-solving skills, verbal reasoning, and mathematics concepts in physical sciences.
• Learn and remember the MCAT physical sciences concepts and how to apply them.
• Extend physical sciences knowledge to biological sciences.

CHAPTER 6

Applied Math Concepts Required for Physical and Biological Sciences
• This chapter provides a quick overview of mathematics concepts for the MCAT.
OPTIONAL

CHAPTER 8

Problem Solving in the Biological Sciences
• Learn how to integrate your study and problem-solving skills, verbal reasoning, and mathematics concepts in biological sciences.
• Learn and remember MCAT biological sciences concepts and how to apply them.
• Recognize advanced concepts in biological sciences.

CHAPTER 9

Full-Length Practice MCAT

Suggestions for Using this Book

The schematic layout briefly describes all chapters and the typical order in which to review them. The way you use this book will depend on your prior experience with the MCAT and your current needs. Suggestions are given both for first-time users of this book and for students who have experience with earlier editions. The schematic layout and steps outlined below will help you develop a self-managed study outline.

If you are using this book for the first time, consider the following steps:

1. Review Chapter 1, Anatomy of the MCAT, and Chapter 2, Study Skills, Verbal Skills, and Problem-Solving Skills for the MCAT, which emphasize MCAT resources, study plans, and learning more about specific components of the MCAT.

2. Skim Chapter 3, Developing Verbal Reasoning Abilities, and Chapter 4, Writing Sample, to become acquainted with verbal reasoning and writing as presented in the MCAT.

3. Skim Chapter 7, Problem Solving in the Physical Sciences, and Chapter 8, Problem Solving in the Biological Sciences, to help you recognize the science topics covered in the physical and biological sciences sections of the MCAT. Understand how each topic is presented as an independent learning unit.

4. Start a formal review of the entire book beginning with Chapter 3; then proceed through Chapter 4.

5. Skim the material presented in Chapter 5, Test-Taking Skills for the MCAT, and review it again more thoroughly after completing a few months of MCAT study or after taking a full-length practice MCAT, such as the one included in the AAMC's *MCAT Student Manual.*

6. Study and practice the material in Chapters 7 and 8 according to your needs. The topics in both chapters are directly linked to the MCAT content outline. Refer frequently to Chapter 2 as a guide to develop a good study schedule and to reinforce newly learned study and problem-solving skills.

7. Chapter 6, Applied Math Concepts Required for Physical and Biological Sciences, is optional and provides a quick overview of math concepts for the MCAT.

If you have prepared for the MCAT before, consider the following steps:

1. Review Chapter 2, focusing on overcoming your weaknesses. Devise a comprehensive study plan before reviewing the other chapters.

2. Use this book with specific goals in mind. For example, if you have difficulty with verbal reasoning, review Chapter 3. Concentrate on verbal reasoning errors and how to correct them.

3. Use this book to learn about experimental and research concepts related to the field of medicine, which are found in the Applied Concepts section at the end of each topic in Chapters 7 and 8. Integrate information from the experimental and research concepts with the comprehensive problem-solving model in Chapter 5. This will provide you with advanced science material to help you handle the difficult sections on the MCAT. Integrate Chapter 5 with Chapter 7 if you are weak in the physical sciences; integrate Chapter 5 with Chapter 8 if you are weak in the biological sciences.

4. Review verbal reasoning in Chapter 3 to improve your understanding of an argument and how arguments are tested for soundness and relevance.

1

Anatomy of the MCAT

Introduction
to the MCAT

The Medical College Admission Test (MCAT) is a day-long test divided into a morning session and an afternoon session (Table 1-1). The morning session includes tests in Verbal Reasoning and Physical Sciences. The afternoon session includes the Writing Sample (two essays) and the Biological Sciences test.

Verbal Reasoning, the first MCAT test of the day, includes 65 questions based on nine reading passages, each 500 to 600 words long (see Chapter 3). Each passage has 6 to 10 multiple-choice questions covering topics in the humanities, social sciences, and areas of the natural sciences not tested in the Physical and Biological Sciences subtests. Because most questions are based on information in the passages, test questions do not require any outside knowledge of topics. You are not tested for subject mastery in the questions that follow the passages.

Physical Sciences, the second morning test, includes 77 questions. All but 15 of these are based on passages, each about 250 words long (see Chapter 7). The remainder are independent of any passage and of each other. This subtest measures comprehensive scientific understanding and reasoning skills in general chemistry and physics. There are about ten problem sets, each having from four to eight questions based on a passage. The emphasis is not on memorization of facts, but on problem-solving skills and knowledge of basic science concepts in physics and physics-related chemistry. You are also asked to demonstrate your ability to interpret information and solve problems based on tables, charts, graphs, and figures. Skills tested may include analyzing and interpreting data, identifying trends and relationships basic to data, determining prior or background knowledge important to the information, and selecting the best means of portraying the data or information.

Writing Sample, the first MCAT test given in the afternoon, consists of two essay topics (see Chapter 4). You will be expected to compose an essay for both topics within one hour (no more than 30 minutes for each essay). Formerly an experimental test, the Writing Sample is now part of the MCAT. It is scored with an alphabetic grade of J through T (J is the lowest score, and T is the highest). Communication skills are important for the medical profession and increased concern has been shown for the deficiency in writing skills among entering medical students. The writing exercise allows examinees the opportunity to demonstrate evidence of their writing and analytical skills and their ability to develop and present ideas.

Biological Sciences, the last test of the day, has the same number and type of questions and passages as the Physical Sciences test (see Chapter 8). This test measures scientific understanding and reasoning skills in biology and organic chemistry. The emphasis on

TABLE 1-1. The MCAT Test Day

Section	Number of Questions	Time Allotted (Minutes)
Verbal Reasoning	65	85
(10-minute break)		
Physical Sciences	77	100
(60-minute lunch break)		
Writing Sample	2	60
(10-minute break)		
Biological Sciences	77	100

TABLE 1-2. Scoring Chart for Verbal Reasoning, Physical Sciences, and Biological Sciences Sections of MCAT*†

Verbal Reasoning Section			Physical Sciences Section			Biological Sciences Section		
Raw Score (correct answers)	Scaled Score	Percentile Rank	Raw Score (correct answers)	Scaled Score	Percentile Rank	Raw Score (correct answers)	Scaled Score	Percentile Rank
65	15	>99	75–77	15	>99.5	75–77	15	>99.5
62–64	14	94–98	68–74	14	98–99	71–74	14	98–99
60–61	13	87–93	61–67	13	94–97	66–70	13	94–97
58–59	12	80–86	56–60	12	91–93	61–65	12	91–93
56–57	11	71–79	51–55	11	82–90	56–60	11	82–90
53–55	10	64–70	48–50	10	70–81	53–55	10	66–81
51–52	9	55–63	46–47	9	60–69	51–52	9	52–65
46–50	8	47–54	44–45	8	45–59	46–50	8	38–51
41–45	7	33–46	41–43	7	32–44	41–45	7	25–37
36–40	6	23–32	36–40	6	20–31	36–40	6	15–24
31–35	5	17–22	31–35	5	15–19	31–35	5	10–14
26–30	4	10–16	26–30	4	10–14	26–30	4	7–9
24–25	3	8–9	21–25	3	7–9	21–25	3	4–6
21–23	2	4–7	11–20	2	3–6	11–20	2	2–3
0–20	1	0–3	0–10	1	0–2	0–10	1	0–1
Mean score: 7.76			Mean score: 7.86			Mean score: 7.93		
Standard deviation: 2.46			Standard deviation: 2.32			Standard deviation: 2.40		

*Drawn from AAMC reports prepared from April 1991 to August 1995. These are not precise MCAT conversions; they are based on the editor's estimates. Total population of examinees: 305,043. Table is based on time-averaged, scaled scores. Tests of several difficulty levels should be used to gauge your progress.

†The median score for the Writing Sample during this time period was the letter O. On average, scores varied between the letters L and Q, which represent the 25th and 75th percentiles, respectively.

basic knowledge of concepts and problem-solving skills parallels that in the Physical Sciences test.

SCORING OF THE MCAT

Use Table 1-2 to estimate your scores when using any practice test materials.

AAMC MCAT Publications

AAMC has published four sets of practice materials for the new MCAT. All practice tests and materials have been tested and used in previous MCATs. A brief introduction to each of these products is given here so that you can determine the ones most useful to you at various stages of your MCAT preparation. Publications are available from AAMC or Williams & Wilkins.

1. *MCAT Student Manual,* 1993. Includes *Practice Test I.* The *MCAT Student Manual* is an excellent starting point for MCAT study, giving detailed outlines and descriptions for the four subtests. The items in *Practice Test I* were tested during the experimental phase of the new MCAT. *Practice Test I* may be used as a "pretest" or diagnostic test in your review program. At this writing, there is no plan to produce a revision of this practice test in the foreseeable future.
2. *MCAT Practice Test II,* 1991. Includes *MCAT Practice Items:* Two booklets: *Verbal Reasoning/Writing* and *Physical/Biological Sciences. Practice Test II* is the full-length MCAT administered nationwide in April 1991. It has been released to the public for a practice test. The *MCAT Practice Items* consist of two booklets containing many practice passages and items in all four subject areas of the exam. The *MCAT Practice Items* booklets should be used during your review of course outlines, class notes, and your textbooks. *Practice Test II* should be used as a diagnostic instrument to assess your weaknesses.
3. *MCAT Practice Test III,* 1995. *Practice Test III* is the most current and most valid instrument in the AAMC series. The practice test presents actual questions used for the MCAT in the past. Questions are classified as easy, moderate, and difficult; graphs are presented so students can determine their weaknesses. This test should definitely be used as a post-test to determine your level of preparedness for the actual MCAT.
4. *Preparing for the MCAT,* 1991. Video (VHS, 25 minutes). The MCAT video should be watched with a copy of the *MCAT Student Manual* at your side. Take quick notes because the video presents quite a few graphic illustrations of problem types and

medical equipment covered on the test. *Preparing for the MCAT* covers all subtests of the MCAT. It provides a quick overview of verbal reasoning and writing sample strategies to be used during your review and practice sessions. It clarifies the structure of the new MCAT passages, illustrating various types of passages and how to interpret information from them. The video is a good illustrative supplement to the *MCAT Student Manual*.

The video and the manual are deficient in presenting a model for passage analysis or a model to learn mathematics concepts required for the science subtests. The video also does not present a comprehensive model for problem solving in biological or physical sciences.

Using the AAMC MCAT Student Manual with the CompPrep

Your MCAT review using *Complete Preparation for the MCAT (CompPrep)* provides what the MCAT requires, but you must continually refer to the *CompPrep* table of contents and to the content outlines in the *MCAT Student Manual* to stay on track. Your use of the practice materials provided in *CompPrep* should be guided by the focus provided from the *MCAT Student Manual*. To enhance the effectiveness of your study program, try to answer the following questions as your MCAT review progresses.

1. Have you worked through the study skills, problem-solving skills, and verbal reasoning skills presented in *CompPrep* Chapters 2 and 3 to prepare you to review the physical and biological sciences in Chapters 7 and 8? Practice and refine the skills first, then attempt the review.
2. Are you regularly referring to the *CompPrep* table of contents, cross-checking it with the content outlines in the *MCAT Student Manual* and other practice tests and materials from AAMC? Make conscious connections between them.
3. Do you continuously review the *MCAT Student Manual* content outlines and look for relationships across disciplines within the outlines? An example would be "work and energy" (physical sciences) related to "enzymes" (biological sciences).
4. By topic and concept, are you able to connect your review to various textbooks, journals, class notes, medical books, science labs, and experiments? All are sources of text and practice problems.

MCAT Verbal Reasoning Passages

The Verbal Reasoning section of the MCAT consists of nine passages derived from several sources in the humanities, social sciences, and natural sciences. Each passage usually presents an argument. The author is generally listed at the end of the passage with source and publication date. Passages may be selected and edited by AAMC test writers to create discontinuity or to mask key phrases. When reading these passages, the student should not use outside knowledge, opinions, or beliefs to determine the validity of an argument. Verbal reasoning skills such as comprehension, evaluation, application, and incorporation of new information are tested through the wording of each question. Each passage should be read to uncover the central thesis and key ideas in each passage. The following reading strategies should be structurally implemented into your verbal reasoning study plan:

1. Learn to skim a passage: read the first and last paragraphs and the first sentence of each paragraph. Do not expect each passage to have a sequential ordering of ideas or events.
2. Learn to skim question statements (test-item stems), marking or noting key phrases or words such as "however," "the author suggests," "the author recommends," "it is implied," "weaken the argument," "reasonable to conclude," "it is likely," and "likely to be least affected." Do not read the four responses or answer choices (A, B, C, and D) yet.
3. Locate and mark the part of the passage to which each question refers.
4. Read the passage top to bottom to determine the connections between paragraphs or ideas. This usually takes about two minutes.
5. Read the first question, paying attention to what is being asked, and locate associative thoughts in the passage. Read the four responses and analyze them for apparently wrong answers (usually two out of four).

SOURCES FOR VERBAL REASONING PASSAGES

MCAT passages may be drawn from books on topics as diverse as agriculture, ethics, China, architecture, or finance. They may be drawn from a wide range of magazines, newspapers, and scientific journals, such as the *Journal of American Medical Education, New England Journal of Medicine, Science, U.S.A. Today*, the *Wall Street Journal, Newsweek*, and design and decorating magazines. Following are some examples of sources used in AAMC practice verbal reasoning passages.

Curtis B. Gans: How to Take the Big Money Out of Politics. *Washington Monthly*, 1985.
Stephen W. Hawking: *A Brief History of Time: From the Big Bang to Black Holes*, 1988.
Jacob Bronowski: *The Reach of Imagination*, MacMillan Publishing Co., 1978.
B.F. Skinner: *Reflections on Behaviorism and Society*, Prentice-Hall, 1978.
Theodore Roszak: Where the Wasteland Ends. *Atlantic Monthly*, 1972.
William K. Hartmann: *Birth of the Moon*. American Museum of Natural History, 1989.
Solar System Exploration Committee of the NASA Advisory Council: *Planetary Exploration Through the Year 2000: An Augmented Program*, 1990.
John P. Reganold, Robert I. Papendick, and James F. Parr: Sustainable Agriculture. *Scientific American*, 1990.
Bruce Stutz: *Hurricanes of the Arctic Nights*, American Museum of Natural History, 1986.
Richard Dawkins: *The Blind Watchmaker*, 1987.
Walter Gropius: *Apollo in the Democracy: The Cultural Obligation of the Architect*, McGraw-Hill, 1968.

MCAT Scientific Passages

Scientific passages are used in both the biological and the physical sciences portions of the MCAT. These passages describe a medically related situation in a few short narrative paragraphs and may be supplemented with data. The data appear in diagrams, charts, tables, or laboratory graphs. Each passage serves as a brief exposure to fairly advanced medical problems. It serves only as a linkage device, or mental bridge, to connect various undergraduate courses to the medical field. The questions following each passage cannot and should not be answered using the information in the passage alone. The passage may touch upon advanced medical concepts only tangentially, and the questions following the passage are either partially or totally unrelated to the advanced concepts. Students should not look for answers in the passage.

To understand the nature of MCAT scientific passages, look at each passage as a source of current, advanced medical concepts (e.g., instruments or experimental methods used in medicine, applications of medical technology, current medical terminology). Each passage is an excerpt or a small unit of medically related information, and is not complete as provided. More information is sometimes provided in the questions, which should be integrated with the passage before answering the question.

UNDERSTANDING MCAT SCIENTIFIC PASSAGES

When taking the MCAT, you have 100 minutes to do the reading and problem solving of these three elements (and mark your answers on the answer sheet). An average of 1 minute per test item would take 77 minutes of your time. This leaves you with approximately 23 minutes to read and understand 10 or 11 passages—about 2 minutes per passage. It is important for you to understand the nature of each passage before answering the questions following it. In order to capture the essence of the passage and be ready to use the information given in the passage, the following tips will help you:

1. Learn to classify the passage by type
2. Learn to classify the subject matter of a passage: biology, inorganic or general chemistry, organic chemistry, physics, or a mixture of various subjects
3. Learn to recognize key words and medical vocabulary associated with MCAT concepts, such as genetic engineering, thermoneutral zone, anomer, and bone stress and strain (see Chapter 2)
4. Learn to classify arguments or statements in a passage by basic scientific reasoning and problem-solving skills, such as hypothesis–conclusion, analysis of a complex chart, evaluation of design and methods presented, or cause–effect analysis (see Chapter 3)
5. Learn to associate a passage with your medical experiences, collected through hospital visits, emergency room visits, reviewing medical literature, talking with friends or relatives with medical problems, discussing topics with your physician or dentist, and other relevant experiences. This helps you find medical applications or look for medical clues in the passage. These medical experiences can be broken down into:
   a. Observing medical instrumentation
   b. Observing and evaluating medical experimentation
   c. Observing and evaluating clinical methods or procedures

TABLE 1-3. AAMC Scientific Passage Classification

	Frequency (%)*	
Passage Type	Physical Sciences	Biological Sciences
Information presentation	26	27
Problem solving	28	27
Research study	27	31
Persuasive argument	19	15

*Frequency data compiled from a review of all current MCAT study materials published by the AAMC.

6. Learn to evaluate a passage as it relates to each question, using associative reasoning to link various parts of the passage to various questions. Although difficult, this step is an efficient tool for solving the problems given in each passage.

PASSAGE TYPES

The *MCAT Student Manual* classifies the passages used in the physical and biological sciences subtests as follows (Table 1-3):

1. **Information presentation**
   a. **Source:** Textbook or journal articles
   b. **Content:** Background knowledge is assumed, but passages may include new information or new uses of basic information
   c. **Skills tested:** Comprehension, application of information
2. **Problem solving**
   a. **Source:** Traditional science textbooks
   b. **Content:** Descriptions of chemistry or physics problems
   c. **Skills tested:** Ability to determine probable causes of events or phenomena using scientific theories, and to select appropriate methods of problem solving
3. **Research study**
   a. **Source:** Research studies (e.g., in microbiology, histology, genetics research, lab reports)
   b. **Content:** Rationale, methods, and/or results of research
   c. **Skills tested:** Ability to understand experimental designs and methods, and to evaluate methods relating to conclusions of experiment
4. **Persuasive argument**
   a. **Source:** Newspaper or magazine articles (e.g., *New York Times, Scientific American, Discover*), dialogue between scientists in a meeting or at a conference
   b. **Content:** Persuasive arguments, advocating one or more points of view, that include pieces of evidence and descriptions of methodologies and biochemical/biomedical products
   c. **Skills tested:** Ability to comprehend arguments and evaluate conclusions; ability to assess the validity of specific methods or evidence used to support arguments

Recognizing and Classifying Passage Types

Students should learn to identify passages in the physical and biological sciences sections of the MCAT according to the AAMC classifications. The source, content, and layout of each passage provide clues to its classification.

Information presentation and **problem-solving** passages usually present material similar to that found in textbooks, lab manuals, and student guides. Students should recognize only relevant information by referring to the questions following the passage. Students should not read these passages in detail. These passages are provided only to stimulate long-term memory and to remind the student of science concepts. Students should not assume that the answers to the questions are in the passage. Relevant information in the passage may include a new premedical term or concept, such as osteoporosis; a Greek symbol, a formula, or a newly defined term, such as frequency of emission spectrograph; or quantitative information, such as units or dimensions. Students should select the information they need from the passage to solve the problems. Watch out for unusual or irrelevant material that can creep into passage construction, especially in information passages from textbooks or encyclopedias.

Research study passages usually can be recognized by introductory phrases such as "the following study was performed to . . . ." Research study passages usually have a clear

TABLE 1-4. Functional Scientific Passage Classification

Passage Type	Frequency (%)* Physical Sciences	Biological Sciences
Descriptive	35	43
Graphic descriptive	15	20
Experimental	26	34
Graphic experimental	1	1
Instrumentation	19	0
Medical instrumentation	1	0
Device-based	3	1
Figure-based (no description)	0	1

*Frequency data compiled from a review of all current MCAT study materials published by the AAMC.

set of hypotheses in the opening lines of the passage and conclusions at the end of the passage, in the form of graphs or statements such as "in lab rats, the rate of immunization depends on. . . ." Students should read these passages carefully and accept the study as described. Apply critical thinking skills linked with prior science knowledge to judge the soundness of experimental work and limitations in the research design.

Persuasive argument passages express arguments made by one or more scientists about a certain process or concept. These passages include biased opinions, beliefs, claims, refutations, or implied statements about a product, methodology, or scientific phenomenon. Students should apply critical thinking to determine the validity of the argument by analyzing supported and unsupported evidence. Physicians constantly read this type of literature from manufacturers such as pharmaceutical companies. Students should analyze this type of passage with an objective to answer questions—not to create a mental debate during the MCAT.

FUNCTIONAL CLASSIFICATION OF MCAT SCIENTIFIC PASSAGES

The science content and current technical information presented in each passage allow a functional classification of each passage. The functional classification will help you link various passages to textbooks, journals, manuals, or laboratory research reports (Table 1-4).

1. **Descriptive.** These passages are basic information passages describing a scientific process, including instruments, in a narrative style.
2. **Graphic descriptive.** These passages usually have a brief narrative accompanied by charts, tables, line graphs from experimental/theoretical studies, diagrams showing a part of a process or system, or a set of equations or a cycle in biology or chemistry.
3. **Experimental.** These passages describe one or more experiments that compare various laboratory results by changing a variable or function in a process. Some experimental passages present unusual research experiments to verify one or more hypotheses in biology or physiology. Formulas or equations may be included in the passage. **Graphic experimental** passages are accompanied by graphics such as tables or graphs.
4. **Instrumentation.** These passages describe a piece of equipment, a laboratory machine, or a household appliance; and usually describe the operation, design, and pros and cons of using the instrument. A schematic diagram is generally included, although the parts are usually not labeled. One reason for including instrumental passages in the MCAT is to check a student's evaluation skills and mechanical ability. **Medical instrumentation** passages involve instruments used only in medical diagnosis or research.
5. **Device-based.** These passages usually illustrate a nonconventional laboratory device created by a scientist to check a concept or to verify a theory. A device is different from medical machines or instruments. Most devices are laboratory tools or simple mechanisms created to manually demonstrate a principle in science.

ANALYSIS OF PASSAGE CONTENT (TABLE 1-5)

An analysis of passage content in AAMC practice materials reveals that some topics appear more frequently than others (e.g., solution chemistry, phase and phase equilibria). In the Physical Sciences test, each passage addressed only one concept or topic, including instrument design and operation. By contrast, in the Biological Sciences test, each passage

TABLE 1-5A. Analysis of AAMC Passage Content in the Physical Sciences*

AAMC Topic	Passage	Functional Classification
Information Passages (26%)		
XX.D	α, β, γ radioactive decay	Desc
IV.C	Physical/chemical allotropes of sulfur	Desc
IV.C	Phases of water, BP & FP, density	Desc
XI.E, F	Dynamic forces on projectiles	Desc
XX.D	Excited states/energy levels of electrons	Desc
XVII.B	EM waves, fields, antennae, E = hf	Desc
IX.A	Electrochemistry, ligands, trans. elements	Desc
VII.A, XVIII.C	Water-heater circuit diagram, calorimeter	Inst
XVI.A	Aerofoil design, fuel, wings, lift, drag	Desc
X.F, XI.E	Projectile motion, Coriolis force, projectiles	Desc
III.B	Molecular formulas and bonds for acids and bases	Desc
III.B, IV.B	Water molecules, bonds, amphoteric compounds	Desc
V.A, IX.A	Solvent extraction of quinine, Pb^{+2}, Zn^{+2} separation	Gr.desc
XVI.A, XVIII.B	Lub. oil tank design with electric heaters, drain plug	Inst
XII.A, XIII	Exercise bike design, basal metabolic rate	Inst
Research Study Passages (27%)		
XIX.B, C; XVII.A	Retroreflecting arrays, pinhole beam splitter	Inst
VII.A	Exothermic reactions	Expt
VII.A, XVIII.C	Water heater, immersion type, Ohm's law, calorimeter	Inst
XIII.C, D; XIV.B, XVII.B	Spring stiffness, oscillations, mag. potential energy	Expt
XVI.A	Water and glycerine flow in pipe; viscosity, density	Expt
X.E, F; XIII.D	Tennis balls, rebound height, microphone, projectiles	Expt
XIV.B, XVII.B	Mag. dipole moment, harmonic oscillator, two magnets	Expt
VIII.B, D, G; V.B	Esterification, equilibrium shift, molar ratio	Gr.desc
IV.A	Mol. wt. of two unknown gases, effusion, vacuum pump	Gr.inst
V.B, IV.B	Volume, temperature, and solubility of KNO_3	Expt
IV.B, C	Four reactions with alum, crystal prep. temperature	Expt
IV.A	Measuring gas constant R with chemical reaction	Devi
VI.A, B; V.B	Adsorption of dye by eggs, vinegar, pH	Gr.expt
XVI.A, V.B	Gasoline separation, glass fibers, selective adsorption	Inst
I.H, III.B	$CaCO_3$ decomposition chemistry	Expt
V.B	Solubility products and properties of nitrates, Pb^{+2}	Expt
Problem-Solving Passages (28%)		
XVII.B, XIII	Electromagnetic railgun	Inst
XVI.A	Open liquid tank with three spheres/floats	Inst
VIII.D, G	Activation energy, reactants/products	Expt
VI.B, IV.A	Titrations, gas laws, reactions	Inst
XI.E, XX.E	Fluorescent lamp, electron accceleration	Inst
XI.F, G	Dynamics on inclined plane with friction	Devi
XVI.A, XV.B, D	Doppler stethoscopes, ultrasound imaging of organs	Med.inst
XII.B, XIV.B	Pendula in series, colliding pendula	Expt
VII.A, VI.A	Styrofoam calorimeter, acid–base reactions	Expt
VII.A, IX.A	ΔG equations, constants, electrochemical reactions	Desc
VII.B	Steam engine, refrigerator function and efficiency	Gr.desc
XVIII.C, E; XVII.A	Silicon wafer, plasma etcher, electric field	Gr.desc
IV.A	Two methods to find N_2 density in laboratory	Expt
XIV.B	Simple pendulum characteristics, $T = K\sqrt{\dfrac{L}{g}}$	Expt
XVI.A	Raft design	Desc
Persuasive Argument Passages (19%)		
VI.B, I.H	Ammonia titration and preparation methods	Expt
V.A, B; I.H, III.B	Soaps, hardness of water	Desc
XX.C	Natural nuclear reactor, fission reactions	Desc
VI.A, III.B, V.B	Rainwater acidity	Desc
XV.A, D; XVI.A	Ultrasonic diagnosis, Doppler blood velocity	Med.inst
XIX.C, D	Hubble telescope, optical detectors	Desc
XII.A, B; XIII.F	Seat belts, collision design, air bags, safety	Desc
XVIII.B, XIV.A, XVII.B	Circuit breaker design, EM waves	Desc
XI.E, XIII.F, XIX.C	Space stations in orbit, solar cells, biological needs	Desc
VI.A, V.B	Buffered solutions, pH–pK_a equations, blood buffer	Desc
VIII.B, D, E	Reaction pathways	Desc
VIII.E, I.H, II.B	$O_3 \rightarrow O_2$ reactions	Gr.desc

*Compiled from a review of all current MCAT study materials published by the AAMC.

TABLE 1-5B. Analysis of AAMC Passage Content in the Biological Sciences*

AAMC Topic	Passage	Functional Classification
Information Passages (27%)		
IV.C, I.B, VI.A	Oxyhemoglobin/PO_2 graphs, ligands, genetics	Gr.desc
XIII.A, D	Bimolecular rate constants, nucleophiles, S_N2	Desc
VI.A, IX.A	Carbaminohemoglobin, haldane, respiration	Desc
X.A, C; XI.A	Ectopic pregnancy, hCG, tubal pregnancy	Desc
IX.B, XI.B	Sweating, salt regulation	Desc
I.B, XI.A	Molecular genetics of inherited human vision	Desc
XII.A, III.D	Signal peptides	Desc
VI.C, II.A, I.B	Antigenic shifts on virulence, influenza	Desc
II.A, B; IV.B, VIII.A	Tetanus infection, spore germination	Desc
II.A, B, C; I.B, XII.A	African sleeping sickness, various surf glycoproteins	Desc
XI.B, I.B, III.D, E	Cystic fibrosis, molecular hybrids, DNA/RNA test	Desc
III.C, VI.A, IV.B	Hypovolemic shock, hemorrhage, Na^+/K^+ pump	Desc
VIII.B, III.D	Stress/strain in bones, bone fracture, osteoblasts	Desc
VII.A, B; XII.A	Digestion in rabbits, cows (cecum, rumen, omasum)	Desc
VIII.A, IV.B	Vertebrate smooth muscle	Desc
II.A, I.B	Vaccinia, AIDS virus	Desc
III.D, E; III.C	Mitotic spindle, kinetochore microtubules	Gr.desc
Research Study Passages (31%)		
III.C, IV.B, VI.A	Na^+ pump, erythrocytes, ATP	Expt
I.A, XII.B	Photosynthesis cycle, Calvin cycle	Gr.desc
II.A	Bacteriology of aerobic genus implants	Expt
I.A, X.A, V.C	Nonshivering thermogenesis, pineal gland	Expt
XIII.A, B, C, F; XVII.D	Soluble/insoluble organic compounds	Gr.desc
VIII.B, V.C	Osteoclasts, PTH binding, Ca^{2+}, UV light, calcitonin	Expt
X.A, I.B, XI.A	RNA/radioactive protein, haploid cells, fungus mutation	Expt
II.A, I.B, III.E	Ames test for mutagens/carcinogens in air	Expt
XVIII.B, A; XVII.A, C	Antifungal chemicals, separations	Expt
XIII.D, XII.C	Iodonium ion, unsaturated fats	Expt
XVII.B, XII.A	Protein separation by gel, ion-exchange chromatography	Expt
XIII.D, A; XIV.C	Alkyl halides produced from alcohols	Expt
I.B, XII.A	Guanosine, adenosine	Expt
II.A, VI.A, C	Potomac horse fever, rickettsia, blood serum study	Expt
I.B, II.A	DNA repair using bacteriophage assay	Expt
XV.B, XVI.C	Butene isomers, reaction mechanisms and kinetics	Expt
XVIII.A, XVII.A	^{1}HNMR and IR spectra and separation experiments	Expt
Problem-Solving Passages (27%)		
XV.B, XVI.C	Conjugated dienes, electrophilic addition	Desc
I.A, XII.A	Proposed catalytic hydrolysis steps, chymotrypsin	7 Figs.
VI.A, IV.B, III.D	Basophilic/acidophilic cardiac muscle cells	Desc
I.A, II.A, XII.C	Biokinetic microbial activity in sludge	Gr.desc
III.C, VII.B	Vasopressin, osmolarity, ADH, plasma, kidneys	Desc
I.A, V.C	Alcohol dehydrogenase, drinking, Krebs cycle	Desc
XII.A, B, C; I.B	Biotin, biotinidase deficiency, biotin cycle	Gr.desc
II.A, I.B	λ bacteriophage	Gr.desc
VI.C, V.C	Radioimmunoassay assayed antigen	Gr.desc
II.A, XII.B	Growth kinetics of bacteria, lactose	Gr.expt
X.C, II.B, I.B	Binary fission reproduction, costimulation, buffer	Expt
I.A, XII.A	Angiotensinogen, pK_a, histidine, ACE enzyme	Gr.desc
XVII.A, D; XVI.C	Albuterol synthesis in lab, asthma	Expt
XII.B, XIII.B	Hydrolysis of glycosides, temperature–rate table	Expt
III.C, X.C	Chorioallantois, diffusion	Desc
IX.B, VI.A	Oxygen consumption/temperature in various animals	Gr.desc
XI.A, B; IV.A; V.A	Synaptic transmission of nerve impulse, synapsin	Gr.desc
XII.A, I.A, X.A	ACTH, reproductive enzymes, adrenocortical hyperplasias	Gr.desc
Persuasive Argument Passages (15%)		
VI.C, II.A, I.B	AIDS, AZT, T-lymphocytes, cancer cells	Desc
XVI.C, XVIII.A	Reaction mechanisms, IR spectra, kinetics	Expt
VI.C, XI.A	Factor VIII, hemophilia, genetic linkage	Desc
III.C, D; II.A	Crawling cells, force mechanism types	Desc
IV.B, VIII.B	Ca^{2+} in contraction of smooth muscle, myosin	Desc
XIII.D, A; XIV.C	Alkylation of carbanion	Expt
XIII.C, XII.C	Phosphoglycerides, esters (properties and structure)	Desc

*Compiled from a review of all current MCAT study materials published by the AAMC.

sometimes included four to five concepts or topics from biology with only one concept in organic chemistry. The test items were more difficult compared to those in the Physical Sciences test, and more concepts were mixed within biology than in traditional organic chemistry. The biological sciences passages included quite a few descriptions of experimental projects or research projects with multiple experiments (two or three) in each passage.

This analysis also reveals that medically related content is selected more often than traditional undergraduate topics. Students should realize that links to medicine are quite apparent in the format of the MCAT. The passages test skills in relation to medical knowledge, familiarity with current medical practices and medical terminology and, above all, the student's problem-solving abilities as a medical novice. The idea is to see how a newcomer in medical school will apply knowledge of biology, chemistry, and physics in solving problems. Advanced medical school courses such as biochemistry, microbiology, and human physiology are used to construct some questions.

UNIVERSAL PASSAGE CLASSIFICATION

Following is a list of scientific passage types that combines the AAMC classification system with the functional classification system.

- Descriptive information passages
- Descriptive information passages with diagrams
- Instrument information passages
- Descriptive problem-solving passages
- Descriptive problem-solving passages with diagrams
- Instrument problem-solving passages
- Problem-solving passages using laboratory devices
- Problem-solving passages with diagrams
- Experimental problem-solving passages
- Experimental problem-solving passages with diagrams

- Research study passages with diagrams
- Instrumental research study passages
- Research study passages using laboratory devices
- Experimental research study passages
- Research study passages with persuasive arguments
- Descriptive persuasive argument passages
- Persuasive argument passages with diagrams
- Experimental persuasive argument passages
- Persuasive argument passages using medical instruments

SCIENTIFIC PASSAGE SOURCES

Scientific passages are fairly easy to find, starting with your college textbooks, laboratory manuals, and workbooks. For your own skills development, we advise you to select long and difficult paragraphs from textbook chapters not studied in class. These provide you with the basic training to relate to passages and also acquaint you with unfamiliar topics and concepts. More extensive training in passage reading and analysis should be done at the library. Look for encyclopedias, scientific journals, and magazines. Literature sources, including catalogs from medical technology organizations, pharmaceutical manufacturers, and hospital equipment and research companies also include medical passages of a type to be found on the MCAT. Develop a glossary covering technological terms and their usage. Based on a review of both physical and biological science passages, the AAMC uses quite a few resources, which may include:

- Medical encyclopedias
- Medical terminology books
- Medical instrumentation books
- Basic science textbooks (e.g., anatomy, physiology, microbiology, histology)
- Physics laboratory reports
- Engineering mechanics laboratory reports

- Bioengineering/biophysics books
- Technology review magazines
- Chemical engineering books
- Technical manuals
- Engineering textbooks
- Wastewater/water supply books
- Electrical appliance manuals

MAJOR TOPICS OF SCIENTIFIC PASSAGES

Following is a complete list of all major topics for physical and biological sciences as given in the *MCAT Student Manual*. The *MCAT Student Manual* breaks each topic into further subdivisions.

Physical Sciences

   I. Stoichiometry
  II. Electronic Structure and the Periodic Table
 III. Bonding

IV. Phases and Phase Equilibria
V. Solution Chemistry
VI. Acids and Bases
VII. Thermodynamics and Thermochemistry
VIII. Rate Processes in Chemical Reactions: Kinetics and Equilibrium
IX. Electrochemistry
X. Translational Motion
XI. Force and Motion, Gravitation
XII. Equilibrium and Momentum
XIII. Work and Energy
XIV. Wave Characteristics and Periodic Motion
XV. Sound
XVI. Fluids and Solids
XVII. Electrostatics and Electromagnetism
XVIII. Electric Circuits
XIX. Light and Geometrical Optics
XX. Atomic and Nuclear Structure

Biological Sciences

I. Molecular Biology
II. Microbiology
III. Generalized Eukaryotic Cell
IV. Specialized Eukaryotic Cells and Tissues
V. Nervous and Endocrine Systems
VI. Circulatory, Lymphatic, and Immune Systems
VII. Digestive and Excretory Systems
VIII. Muscle and Skeletal Systems
IX. Respiratory and Skin Systems
X. Reproductive System and Development
XI. Genetics and Evolution
XII. Biological Molecules
XIII. Oxygen-containing Compounds
XIV. Amines
XV. Hydrocarbons
XVI. Molecular Structure of Organic Compounds
XVII. Separations and Purifications
XVIII. Use of Spectroscopy in Structural Identification

Study Skills, Verbal Skills, and Problem-Solving Skills for the MCAT

PART 1
General Study Skills

MCAT: A Test of Analysis and Synthesis

The MCAT is designed to help medical schools choose the best possible candidates. In addition to testing science knowledge, the MCAT measures students' skills in areas identified as fundamental to success in medical school, such as verbal skills, math skills, and problem-solving skills.

Because the most successful medical students tend to be those who can effectively analyze and synthesize large amounts of theoretical and research-related information, the MCAT also tests students' ability to perform these tasks. Therefore, students preparing for the MCAT must incorporate analysis and synthesis in their study approach.

What are analysis and synthesis? **Analysis** is the ability to break something down into parts. **Synthesis** is the ability to combine or unify individual pieces of information into a meaningful whole. Synthesis occurs when you summarize what you read, explain the solution to a problem in your own words, or apply what you learned in biology today to what you learned in organic chemistry last week. The most prepared premedical students are those who make connections between the physical and biological sciences, seeing them as different pieces that fit into a complete picture. For example, understanding the structure and functions of the lungs involves understanding the relationship between the physical, chemical, and biological characteristics of lungs. Figure 2-1 presents two additional examples of synthesis.

SKILLS ASSESSMENT INVENTORY

Because many students acquire their skills sporadically throughout their undergraduate careers, they are often unprepared for the MCAT. Before launching into a plan for MCAT preparation, take time to assess your typical study strategies. Note that the key word here is *typical*. In preparing for the MCAT, students often take preparation courses or read preparation guides for advice on effective study strategies. These strategies then become part of their preparation approach for the MCAT. But newly acquired strategies do not always represent your typical approach to medical course work. Examining how you typically study will enable you to make changes to your study approach that will carry you through the MCAT and beyond.

Using the the following skills assessment inventory (Figure 2-2), evaluate your habits critically. This assessment will help you identify your strengths and weaknesses and assist you in setting goals for improvement.

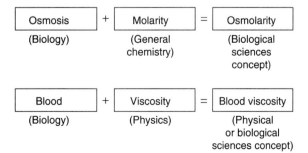

Fig. 2-1. The synthetic process.

Study Skills:	I do	I do not
Break time into manageable units to increase productivity	_____	_____
Pace study to allow adequate time for reviewing and memorizing	_____	_____
Memorize only after understanding information	_____	_____
Reinforce information through timely repetition at intervals ranging from the same day to several weeks later	_____	_____
Use organized system for learning new vocabulary words	_____	_____

Note-taking Skills:	I do	I do not
Listen for speaker's organizational structure during lecture	_____	_____
Take notes during lecture	_____	_____
Identify central ideas in textbook passages	_____	_____
Use a system that shows the relationship among facts rather than a list of facts	_____	_____
Vary the format of taking notes according to the content of the material	_____	_____
Consolidate information taken from several sources into a master set of notes	_____	_____
Consistently update and summarize the information learned	_____	_____

Fig. 2-2. Skills assessment inventory.

Problem-solving Skills:	I do	I do not
Determine the intent of a problem and the accompanying passage	_____	_____
Identify components of a problem	_____	_____
Clarify unfamiliar or vague terms	_____	_____
Consider multiple paths to problem solution	_____	_____
Distinguish fact from opinion and claims from arguments in the passage	_____	_____
Attempt to reason through a problem, even when uncertain	_____	_____
Apply a systematic reasoning process through entire problem	_____	_____
Rely on reasoning rather than feelings or impressions	_____	_____
Determine similarities and differences among concepts and details	_____	_____
Select appropriate data to be used in problem solution	_____	_____
Draw diagrams, when appropriate, to clarify ideas	_____	_____
Test answers for relevancy to a problem	_____	_____
Integrate new information in a problem with previous knowledge from the passage	_____	_____
Establish relationships across subjects as well as within	_____	_____

BUILDING DISCIPLINE FOR MCAT REVIEW

You must be as disciplined in studying for the MCAT as you need to be in taking it. For example, many students don't like organic chemistry. If this is true for you, you may avoid studying organic chemistry and, on the test itself, you may be reluctant to get to that portion of the test. As a result, you may spend a longer time on the biology questions in the Biological Sciences test, because you feel more comfortable about them, and defer the organic chemistry questions to the point that you do not leave yourself enough time to answer all the questions. A disciplined approach acquired through efficient study tactics can help build your confidence in the subjects you like least.

Test-taking Skills:	I do	I do not
Try to predict test questions while studying	_____	_____
Read test instructions carefully	_____	_____
Read questions carefully and identify key terms	_____	_____
Attempt to define key terms in a question before working through the question	_____	_____
Determine the intent of the test question without over-interpreting it	_____	_____
Evaluate all information before choosing an answer	_____	_____
Use a problem-solving strategy rather than guessing when uncertain of an answer	_____	_____
Apply consistent logic to answer choice options within a test question	_____	_____

Now take a moment to review your answer patterns and record your observations in the spaces below. Where are your strengths and weaknesses? As you work with this book, you will want to pay particular attention to those suggestions that address your weaknesses. As you make changes in your approach, however, take care not to lose track of your areas of strength and instead take advantage of them.

Strengths

_____
_____
_____
_____
_____
_____

Weaknesses

_____
_____
_____
_____
_____
_____

Goals

_____
_____
_____
_____
_____
_____

Fig. 2-2.—continued

Incorporating Analysis and Synthesis Into Your Study Approach

To be prepared for the MCAT, you must think like the MCAT test-makers. Because the MCAT tests the ability to analyze and synthesize, you must incorporate these strategies into your study approach. Mere memorization is not enough. You must be able to break a topic down into its component parts and must also see the interdisciplinary connections between topics.

The content topic outline in the *MCAT Student Manual* lists 9 topics in general chemistry, 11 topics in physics, 20 topics in physical sciences, 12 topics in biology, 6 topics in organic chemistry, and 18 topics in biological sciences. All of these topics can be further broken down into smaller components. In addition, approximately 700 interdisciplinary connections can be made between these topics.

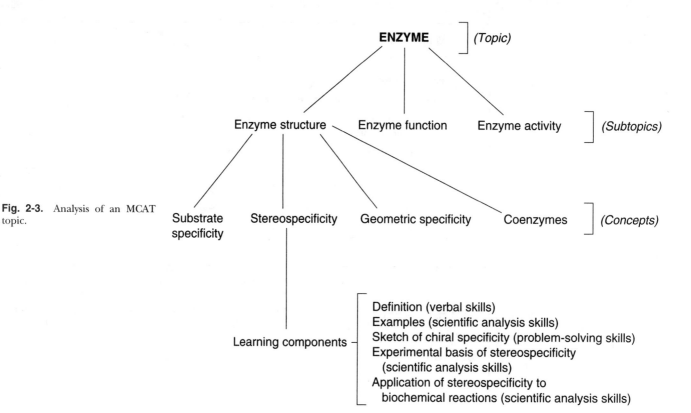

Fig. 2-3. Analysis of an MCAT topic.

The following section details how to incorporate analysis and integration into your study approach. Immediately following this section is a general game plan for preparing for the MCAT. Devising a game plan is half the battle in studying for the MCAT. Once you know what you have to do, the task of actually studying becomes easier because you know the parameters of the endeavor. Seeing the "big picture" laid out before you can lessen your anxiety and provide you with precise starting and end points.

ANALYSIS

Your study approach should include analysis of all the topics contained in the *MCAT Student Manual's* topic outline. To analyze a topic, break it down into its component parts (Figure 2-3):

1. Divide major topics into subtopics. For example, enzymes, a major topic in molecular biology, can be divided into subtopics of structure, function, and activity.
2. Divide subtopics into concepts. For example, enzyme structure can be divided into concepts of substrate specificity, stereospecificity, geometric specificity, and coenzymes.

The goal of analysis is to break down large pieces of content into smaller, more manageable parts. Dividing a topic into smaller parts allows you to organize and focus your study approach. It also ensures that you will not overlook important concepts inherent in specific topics.

But breaking a topic into smaller parts is not enough. Look again at Figure 2-3. You can see that concepts are further broken down into **learning components.** Each learning component is associated with different skills, such as verbal skills, scientific analysis skills, problem-solving skills, instrument analysis skills, and math skills.

The process of breaking down concepts into learning components is crucial in your review because the MCAT tests your ability to apply different skills to different concepts. In performing this step, your main goal should be to examine how one concept can be approached from a variety of angles. For example, Figure 2-3 shows how the concept of enzyme specificity can be studied using verbal skills, scientific analysis skills, and problem-solving skills.

SYNTHESIS

During the analytical process you divided MCAT topics into concepts and learning components. Now is the time to synthesize topics, or combine them across disciplines (Figure 2-4).

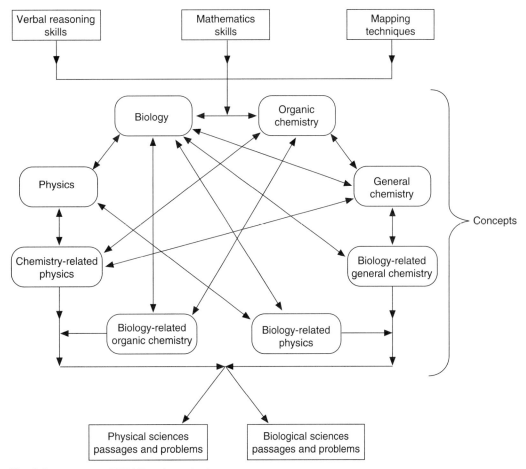

Fig. 2-4. Diagram of MCAT topic synthesis.

For example, let's assume you have divided the topic of reaction rates of chemical reactions into the following concepts: activation energy, reaction rate law, and temperature dependence of reaction rate. All of these concepts deal with general chemistry. Next, relate these concepts to general biology concepts; for example, reaction rate law for coenzymes and activation energy and substrate specificity of chymotrypsin.

To test your ability to synthesize topics, make interdisciplinary connections between the following topics. Use the content topic outline in the *MCAT Student Manual.*

1. Bonding and hydrocarbons
2. Wave characteristics and periodic motion in fluids and solids
3. Equilibrium and momentum of biological molecules
4. Microbiology of the nervous and endocrine systems
5. Use of spectroscopy in structural identification of acids and bases

If performed correctly, the synthetic process reveals that each topic contained in the *MCAT Student Manual* topic outline can be connected to other topics in the outline. To illustrate how effective synthesis reveals these connections, the following examples examine some of the interconnections that can be made for two broad topics: microbiology and general chemistry. See if you can answer the questions listed under each topic. If you can, you have already discovered many of the interdisciplinary connections for each of these two topics.

Biology Topics: Microbiology

1. Assume a research paper examines various AIDS-related viral studies and conceptualizes the kinetic or thermodynamic control studies needed to develop an AIDS vaccine. Would laser microscopic studies have been carried out in the experiments discussed? (Chemistry-related physics concepts)
2. Do you understand the chemical structure of the HB2-g virus and how the chemical structure affects its life cycle? (General chemistry concepts)

General Chemistry Topics: Stoichiometry and Rate Processes in Chemical Reactions

1. Can you quickly and accurately do stoichiometric calculations of kinetically controlled or thermodynamically controlled reactions? (Physics concepts)
2. Can you apply and extend concepts learned in stoichiometry to one or more experimental situations using enzymes as catalysts for metabolic pathways, with special emphasis on compare-contrast relationships among various experiments? (Biology concepts)

A General Approach to Studying for the MCAT

Now that you understand how important analysis and synthesis are to MCAT preparation, you're ready to devise a plan of attack for review. As you've learned, review doesn't mean simply reading and memorizing. Review involves analyzing topics and drawing connections between topics. You must design an approach that allows you to both analyze and synthesize all the topics contained in the topic outline.

The prospect of MCAT review can be daunting, but an organized plan can help lessen your apprehension. First, set goals for your review. Second, divide the review into manageable study sessions. Third, determine goals for each study session. Finally, set aside time for the periodic review of material you've already covered.

SET GOALS

The topic outline in the *MCAT Student Manual* is your road map to your study approach. For each topic listed in the outline, set study goals for each area. Your review will be more focused if you write out exactly what you want to accomplish. Use the worksheet provided in Figure 2-5 to construct an outline of your goals, adding as many pages as you need to complete the task.

Notice that the review worksheet requires you to analyze a topic by breaking it down into smaller concepts. By filling out review worksheets, you've already begun the process of analysis. Your review worksheets for each topic should also include the learning components, or skills, for each concept.

ESTABLISH AN AGENDA FOR EACH STUDY SESSION

Your next task is to divide your review into study sessions and establish an agenda for each session. Use your review worksheets. It's a good idea to estimate, in hours, how long each review worksheet will take to complete. Then, based on the number of hours you've designated for each worksheet, decide how many study sessions you should devote to each worksheet. For instance, one worksheet on a small topic might require one study session. Worksheets for more complex topics may require several study sessions.

How long should each study session last? The duration of each session depends on your ability to concentrate. Concentration requires both endurance and discipline. Consciously limiting the time you spend on each topic may help you concentrate. Avoid open-ended study sessions—the kind where you say "I'm going to work on this organic chemistry until I've finished it, all night if I have to." Open-ended study sessions give permission to daydream. Tell yourself instead, "I have exactly 1½ hours to finish this organic chemistry. If it isn't finished by then, too bad." At the end of 1½ hours,

---

Topic: *Molecular Biology*

Subtopic: Enzymes

Concepts: General function and importance in catalyzing biochemical reactions ⎫
Basic principles of enzyme specificity ⎬ *Example*
Enzyme cofactors ⎪
Feedback inhibition ⎭

Topic: _____

Subtopic: _____

Concepts: _____

_____

_____

_____

Fig. 2-5. Sample worksheet for setting review goals.

stop. Limitless sessions tend to encourage a lack of focus. Limiting the time in advance encourages you to concentrate harder.

Ask yourself these questions: What topics are the hardest to concentrate on? What time of day is best for concentration? Worst? Does the kind of food you eat affect your concentration? How about background noise or lack of it? Does stress in school, job, or personal relationships affect your concentration? Does your workplace or study area affect your concentration? Self-awareness gained by paying attention to these issues can help circumvent obstacles that impair your powers of concentration.

DEVELOP A PLAN OF ATTACK

As noted above, open-ended study sessions are not productive. To make the most of your time, form a plan of attack for each session. Each session should include the following steps:

Review

First, determine what you remember instead of going immediately to a text or notes. Start with a blank sheet of paper and brainstorm on the topic for 5 to 10 minutes. What main subdivisions of the topic do you recall? Write them down. Now look at your divisions of the topic and jot down as much detail about them as you can remember. Even if you think you do not remember very much, push yourself to put down as much as you can. Now evaluate your relative strengths and weaknesses on the topic.

What did you find? Chances are that you remembered a lot of information in some areas, a modest amount in others, and very little in the remaining areas. However, you will have accomplished a great deal by going through this exercise. This highly active process helps you to quickly achieve a high level of concentration so that you avoid wasting time getting warmed up. You also know how to best distribute your time, because you have identified those areas needing only a quick review and those that require more time.

Selectively Re-Read

Selectively re-read according to your content strengths and weaknesses. In areas where your recall of information was good, skim over the information in your text or notes to confirm accuracy and to make sure you did not forget something important. Slow down and read more carefully in places where your recall was incomplete. You will find that any re-reading you do at this point tends to go much faster. Selective re-reading after brainstorming saves time because you are actively looking for specific information to fill in gaps in your knowledge.

Stop and Summarize

Periodically, stop reading and summarize what you have just read. Talk to yourself and actually put into words what you think is important. Include a statement of the main idea, as well as relevant details that develop the main idea. If information is missing in the notes you jotted down while brainstorming, add it to your notes at this time.

Ask Yourself Questions

To confirm your understanding and to consider the information from a different perspective, try to predict test questions you think a professor might ask and then try to answer them.

As you can see, this approach is designed to maximize your time. Rather than focusing on material you already know, this approach allows you to concentrate your efforts on material you do not know.

PERIODICALLY REVIEW MATERIAL

It's important that you go over topics that you've studied in previous study sessions. Otherwise, you may forget the concepts you've learned in your zeal to make it through your review worksheets. Here's how to periodically review what you've learned:

1. Each day, spend 5 – 10 minutes reviewing the previous day's topic by quickly reconstructing your notes from memory. Because the greatest loss of newly acquired information occurs during the first 24 hours, repetition of the previous day's information is very important. If you do not include this step, you will find yourself having to rebuild a significant portion of your foundation when you finally come back to review.
2. On weekends, summarize what was important from the week. If you keep to this schedule, your review will go quickly because information you studied during the week will still be fresh in your mind.

Study Tools

Now that you have a plan, you're ready to review. This section discusses various tools that will make your review more efficient.

STUDY PARTNERS

Studying with a partner can be extremely useful when preparing for the MCAT. Explaining difficult material to someone else is a good way to make sure you understand what you read and memorize. Choose study partners who are strong in areas where you are weak and whose weaknesses complement your strengths. When your study partner has difficulty, you can act as a critical listener. The job of the critical listener is to make sure that what the speaker says is accurate, complete, precise, and to the point. Working with others provides a less punitive check than waiting to test your knowledge on the exam day itself. Have textbooks, reference materials, and course objectives handy to redress any differences of opinion about facts or interpretations.

NOTE-TAKING

Regardless of the note-taking system you use, a number of techniques can optimize your performance.

1. Date all notes and number the pages.
2. Try writing in erasable ink. Notes written in pencil can smudge. Erasable ink is easier to read and corrections can still be made.
3. Look up vocabulary that is not fully defined or that you don't know.
4. Determine the organizational patterns used to develop the material you are studying.
5. Use time-savers such as mnemonics, standard abbreviations, simplified indented format, and your own shorthand style. Beware, however, of inventing abbreviations that you may not be able to interpret when reviewing at a later time.
6. Keep notes on similar topics together by using tabbed page dividers and a loose-leaf notebook. Incorporate class handouts into the appropriate sections (you'll need a three-hole punch). Grouping similar topics together saves valuable study time by preventing fruitless searches of related bits of information.
7. Keep facts and opinions separate in your notes. You might enclose your opinions in parentheses or brackets.
8. When formulas are used, solve problems using derivations as well as the basic formula.
9. When examples are worked by the professor, record all steps of the explanation in your notes.
10. To reduce internal distractions, avoid daydreaming, doodling, and writing notes to yourself on other topics.
11. Review your notes within 24 hours to reinforce short-term memory. Distributed practice is an effective way to increase long-term memory.
12. Keep all your notes in an ''MCAT Concepts'' notebook for repeated review.

FLASH CARDS AND CONCEPT CARDS

With the large amounts of information you are learning in your classes and labs, you need to develop a method for efficiently analyzing and synthesizing the information (Figure 2-6). Developing flash cards and concept cards is one way to manage information. A flash card contains brief information, such as definitions. A concept card contains detailed information, such as the key points of a concept.

To construct flash cards and concept cards, begin by reviewing the *MCAT Student Manual* outline that pertains to the topic you are studying, such as molecular biology. Review your molecular biology textbook, your molecular biology class notes and lab notes, and any additional information you read independently about molecular biology in journals, newspapers, and magazines. Segregate the topic into the key points as listed in the *MCAT Student Manual* molecular biology outline, and write these key points on a summary sheet. When you have completed this task, construct flash cards for vocabulary and concept cards for concepts. On a flash card, write the word on one side and the definition on the other side. On a concept card, write the concept on one side; then highlight integrated areas of the subject and/or relevant experiments on the other side, listing the key points about the subject.

READING AND WRITING PRACTICE

Do not concentrate exclusively on science review. Remember, the MCAT not only tests basic science knowledge, it also tests your verbal reasoning and writing skills. Set aside time each day to include practice in reading and writing. You can warm up at the beginning of each study session by practicing your reading and writing. Or, use reading and writing practice to break up your science studies.

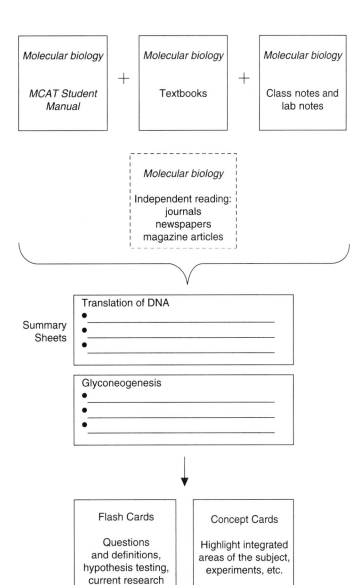

Fig. 2-6. Constructing flash cards and concept cards.

Active Reading

To read effectively, become an "active" reader. In other words, as you read, actively participate in the information being presented. Active reading involves the following activities:

- When you read an article in a scientific journal or a magazine, always read the first paragraph and stop. Close the journal and think about the author's primary purpose or hypothesis for writing the article. See if you can predict any scientific conclusions that the author will make.
- Consult your textbooks or classnotes that relate to the article. Can you find a connection between the journal article and your textbooks? Compare classnotes, textbooks and research articles to understand applications of MCAT concepts.
- Now return to the second paragraph and read the journal article to the end. Using short sentences, write down the MCAT concepts that are covered in the article. Check your textbooks and classnotes to see if you learned these concepts in class. Make notes on any new concepts or skills that are included in the article.
- If you find scientific theories, hypotheses or scientific terms that you have not encountered in your studies, record them in the corresponding sections of the *Comp-Prep* for future review.

USING TEST ITEMS FOR REVIEW

Sample MCAT test questions can be found in a variety of MCAT practice books (including this one). When working test items, practice on only a small number at one time (one passage and its follow-up questions, or ten indendepent test items in any of the other areas). Avoid marathon test sessions. Practice test sessions should be short and concentrated, and should include a systematic analysis of errors.

Error analysis is important because it requires you to examine the reasoning you used as you worked the problem. To analyze your errors, check your answers against the answer key first. If your answer is wrong, analyze the reasoning you used to solve the problem, and see if you can find the reasoning error you made along the way. If you cannot understand why your answer is wrong, then use the explanations provided with your practice test.

Keep a written record of your errors. Your errors can be classified in a number of ways. For example, specific content errors (e.g., genetics problems in the biological sciences) or specific question format errors (e.g., multiple-choice) may give you trouble. An "error journal" will help you use your time efficiently because it identifies the areas in which you need more intense review or the kinds of problems that give you the most trouble.

An additional benefit of working sample test items is that you can get an idea of what topics the MCAT emphasizes. For example, you may find that the sample test questions emphasize genetics, so time spent reviewing Mendelian genetics and application of the Hardy-Weinberg principle will repay the effort. Conversely, you do not need to take an entire course just so you can answer a single obscure question from a topic that only appears once. The *MCAT Student Manual* and Chapter 1 of this book also provide information about which topics are important.

Another way to use test questions in your study approach is to formulate your own MCAT-type questions while you study or read. Develop four response choices to each test question you write, considering what is false or the exception as well as what is true. Formulating your own questions helps you to think like a test-maker and develops your ability to anticipate what the test-maker will ask about for specific areas of content.

As you work through test questions, you may identify and review topics that you did not list on your review worksheets. Take time to address these topics if you find your information base is weak. Also consider the pattern of your content weaknesses. If you have determined that you are spending too much time on basic concepts and not enough time on details, modify your strategies to obtain better balance. You may want to work additional practice questions to monitor your progress as you make changes to your study approach.

DEVELOPING LONG-TERM MEMORY

Learning the circulatory system well is a long-term memory task; it requires you to understand what happens at each step as the blood enters and leaves the heart. As you discuss or draw the parts of the circulatory system, you are storing the information in your long-term memory.

A variety of other techniques can help you develop long-term memory. You could go to physiology or anatomy labs and carefully examine models of animal organs, such as the heart and kidneys. You may have the opportunity to observe and feel actual organs, holding each one under a water faucet where you can observe the flow of water through each organ and observe its texture. When you visit a drugstore, look at the labels of prescription and nonprescription drugs. This exercise can help you remember chemical names, symbols, and units of measure for chemical compounds. For example, what are the ingredients in aspirin? Can you draw the molecule or structure of the ingredients?

Repetition and drawing are keys to long-term learning, as is anything that encourages retention of visual images. Visual props can be especially helpful. For example, for organic chemistry, plastic models of molecules may help you understand the three-dimensional structure of molecules.

Using many different approaches to understanding a topic helps you retain the details as well as reinforce the concepts. Look for opportunities to develop long-term memory as you study for the MCAT.

DEVELOPING SHORT-TERM (OPERATIONAL) MEMORY

Short-term memory items are used and then forgotten, unlike long-term memory items, which are developed by focusing on conceptualization, not by memorizing details. Three months before the MCAT, do not waste time memorizing seldom-used equations or short-term information, such as a comparison of smooth, skeletal, and cardiac muscles. When working practice test items that require short-term memory information, solve the problem with the information in front of you. During the last few days of your study time and just before taking the MCAT, commit to memory what you have identified as short-term memory tasks. On the day of the test, take a few minutes after the exam begins to write out some of those short-term items in the margins of the test booklet so that you have them to use without having to hold them in your memory.

PART 2
Verbal Skills

The MCAT tests students' ability to read and understand complex scientific information. The test is based on passages, or excerpts, of scientific material culled from scientific books and journals. On the MCAT, you will be asked to analyze and synthesize the scientific information contained within these passages.

We've already covered how to become a more active reader. In the following section, you will learn how to construct various types of maps and diagrams to help you visualize a topic. You will also learn how to develop specific verbal skills for understanding scientific instruments, experiments, and vocabulary.

Visual Imaging: Using Maps and Diagrams

Maps and diagrams provide a visual image, or "snapshot," of a passage. When you map or diagram a passage, you tease out the various concepts presented in the passage. Maps and diagrams also allow you to make interdisciplinary connections between concepts. In effect, maps and diagrams are powerful tools for analyzing and synthesizing passages.

In the following section, we discuss four such tools that can help you visualize a passage: concept maps, process maps, classification maps, and Venn diagrams.

CONCEPT MAPS

If you've filled out review worksheets illustrated in Figure 1-5, you have already broken down the topics listed in the *MCAT Student Manual* topic outline into concepts. Concept maps allow you to probe a concept in more detail. To construct a concept map for each concept, analyze it according to the D-E-F-IN-E model (Figure 2-7). Use Figure 2-8 to apply the D-E-F-IN-E model to an example, such as obligate anaerobe.

Following these examples, use the blank D-E-F-IN-E model sheet in Figure 2-9 to analyze the following concepts:

1. Osmolarity
2. Nephron
3. Enantiomers
4. Isomers
5. Glycogenolysis

The D-E-F-IN-E model can be applied to advanced biological concepts, as well. Apply the model to the following:

1. Active transport of amino acids in the intestine
2. Cushing's syndrome
3. Glycogenolysis and glycogenesis

Hints:

1. **D:** This concept includes amino acids, active transport process, and transport through intestinal membranes. **F:** Include a sketch showing active transport. **IN:** Include the organic and physical aspects of typical amino acids. **E:** Include an explanation of the transport model or mechanism that should be explained.

D	**Define** or describe the concept
E	**Example** of the concept
F	**Formulate** an equation or sketch for the concept
IN	**Investigate** the concept in detail
E	**Expand** your conceptual horizon by application

Fig. 2-7. The D-E-F-IN-E model.

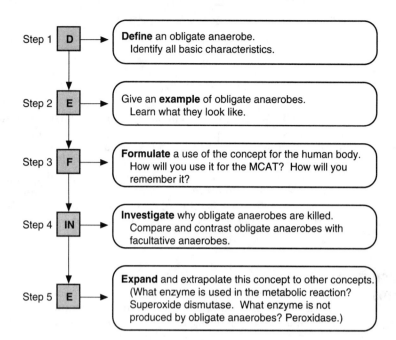

Fig. 2-8. D-E-F-IN-E: Obligate anaerobe.

Step 1 **D** → **Define** an obligate anaerobe. Identify all basic characteristics.

Step 2 **E** → Give an **example** of obligate anaerobes. Learn what they look like.

Step 3 **F** → **Formulate** a use of the concept for the human body. How will you use it for the MCAT? How will you remember it?

Step 4 **IN** → **Investigate** why obligate anaerobes are killed. Compare and contrast obligate anaerobes with facultative anaerobes.

Step 5 **E** → **Expand** and extrapolate this concept to other concepts. (What enzyme is used in the metabolic reaction? Superoxide dismutase. What enzyme is not produced by obligate anaerobes? Peroxidase.)

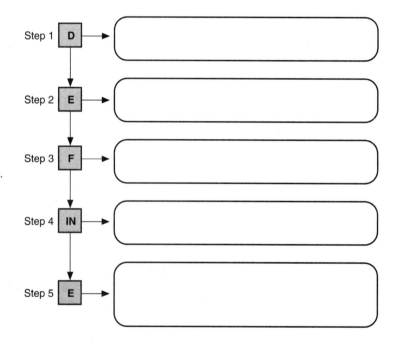

Fig. 2-9. D-E-F-IN-E worksheet.

Step 1 **D** →

Step 2 **E** →

Step 3 **F** →

Step 4 **IN** →

Step 5 **E** →

2. **D:** This syndrome should be classified as a hormonal disorder. **E:** Include its causes and symptoms. **IN:** include the glands that are affected.
3. **D:** Glycogenolysis refers to the intracellular breakdown of glycogen, whereas glycogenesis is the intracellular synthesis of glycogen. **IN:** Analyze activity of the muscle and liver cells for each process. **E:** Investigate the structural changes that take place in the muscle and liver cells.

The same process works for physical sciences concepts. Figure 2-10 applies the D-E-F-IN-E model to a physical sciences concept, free-body diagrams. Following this example, use the blank D-E-F-IN-E worksheet to analyze the following concepts:

1. Refraction index
2. Capacitance

3. Shadows
4. Angular torque
5. Density

PROCESS MAPS

The primary goal of the process map is to analyze how something functions or evolves. Process maps present an orderly or prescribed series of steps or operations that lead to a result or product. Most process maps resemble a chain of events in which the result of one step becomes the cause of another (Figure 2-11). Figure 2-12 depicts a process map for making butter. Each step in this map leads logically to the next step. Notice that step four contains two substeps.

Process maps are useful for MCAT questions that present the steps of a process, except one step will not be described. These questions require you to supply the missing step. Sketching a process map allows you to see the entire process as a whole and to easily fill in the missing step.

Exercise: Construct a process map for an acid–base titration (titrating NaOH against HCl), using your general chemistry lab manual and textbook.

CLASSIFICATION MAPS

In science, classification systems are used to organize groups with varying characteristics. Classification systems can be based on demographics, phyla, behavioral traits, family trees, etc. Some MCAT questions probe your ability to classify. For instance, classification questions frequently name the classification category for a group of objects, but in order to determine the correct answer, you must consider whether an additional concept fits into the designated classification.

Classification maps can be used to show complex relationships between groups. They are especially useful in showing the development of a cell type, tissue, or organ. The basic structure of classification maps resembles that of a "family tree," in which the "branches" designate different subgroups (Figure 2-13).

Figure 2-14 is a classification map constructed for the concept "connective tissue." Notice that this map not only lists the kinds of connective tissue, but some of the differentiating characteristics, as well. When constructing these maps, feel free to include as much information as you think is appropriate to help you understand the concept.

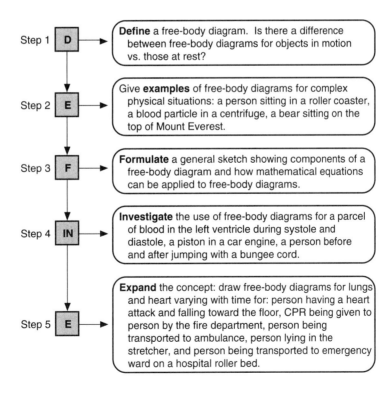

Fig. 2-10. D-E-F-IN-E : Free body diagram

Step 1 **D** — **Define** a free-body diagram. Is there a difference between free-body diagrams for objects in motion vs. those at rest?

Step 2 **E** — Give **examples** of free-body diagrams for complex physical situations: a person sitting in a roller coaster, a blood particle in a centrifuge, a bear sitting on the top of Mount Everest.

Step 3 **F** — **Formulate** a general sketch showing components of a free-body diagram and how mathematical equations can be applied to free-body diagrams.

Step 4 **IN** — **Investigate** the use of free-body diagrams for a parcel of blood in the left ventricle during systole and diastole, a piston in a car engine, a person before and after jumping with a bungee cord.

Step 5 **E** — **Expand** the concept: draw free-body diagrams for lungs and heart varying with time for: person having a heart attack and falling toward the floor, CPR being given to person by the fire department, person being transported to ambulance, person lying in the stretcher, and person being transported to emergency ward on a hospital roller bed.

Fig. 2-11. Process map.

□ → □ → □ → □

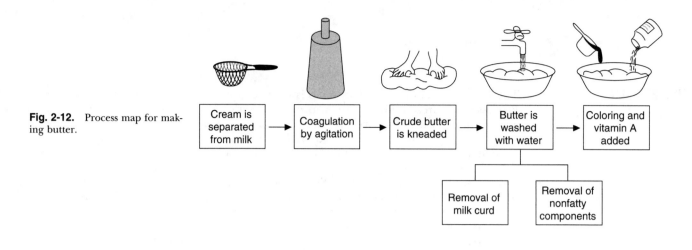

Fig. 2-12. Process map for making butter.

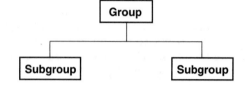

Fig. 2-13. Classification map.

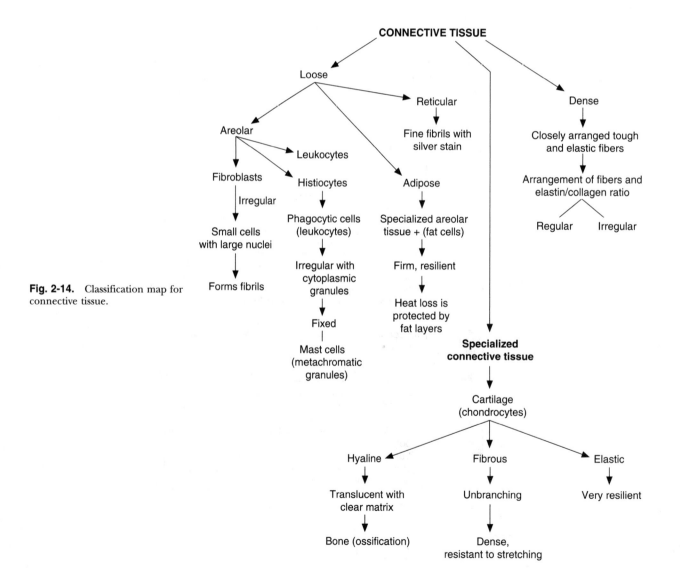

Fig. 2-14. Classification map for connective tissue.

Exercise: Construct a classification map for stereoisomers, using your organic chemistry lab manual and textbook.

VENN DIAGRAMS

Venn diagrams, or association diagrams, can be useful for questions that emphasize differences between things. They are useful for determining what should be and should not be included in analyzing information. In contrast to maps, Venn diagrams are used to visually represent **statements** rather than concepts.

Consider the following illustration: The statement, "all roses are red" can be broken down as follows:

- Things that are red
- Roses (all are red)
- Things that are red, but are not roses

This is illustrated in Figure 2-15.

In a Venn diagram, a circle entirely contained within another circle means that all the members of the inner group belong in the outer group as well. In Figure 2-15, the inner circle denotes roses (all of which are red) and the outer circle denotes "things that are red." The space inside the larger circle (but outside the smaller circle) represents all those things that are red but are not roses.

The statement "some roses are red" is diagramed in Figure 2-16. If you look at the lines of the circles, you can see the relationship between red things and roses, only some of which are red. But if you look at the spaces rather than the lines, you see the relationships between three categories:

- roses that are not red
- some roses, which are red
- red things that are not roses

The statement "no roses are red" is diagramed in Figure 2-17.

Verbal Skills to Understand Scientific Instruments

Questions containing references to scientific instrumentation appear on the MCAT. The MCAT requires that students be familiar with reading information describing instruments, such as a user's manual or operations manual. The following section on instruments should be included as exercises in your review and linked to your study of the physical and biological sciences in chapters 7 and 8 of this book (Figure 2-18).

The following is a list of experimental and medical equipment that you should be familiar with. These are discussed in the AAMC video *Preparing for the MCAT* (see Chapter 1).

- Pressure gauges, manometers, pressure transducers
- CATSCAN machine, dynamic spatial reconstruction (DSR) machine
- X-rays used in graphic analysis as obtained in radiology with lighted background
- Human skeleton (3D) model, heart model, advanced microscopes
- Surgery room equipment: overhead flood lights, blood pressure monitors, EEG/EKG monitors, pulse rate monitors
- Small flashlight used by nurse to check a baby's eye in pediatrics
- Electron microscope used in neurosurgery
- Dissection tools for use during surgery
- Chemistry laboratory equipment, including volume-measuring flasks, cylinders, etc.
- Instruments used in a chemical separations and purifications laboratory

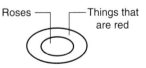

Fig. 2-15. Venn diagram: "all roses are red."

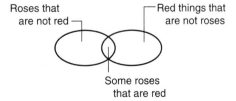

Fig. 2-16. Venn diagram: "some roses are red."

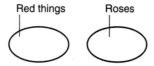

Fig. 2-17. Venn diagram: "no roses are red."

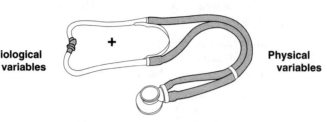

Fig. 2-18. Linking instrumentation to the physical and biological sciences.

Here are some activities that will enhance your understanding of clinically relevant instruments and procedures.

- Learn to read a complex sketch or drawing (look at the size, position, shape, and name of each part)
- If an instrument is described but not illustrated, draw a representative schematic of the instrument showing its structure and function
- Relate principles of biology, chemistry, or physics to an explanation of the instrument
- Interpret the functions of the instrument from its description
- Connect the application of an instrument to medical technology (i.e., its use in a laboratory or hospital)
- List possible sources of malfunction of the instrument
- Find scales of measurement and range for precision and accuracy of the instrument from the manufacturer's label or instructions. If applicable, find any precautions associated with the instrument
- Compare and contrast the parts of an instrument and the function of each in its operation

Verbal Skills to Analyze Scientific Experiments

You should evaluate scientific experiments from a critical standpoint. As you read the details of a scientific experiment, evaluate the hypothesis, look for explicit and implicit assumptions, and propose direct and indirect conclusions based on experimental data, graphs, and other observed evidence.

Usually, ten components are included in the laboratory report of a scientific experiment. Some MCAT passages that describe experiments include tabulated observations, but give only a few of the other experimental components. Students should know the list of components well enough to detect when some are missing from MCAT passages and why they are important for answering the test questions. In the following list of components, those shown with an asterisk are usually provided in MCAT questions.

1. Purpose or scope of the experiment
2. * Introduction and background material
3. Equipment, instruments and chemicals list
4. Sequential setup and skills in the overall procedure
5. * Procedural sketch or schematic of experiment
6. * Data collected and observations
7. * Calculations and results, including graphs
8. Precautions observed during experiment
9. Comments, including sources of errors
10. Questions and problems to be solved by the experiment

As you study, pay particular attention to presentations of experiments. When reading physical sciences materials, work on understanding graphs drawn in physics and chemistry labs and the design and operation of laboratory equipment as it applies to physics and

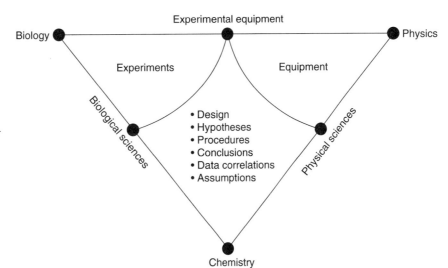

Fig. 2-19. Schematic depicting the analysis of an instrument or experiment, using integrated concepts in biology, chemistry, and physics.

general chemistry concepts. For biological sciences, read and analyze research articles in journals on biology, organic and molecular biochemistry, and physiology. Understand how several variables are shown in tables and graphs. In addition, study how researchers accept and reject various research hypotheses.

Premedical students often do not apply critical thinking skills to experimental equipment or experimental procedures. However, critical thinking is essential in clinical work. Figure 2-19 provides a schematic of how integration of concepts in biology, chemistry, and physics can lead to better analysis of equipment or an experiment using logical steps of exploration. For example, understanding the physical principles (such as gravity) applied to the solution in a glass burette will lead students to understand errors in volume measurement, speed of a falling drop of a titrant, and better observations of the optical meniscus to observe liquid levels.

Developing Vocabulary During MCAT Review

Good ways to learn vocabulary are constructing flash cards and keeping a vocabulary notebook for writing down unfamiliar terms that you encounter in your reading. Whether you use flash cards, a notebook, or both, it is important that you review vocabulary regularly. Regular review will reinforce your working vocabulary significantly.

Vocabulary review is essential when studying for the MCAT because difficult words and technical terminology can cause trouble. The MCAT assesses your ability to handle definitions of technical or difficult words in three areas:

1. distinguishing between unfamiliar technical terms that are closely related
2. distinguishing between words that sound alike
3. demonstrating your understanding of the issues involved in defining a concept in an extended definition

DISTINGUISHING BETWEEN CLOSELY RELATED TERMS

In some problems or passages, you are presented with an unfamiliar topic or an advanced concept. The passage will resemble an introduction to an article and will present basic scientific terminology. To answer the question, you might be asked to distinguish between related subgroups within the topic area. For example, you might be asked to distinguish between different kinds of immune disorders presented in the passage. Students often have difficulty reading this kind of passage for any one of the following reasons:

1. Lack of precision in distinguishing one term from another,
2. Anxiety related to the time it takes to understand such unfamiliar material,
3. Failure to have an available strategy for dealing with the difficulty.

When reading and answering questions, learn to recognize whether the form of the passage is definitional. This recognition provides insight into the purpose of the passage and alerts you to what you will likely be asked to do in answering the questions. As you read, it is helpful to make a note in the margin wherever you have identified a definition.

DISTINGUISHING BETWEEN WORDS THAT SOUND ALIKE

If "affect" and "effect" caused you trouble in high school English, the distinction between "astronomy" and "astrology" may be likely to cause confusion on the MCAT, and the terms "afferent" and "efferent" will undoubtedly cause you some difficulty in medical school. Counter this difficulty by employing a specific strategy for dealing with terms that are confusing simply because of acoustic similarities.

As you study, collect words that you typically confuse with each other. Write them on flash cards and practice them often. Develop mnemonics to help distinguish between them. For example, associate "exit" and "efferent." A more complex mnemonic for distinguishing between "afferent" and "efferent" would be SAME and DAVE. SAME reminds you that sensory and afferent go together, as do motor and efferent. DAVE reminds you that dorsal and afferent belong together, as do ventral and efferent. Words with similar-sounding but different prefixes may also cause trouble, such as homogeneous and heterogeneous, and intercellular and intracellular. Construct flash cards for these terms as well.

UNDERSTANDING EXTENDED MEANINGS USED IN PASSAGES

You may have problems with MCAT passages that present an extended definition of a word. The word can be a technical term that requires a thorough extended discussion, such as *psychosis*. Unlike passages that introduce completely new but specific terminology, extended-definition passages often define a broad term with which you are somewhat familiar, but understand imprecisely. Often, the purpose of the extended definition passage is to refute a commonly held definition in favor of the author's own view. In effect, these questions ask you to understand and follow another person's argument.

You may find extended-definition passages difficult either because you fail to recognize that the discussion is an argument, or because you answer the questions based on your own view, which is not necessarily that of the author. Remember that all definitions are open to examination and modification. For example, astronomers are currently debating the precise definition of "planet" because new data seem to require a revised one. The key to answering these types of questions is to recognize that the question is not about a definition but about argument and persuasion.

PART 3
Problem-Solving Skills for the Sciences

No part of the MCAT causes students more concern than the inclusion of problem-solving within the context of the sciences. Yet, if you were not interested in solving medical problems, you would not be seeking admission to medical school. Problem-solving can be difficult and frustrating, but it is also exciting, satisfying, and fun. View problem-solving as a competitive game: you versus the test-maker. Think of the question writer as a villain to be vanquished or a puzzler to be outfoxed. Remember that the rules of this game have been defined by the test-maker and that your task is to win working within those rules. The first order of business in perfecting your problem-solving skills is to learn these rules.

Problems based on passages in the MCAT frequently contain unfamiliar or unexpected material. Familiar knowledge may be cast in unusual circumstances or combined with knowledge from a different discipline. You may need to apply both biology and physics to answer a single question. To build your confidence in solving passage-based problems in the MCAT, you will need to work with the unfamiliar and the unexpected, with unusual research studies, and with the demands of combined and separate disciplines. In the remainder of this section, we will systematically help you construct an approach to conquering these challenges.

Many students develop problem-solving skills in a hit-or-miss fashion because most schools teach these skills in a random or unorganized way. This section will help you develop your problem-solving skills and give you practice and confidence in answering science problem questions within a conscious problem-solving framework. When working science problems, be precise and work quickly. Be sure you fully understand each problem; read carefully and think actively. You must recall facts, but you should be able to apply scientific concepts. The more precisely you can apply these concepts, the greater your mastery of the information.

Problem-Solving Practice for Passage-Based Problems

Problem-solving always requires background knowledge. Some background knowledge will come from what you have already learned in your college courses and some will be given to you in charts or passages that precede the problem statement. The approach outlined below will serve you well if you apply it to each passage:

1. Where is this passage taken from (e.g., book, laboratory research report, encyclopedia)?
2. Which branches of science are discussed in this passage?
3. What topics does the passage discuss in detail?
4. What is given in the passage about a topic?
5. What is it about the topic that is not given in the passage? Why not?

The passages that precede problem statements in the MCAT come from a variety of sources. These include college textbooks, scientific publications, and research reports. Your college courses teach the background knowledge required for problem-solving, and scientific journals and books display the form and content of the material on which MCAT passages are based. Become familiar with the style, form, and vocabulary used in these sources. The more familiar you are with these sources before you take the test, the more comfortable you will be working problems based on these sources.

Another important resource for developing problem-solving skills can be found in the graphic representation of scientific data. Most research publications and medical books present scientific data in compact representations that may require considerable effort to convert to a form useful in problem solving. A frequently used form of data presentation is the continuous line graph representing a functional relationship. The task is to identify the functional relationship and check its validity; for example, viscosity versus temperature, nitrogen concentration versus volume (exhalation), and myogram (force versus time) of a typical muscle.

Reading Practice for Problem Solving

Now is an appropriate time for you to experience a typical MCAT passage containing new information. As you read the passage, actively mark your passage to highlight important points. Use your reading comprehension skills, including analysis, synthesis, and visual imagery. The passage presented here is a classification-type passage similar in format and style to passages found in the actual MCAT. Consider using the following techniques during this reading exercise:

1. Skim the passage for approximately 30 seconds. Decide what the passage is about.
2. Read the questions that follow this passage.
3. Take 3 to 5 minutes to read the passage.

Passage: Connective Tissue: General Characteristics and Functions

Connective tissue allows movement and provides support. In this tissue there is an abundance of intercellular material called matrix, which is variable in type and amount and is one of the main sources of difference between the types of connective tissue. It consists of various fibers embedded in a ground substance.

Loose Connective Tissue

The fibers of loose connective tissue are not tightly woven. The tissue, filling space between and penetrating into the organs, is of three types: areolar, adipose, and reticular.

Areolar Tissue. The most widely distributed connective tissue is pliable and crossed by many delicate threads; yet, the tissue resists tearing and is somewhat elastic. Areolar tissue contains fibroblasts, histiocytes (macrophages), leukocytes, and mast cells.

Fibroblasts are small, flattened, somewhat irregular cells with large nuclei and reduced cytoplasm. The term fibroblast refers to the ability of a cell to form fibrils. Fibroblasts are active in repair of injury. It is generally believed that suprarenal steroids inhibit and growth hormones stimulate fibroblastic activity. Histiocytes are phagocytic cells similar to leukocytes in blood; however, they perform phagocytic activity outside the vascular system. The histiocyte is irregular in shape and contains cytoplasmic granules. The cell is often stationary (or "fixed"). Mast cells, located adjacent to small blood vessels, are round or polygonal in shape and possess a cytoplasm filled with metachromatic granules. Mast cells function in the manufacture of heparin (an anticoagulant) and histamine (an inflammatory substance responsible for changes in allergic tissue). Depression in mast cell activity results from the administration of cortisol to patients. Areolar tissue is the basic supporting substance around organs, muscles, blood vessels, and nerves forming the delicate membranes around the brain and spinal cord and comprising the superficial fascia, or sheet of connective tissue, found deep in the skin.

Adipose Tissue. Adipose tissue is specialized areolar tissue with fat-containing cells. The fat or lipid cell, like other cells, has a nucleus, endoplasmic reticulum, cell membrane, mitochondria, and one or more fat droplets. Adipose tissue acts as a firm yet resilient packing around and between organs, bundles of muscle fibers, nerves, and supporting blood vessels. Since fat is a poor conductor of heat, adipose tissue protects the body from excessive heat loss or excessive rises in temperature.

Reticular Tissue. Reticular fibers consist of finely branching fibrils taking a silver stain as observed under the microscope. The primary cell of the reticular fiber is the reticular cell. Reticular fibers form the framework of the liver, lymphoid organs, and bone marrow.

Dense Connective Tissue

Dense connective tissue is composed of closely arranged tough collagenous and elastic fiber. It can be classified according to the arrangement of the fibers and the proportion of elastin and collagen present. Examples of dense connective tissue having a regular arrangement of fibers are tendons, aponeuroses, and ligaments. Examples of dense connective tissue having an irregular arrangement of fibers are fasciae, capsules, and muscle sheaths.

Specialized Connective Tissue

Cartilage. Cartilage has a firm matrix consisting of protein and mucopolysaccharides. Cells of cartilage, called chondrocytes, are large and rounded with spherical nuclei. Collagenous and elastic fibers are embedded in the matrix, increasing the elastic and resistive properties of this tissue. The three types of cartilage are hyaline, fibrous, and elastic.

In utero, hyaline cartilage, the precursor of much of the skeletal system, is translucent with a clear matrix caused by abundant collagenous fibers (not visible as such) and cells scattered throughout the matrix. Hyaline cartilage is gradually replaced by bone in many parts of the body through the process of ossification; however, some remains as a covering on the articular surfaces. The hyaline costal cartilages attach the anterior ends of the upper seven pairs of ribs to the sternum. The trachea and bronchi are kept open by incomplete rings of surrounding hyaline cartilage. This type of cartilage is also found in the nose.

Fibrous cartilage contains dense masses of unbranching, collagenous fibers lying in the matrix. Cells of fibrous cartilage are present in rows between bundles of the matrix. Fibrocartilage is dense and resistant to stretching; it is less flexible and less resilient than hyaline cartilage. Fibrous cartilage, interposed between the vertebrae in the spinal column, is also present in the symphysis pubis, permitting a minimal range of movement.

Elastic cartilage, which is more resilient than either the hyaline or the fibrous type because of a predominance of elastic fibers impregnated in its ground substance, is found in the auricle of the external ear, the auditory tube, the epiglottis, and portions of the larynx.

Bone is a firm tissue formed by impregnation of the intercellular material with inorganic salts. It is living tissue supplied by blood vessels and nerves and is constantly being remodeled. The two common types are compact, forming the dense outer layer, and cancellous, forming the inner lighter tissue of the shaft of a long bone.

The dentin of teeth is closely related to bone. The crown of the tooth is covered by enamel, the hardest substance in the body. Enamel is secreted onto the dentin by the epithelial cells of the enamel organ before the teeth are extruded through the gums. Dentin resembles bone but is harder and denser.

Blood and Hematopoietic Tissue. Marrow is the blood-forming (hematopoietic) tissue located in the shafts of the bones. The red blood cells (erythrocytes) and most white blood cells (leukocytes) originate in the capillary sinusoids of bone marrow. Some leukocytes are formed in the lymphoid organs.

Blood is a fluid tissue circulating through the body, carrying nutrients to cells, and removing waste products.

Lymphoid tissue is found in the lymph nodes, thymus, spleen, tonsils, and adenoids. The germinal centers of lymph tissue produce plasma cells and lymphocytes. Lymphoid tissues function in antibody production.

Connective tissues perform many functions, including support and nourishment for other tissues, packing material in the spaces between organs, and defense for the body by digestion and absorption of foreign material.

Reticuloendothelial system. Connective tissue cells, carrying on the process of phagocytosis, are frequently referred to as the reticuloendothelial system. The cells ingest solid particles similar to the manner in which an amoeba takes in nourishment. Three types of phagocytic cells belong to this classification; reticuloendothelial cells lining the liver (Kupffer's cells), spleen, and bone marrow; macrophages, termed tissue histiocytes or "resting-wandering" cells; and microglia, located in the central nervous system. The reticuloendothelial system is a strong line of defense against infection.

Synovial membranes. Synovial membranes line the cavities of the freely moving joints and form tendon sheaths and bursae.

In order to better understand passage-based problems, answer the following questions for yourself before moving to the marked-up passage in Figure 2-20.

1. How much time did it take to read the passage?
2. What is the main idea conveyed in the passage?
3. Did you mark up the passage to extract information?
4. Do you remember 20 new or difficult terms? (do not re-read passage)
5. Write a short summary of the passage.
6. Which parts of the passage were most difficult?
7. Is there irrelevant information in the passage?

The marked-up passage illustrates active reading. Important points are marked by underlines, circles, and other notations. Compare your markup of the passage with the sample markup. How accurate were you in marking the various key points?

Answers to Questions 1 Through 7:

1. You should spend no more than 5 minutes reading this kind of passage. Furthermore, passage reading time should be only half the time spent reading and answering the questions.
2. If you made a classification map (see Figure 2-14), you know the passage is about structure, function, and types of connective tissue. The classification map is also a visual index to the passage that helps identify items for later reference.
3. Marking the passage helps you remember details. Use long arrows or leaders to connect terms that repeat in the passage (e.g., arrows connecting words such as fibroblasts and histiocytes).
4. Use your classification map to find 20 terms, including: loose tissue, dense tissue, areolar, adipose, reticular, fibroblasts, fibrils, histiocytes, cytoplasmic granules, mast cells, metachromatic granules, hyaline, ossification, cartilage, chondrocytes, fibrous cartilage, elastic cartilage, elastin/collagen ratio, phagocytic cells, leukocytes, resilient. Add any new terms to your vocabulary notebook.
5. You should be able to write a one- or two-paragraph summary based on your marked-up passage and classification map. A summary repeats important things in a passage and improves your short-term memory of its content.
6. The most difficult part of a passage has the most details. A classification map will help you to remember the details because they are written down.
7. Information that you do not use to answer questions is unused information, but do not consider it irrelevant. Irrelevant information is usually limited in MCAT passages.

Modes of Reasoning

The MCAT tests your level of mastery of many scientific concepts. For each concept you study, ask yourself the following questions. Do you fully understand the concept or have you merely memorized what you need in order to pass? Applying something you learned in one way, can you solve a problem that is unlike anything you have seen before? In your own words, can you explain the concept to a colleague who is having trouble understanding it? If you find yourself saying, "I know that material, but I just can't put it into words," you have not mastered the information.

Content mastery can be tested by asking you to use skills developed throughout your academic life in analytical reading, logical reasoning, quantitative reasoning, perceptual reasoning, and problem-solving. These skills are like tools in a toolbox. For efficiency and effectiveness, you need to be able to use them all, and it is better to do so consciously than to fumble around in a hit-or-miss fashion.

① control passage as it branches from the intro. paragraph →
keep looking for differences in structure (S) and function (F)
② develop a mental layout of passage as it expands
in content

(approx. 500 words)

Connective Tissue: General Characteristics and Functions

Connective tissue allows movement and provides support. *F* In this tissue there is an abundance of intercellular material called matrix, *S* which is variable in type and amount and is one of the main sources of difference between the types of connective tissue. It consists of various fibers embedded in a ground substance.

Loose Connective Tissue

The fibers of loose connective tissue are not tightly woven. The tissue, filling space between and penetrating into the organs, is of three types: areolar, adipose, and reticular.

Areolar Tissue. The most widely distributed connective tissue is pliable and crossed by many delicate threads; yet, the tissue resists tearing and is somewhat elastic. *S* Areolar tissue contains fibroblasts, histiocytes (macrophages), leukocytes, and mast cells.

Fibroblasts are small, flattened, somewhat irregular cells with large nuclei and reduced cytoplasm. The term fibroblast refers to the ability of a cell to form fibrils. Fibroblasts are active in repair of injury. It is generally believed that suprarenal steroids inhibit and growth hormones stimulate fibroblastic activity. **Histiocytes** ar phagocytic cells similar to **leukocytes** in blood; however, they perform phagocytic activity outside the vascular system. The histiocyte is irregular in shape and contains cytoplasmic granules. The cell is often stationary (or "fixed"). **Mast cells** located adjacent to small blood vessels, are round or polygonal in shape and possess a cytoplasm filled with *S* metachromatic granules. Mast cells function in the manufacture of heparin (an anticoagulant) and histamine (an inflammatory substance responsible for changes in allergic tissue). Depression in mast cell activity results from the administration of cortisol to patients. Areolar tissue is the basic supporting substance around organs, muscles, blood vessels, and nerves forming the delicate membranes around the brain and spinal cord and comprising the superficial fascia, or sheet of connective tissue, found deep in the skin.

Adipose Tissue. Adipose tissue is specialized areolar tissue with fat-containing cells. The fat or lipid cell, like other cells, has a nucleus, endoplasmic reticulum, cell membrane, mitochondria, and one or more fat droplets. Adipose tissue acts as a firm yet resilient packing around and between

↑
remember elasticity and spring from Physics (Are density and elasticity related?)

organs, bundles of muscle fibers, nerves, and supporting blood vessels. Since fat is a poor conductor of heat, adipose tissue protects the body from excessive heat loss or excessive rises in temperature.

heat eqn. ⇒

Reticular Tissue. Reticular fibers consist of finely branching fibrils taking a silver stain as observed under the microscope. The primary cell of the reticular fiber is the reticular cell. Reticular fibers form the framework of the liver, lymphoid organs, and bone marrow.
where?

Dense Connective Tissue

Dense connective tissue is composed of closely arranged tough collagenous and elastic fiber. It can be classified according to the arrangement of the fibers and the proportion of elastin and collagen present. Examples of dense connective tissue having a regular arrangement of fibers are tendons, *where?* aponeuroses, and ligaments. Examples of dense connective tissue having an irregular arrangement of fibers are fasciae, capsules, and muscle sheaths.
where?

Specialized Connective Tissue

A

Cartilage. Cartilage has a firm matrix consisting of protein and mucopolysaccharides. Cells of cartilage, called chondrocytes, are large and rounded with spherical nuclei. *S* Collagenous and elastic fibers are embedded in the matrix, increasing the elastic and resistive properties of this tissue. The three types of cartilage are hyaline, fibrous, and elastic.

In utero, **hyaline cartilage**, the precursor of much of the skeletal system, is translucent with a clear matrix caused by abundant collagenous fibers (not visible as such) and cells scattered throughout the matrix. Hyaline cartilage is gradually replaced by bone in many parts of the body through the process of ossification; however, some remains as a covering on the articular surfaces. The hyaline costal cartilages attach the anterior ends of the upper seven pairs of ribs to the sternum. The trachea and bronchi are kept open by incomplete rings *where?* surrounding hyaline cartilage. This type of cartilage is also found in the nose.

Fibrous cartilage contains dense masses of unbranching, collagenous fibers lying in the matrix. Cells of fibrous cartilage are present in rows between bundles of the matrix. Fibrocartilage is dense and resistant to stretching; it is less flexible and less resilient than hyaline cartilage. Fibrous cartilage, interposed between the vertebrae in the spinal column, is also present in the symphysis pubis, permitting a minimal range of movement.
Physics

experimental procedure

any connections?

physiology → inhibit and stimulate (examine cause and find effects)

biochemistry → visualize and relate structure + functional groups for histamines/heparin

where?

where?

anatomy of a fat cell

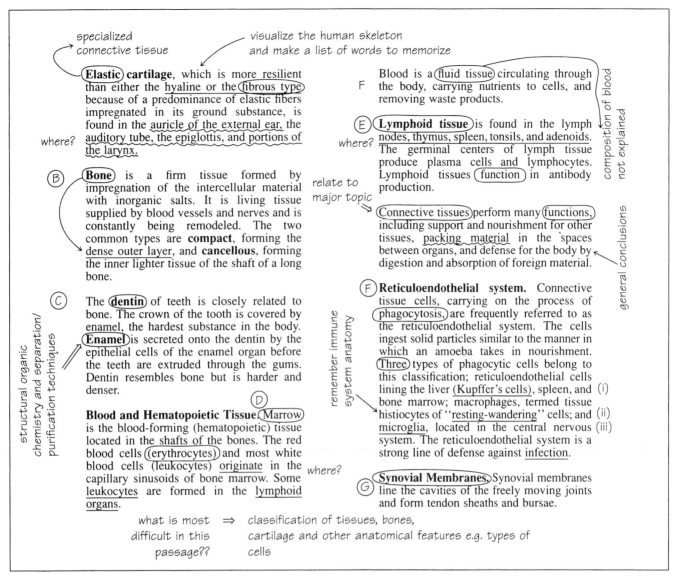

specialized connective tissue

visualize the human skeleton and make a list of words to memorize

Elastic **cartilage**, which is more resilient than either the hyaline or the fibrous type because of a predominance of elastic fibers impregnated in its ground substance, is found in the auricle of the external ear, the auditory tube, the epiglottis, and portions of the larynx.

where?

Ⓑ **Bone** is a firm tissue formed by impregnation of the intercellular material with inorganic salts. It is living tissue supplied by blood vessels and nerves and is constantly being remodeled. The two common types are **compact**, forming the dense outer layer, and **cancellous**, forming the inner lighter tissue of the shaft of a long bone.

Ⓒ The **dentin** of teeth is closely related to bone. The crown of the tooth is covered by enamel, the hardest substance in the body. **Enamel** is secreted onto the dentin by the epithelial cells of the enamel organ before the teeth are extruded through the gums. Dentin resembles bone but is harder and denser.

Ⓓ **Blood and Hematopoietic Tissue.** **Marrow** is the blood-forming (hematopoietic) tissue located in the shafts of the bones. The red blood cells (erythrocytes) and most white blood cells (leukocytes) originate in the capillary sinusoids of bone marrow. Some leukocytes are formed in the lymphoid organs.

structural organic chemistry and separation/purification techniques

F Blood is a fluid tissue circulating through the body, carrying nutrients to cells, and removing waste products.

Ⓔ **Lymphoid tissue** is found in the lymph nodes, thymus, spleen, tonsils, and adenoids. The germinal centers of lymph tissue produce plasma cells and lymphocytes. Lymphoid tissues function in antibody production.

where?

composition of blood not explained

Connective tissues perform many functions, including support and nourishment for other tissues, packing material in the spaces between organs, and defense for the body by digestion and absorption of foreign material.

relate to major topic

general conclusions

Ⓕ **Reticuloendothelial system.** Connective tissue cells, carrying on the process of phagocytosis, are frequently referred to as the reticuloendothelial system. The cells ingest solid particles similar to the manner in which an amoeba takes in nourishment. Three types of phagocytic cells belong to this classification; reticuloendothelial cells lining the liver (Kupffer's cells), spleen, and bone marrow; macrophages, termed tissue histiocytes of ''resting-wandering'' cells; and microglia, located in the central nervous system. The reticuloendothelial system is a strong line of defense against infection.

(i)
(ii)
(iii)

remember immune system anatomy

Ⓖ **Synovial Membranes.** Synovial membranes line the cavities of the freely moving joints and form tendon sheaths and bursae.

where?

what is most difficult in this passage?? ⟹ classification of tissues, bones, cartilage and other anatomical features e.g. types of cells

Fig. 2-20. Sample marked-up passage on connective tissue.

A conscious awareness of reasoning skills can improve your understanding of the material you study and result in improved test performance. As you read this section, concentrate on the similarities and differences between the various reasoning patterns. Anticipate how test questions could be formulated to assess particular reasoning skills, and consider how passages that precede test questions may be structured around various reasoning patterns.

ANALYTICAL REASONING

Analysis involves breaking something down into its component parts. This is as true of reading analysis as it is of chemical analysis. Analysis involves identifying primary and secondary pieces of information and then, by reasoning, determining the relationship between them. An important part of analysis is separating relevant information from irrelevant information.

For example, you are practicing analysis as you take notes in class. You are selecting the main points (the primary information) and the supporting details. When you outline, you are indicating the relationship between primary and secondary information. Underlining is also a tool for analyzing text, if used appropriately. The effective student reads first, and then selectively underlines key words. At the same time he or she makes notes in the margin or uses numbers to indicate the relationship of one piece of information to another and, especially, how both relate to the whole. Venn diagrams and maps are graphic analytical tools that you can use to analyze complex passages.

If analysis involves identifying primary and secondary information, analytical reasoning often requires a focus on words that are important in relating pieces of information to each other. The careless or hurried reader may overlook qualifying words, such as *always, some, and, or, for example, most likely, probably, however, consequently,* and *as a result of.* These words should serve as red flags. As you read practice passages, circle qualifying words and think about what they are telling you.

Analytical Reasoning Exercises

Exercise 1: Four doctors—Harry, Louise, Kate, and Bob—collect automobiles. Among them are owned 20 cars, of which 12 are vintage. Harry has three new cars and Louise has the same number of vintage autos. Louise has one more car than Harry, who has five. Kate has three more vintage cars than new ones and the same number of new ones as Bob. How many vintage cars does Bob have?

Exercise 2: Make a Venn diagram to illustrate the relationship between the following words: *mothers, daughters, grandmothers, aunts.* (Hint: These relationships are difficult to diagram. Start with mothers and daughters only, and remember that any circle that is contained within another circle means that all its members belong to both groups. When you have that relationship represented by Venn diagrams, add a circle for grandmothers, and then add aunts.)

As with any skill, it is important to practice the process of visually representing and summarizing concepts. Maps and diagrams can be used on the MCAT as a "sorting" tool to organize and analyze content.

Exercise 3: Develop a sketch based on the following biological sciences passage.

The eye is a layer of photoreceptor cells and associated neurons packaged within a fibrous, rubberlike protective globe that is transparent in front. The eyeball is almost spherical in shape, about 2.5 cm in diameter, with three concentric coats, or tunics, surrounding the refractive media. These coats are the fibrous coat, the vascular coat, and the nervous coat.

The fibrous tunic is the outermost coat and consists of the sclera and the cornea. The sclera (meaning *hard*) is a tough, white, supporting tunic. It covers the posterior five-sixths of the eye. The cornea (meaning *horny*) covers the anterior one-sixth and is continuous with the sclera. The radius of the cornea is less than that of the sclera; that is, it has a greater curvature, so it bulges somewhat. In addition to transmitting light, the cornea also is a refractive medium and focuses light rays.

The middle coat, or vascular tunic, is divided into the iris, the ciliary body, and the choroid. The iris forms a diaphragm between the cornea and the lens and is like a curtain with a central perforation, the pupil. The diameter of the pupil may be altered by the muscles in the iris that are oriented in two directions. One set of muscles pulls the iris back toward the ciliary body to dilate the pupil. The other muscle draws the iris down around the front of the lens to constrict the pupil. The color of the iris is largely a function of the amount of pigment within. The ciliary body is ring-shaped with protrusions or folds on the internal surface that are responsible for the secretion of aqueous humor. The choroid, chiefly composed of blood vessels and pigment, lines the posterior part of the sclera. This vascular, highly pigmented layer absorbs light and prevents scattering.

The innermost tunic is the retina, which is the light-sensitive layer of the eye. It consists of several layers of cell bodies and fibers. One of these layers consists of photoreceptor neurons called rods and cones. The rods are highly sensitive to light and insensitive to color, whereas the cones are sensitive to color and provide the highest visual acuity.

Exercise 4: Construct a Venn diagram based on the following biological sciences passage. Diagram these terms: *carbohydrates, monosaccharides, disaccharides, starch, lactose, glucose, polysaccharides, fructose, sucrose, maltose, cellobiose, glycogen, cellulose.*

Carbohydrates have the general formula $Cn(H_2O)m$, in which n and m are whole numbers. Monosaccharides are the basic units of carbohydrates. They are classified by the number of carbons they contain, such as hexoses (C6) and pentoses (C5). Hexoses and pentoses exist predominantly in ring forms called pyranoses (six-membered rings) or furanoses (five-membered rings) in equilibrium with open-chain forms. Ring forms are hemiacetals; open-chain forms are polyhydroxyl aldehydes. In the ring forms, α or β anomers are possible. The pyranoses exist in the stable chain conformation with most, if not all, of the hydroxyls in equatorial positions. When two monosaccharides differ by the configuration of one hydroxyl group, they are called epimers. If n is the number of asymmetric carbons, then $2n$ is the number of optical isomers (based on open-chain).

In hexoses, usually $n = 4$; in pentoses, usually $n = 3$. Sugars are given a relative configuration on the basis of the orientation of the next-to-last carbon's hydroxyl group as compared to D-glyceraldehyde. Most naturally occurring sugars have the D configuration. A ketose is a carbohydrate with a ketone group; aldose has an aldehyde group.

Monosaccharides join together to form disaccharides. The new bond is called a glycosidic bond, and is between the hemiacetal carbon and a hydroxyl group of the other sugar; water is released when the bond is formed. Hydrolysis (breaking) of the bond requires water. The glycosidic bond is an acetal grouping. Sucrose (common sugar) is made of glucose and fructose. Lactose (milk sugar) is made of galactose and glucose. Maltose (α-1,4 bond) is made of two glucose units and is a hydrolysis product of starch or glycogen. Cellobiose (β-1,4 bond) is also made of two glucoses, and it is the breakdown product of the cellulose.

Polysaccharides are many monosaccharides joined by glycosidic bonds; they may be branched also. Starch (plant energy storage), glycogen (animal short-term energy storage), and cellulose (plant structural component) are all made from glucose. Cellulose has β-1,4 bonds not found in the other two. Starch and glycogen both have α-1,4 bonds, but differ in the frequency and position of branch points (α-1,6 bond).

Insulin is a polymer of fructose.

Exercise 5: Here are three more Venn diagram exercises. The more you practice, the more proficient you will become. First, decide what information belongs in the diagram to help you remember the concept. Then, be as careful and precise as possible. Check especially what each space represents. These exercises may be done along with your reading of related sections in Chapter 8. Remember, problem areas present opportunities for learning. Use your textbook or other resources to clarify any word or term that is difficult for you.

1. Draw a Venn diagram illustrating the characteristics of eukaryotic cells and prokaryotic cells.
2. Draw Venn diagrams that illustrate the relationship between isomers, stereoisomers, and enantiomers.
3. Draw Venn diagrams to illustrate the relationship between diastereomers and meso compounds.

SYNTHETIC REASONING

If all reasoning were analytical, we would understand only how pieces are derived from the whole. In synthetic reasoning, the opposite process occurs; individual pieces are recombined in a way to form a larger integrated piece. For example, three individual slices of apple pie and three individual slices of peach pie together form a complete apple–peach pie of six slices.

An example of synthetic reasoning is the construction of summaries, or maps. Another is explaining the relevant information covered in a lecture to a classmate. Both of these activities involve constructing meanings from a body of information. The MCAT is particularly interested in your ability to synthesize facts from various subjects to construct new possibilities; for example, your understanding of human physiology in light of what you have learned in physics, chemistry, biology, and math. Synthetic reasoning often involves creativity in devising ways to integrate content information and in constructing frameworks.

Synthetic reasoning can also be called integrated reasoning. Understanding the biology of bone involves studying bone matrix at a cellular level; understanding the physics of bone involves studying stress, forces on bones, and elasticity of bones. Integration of biology and physics results in the biophysics of the bone.

The importance of synthetic reasoning to the MCAT is reflected in the combination of science disciplines into the MCAT subtests. The Physical Sciences subtest contains physics and general chemistry; the Biological Sciences subtest contains biology and organic chemistry. The problems presented in the MCAT, especially the passage-based problems, require integration of concepts and principles from across science disciplines. Students should master the process of combining topics from all the natural sciences to gain proficiency in synthetic reasoning.

Synthetic Reasoning Exercises

Exercise 6: Complete this sequence and describe the pattern it follows.
  1000, 1500, 1450, 1950, 1900, 2400, 2350, _____, _____, _____

Exercise 7: Complete the following sequence and explain how it is formed:
12, ⁻6, 3, ⁻1.5, _____, _____, _____

Exercise 8: Derive a rule concerning the sum of a fraction and its reciprocal.

Exercise 9: *A* travels 20 miles a day; *B* starts 3 days later and travels 8 miles the first day, 12 the second, and so on, in arithmetical progression. In how many days will *B* overtake *A*?

ASSOCIATIVE/ANALOGIC REASONING

Associative, or analogic, reasoning enables a transfer of concepts from one subject to another using the principle of similarity. Biological concepts can often be explained in terms of physics or chemistry. For example, consider how the movement of blood inside veins and arteries relates to the concept of fluid flow in physics.

Analogic reasoning uses associations in a particular way. In analogic reasoning, a difficult concept is compared to something easier to understand in order to develop better understanding. Analogy is often a creative tool used by scientists. The structure of DNA, for example, is often presented using a visual analogy of two ladders, with the base-pairs as the "rungs" of the ladders.

The terms analogic and associative are important because they imply a linkage between key words. This kind of reasoning is useful in establishing connections and analyzing similar situations. Analogic reasoning can also be a powerful tool in memorization. For example, if you want to remember Boyle's law, you might associate it with the action of pushing on the accelerator while driving a car. In Boyle's law, pressure is inversely proportional to volume. When you push down on the accelerator, you are decreasing the volume and increasing the pressure in the piston. Conversely, when you let up on the accelerator, the volume in the piston increases and the pressure decreases.

In many textbook charts and tables, the data included are examples of associations. Charts and tables should be studied for the relationships between given information, but constructing your own associations is a powerful exercise for clarifying your reasoning and assisting in your memorization. You should develop analogies between laboratory experiments and knowledge of theories, principles, and laws as part of your study approach for the MCAT.

Analogic Reasoning Exercises

Exercise 10: The number 60 is to 10 as _____ is to _____:

A. 120, 20
B. 20, 5
C. 150, 100
D. 5, 20

Exercise 11: Acorn is to oak as _____ is to _____:

A. nut, crack
B. cone, hemlock spruce
C. squirrel, nut
D. spruce, cone

Exercise 12: Hand is to shoulder as _____ is to _____:

A. foot, hip
B. head, neck
C. toes, finger
D. toes, foot

COMPARATIVE REASONING

Associative reasoning leads naturally to comparison and contrast. Comparison is noting the similarities between things, while contrasting is noting the differences. We tend to compare and contrast things that are similar in some ways, yet dissimilar in others. No

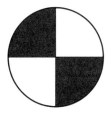 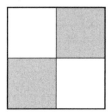

Fig. 2-21.

one bothers to compare an orange and a truck, but one would compare and contrast smooth and skeletal muscles, or afferent and efferent nerves. When reading about how two things are different, remember that they are being contrasted because they also have similarities.

In order to distinguish adequately between similarities and differences, it is necessary to organize information so that these distinctions are discernible. For example, it is easy to confuse the functions of the liver with those of the spleen. A table that compares and contrasts the functions of these two organs will speed up your review and make it more detailed.

Comparative Reasoning Exercises

Exercise 13: Compare and contrast the two drawings in Figure 2-21. List 10 similarities and 10 differences.

Exercise 14: For the following compare–contrast exercises, list aspects that are shared or are not shared by each set of items. Then check your list against information in your textbook or other references.

1. Electrolytic, galvanic, and concentration cells
2. Heterozygous and homozygous genes
3. Period and group for the atomic table
4. Entropy and enthalpy
5. Capacitors and resistors

INTUITIVE REASONING

Intuitive reasoning (also called creative or abstract reasoning) is a creative use of the imagination to solve problems. This form of reasoning is rarely mentioned in the classroom because we know neither how to teach it nor how to test it. A creative imagination makes an intuitive leap that is not logically apparent. Thus, a doctor may make a preliminary diagnosis based on intuition. The diagnosis is then systematically and carefully checked with further questions, examinations, tests, etc. The scientist who discovered the way stars age did so by making an intuitive connection between aging stars and humans.

Intuitive Reasoning Exercises

Exercise 15: The electric knife and electric spoon exist. How could an electric fork be used?

Exercise 16: How long would it take to skateboard from Seattle to Maine?

Exercise 17: You are a passenger on a train. How could you calculate its speed? Repeat this problem for a subway and an airplane.

Exercise 18: Prove that light travels in straight lines without using any equipment.

VISUAL REASONING

Experimental evidence shows that infants can reason well visually before they acquire language. Although the ability to reason visually is the key to solving many science problems, some students find they have neglected their visual reasoning skills.

Visual reasoning skills can help you solve physics problems such as those concerned with the flow of water through pipes of different diameters. (As a doctor, you will be concerned with the flow of liquids through the "pipes" of living beings.) Picture a first floor apartment and a sixth floor apartment in the same building. Which apartment is likely to have better water pressure in the shower? Why? Which apartment is likely to have the better bathtub drainage? Why? How could you improve water pressure or drainage?

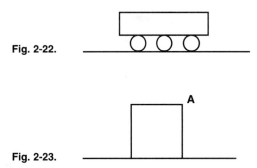

Fig. 2-22.

Fig. 2-23.

Visual reasoning involves the process of representing concepts in such a way that relationships become apparent. For example, in geometry, the parts of the problem must often be sketched so that the relationships are evident. On the MCAT, the ability to reason visually is an important key to solving many problems in both the science and verbal reasoning sections. Often, a quick diagram or sketch can be an important tool in establishing relationships.

Visual Reasoning Exercises

Notice in the following exercises that in addition to picturing objects, you must also be able to imagine how they move.

Exercise 19: A box is set upon a series of cylinders, each of which has a circumference of 3 feet (Figure 2-22). The cylinders, which are not attached to the box, lie on level ground. If the box is pushed, causing the rollers to make one revolution, how far does the box travel with respect to the ground (assume no slippage occurs)?

Exercise 20: Draw a schematic or a clear sketch that demonstrates your mastery of the following concepts:

1. Visualize the Doppler effect. Can you explain in one sentence what causes it?
2. Draw the molecules of epimers and anomers to help you conceptualize them in your mind. (Use straight lines.)
3. Sketch the filtration process that takes place in the glomerulus and nephron of a human kidney.

Exercise 21: Describe the trace of corner *A* as the square in Figure 2-23 turns end-over-end along level ground.

LOGICAL REASONING

Logical reasoning provides a systematic means for testing or proving a hypothesis or conclusion. Because it is concerned with proof, logical reasoning is a way of thinking associated with the development of science and the scientific method. Conclusions can be valid or invalid, and can have three degrees of certainty: hypothesis, conclusion suggested, and conclusion confirmed. In addition to understanding the rules of formal logic, it is also important to know fallacies of reasoning, because they can pinpoint errors in thinking patterns.

Many books are available that discuss formal rules of logic and exercises to practice them. We recommend that you use these books to improve your logical reasoning ability.

Logical Reasoning Exercises

Exercise 22: If some teacups are olimunds and all olimunds have handles,

A. Do all teacups have handles?
B. Do some teacups have handles?

Exercise 23: Make a Venn drawing showing the following relationships:

A. All apples are brown
B. No brothers are crazy
C. Some colas are diet

Exercise 24: The town clerk of Mudville needs to mail license renewal notices to all residents who own one or more dogs and to all gun owners. Using these statistics, how many people must be contacted?

A. Gun owners: 500
B. Dog owners: 850
C. Gun owners with dogs: 350

QUANTITATIVE REASONING

Quantitative reasoning involves choosing a reasonable mathematical method to solve a problem. It involves distinguishing the known from the unknown and applying the information to a mathematic process or formula. It might also involve estimating and judging the appropriateness of an answer. For example, in solving for the leg of a right triangle, all answers could be eliminated which are longer than the hypotenuse.

Quantitative skills are used when you quickly and precisely carry out mathematical operations in your head. For example, multiply 41 by 41. Quantitative reasoning is also used to translate words to numbers and numbers to words. For example, looking only at a graph or chart in a newspaper, can you tell what the accompanying story is about? Conversely, can you read the article and then picture a graph or chart to accompany it?

The MCAT tests your quantitative reasoning indirectly through mathematical problems in physical and biological sciences. The application of mathematics concepts to problem solving is required and mastery of these concepts is essential. In this book, the MCAT mathematics review (Chapter 6) is organized by concept, and each concept is followed by conceptual examples and exercises.

Quantitative Reasoning Exercises

Exercise 25: Distribute $3 among Tom, Dick, and Harry so that Tom and Dick each have twice as much as Harry.

Exercise 26: Arrange in order of magnitude: 9 times the square root of 3, 6 times the square root of 7, 5 times the square root of 10.

Exercise 27: Which statement is correct?

A. $\dfrac{0.7}{7} > \dfrac{7}{0.7}$

B. $\dfrac{0.7}{7} = \dfrac{7}{0.7}$

C. $\dfrac{0.7}{7} < \dfrac{7}{0.7}$

Exercise 28: A technician counts a quantity of syringes that he knows is between 50 and 60. When he counts them three at a time, there are 2 left over; when he counts them 5 at a time, there are 4 left over. How many are there in all?

Exercise 29: Which is greater, m × m + m or m^3 + 1, given m is positive.

PROPORTIONAL REASONING

Proportional reasoning is often used to measure changes in one variable relative to changes in another, as in problems applying Boyle's law. Proportional reasoning may also be used to solve problems in physics and chemistry, such as velocity of moving particles and acid–base concentrations. It may also be useful in answering questions that relate to population tables and charts.

Proportional reasoning is important to both physical and biological sciences and, therefore, is worth additional emphasis. In contrast to additive reasoning, in which one asks, "what do I add to (or subtract from) *x* in order to get *y*?," in proportional reasoning one asks, "what do I multiply *x* by to get *y*?" The easiest method to find this unknown is to divide y by x; if these numbers are in proportion, the result will be a constant number no matter which set of (x,y) pairs is used. For example, the length of the circumference (C) of a circle is in direct proportion to the length of that circle's diameter (D). If we divide the circumference by the diameter, we will always get the number pi (π). (There is no one number that you can add to the diameter that will always yield the circumference.) In proportional problems we often leave out the constant and equate two pairs of numbers: C1/D1 = C2/D2. The fact that both ratios are equal to pi is what makes it possible to equate them.

It is often useful to visualize the proportion. To visualize a proportion, sketch the two quantities. One is usually larger than the other. The factor (constant number) obtained by dividing the larger quantity by the smaller tells you how much to inflate the smaller to get the larger.

Proportional Reasoning Exercises

Exercise 30: Two numbers have a ratio of 3:4. The ratio of their sum to the sum of their squares is 7:50. Find the two numbers.

Exercise 31: The speeds (or rates) of a bicycle and a tricycle have a ratio of 5:4. In a one-mile race, the tricycle had a half-minute head start but was beaten by $\frac{1}{10}$. Find the rate of each.

Solutions to Exercises

Analytical Reasoning

1. For this type of problem it is useful to make a table. The table in Figure 2-24 shows information that is given in the problem.

	New	Vintage	Total
Harry	3		5
Louise		3	5 + 1
Kate	n	n + 3	
Bob	n	?	
		12	20

Fig. 2-24.

Next, work with the rows and columns to figure the missing elements (Figure 2-25).

It is clear that n = 1, hence Kate has five cars; therefore Bob must have four cars, of which only one is new. Bob owns three vintage cars.

	New	Vintage	Total
Harry	3		5
Louise	3	3	5 + 1
Kate	n	n + 3	
Bob	?	?	
	8	12	20

Fig. 2-25.

2. In the left-hand drawing in Figure 2-26, the outer circle is daughters because all mothers are daughters, but daughters are not all necessarily mothers. The space between the circles becomes "daughters who are not mothers." In the drawing on the right, all mothers and grandmothers are daughters and all grandmothers are mothers. While all aunts are daughters, the drawing shows that some aunts are grandmothers and mothers.

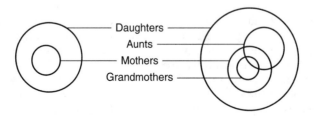

Daughters
Aunts
Mothers
Grandmothers

Fig. 2-26.

3. See Figure 2-27.

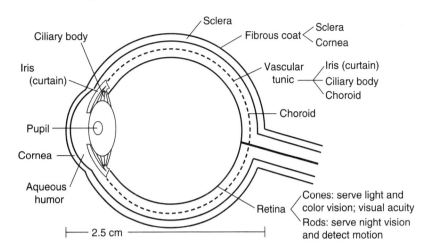

Fig. 2-27.

4. See Figure 2-28.

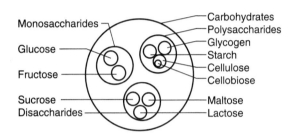

Fig. 2-28.

5. These exercises should be done using information provided in Chapter 8.

Synthetic Reasoning

6. The additive jumps are: 500, ⁻50, 500, ⁻50, 500, ⁻50. The next elements will be: 2850, 2800, 3300.

7. Additive changes don't seem to work; try multiplicative changes. The sign keeps changing so try a negative number; the size keeps reducing, so try a fraction. The factor is ⁻½. The next three elements are: ¾, ⁻⅜, ³⁄₁₆.

8. What is the sum of $1/x + x$? Try some examples.

$$\frac{1}{2} + 2 = 2\frac{1}{2} = \frac{5}{2} = \frac{(4 + 1)}{2}$$

$$\frac{1}{3} + 3 = 3\frac{1}{3} = \frac{10}{3} = \frac{(9 + 1)}{3}$$

$$\frac{1}{4} + 4 = 4\frac{1}{4} = \frac{17}{4} = \frac{(16 + 1)}{4}$$

$$\frac{1}{x} + x = \frac{(x2 + 1)}{x}$$

9. Drawing a diagram may be useful (Figure 2-29). *B* will overtake *A* after 13 days or 260 miles.

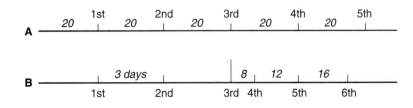

Fig. 2-29.

Analogic Reasoning

10. A. The simplest operations to get from 60 to 10 and 120 to 20 is to divide by 6.

11. B. Acorns are the fruit of an oak; cones are the fruit of a hemlock spruce.

12. A. The hand is at the end of the limb that starts at the shoulder; the foot is at the end of the limb that starts at the hip.

Comparative Reasoning

13. Some examples of similarities and differences: both figures are divided into quarters with half of the area shaded. The left figure is round while the right figure is square; the first and third quadrants of the right figure are shaded, whereas on the left figure these quadrants are clear.

14. The compare–contrast exercises should be done using the information presented in Chapters 7 and 8.

Intuitive Reasoning

15. Answers will vary depending on how you use an electric spoon and knife.

16. Estimate the distance, perhaps 4000 miles. Think how far one can skateboard in an hour, remembering that some roads may not be as easy to skateboard on. It is probably quicker than a fast walk, maybe 6 miles per hour. If you cover 40 miles per day, it will take 100 days.

17. For the train, measure how many seconds between the telephone poles, and then estimate the spacing of the poles. For the subway it is much harder to find a repetitive object with an even spacing from which you can estimate, but there may be one if you look for it. For the plane, you may be able to use the wing edge to measure how long it takes to cross a field, but estimating the field size could prove difficult. If you cannot see the ground, the problem is much harder; you might find the average speed for the trip using the flight time and estimating the distance using the map in the flight magazine.

18. The phenomenon that "light travels in straight lines" can be demonstrated by holding an object in front of a light source. Watch sunrise and sunset and how sun rays filter in straight paths through branches of trees. On a partially sunny day the sun rays travel through clouds in straight lines.

Visual Reasoning

19. This question may require that you actually try the problem with a model. The box will move forward one circumference with respect to the cylinders and the cylinders will move forward one circumference with respect to the ground. The box therefore moves two circumferences, or 6 feet.

20. Use the information provided in Chapters 7 and 8 to construct these diagrams.

21. See Figure 2-30.

Fig. 2-30.

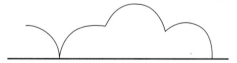

Logical Reasoning

22. A. Maybe, if all these teacups are olimunds.
    B. Yes

23. See Figure 2-31.

24. A Venn diagram may be useful. Answer: 1000 people.

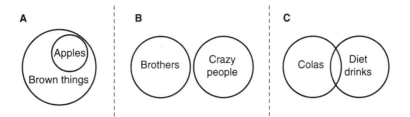

A | B | C

Fig. 2-31.

Quantitative Reasoning

25. Tom gets 2x, Dick gets 2x, and Harry gets x:

    $2x + 2x + x = \$3.00$ (or $5x = \$3.00$) and $x = .60$

    (Tom = \$1.20, Dick = \$1.20, Harry = \$.60)

26. To arrange these numbers in order: $9\sqrt{(3)}, 6\sqrt{(7)}, 5\sqrt{(10)}$, one can square each number to remove the square roots: $81 \times 3 = 243$, $25 \times 10 = 250$, $36 \times 7 = 252$.

27. C

28. The given information is: $3x + 2 = 5y + 4$; or, $x = (5y + 2) \div 3$. We also know that $3x + 2$ must fall between 50 and 60. Therefore, x must be less than 20. Try values for y that might generate such an x. Begin by choosing values of y, which, when multiplied by 5, yield a number between 50 and 60. The first such number is 10, but this does not work in the equation above. The next number, 11, yields an answer of 59 ($5y + 4$), which is also equal to $3x + 2$ when $x = 19$.

29. Make a table: m   m × m + m   m × m × m + 1

    | 1 | 2 | 2 |
    | 2 | 6 | 9 |
    | 3 | 12 | 28 |
    | 4 | 20 | 65 |

    $m^3 + 1$ is larger for values of m larger than 1.

Proportional Reasoning

30. Two numbers that are in the ratio of 3:4 are 3x and 4x. The rest of the problem says that:

    $$\frac{(3x + 4x)}{(9 \times 2 + 16 \times 2)} = \frac{7}{50}$$

    $$\frac{7x}{25 \times 2} = \frac{7}{50}; \text{ hence, } x = 2.$$

    The two numbers are 6 and 8.

31. See Figure 2-32.

	Distance	Rate	Time	Distance = Rate x Time
Bicycle	1	(5/4)R	t - 1/2	Therefore, Rate = $\frac{\text{Distance}}{\text{Time}}$
Tricycle	9/10	R	t	

Bicycle:
Tricycle: $\dfrac{5}{4} = \dfrac{\dfrac{1}{t - 1/2}}{\dfrac{9/10}{t}}$ $\left(\dfrac{\text{Distance}}{\text{Time}} \text{ for bicycle}\right)$ $\left(\dfrac{\text{Distance}}{\text{Time}} \text{ for tricycle}\right)$

$t = 9/2$ minutes (the time the tricycle spends racing)

Tricycle rate: $\dfrac{9/10}{t} = \dfrac{9/10}{9/2} = \dfrac{9}{10} \times \dfrac{2}{9} = \dfrac{1}{5}$

Bicycle rate: $\dfrac{5}{4} R = \dfrac{5}{4} \times \dfrac{1}{5} = \dfrac{1}{4}$ mile/minute

Fig. 2-32.

Problems 25–31 were selected from a standard high school algebra book that was in use over 100 years ago.

EXERCISES IN INTEGRATED REASONING

No problem can involve only one kind of reasoning, nor is it possible to solve a problem using only reasoning and no facts. MCAT problems are designed to assess how well you can coordinate several different kinds of reasoning while working with the knowledge you gained from your undergraduate science courses. As you work the following problems, identify the types of reasoning you use.

Use Figure 2-33 to answer questions 1–5.

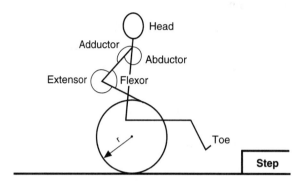

Fig. 2-33.

1. Which pattern of muscle activity will have the effect of moving the wheelchair forward?

   A. Stimulate the extensor and abductor, inhibit the flexor and adductor
   B. Stimulate the abductor and adductor, inhibit the flexor and extensor
   C. Inhibit the flexor and abductor, stimulate the extensor and adductor
   D. Inhibit the extensor and abductor, stimulate the flexor and adductor

2. The maximum technical advantage is found in

   A. The adductor or the abductor
   B. The flexor or the adductor
   C. The extensor
   D. The wheel

3. The force applied to the wheel is directed along a tangent to the wheel at an angle of about 45 degrees in the horizontal. In which of the following directions could the force be applied to obtain an equally efficient or a more efficient effect? There may be more than one correct answer.

   A. Tangential to the wheel, applied closer to the hub
   B. Tangential to the wheel, applied horizontally
   C. Any horizontal force, whether or not it is tangential
   D. A force applied at 30 degrees to the horizontal plane

4. When the wheelchair reaches the step indicated in the diagram, the extra force needed will be equal to

   A. W (the weight of the chair and the occupant)
   B. W/r (W divided by the radius of the wheel)
   C. $W/2\pi r$
   D. W/2

5. The wheelchair comes to a smooth up-ramp with railing. It can negotiate the ramp without having the wheels slip. Will more force need to be applied pulling on the railings, or pushing on the top rim of the wheel?

   A. More on the railings
   B. More on the wheels
   C. The same on each
   D. Depends on the slope of the ramp

   Use Figure 2-34 to answer questions 6–8.

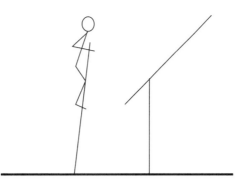

Fig. 2-34.

6. The ladder in the diagram starts to swing out to the left. In order to return to the house, which of the following actions should the man take? More than one answer may be correct.

    A. Swing his arms clockwise
    B. Swing his arms counterclockwise
    C. Lean forward
    D. Lean backward

7. The man will have less leeway in time to react if (indicate all correct responses):

    A. The ladder is long
    B. The ladder is short
    C. He recently had two shots of alcoholic beverages
    D. He is over 40 years old

8. As the ladder continues to swing left (indicate all correct responses):

    A. The man's heart rate will increase and he will begin to lose heat rapidly
    B. The man's vision will blur
    C. The man's angular momentum will be conserved
    D. The concentration of CO^2 in his exhaled breath will decrease

Solutions to Exercises in Integrated Reasoning

Exercises 1–5

1. A. Extensor increases the angle at joint; abductor moves bone away toward midline

2. D. All muscles work at a fractional mechanical advantage

3. B. Tangential to the wheel applied at rim

4. D. The wheel will act as a lever of length 2r with the weight concentrated at its center

5. A. You can think of the wheel as a lever or consider the distance through which the forces are applied. When the rail is pulled, the force is applied through the same distance as the chair moves. But when pushing on the rim of the wheel, the force is applied through twice the distance as the chair moves. This is not easy to see. One revolution of the wheel produces a forward movement of one revolution. The point of force application at the top of the wheel moves forward both by the forward motion of the entire chair and by the rotation of the wheel.

Exercises 6–8

6. B and D, if ladder swings to right; A and C, if ladder swings to left. The counter torques (caused by swinging of arms and leaning) should resist the torque of the falling ladder. Note: Center of mass of the man and ladder, and friction between ladder and ground, should be considered in your analysis.

7. B, C, and D. The period of swing decreases with length; therefore, the longer the ladder, the longer it will take the ladder to move, giving the man more time to respond. Age and alcohol both increase human reaction times, making it much harder to respond in time.

8. A, C, and D. The fright response includes increased heart rate, sharper vision, faster blood flow, and increased rate of breathing. Faster blood flow and rapid movement through the air would increase heat loss. Faster breathing without strenuous exercise would decrease the concentration of CO_2 in each breath.

Model for Passage-Based Problem Solving

The following problem-solving model can help you solve almost any physical and biological science problem on the MCAT. This model has been tested on many different audiences, including students, assistant faculty, counselors, and other health professions candidates. You are urged to develop confidence with this model by using it over and over again.

Step I: Complete understanding by reading: what is given?

This step includes a full understanding and total comprehension of the passage and the accompanying problem. The step may be subdivided into the following substeps.

SUBSTEP 1. Interpret passage by content. Include recall of related concepts, and ask yourself questions as you read the passage.

SUBSTEP 2. Interpret passage stressing data presented or given in graphs, diagrams, or designs. Watch for graphic details.

SUBSTEP 3. Interpret passage to understand research procedures or experimental findings. Look for most probable causes, discern underlying cause–effect relationships, and develop familiarity with new information.

SUBSTEP 4. Look for relationships among several variables or methods. This substep helps you choose the appropriate problem-solving method or strategy.

SUBSTEP 5. Check your comprehension of new technical terms. Do not make assumptions about the meaning of new terms; instead, find their contextual meaning by association with the surrounding text.

SUBSTEP 6. Guess the source of the passage (i.e., journal, textbook, or other source) to discover why the passage is written. This substep can help you distinguish relevant from irrelevant information.

SUBSTEP 7. The above substeps lead you to the following question: "What is given in the passage and in the problem?" Detailed understanding and comprehension eventually help you to dissect all the given information.

Step II: Preparing a perceptive model of given information: how can the given be used?

This step is creative and requires a higher level of concentration. Because it involves organization and assembling of pertinent information, a rough sketch or a flow diagram based on the given information may help you complete this step. A graphical representation of the given information is easier to use than textual information. The following substeps will help you keep your attention focused:

SUBSTEP 1. Use similar situations to draw a simple sketch. Use analogic, analytical, and logical reasoning methods to help you mentally see the given information.

SUBSTEP 2. Reread some sections or parts of the passage slowly. Underline or circle cues that link the given information to concepts you already know. Sketch what you see (a mental picture is acceptable, but a rough picture on paper is more convenient to use). This substep helps you resolve any doubts that stem from superficial familiarity with the passage.

Step III: Understanding the problem: what is the question?

This step is critical before you solve the problem. Ask yourself, "What question is really being asked?" The following substeps will help you.

SUBSTEP 1. Condense the question as much as possible in order to comprehend the nature of the question. Check to see if the question is complete and directly stated. A word of caution: Do not rephrase the question according to a simpler or easier version that you have seen before. Do not assume or pretend that if you can answer a simpler question, you also know this problem equally well. The test-maker may have considered the simpler option and included a response to check your precision in understanding the question.

SUBSTEP 2. Isolate and examine the limitations and assumptions inherent in the question. Isolating the limitations of the question allows you to eliminate wrong answers from multiple choice responses.

Step IV: Finding the appropriate problem-solving method: how do you solve it?

This step is time-consuming because it integrates the earlier steps. You could waste time in this step if you do not know which way to go. It is important to mention here that MCAT problems are not mechanical—you should not plug any numbers into any equation unless you are sure. Each calculation that you carry out uses up precious time.

It is always worthwhile to break a complex or long problem into simpler and more easily managed units, and then choose an approach to manage each unit. A few fundamental approaches are suggested to help you pick the right one. MCAT problems require a mixture of approaches to solve various parts of a problem. Do not be discouraged if the answer is not obvious. You should not sacrifice a systematic approach in problem solving for a shortcut. Use the following approaches as you need them:

1. Apply concepts that you have already learned to fill in the gaps from information provided in the passage. Only use principles, definitions, equations, theories, and laws to fill in the gaps. Information given in problems should be integrated with the passage.
2. Apply the newly learned concepts from the passage as appropriate after you have gained a thorough understanding.
3. When working with mathematic problems, watch for consistency in units and conventions, and always start from the given data (see Step II).
4. Use only the relevant facts.
5. Do not erase or write over your calculations. Performing mathematical operations in small spaces can be a frustrating experience. Write carefully and clearly.
6. Do not expect formulas and equations (except the *MCAT Student Manual* formulas) to be provided during the test. You must memorize important formulas.
7. Use proportional reasoning as required to compare various options.
8. Evaluate designs, methods, and phenomena; and their effects, in a logical and systematic way. Do not be swayed by the writer's arguments if you discover technical flaws or problems. Solving these problems may not require any mathematical operations; analytical or logical reasoning may suffice.
9. Use integrated reasoning to look at pieces of evidence, parts of instruments, steps in procedures, and various actions in phenomena. Evaluate and interpret particular perspectives, including technical views and opinions.
10. Always try to get the answer in the form presented, especially in data analysis problems. Organize and interpret your data so they are directly linked to the format of the answers presented.
11. Check the four test responses against your answer.
12. Use various strategies and approaches to solve the problem in any order, as long as the strategies are well connected and sequential in solving the problem.

Step V: Evaluating the solution given and your solution: is your solution accurate?

All the above steps will be useless if you did not obtain an accurate solution. Hasty calculations or reading may lead to an incorrect response. Always check your solution against the responses. You should be able to go back if your solution and the given solutions do not match. Check each response as an argument and see if it is valid. Do not sacrifice accuracy at any cost (including speed or reasonable guessing). Unreasonable answers should be thoroughly cross-examined by using another solution method. Your previous knowledge in the subject should provide you with a ballpark estimate to lead you in the right direction.

Step VI: Evaluate your experience with passage-based problems: what did you learn?

You cannot perform this step on the actual MCAT, but it is good exercise while preparing for the test and should be an integral part of your review process. Problem solving comes by experience, and experience is gained by problem solving. The following questions should be asked for each practice exercise:

1. Was the passage difficult? If so, why?
2. Was the problem difficult? If so, why?
3. Were the four responses hard to understand? If so, why?

Figure 2-35 shows how to apply this problem-solving model to an MCAT passage.

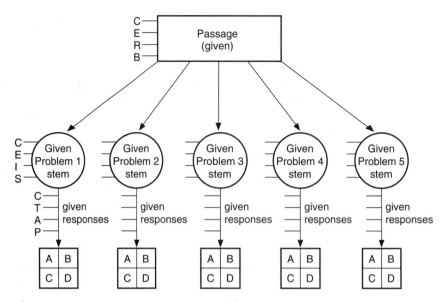

Fig. 2-35. Application of the problem-solving model to the MCAT. C = comprehension of given information in the passage, problems, and responses. I = any new information provided to problems from the passage and the problems. E = evaluation of given information. B = bringing knowledge-based concepts from various disciplines into the passage and trying to make sense of them. R = understanding the direct or hidden relationship or link between the passages and the problems. S = solving problems using one of several available methods. T = testing and checking each response as a possible solution. A = application of elimination procedures to cross out irrelevant information. P = picking the best response, not the almost correct response.

Exercises in Using the Problem-Solving Model

The following exercises provide the practice you need to move from theory to real problems. Do the following example problems now and complete them before you read further in the book. As you work the problems, write out all the steps and draw diagrams as needed.

Exercise 1: To test your mastery of the nervous and endocrine systems, try the following tasks, referring to textbooks only when you need help.
1. **List** the major structures of the nervous system. A drawing or diagram will help.
2. **Describe** the characteristics of the major structures (i.e., location and functions).
3. **Define** the parts of the nervous system. (If you were given a definition, could you name the part?)
4. **Describe** basic nerve cell structures.
5. **Discuss** the concept of action potential.
6. **List** the endocrine glands and describe the characteristics of each.
7. **Discuss** the effects of hormonal products on target tissues.
8. **Discuss** how the feedback loop works.
9. **Compare and contrast** different parts of the endocrine and nervous systems.

When you complete the above exercise, check your work in Chapter 8 of this book, and review the nervous and endocrine systems. Is there anything you missed or do not fully understand? If something still seems unclear, consult a textbook (preferably one you have not used before) and work to clarify the concept. You could also ask a professor or fellow student for help. Now is the time to master what may have been imperfectly learned before. A thorough approach will pay off in the MCAT and, more importantly, in medical school, where the pressure of time frequently prevents review or clarification of previously learned materials.

Exercise 2: Mirages are considered optical illusions. What causes a mirage? Is it reflection, refraction, diffraction, or polarization of light? Hot air rises because it is lighter. A mirage is caused by refraction of light rays passing through various heated layers of air, all having different densities. In order to perform experiments on optical illusions and to understand solar and lunar eclipses, a man 2 m tall stands 3 m from an intense source of light that is at the level of his feet. The man's shadow appears on a wall 15 m from the source of light. How tall is the shadow?

Poorly proportioned

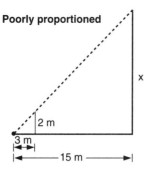

Well proportioned

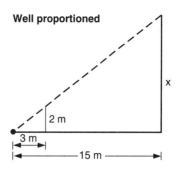

Fig. 2-36. Exercise 2: (*left*) A poorly proportioned sketch that could yield a wrong answer to this exercise. (*right*) A well-proportioned sketch.

A. 6 m
B. 10 m
C. 12.5 m
D. 17.5 m

If you recognize that the problem involves two similar triangles, solving the problem is easy because you can **carefully** construct a proportional diagram according to the rule that allows you to compare similar triangles: $\frac{3}{15} = \frac{2}{x}$. You should also note that extra or irrelevant information is given to distract.

The word *carefully* is emphasized in the paragraph above because the test-maker, who knows that some students will do this step carelessly, has included a distractor that could fit if you calculate incorrectly. For example, if your answer was 6, you probably put 12 in place of the 15 in the ratio.

Many students don't have the patience or confidence to work through all the steps to solve this problem; they take shortcuts and make errors. For example, some students draw the picture accurately and then try to solve for the hypotenuse—a complicated and time-consuming task that fails to yield the correct answer, although, once again, the test-maker has included a distractor that would fit.

Solving the problem is elementary only if you have correctly recognized that the problem involves proportion and if you have drawn a correctly proportioned diagram (Figure 2-36). This problem is not especially difficult either in content or mathematics, but in order to solve it correctly, you must think carefully and be precise. These are the qualities of a good problem solver. In fact, these are also the qualities we want in our doctors as well.

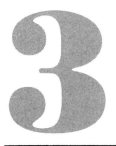

Developing Verbal Reasoning Abilities

Reading Comprehension, Verbal Reasoning, and Critical Thinking

The MCAT is designed to assist medical schools in selecting candidates who have breadth and flexibility in their thinking and who exhibit competent analytic skills when faced with the demands of long, complex materials. The current MCAT covers basic reading comprehension, or verbal reasoning, as well as higher level thinking, or "critical thinking skills," with nine prose passages from the humanities, social sciences, and natural sciences.

Because the MCAT assesses levels of critical thinking, it tests factual knowledge as well as your ability to handle inference and argument. It also will test your ability to comprehend, evaluate, apply, and incorporate new information. This chapter presents the most widely used MCAT verbal reasoning question formats, as well as some variations found in medical school examinations. This broad-based approach is provided through a range of practice examples to help you develop critical thinking skills.

Patterns in reasoning that you may not be using consciously can be honed to your advantage for the MCAT and beyond. This chapter and the following chapter on problem solving (Chapter 4) present those patterns in the form of study materials and exercises that can help you build more effective analytical reasoning skills.

Verbal Reasoning Skills Assessment

If you want to go to medical school, you should ask yourself the following two questions relative to your background in reading and your achievement on the MCAT:

1. Has your practice of reading skills led to a standard that ensures your success in medical school?
2. Can practice that is directed to reading and critical thinking improve academic performance?

In addressing these questions, begin by completing the Verbal Reasoning Skills Assessment in Table 3-1. The information you gather from this inventory will give you an idea

TABLE 3-1. Verbal Reasoning Skills Assessment

Type of Skill	I Do	I Do Not
Basic Reading Skills		
Establish the purpose of the information	————	————
Scan information for sense of organization	————	————
Understand main concepts after reading information one time	————	————
Determine details relevant to the development of the main idea	————	————
Critical Thinking Skills	————	————
Identify relationships among the facts	————	————
Prioritize relevant information	————	————
Apply information to new situations	————	————
Determine relevant interpretations	————	————
Infer from given information	————	————
Differentiate premises from conclusions in arguments	————	————
Draw logical conclusions	————	————
Evaluate strength of conclusions	————	————

of how well you have developed your verbal reasoning skills, and it can act as a basis for setting your goals for improvement. As you complete the skills assessment, pay attention to whether you find yourself thinking "I sometimes do that" or "I should do that."

Positive changes occur when students learn strategies to sharpen the way they think about concepts and ideas. Reading can serve as an important vehicle for practicing these thinking skills.

Reading Comprehension Skills for Scientific Text

Comprehension means that you retain enough information from reading to make connections. Although the ability to comprehend what you read depends somewhat on your concentration and your interest in and familiarity with the subject matter, having difficulty with a passage usually stems from problems with content (new information) and vocabulary.

BROADEN YOUR READING BASE

The MCAT requires you to read, organize, and analyze new information from a broad reading base. MCAT verbal reasoning passages range in length from 500 to 600 words, accompanied by 6 to 10 questions, each based on information in the passage. According to the Association of American Medical Colleges (AAMC) *MCAT Student Manual*, passages are selected from a range of subjects in 26 major fields: anthropology, archaeology, architecture, art and art history, astronomy, botany, business, computer science, dance, ecology, economics, ethics, geology, government, history, literary criticism, meteorology, music, natural history, philosophy, political science, psychology, religion, sociology, technology, and theater.

You are not expected to have a detailed knowledge of these subjects. Instead, it is expected that your reading and related skills enable you to answer questions based on the information given in the passage. A familiarity with the vocabulary of various disciplines is most helpful; therefore, you should read regularly from a diverse number of sources.

Make a habit of reading from a wide range of sources on a regular basis, including daily newspapers (e.g., the *New York Times, USA Today*), magazines (e.g., *Scientific American, Discover, American Scientist*), professional journals (e.g., the *New England Journal of Medicine*), and reference works (e.g., *Encyclopedia Britannica*).

DEVELOP YOUR VOCABULARY

A strong vocabulary is a useful tool in decoding MCAT passages and test items. Vocabulary expansion should be an active part of your MCAT preparation, especially if you encounter or even use words that you cannot define. Construct a vocabulary notebook. Record daily any new words you come across, and as a regular part of your study approach ask yourself the meaning of even the most routinely used terms. When preparing for the MCAT, check all definitions of words that you are unsure about, using resources such as a general dictionary, a medical dictionary, a glossary of medical terminology, and thesauri in biology, physics, and chemistry.

The better your vocabulary, the better equipped you will be to answer the MCAT questions. As an example, consider the following puzzle: A tree stands at each corner of a square, man-made lake (Figure 3-1). How can you double the area of the lake, still keeping it square, without disturbing the trees?

Invariably, the first answer is, "Dig the lake deeper." If that was your answer, you have insufficiently comprehended the distinction between "area" and "volume"—a definition problem—and this difficulty may adversely affect your solutions to physics problems. Review basic definitions, even of those terms you use quite regularly, and enter them in your notebook. (The answer to this problem is shown in Figure 3-2.)

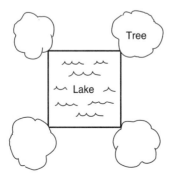

Fig. 3-1.

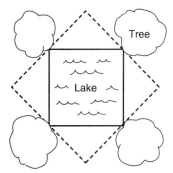

Fig. 3-2.

In addition to working with the correct resources, you should develop a systematic approach for learning new definitions. For efficient learning, you should memorize definitions as groups of words that belong together. For example, the definition of *synapse* in a biology thesaurus includes several other technical words (e.g., neuron, axon, dendrite, effector organ). All of these terms belong together and are located in the section on the nervous system.

You will find that learning a term as part of a matrix of related terms helps you answer multiple-choice questions correctly. For example, if the term *synapse* appears in a question stem, the correct answer choice is likely to include one of the other terms (i.e., axon, neuron, dendrite) that belongs with it. In addition, you know that the term *synapse* is part of the nervous system, so if *synapse* appears in a question stem, you would not expect the correct answer choice to be part of the endocrine system. Classifying and sorting large amounts of information is easier when definitions are used.

Consider the following problem:

When you touch a hot item, you immediately pull your hand away from that object. This is an example of:

A. irritability.
B. a feedback loop.
C. conscious nervous control.
D. a reflex arc.

Most students eliminate choices A and C, but then they have to think about choices B and D. However, if you studied with the biology thesaurus, you know that choice B is found in the section on the endocrine system and would not apply, whereas choice D is a term found in the section on the nervous system and, therefore, is the best answer choice.

Note that both the correct answer and the most likely distractor came from two systems that are often paired together in textbooks. The endocrine system and the nervous system are the two systems that modulate, integrate, and control the activities of the body, and test-makers know that students often confuse the details of these two systems. Always review your material with the test-makers in mind.

Studying from a page of connected words in the biology thesaurus helps you synthesize facts around a central topic, similar to a reading passage. Working toward this synthesis will improve your comprehension, problem-solving ability, and most fundamentally your ability to retain a great deal of information. Remember to consider the total concept as well as the details when distinguishing between the almost-correct answer and the correct answer in problem solving.

In working with definitions, students tend to focus only on technical terms. However, general vocabulary is also important to your performance in the Verbal Reasoning and Physical and Biological Sciences sections of the MCAT. If you do not read extensively outside assigned texts, or if your scores on the verbal portions of the SAT and ACT examinations were low, you may want to assess and review your basic reading vocabulary. Even if you do command a strong reading vocabulary, you still need to focus on the uses of definitions for the MCAT. Scientific writing is replete with definitions embedded in sentence and paragraph structure to establish a word's precise meaning in a particular context.

In learning definitions of important terms, there are two types of definitions to consider: defining by synonym and defining by genus.

Defining by Synonym

Can you define *pleasant?* If your answer was *agreeable* or *nice,* you were defining by synonym. It is useful to think about synonyms, both to improve your memory and to gain more versatility in solving problems.

Scientists attempt to use words very precisely, almost mathematically. They want one term to have one meaning. Therefore, science teachers often tell students that scientific terms have little or no correspondence to the same words used in ordinary life, or even in other disciplines. Sometimes, of course, this is true. However, in general, the scientific word often does have a relationship to ordinary English usage that is found in the etymology. For this reason, a glossary of medical terminology is recommended as you prepare for the MCAT.

In understanding and remembering precise scientific meaning, it may be useful to work from the common meaning. For example, consider the term *intercostal muscles.* Partridge's *A Short Etymological Dictionary of Modern English Origins* shows that *costal* and *coastal* are related terms; *intercostal* would appear to mean "between the coasts" or "between the ribs." Similarly, in the biological term *parallel evolution,* the word *parallel* has a relationship to *parallel* as it is used in geometry.

Making connections, or synthesizing and cross-referencing language and ideas, will aid your understanding, memory, flexibility, and application of words in solving MCAT problems. In particular, it will help you analyze passages and develop connections between topics in the passage. For example, when faced with the terms *interstitial fluids* and *hormones,* you will know that the physics of fluids is linked to the diffusion of hormones in various biological entities, such as tissues or organs.

Defining by Genus

Scientific definitions most commonly include genus and difference. The ability to define indicates a specific rather than a global or diffuse understanding of terms. Definitional knowledge is important to your performance on the MCAT, because it provides you with a broad base of information to use in problem solving during the test. Definitional knowledge in science includes knowing not only how to formulate a definition, but also determining the essential characteristics of the term—that is, its function, location, structure, example, and so on. Consider the definition of *northwest* as "a point on the compass equidistant between north and west." The first part, "a point on the compass," tells you the genus, or broad definition. The second and more specific part of the definition, "equidistant between north and west," tells you how this particular word is different from others in its genus. Similarly, if you define *heart,* you would want to give its genus as "a major organ of the body," as well as the way it differs from other organs, which in biology tends to be its location and functions.

Definitional test items can be played both ways: you may have to identify a term based on a given definition, or be able to define a specific term. To prepare for these questions, it is a good idea to develop the habit of keeping definitions on index cards, with the term on one side and the definition on the other. Practice thinking both from term to definition and from definition to term.

APPLY ANALYTICAL REASONING

Analytical reasoning can help you become a more discriminating reader. Using analytical reasoning, the reader approaches a complex passage by breaking it into short, understandable parts:

1. Find the central idea
2. Identify cause-and-effect statements
3. Develop interrelationships in the text
4. Recognize comparison–contrast shifts
5. Uncover assumptions—direct or stated and indirect or unstated
6. Determine conclusions—direct or obvious and indirect or implied
7. Learn to analyze your error patterns and determine how to avoid them (see Chapter 5, Strategy 6)

MASTER SIGNAL WORDS AND TRIGGER WORDS

For a careful reader, words act as both "signals" about new information to come and "triggers" that distinguish subtle shades of meaning.

Signal Words

Signal words are often basic to an understanding of structure, which in turn helps you comprehend an author's ideas. Signal words help you predict what you will read. For example, the word *but* indicates that the discussion or argument is about to take a turn in direction; for example, "She usually scored very well on tests, but she was not herself that morning." As you read the passages in the practice exercises, circle or underline the signal words presented in Table 3-2.

TABLE 3-2. Sample Signal Words and Their Meaning

Indicated by Signal	Signal Words and Phrases		
A continuous thought	also first besides next furthermore	then in addition (to) one reason likewise another reason	similarly for example moreover for instance
A shift in direction (usually opposite)	although on the contrary but otherwise	despite rather however whereas	in spite of yet on the other hand nevertheless
A list or pattern	many a few much a number of	several most another besides	also furthermore too in addition one (two, three)
Material in order of importance	next first (second, third) then soon later	after finally subsequently at last ultimately	begins ends more, most less, least worse, worst better, best
Ideas compared	like as	again still	likewise same similarly
Ideas contrasted (ideas that are different from one another)	but on the other hand however	on the contrary rather in comparison	different in contrast instead
Cause-and-effect relationships	because since therefore consequently so effects	brought about is the outcome of determines if then results	affects resulted in as a result (of) for this reason leads to thus either/or

Adapted with permission from Quinn S, Irving SF: *Active Reading*. Boston, Houghton Mifflin, 1986.

Trigger Words

Trigger words are another set of clues to help you understand the shades of meaning that distinguish the definite from the conditional.

It is vital for you to be sensitive to the nuances of word usage in the MCAT passages. By changing one word, the entire meaning of a passage can be dramatically changed or an otherwise acceptable answer choice can be disqualified, particularly with answer choices that are similar in meaning.

Trigger words can give cues for recognizing the *best* answer to an ambiguous question. For example, "I will come" has a different meaning than "I may come." In quantitative terms, the first statement indicates a 100% probability, whereas the latter indicates only a partial probability; *will* is definite, and *may* is conditional.

When you read a passage, mark the trigger words it contains. Table 3-3 presents selected trigger words, classified as definite and conditional, to give you a sense of the difference between the two.

These suggestions are not intended to be applied mechanically. Rather, a familiarity with the nuances of vocabulary will enable you:

- To sort through the information presented in a passage
- To identify the key ideas
- To recognize when an argument may switch direction
- To quickly refer to the passage to answer questions

TABLE 3-3. Trigger Words: Definite and Conditional

Definite		Conditional	
shows	same	suggests	extensive
establishes	only	usually	similar
proves	will	most	typical
confirms	is	often	usually
concludes	every	occasionally	can
always	each	largely	might
never	constant	rarely	probably
none	essential	some	seems
all	indispensable	most	most
any	necessary	prevalent	usually
		principally	normally
			primarily

Reading Like a Detective

It may be useful to consider the familiar process of reading from a new perspective. A reader is like a detective involved in cracking an important case. What attributes do you bring to your task? Curiosity? Observation? Guidelines and procedures? To be an effective reader, you need to develop these detective skills and practice them until you feel competent.

A common error in taking the MCAT is reading too quickly and answering questions based on incomplete knowledge. You may be tempted to rush through the passages and then grab at responses that appear correct on the surface. If a detective operated this way and a suspect were indicted by such hastily gathered, circumstantial evidence, the case would probably be thrown out of court. Always try to uncover the relevant information hidden in all the pieces of evidence. You can discard the irrelevant information to avoid confusion.

To get the most out of the evidence in a passage, study the techniques of good investigation and apply them to the reading process.

STEPS FOR ACTIVE CRITICAL READING

Rule 1: Survey the Passage

In the same way that a detective surveys the scene and becomes actively involved, you should scan a reading passage and note its length, whether tables or graphs are included, the presence or absence of a summary, and unusual vocabulary (Figure 3-3). This does not take long, but it does provide a reference point for beginning to assemble the passage clues.

Rule 2: Determine the Purpose

Following your initial survey, determine the purpose of the passage (see Figure 3-3). You may find that the purpose is to inform, to present an opinion, or to present a controversial view or idea. Usually, a quick check of the first and last paragraphs will indicate the purpose of the passage. Based on a closer reading of the passage, however, you may later need to refine your initial observations.

Rule 3: Identify the Main Idea

Unless you are reading dialogue, virtually every paragraph on the MCAT will have a "smoking gun"—a clue so central to the passage that it cannot be ignored. The MCAT test-makers are going to want to know if you read in-depth enough to understand the fundamental elements of the passage. They may use various question formats; for example, "Which of the following phrases best describes the central idea of the passage?" or "The main topic of this passage is . . ." or "The author's primary emphasis is upon . . ."

How do you practice this skill? Try the following: First, look in the obvious places and check or circle those points that seem to contain the main idea (see Figure 3-3). The author may place the main idea in the beginning, middle, or end of each paragraph in the passage. Second, after you read the passage, ask yourself, "What is the most important thing I need to remember?"

Rule 4: Look for the Writer's Method

After you have identified the main ideas of the paragraphs, it is essential to analyze the manner in which these ideas are linked together. On the MCAT, don't skip directly from identifying the main idea to answering the questions, because you won't be prepared for

Passage 3 (Questions 12–15)

The conventional interpretation of the (Cuban) missile crisis has changed dramatically over the past decade. For many years, it has been argued that the Kennedy administration's handling of the crisis—its ability to calibrate the level of tension and thus to strike just the right balance between firmness and flexibility—had demonstrated that there was a kind of art of crisis management. But by 1987 it had become clear that the standard interpretation had changed. The argument now was that crises between nuclear powers are inherently unmanageable.

Main idea → ✓

This was certainly the view of certain key officials of the Kennedy administration who gathered on a number of occasions to look back and reflect on the crisis. Former Secretary of Defense Robert S. McNamara, for example, argued repeatedly that no one can with any confidence predict how events in a nuclear crisis would unfold, especially if military force is actually used. The way a crisis runs its course would be dominated by such factors as "misinformation, miscalculation, misjudgment and human fallibility." It was therefore "not possible," he said, "to manage a crisis in the nuclear age," in the sense of being able to exercise strong control over how the confrontation works itself out.

Tables and charts

Main idea → ✓

Unusual vocabulary

For McGeorge Bundy, President Kennedy's national security adviser in 1962, the missile crisis appeared in retrospect not as an exercise in successful crisis management; it looked more like a "battle of blunders," and had resulted mainly from a kind of communication failure: "With more foresighted and better informed governments, more able to communicate with each other openly and honestly, the Cuban missile crisis need never have happened." The same sorts of arguments were made by other commentators on the crisis—by Raymond Garthoff, for example, and by Daniel Ellsberg and Seymour Hersh. Greiner here takes a similar line.

Main idea → ✓

Check passage length

Check purpose

Chart — y-axis: Percent of federal health spending (0, 25, 50, 75, 100); x-axis: Fiscal year (1960, 1970, 1980, 1990, 2000). Legend: Medicare, Retirement, Disability, Other health.

the variety of questions that require you to understand the connections among the ideas in the passage. Instead, you may want to consider which pattern is being used to organize the information.

Specific passage format patterns arise most typically on tests. You should now be able to identify them quickly. They are:

- Cause and effect
- Classification
- Comparison and contrast
- Word usage (definition)
- Process
- Reasoning
- Spatial or geographic
- Time order

Another difficult task is to deal with nuance and ambiguity while you sort through unfamiliar information. Remember that your objective is to answer questions about the passage; you are not trying to understand and remember the material for a future test. Do not spend time memorizing lists, names, or other kinds of specifics from the passage. If a question calls for detailed information, look back at the passage and retrieve it. Rather than remembering details, try to get an overall sense of how the author presents and organizes information. A key to the author's organization can often be found in language clues such as signal words.

Rule 5: Identify and Evaluate the Writer's Arguments

The MCAT requires you to comprehend quickly the subject of the passage, the author's position (if any) on the subject, and the implications of the author's point of view. You may not agree with the author's arguments, but you need to resist the temptation of superimposing or adding your own point of view or knowledge into the passage. You must differentiate how the author thinks about a subject and how you connect it to various test items.

What are the writer's arguments regarding a point of view expressed in the passage? You can judge the soundness of the author's arguments against the following:

- Generalizing from limited experience
- Begging the question
- Avoiding the question
- Arguing against the person rather than the issue
- Setting up a false dichotomy

Rule 6: Assess Credibility of the Evidence

Both the careful detective and the careful reader must constantly ask whether the evidence gathered and the conclusions made are logical and truthful. Without these vital skills of critical thinking, many serious errors could be made due to judgments based on incomplete or false assumptions.

Rule 7: Look for a Verbal Reasoning Skill in Question Stems

To answer questions efficiently, identify which verbal skill is being tested. The list of 24 verbal skills from the MCAT is in Table 3-4. Understanding the skill behind the question will provide a quick clue to its answer.

What Are Arguments?

It is beneficial to review the structure of logical thinking in order to handle the MCAT passages that involve argument analysis. For our purposes, an argument is a reasoning process based on elements of logic. Arguments consist of statements called propositions, which can be either true or false and can be used as premises or conclusions.

Here is an example of an argument:

Poodles do not shed. (First proposition.)
Joan's dog is a poodle. (Second proposition.)
Therefore, Joan's dog does not shed. (Conclusion.)

In the poodle example, the two propositions serve as premises leading to a conclusion. Signal words can help you to discriminate premises from conclusions. Premises might be indicated by words such as *in addition to, and, because, but, since,* and *for that reason.* Conclusions may be indicated by *therefore, thus, as a result, consequently,* and *finally.*

At times you may sense a gap in a passage between the premise and the conclusion. In these cases, there may be an unexpressed premise. For example, the statement "Sue's third set must have won the tennis match" clearly indicates that an underlying assumption—or unstated premise—must be identified.

Stated premise: Sue won the third set.
(Unstated premise: If a three-set tennis match goes into the final set, the winner of the set will win the match.)
Conclusion: Sue won the match.

As you work through longer examples, it is also important to differentiate the premise and premise support from the conclusion. Consider the following:

Argument 1: Some coaches and administrators say that athletic shoe companies, through promotional deals with coaches, are exerting too much influence on college sports. Therefore, promotional endorsements should be eliminated.

Argument 2: Some coaches and administrators say that athletic shoe companies, through promotional deals with coaches, are exerting too much influence on college sports. In some cases, prospective college students choose a school that is inappropriate for them, based on the coach's connections with these companies. Therefore, promotional endorsements should be eliminated.

TABLE 3-4. Verbal Reasoning Skills for Item Analysis on the MCAT

Statement of Skill	Skill Performance Area
1. Identify thesis	Comprehension
2. Identify reasons to support thesis	Comprehension
3. Identify background knowledge	Comprehension
4. Determine meaning of significant vocabulary	Comprehension
5. Identify assumptions (stated or unstated)	Comprehension
6. Judge credibility of source	Evaluation
7. Identify a general theory or model	Application
8. Recognize a paraphase of complex information	Comprehension
9. Identify comparative relationships	Comprehension
10. Recognize questions of clarification	Comprehension
11. Judge soundness of argument or a reasoning step	Evaluation
12. Predict result based on content and specific facts	Application
13. Judge if reason leads to a given conclusion	Evaluation
14. Use information to solve problem	Application
15. Identify probable cause of event or result	Application
16. Recognize scope of application of hypotheses and conclusions	Application
17. Appraise strength of the evidence	Evaluation
18. Distinguish between supported and unsupported claims	Evaluation
19. Judge relevant information related to argument	Evaluation
20. Determine implications of conclusions or results	Application
21. Recognize alternative hypotheses or solutions	New information
22. Determine how to modify conclusions to incorporate new information	New information
23. Judge the effect of new evidence on conclusions	New information
24. Recognize methods or results that challenge given models, hypotheses, or theories	New information

Adapted from the *MCAT Student Manual*.

In argument 1, the premise—regarding the influence of promotional deals with coaches—is linked with the conclusion that these arrangements should be ended. In argument 2, specific support is given for the premise, which is that the relationship between the coaches and promotional contracts is affecting a student's choice of school. In evaluating arguments, it is important to judge the strength of support given for the premises as additional evidence for the conclusion.

TYPES OF ARGUMENTS

Arguments are constructed using either inductive or deductive reasoning. *Inductive reasoning* begins with specifics, which in combination lead to a general conclusion. By contrast, *deductive reasoning* begins with a conclusion, and the supporting evidence must be constructed. An example of an inductive argument would be: ''Columbus did not fall off the edge of the earth (specific observation); therefore, the earth must be round (general conclusion).'' In contrast, a deductive argument would be: An attorney knows the general charge made against a client (general conclusion), and must construct an explanation of innocence (specifics).

If, while reading the MCAT verbal reasoning passages, you can determine whether the author is using inductive or deductive argument, you will be in a better position to answer the questions. The process of reasoning dictates the form and direction of the argument as well as the best evaluation approach. When evaluating a deductive argument, you must test the inevitability of the conclusion; in an inductive argument, you focus on the probability of the conclusion.

Recognizing trigger words will also help you distinguish a deductive from an inductive argument. *Definite* trigger words are associated with deductive reasoning, because they indicate that the author is starting with a definite conclusion. *Conditional* trigger words are indicative of an inductive argument, in which specific suppositions are made in order to draw a probable conclusion.

CONTENT OF ARGUMENTS

At least one of the MCAT passages usually contains an argument. You should examine the content of each argument while keeping the premises, evidence (supporting statements), and conclusions in mind. Ask yourself the following four questions:

1. What is the key issue and what is the author's point of view?
2. Does the passage reveal all the pertinent information required to understand the argument?

3. Is there enough presented or implied evidence to verify claims in the argument?
4. What type of evidence will make the author's position weaker or stronger?

STRUCTURE OF ARGUMENTS

In an argument, a writer takes an explicit or implicit position on an issue and provides support for that position. The writer's position can be called a claim, thesis, proposition, assertion, or conclusion. Writers often give their readers clues by prefacing their claims with signal words and phrases such as *therefore, hence, so, thus, consequently, then, it follows, in summary, as a result,* and *proving/suggesting that.*

To substantiate a position, a writer offers examples, definitions, descriptions, comparisons, contrasts, classifications, and/or statements of cause-and-effect relationships. These writing devices are referred to as premises, backing, appeals, evidence, reasons, data, support, or opinion. A number of words provide clues that substantiate an author's position, including, *because, for, since, if, given that, as shown by, in the first place,* and *whereas.*

A writer often provides information in addition to a claim and support for that claim. For example, an argument may be strengthened if the writer acknowledges that there is another side to the issue. In effect, the writer states the counterargument, rebuttal, or opposing viewpoint. Assumptions, generalizations, or warrants underlie the writer's position and may or may not be included in the argument.

Detecting Fallacies

The basis for evaluating arguments is the *fallacy*. When the premises of an argument are true and the reasoning process is sound, then the argument is considered valid. However, sometimes the premise or the reasoning is fallacious, as shown in the following examples:

Fallacy of premise: All men can cook. John is a man. Therefore, John can cook.
Fallacy of logic: Many mothers have a nurturing instinct. Betty is a mother. Betty must have a nurturing instinct.

In the fallacy-of-premise example, the initial premise is invalid. In the fallacy-of-logic example, the conclusion is not supported by the information presented. Thus, fallacies can be identified within single sentences ("All men can cook") or within the context of passages, as in the first example. Also, fallacies can occur either in the structure of the argument (even when the premises and conclusions are true) or in the reasoning process itself, as in the second example.

Authors writing in the field of critical thinking have identified many types of fallacies. For the purpose of studying for the MCAT, the following 10 fallacies should be reviewed:

1. **Appeal to authority**—use of an inappropriate authority figure to give credibility
2. **Appeal to tradition**—support based on long-held beliefs and notions, rather than on facts about a topic
3. **Argument from analogy**—an analogy in which there are not enough points of similarity or difference to substantiate a comparison
4. **Begging the question**—circular argument in which the premise and the conclusion contain the same information
5. **Either-or**—forced choice when other alternatives are possible
6. **Equivocation**—intentionally vague language
7. **Hasty generalization**—conclusions drawn from insufficient information
8. **Non sequitur**—irrelevant premise used as a basis for a conclusion
9. **Semantical ambiguity**—words used with multiple meanings or in an unclear manner
10. **Slippery slope**—one event precipitously leading to others

Analysis of Arguments and Passages

In the process of evaluating an argument, you have to ascertain whether the writer did or did not use fallacious reasoning. For the MCAT you will not have to name any fallacies. However, you may be asked to consider a line of reasoning that would weaken an argument. You could evaluate each option by asking yourself whether the statement is ambiguous, introduces irrelevant information, or whether it presumes too much. (Note that this discussion of argument evaluation is intended only to orient you to the passages you will read on the MCAT; it is not a substitute for a course in logic or rhetoric.)

MCAT verbal reasoning passages are selections from published works. You will find a citation at the end of each one that tells you who wrote the passage, in what year, where it was published, and for which audience. Don't ignore this information. Your understanding of the passage—and your ability to evaluate the argument put forth by its author—is enhanced by knowing when the passage was published and the audience for which the author was writing. Once you have identified an argument in an MCAT verbal reasoning passage, evaluate it by following these four steps:

1. Evaluate factual and inferential claims
2. Check whether the premises and/or conclusions are true or false
3. Differentiate between sound and unsound reasoning—thinking that is cogent and thinking that is not cogent—in evaluating an argument
4. Classify an argument as deductive or inductive, and test the author's claims—a deductive argument may be valid and sound, valid but unsound, or invalid (unsound) and an inductive argument may be strong and cogent, strong but not cogent, or weak (not cogent)

Changing Reading Behaviors

Your biggest potential problem when taking the MCAT is resorting to old habits under pressure of time and uncertainty. Therefore, if you are to improve your reading and verbal reasoning skills with the certainty that they will be natural to you on the day of the test, you must develop and practice an approach that is both comfortable and adaptable. Practice often well in advance of the MCAT so you can concentrate on the passages you confront rather than on the process. Emphasize the transference of skills learned when practicing with different types of content.

PRACTICE EXERCISES

The remainder of this chapter is devoted to practice exercises. Before beginning the practice exercises, review this chapter and refresh your memory on the patterns of reasoning and the process recommended for critical thinking (see Chapter 5). From this information, you should be able to determine the personal skills you want to develop to improve and synthesize reading approaches that are most effective for the MCAT.

Tips for Becoming a Critical Reader

- Read at least two pieces of lengthy and complex materials each week

- Treat reading as an analytical exercise

- Be aware of the tone of the passage and/or the author's attitude toward a particular idea

- Detect implied or expressed assumptions involved in an argument or a specific chain of reasoning

Recognize how conflicting facts or arguments are resolved

Verbal Reasoning Passages

The following are 12 verbal reasoning passages in MCAT format. They provide exercises in critical thinking and reasoning skills, based on the skills listed in Table 3-4. Some of these passages have fewer than 6 to 10 questions. For those passages, construct questions of your own. This is an excellent way to improve passage analysis and develop an understanding of critical thinking skills required for the MCAT.

Passage I (Questions 1–5)

The archaeological dig on the Hanson Trust site by Southwark Bridge in London has found an entrance to the original Globe. How far past the entrance it will be possible for archaeologists and theatre historians to go will depend in large part on what judgment the British government makes about the value that the site may have. The dig has confirmed what was always suspected, that nearly half of the theatre's original site is under Southwark Bridge Road, and most of what has survived subsequent rebuilding is under the row of late eighteenth-century houses, until recently offices for the brewery which owned the site, now known as Anchor Terrace. The level of the cellar floors in Anchor Terrace is about three feet above the grade level where a cross section of the Globe's remains might be found, so there is a good chance that in the end more than forty percent of the Globe's original circuit could be excavated. But Anchor Terrace has a preservation order on it, and it already leans some way from the vertical. Heavy digging in its cellarage might imperil the building, not to mention the archaeologists, and digging up Southwark Bridge Road would certainly have a distinct effect on London's traffic-flow; thus the question of whether to dig for the rest of the Globe becomes complicated and political.

The exploratory dig by the Museum of London team of archaeologists has found a lot more than just the theatre's precise location and a small slice of its perimeter walls. Essentially, what the dig has found is a stair turret. This means a great deal to the scholars who have been trying to work out what its structure was just from the pieces of paper that comprised all the evidence previously available. Wenceslas Hollar's drawing of the second Globe, from which his "Long View" was made, shows a building about one hundred feet in outside diameter, with two stair turrets for access to the galleries opposite the stage, located more or less on the east-northeast and north-northeast flanks of a seemingly round structure. What the initial dig seems to have turned up is the foundations of the stair turret on the east-northeast side and sections of the related foundations . . .

The existence of the stair turret is important not just for its design details but because it differentiates the Globe from the Rose and confirms the conjecture that admission to the Globe was markedly different from the system of admission built into the earlier playhouses. References in contemporary accounts indicate that the Rose and the Theatre had an entry system like that described by William Lambarde in 1596, where audiences "first pa(id) one pennie at the gate, another at the entrie of the Scaffold, and the thirde for a quiet standing." Admission in the early playhouses was first by a gate into the yard, where the "gatherer" collected the first penny.

Those who wanted a seat and a roof over their heads paid a second and sometimes a third charge to get into the galleries. Access into these galleries was internal. It went from the yard, most likely by steps like those marked "ingressus" in De Witt's drawing of the Swan . . .

The Globe opened as the first players' co-operative, with the leading sharers, Shakespeare included, taking yard income as players and gallery money as landlords. Separate gatherers for the different sorts of income may not have been necessary. Possibly the introduction of the stair tur-

rets, if it was an innovation at the Globe, came as a development out of the new system of financial management at the new theatre. But it would be safer to be more pragmatic. By cutting out the gangways needed for internal access up each gallery bay, stair turrets did allow more seating space.

Andrew Gurr, "Notes: A First Doorway into the Globe," *Shakespeare Quarterly* 41 (Spring 1990): 98–100. Reprinted by permission.

1. The Globe Theatre lies under which of the following?

   I. Southwark Bridge Road
   II. 18th century houses
   III. Museum of London
   A. I only
   B. I and II only
   C. II and III only
   D. I and III only

2. The author implies that a major benefit of finding the location of the stair turret was that it:

   A. allowed for better measurement of the Globe.
   B. helped identify the original structure of the first Globe Theatre.
   C. helped archaeologists uncover the other turrets.
   D. permitted interpretations on audience payment procedures.

3. According to paragraph three, which of the following had similar entry systems?

   I. Rose
   II. Globe
   III. Theatre
   A. I only
   B. I and II only
   C. II and III only
   D. I and III only

4. The author states that the finding of the turret primarily indicates:

   A. the Globe had more seating capacity than previously estimated.
   B. the Globe was built like the Swan.
   C. there were financial payment innovations.
   D. those who entered had to pay three times.

5. Which one of the following statements regarding further excavation of the Globe is true?

   A. Political and economic issues outweigh the archaeological benefits.
   B. Further excavation will be determined by whether or not it will jeopardize the Anchor Terrace.
   C. The government does not support further excavation.
   D. Making the decision to excavate will not be easily resolved.

Passage II (Questions 6–9)

The conventional interpretation of the (Cuban) missile crisis has changed dramatically over the past decade. For many years, it had been argued that the Kennedy administration's handling of the crisis—its ability to calibrate the level of tension and thus to strike just the right balance between firmness and flexibility—had demonstrated that there was a kind of art of crisis management. But by 1987 it had become clear that the standard interpretation had changed. The argument now was that crises between nuclear powers are inherently unmanageable. The missile crisis, it was claimed, was a good deal more dangerous than people had realized. There were so many things that did go wrong, and so many more that could have gone wrong, especially once military action had begun, that the crisis could very easily have gotten out of hand.

This was certainly the view of certain key officials of the Kennedy administration who gathered on a number of occasions to look back and reflect on the crisis. Former Secretary of Defense Robert S. McNamara, for example, argued repeatedly that no one can with any confidence predict how events in a nuclear crisis would unfold, especially if military force is actually used. The way a crisis runs its course would be dominated by such factors as "misinformation, miscalculation, misjudgment and human fallibility." It was therefore "not possible," he said, "to manage a crisis in the nuclear age," in the sense of being able to exercise strong control over how the confrontation works itself out. For McGeorge Bundy, President Kennedy's national security adviser in 1962, the missile crisis appeared in retrospect not as an exercise in successful crisis management; it looked more like a "battle of blunders," and had resulted mainly from a kind of communication failure: "With more foresighted and better informed governments, more able to communicate with each other openly and honestly, the Cuban missile crisis need never have happened." The same sorts of arguments were made by other commentators on the crisis—by Raymond Garthoff, for example, and by Daniel Ellsberg and Seymour Hersh. Greiner here takes a similar line. He speaks, for example, of the Soviets losing "control over military decision-making in Cuba." The dangers inherent in such a situation, he says, were not really understood, and only at the last minute did Khrushchev realize "how close both sides had come to the brink of war."

This new interpretation did not take shape as people tried to come to terms with the new evidence on the crisis that became available over the past decade. Indeed, that evidence should have had the opposite effect. The most important point to emerge from these new sources was that President Kennedy was much more willing to compromise on the issue of the Jupiter missiles in Turkey than had previously been thought. This implied that there was more of a "cushion," more room for diplomatic settlement, and less risk than had earlier been assumed.

This was, however, only the most important of many new findings that pointed—or should have pointed—to the basic conclusion that the risks were not as great as people had thought.

March Trachtenberg, "Commentary: New Light on the Cuban Missile Crisis?" *Diplomatic History* 14 (Spring 1990): 242–43. Copyright © 1990 by Scholarly Resources, Inc. Reprinted by permission of Scholarly Resources, Inc.

6. In paragraph three, the author refers to "these new sources." To whom is he referring?

   A. The commentators listed in paragraph two
   B. President Kennedy's presidential papers
   C. Khrushchev's memoirs
   D. Members of President Kennedy's administration

7. If new documents released under the Freedom of Information Act indicated that President Kennedy had been warned of defective firing mechanisms in the missiles in Turkey, what effect would this new insight have upon the author's argument?

   A. It would strengthen the author's argument.
   B. It would weaken the author's argument.
   C. It would neither strengthen nor weaken the author's argument.
   D. It would challenge the Freedom of Information Act.

8. What does the passage suggest about the current unity of President Kennedy's former administration officials?

   A. They have only recently concurred with each other since there has been significant disagreement between them over the years.
   B. They have changed their minds over time.
   C. They have not had an opportunity to talk with each other about the crisis until recently.
   D. They were restrained by the government from discussing the events leading to and during the crisis.

9. The author's conclusion that the Cuban missile crisis was not as risky as previously assumed is based on:

   A. an analysis of the United States' military strike force.
   B. the comments of McGeorge Bundy, President Kennedy's national security advisor.
   C. reanalysis of President Kennedy's range of options.
   D. President Kennedy's skill in crisis management.

Write a question with four responses, based on the passage. Do not base your question on information used in the items above. Use a separate piece of paper.

Passage III (Questions 10–15)

I passed all the other courses that I took at my university, but I could never pass botany. This was because all botany students had to spend several hours a week in a laboratory looking through a microscope at plant cells, and I could never see through a microscope. I never once saw a cell through a microscope. This used to enrage my instructor. He would wander around the laboratory pleased with the progress all the students were making in drawing the involved and, so I am told, interesting structure of flower cells, until he came to me. I would just be standing there. "I can't see anything," I would say. He would begin patiently enough, explaining how anybody can see through a microscope, but he would always end up in a fury, claiming that I could too see through a microscope but just pretended that I couldn't. "It takes away from the beauty of flowers anyway," I used to tell him. "We are not concerned with beauty in this course," he would say. "We are concerned solely with what I may call the mechanics of flars." "Well," I'd say, "I can't see anything." "Try it just once again," he'd say, and I would put my eye to the microscope and see nothing at all, except now and again a nebulous milky substance—a phenomenon of maladjustment. You were supposed to see a vivid, restless clockwork of sharply defined plant cells. "I see what looks like a lot of milk," I would tell him. This he claimed, was the result of my not having adjusted the microscope properly, so he would readjust it for me, or rather, for himself. And I would look again and see milk.

I finally took a deferred pass, as they called it, and waited a year and tried again. (You had to pass one of the biological sciences or you couldn't graduate.) The professor had come back from vacation brown as a berry, bright-eyed and eager to explain cell-structure again to his classes. "Well," he said to me, cheerily, when we met in the first laboratory hour of the semester, "we're going to see cells this time, aren't we?" "Yes, sir," I said. Students to the right of me and to the left of me and in front of me were seeing cells; what's more, they were quietly drawing pictures of them in their notebooks. Of course, I didn't see anything.

"We'll try it," the professor said to me grimly, "with every adjustment of the microscope known to man. As God is my witness, I'll arrange this glass so that you see cells through it or I'll give up teaching. In twenty two years of botany, I—" He cut off abruptly for he was beginning to quiver all over, like Lionel Barrymore, and he genuinely wished to hold onto his temper; his scenes with me had taken a great deal out of him.

So we tried it with every adjustment of the microscope known to man. With only one of them did I see anything but blackness or the familiar lacteal opacity, and that time I saw, to my pleasure and amazement, a variegated constellation of flecks, specks, and dots. These I hastily drew. The instructor, noting my activity, came back from an adjoining desk, a smile on his lips and his eyebrows high in hope. He looked at my cell drawing. "What's that?" he demanded, with a hint of a squeal in his voice. "That's what I saw," I said. "You didn't, you didn't, you didn't!" he screamed, losing control of his temper instantly, and he bent over and squinted into the microscope. His head snapped up. "That's your eye!" he shouted. "You've fixed the lens so that it reflects! You've drawn your eye!"

James Thurber, "University Days," in *My Life and Hard Times* (New York: Harper & Row). Copyright © 1933, 1961 by James Thurber. Reprinted by permission.

10. The author states that the reason he was taking the botany course was because:

    A. he was a premedical student.
    B. he needed it to graduate.
    C. he wanted to see the structure of cells.
    D. it was required of science majors.

11. Based on the passage, it could be inferred that the professor's attitude toward the author was:

    I. encouraging.
    II. disbelieving.
    III. instructive.
    A. I only
    B. I and II only
    C. II and III only
    D. I, II, and III

12. The phrase "lacteal opacity" in paragraph four means:

    A. milky color.
    B. differentiated shadows.
    C. distinct shapes.
    D. darkness.

13. In considering the example provided by the author, the probable outcome of this episode is:

    A. the author failed the course.
    B. the professor gave him another chance.
    C. the student learned from his errors.
    D. the student passed by "faking" it.

14. The primary reason the author had difficulty with the microscope probably was due to:

    A. the fact that he didn't try.
    B. a faulty instrument.
    C. poor instruction.
    D. the professor adjusting it to his own eyes.

15. The tone of this passage could best be described as:

    A. self-congratulatory.
    B. ironic.
    C. degrading.
    D. critical.

Passage IV (Questions 16–19)

Who would dare change the arms of God on the first day of creation? Michelangelo. First he scribed outlines for God's arms into wet plaster with quick strokes of a sharp tool. Then he abandoned those outlines in a flash of brushstrokes. He painted God's left arm so it swept directly overhead, made that arm plunge a divine hand into the turbulent light and wrenched it from the darkness. The Sistine Chapel quivers still with the aftershocks of Michelangelo's daring now even more as nine years of careful cleaning and restoration by Vatican experts come to an end. They have been separating darkness—the accumulated grime of nearly five centuries—from Michelangelo's light. It is a light to amaze the eye and blind the soul.

Yet what a reluctant light it was, for the artist who was cajoled and harassed, forced really, into completing one of the crowning masterpieces of Western civilization.

By age 33 Michelangelo had already made his reputation as a sculptor equal to any ancient Greek or Roman. His marble "Pieta," the crucified Christ lifeless across the knees of a Mary forever young and innocent, transcended grief. His giant "David" glowered fiercer than any Goliath.

Now he had a commission from Pope Julius II to make for him a tomb of sculptures so elaborate and so huge as to confound the imagination. Julius, however, first insisted that Michelangelo paint the ceiling of the Pope's own Sistine Chapel.

Michelangelo did not want the Sistine job he began in 1508. Though trained to the brush, he had painted infrequently. Julius, whose fame came from enlarging the papal domain by the sword, bullied him like a drill sergeant, once hitting him with a cane, once threatening to throw him off the scaffold. The artist grumbled constantly, asking for release, signed his letters: "Michelangelo, sculptor." . . .

The artist was desperate to quit the commission: the Pope was adamant that he continue. The work did not go well at first, partly from inexperience. The fresco of the Flood was soon hazed over by "mildew," the result perhaps of mixing too much water in the surface plaster, or intonaco. Michelangelo complained to the Pope: "Indeed I told your Holiness that this is not my art; what I have done is spoiled." Julius did not relent; Michelangelo must make it his art.

The restorer's credo is like the physician's: First, do no harm. The treatment is to lift layers of Rome's dust, sooty grease from burning candle tallow, and other substances—even the residue of Greek wine used as a cleaning solvent some 275 years ago. All have obscured Michelangelo's Promethean work.

Worst of all were varnishes made of animal glues. Applied in various centuries to brighten the darkening surface, they did so for a time. Then each deteriorated and turned the ceiling darker than before.

Despite its dingy appearance, most of the fresco remained in good condition. The technique of painting on fresh plaster was its own best protection. In the hours after Michelangelo painted, the day's application of fresco dried. As it did, the pigments were chemically bonded in a hardening layer of calcium carbonate. The various glues and gums of centuries did not penetrate the hard carbonate shell.

The glues have, however, shrunk and puckered, and in spots scabs of glue have fallen away, pulling pigment with them. This slow destruction by glue pox, rather than some large and immediate threat, has been the Vatican's principal motivation for cleaning the ceiling now. Water damage from roof leaks since plugged has also infiltrated dissolved salts to the surface, stains that cannot be removed as easily as ordinary grime.

The restoration plan calls for examination of each section of fresco with scientific instruments and assessment of the results with human judgment. Then under exacting procedures, the gentlest effective solvent is applied to overlying grime and both are rinsed away. It seems a nearly magical process to watch.

David Jeffrey, "A Renaissance for Michelangelo," *National Geographic* 176 (December 1989): 688, 696, 699. Reprinted by permission.

16. According to the passage, the relationship between Pope Julius II and Michelangelo could be described as:

   A. tempestuous.
   B. collegial.
   C. defamatory.
   D. ecclesiastical.

17. It can be inferred from the passage that Michelangelo signed his name with the word *sculptor* because:

   A. he wanted to begin the tomb of sculptures for the Pope.
   B. he wished to annoy the Pope.
   C. he wanted to get permission to finish his sculpture "David."
   D. he saw it as a way to annoy Pope Pius II.

18. A church in England had a painted ceiling that had darkened with time. As the restorers attempted to lift the grime, the paint also was lifted off. The probable difference between this ceiling and the one in the Sistine Chapel is that for the English ceiling:

   A. the varnishes were made of animal glue.
   B. paint was not applied to fresh plaster.
   C. the ceiling had glue pox.
   D. the solvent was not rinsed away.

19. The author infers that Michelangelo's artistic process included:

   A. copying his designs from preliminary plans onto the ceiling.
   B. the use of outline drawing with artisans filling in detail.
   C. creative changes as he worked.
   D. meticulous detail with fresco added as a stabilizer.

Write a question with four responses, based on the passage. Do not base your question on information used in the items above. Use a separate piece of paper.

Passage V (Questions 20–24)

Although every planet in our solar system, with the possible exception of Mercury, has an atmosphere, the earth's atmosphere is probably the only one that is composed entirely of nitrogen and oxygen. Mars and Venus have atmospheres composed mostly of carbon dioxide, while Jupiter's and Saturn's atmospheres contain mostly hydrogen, helium, and compounds of hydrogen, such as methane and ammonia. The origin of the earth's particular kind of atmosphere is still the subject of much speculation. However, one thing seems fairly certain—when the earth was formed five billion years ago, it was probably too hot to retain any atmosphere that it may have had to begin with. This is because high temperature implies high molecular speeds. What keeps the moving gas molecules from escaping from a planet is gravitational attraction, which depends on the mass of the bodies. Thus, small, hot planets such as Mercury can hold only the most massive molecules. The release of gases from the earth's interior is generally thought to be the process that produced our atmosphere. Most of the lighter gases produced in this way have since been lost, but the earth is massive enough and cool enough at the present time to retain the thin envelope of gases that remain. The atmospheres of extremely massive planets such as Jupiter and Saturn are probably much the same today as they were at the time of their origin.

At the outer limits of the earth's atmosphere, a slow seepage of molecules to outer space continues. At levels above 600 km, the gases are thin enough and hot enough so that some of the lighter, faster molecules can escape the gravitational pull of the earth. Because the upward escape velocity required for a particle to escape from the earth is quite high—about 11.3 km/s (compared to 2.4 km/s for the much smaller moon)—only the very light gases, such as hydrogen and helium, can leave the earth at a significant rate.

At the beginning of Earth's existence, the original atmosphere was probably composed chiefly of a mixture of methane (CH_4) and ammonia (NH_3), which are even now important constituents in the atmospheres of Jupiter, Saturn, Uranus, and Neptune. It is fairly certain that the first atmosphere was devoid of free oxygen.

According to one theory, the earth's present atmosphere did not evolve until much of the original one had been driven off and the earth had started to cool. This new atmosphere was created when gases that had been dissolved in the molten rock bubbled out of the surface, a process called outgassing. As cooling continued, the water vapor condensed to form the great oceans. The liquid water gradually absorbed most of the atmosphere's carbon dioxide, thus leaving nitrogen as the predominant gas. The oxygen in our atmosphere is believed to have appeared only after primitive plant life developed (about three billion years ago?) and began acting on carbon dioxide through photosynthesis to form oxygen. The concentration of oxygen in the atmosphere probably increased very slowly at the outset, since much of the oxygen was consumed in the oxidation of the earth's surface materials, and the present level was probably not reached until a few hundred million years ago.

Albert Miller and Jack Thompson, *Elements of Meteorology*, 4th ed. (Indianapolis: Merrill, 1983). Reprinted with permission of Merrill, an imprint of Macmillan Publishing Company.

20. Gas molecules that escape the earth's atmosphere include:

  A. fast-moving molecules.
  B. slow-moving molecules.
  C. lightweight gases.
  D. heavyweight gases.

21. In the first phase of the earth's development, its atmosphere was a direct result of:

  A. release of gases from inside the planet.
  B. the ratio of oxygen and carbon dioxide.
  C. weak gravitational force on heavy molecules.
  D. the retention of gases within the planet.

22. If the earth were subject to global warming, which of the following would occur?

  I. Gas molecules would move faster.
  II. Lighter gases would escape at a greater rate.
  III. Gravitational force would be less upon the lighter molecules.
  A. I and II only
  B. II only
  C. I and III
  D. I, II, and III

23. The second and third stages of the earth's atmosphere are characterized by:

  I. a vacuum created by lack of oxygen.
  II. carbon dioxide being broken down by photosynthesis.
  III. the cooling of water vapor to form the seas.
  A. I and II only
  B. II only
  C. II and III only
  D. I, II, and III

24. What is the ratio comparing the age of the earth to the length of time oxygen has been in enough quantity to sustain life (assuming the earth began to support life two billion years ago)?

  A. 5:2
  B. 2:50
  C. 50:2
  D. The answer cannot be determined from the information in the passage.

Write a question with four responses, based on the passage. Do not base your question on information used in the items above. Use a separate piece of paper.

Passage VI (Questions 25-28)

What do crabs, sea urchins, earthworms, malaria parasites and corals have in common? In fact, these very diverse groups share very little, apart from the fact they all lack a backbone. Of the 1,071,000 or so known species of animals about 1,029,300 are invertebrate; that is, over 95 percent are animals without backbones. Invertebrates make up the bulk of animals, measured both in terms of numbers of species recognized and numbers of individuals. Some invertebrates, like garden snails and earthworms, are conspicuous and familiar animals, while others, although abundant, pass unnoticed by most people.

Invertebrate body forms range in size from the lowly microscopic Amoeba, which may be just one micrometer in diameter, to the Giant squid, 18m (59 ft) in length, a ratio of 1:18,000,000. They include life forms as diverse as the Desert locust and the sea anemones. They inhabit all regions of the globe, and all habitats, from the ocean abyss to the air. Life almost certainly originated in the seas, and virtually all the major invertebrate groups (phyla) have marine representatives. Somewhat fewer (almost 14 phyla) have conquered fresh water. Fewer still (about 5 phyla) live on land and of these only the jointed-limbed groups (arthropods) have mastered the air and really dry places. Most numerous among arthropods are the uniramians (e.g., insects, millipedes, centipedes) and the chelicerates (e.g., scorpions, spiders, ticks, mites).

Many invertebrates, like slugs (whether of the garden or sea), are free living; others, such as barnacles, are attached to the substrate throughout their adult life; yet others live as parasites in or on the bodies of plants or other animals. Some invertebrates are of great commercial significance, either as direct food for man (e.g., prawns and oysters), or as food for man's exploitable reserves (e.g., the planktonic copepods on which herring feed). Others (e.g., earthworms) are much appreciated because they improve the soil for agriculture. Many invertebrates live as parasites, either in man himself or in the bodies of domestic animals and plants, where great damage may be wrought, and so are of great medical or agricultural importance.

This great diversity of form and life-style in animals has led zoologists to sort out, or classify, animals according to type and evolutionary connections. To be certain that they are speaking of the same animals, they give each species a unique scientific name (e.g., *Lumbricus terrestri*, the common earthworm). Every species is classified into one of the major groups, or phyla. A phylum comprises all those animals which are thought to have a common evolutionary origin. According to their understanding of the probable evolutionary processes involved, zoologists may recognize some 39 animal phyla. With one exception, they are made up exclusively of invertebrate animals. The phylum Chordata includes all animals with a hollow dorsal nerve cord. Nearly all—including fishes, amphibians, reptiles, birds—have a backbone, but some are invertebrate, such as the sea squirt.

The technical classification that zoologists employ leads from the most primitive and simple animal types to the most complex and advanced. In order to achieve some form of system, various levels of organization are recognized which give clear distinctions between phyla. The most fundamental of these lies in the number of cells in the body. A cell is the smallest functional unit of an animal, governed by its own nucleus which contains genetic material, known as DNA.

Keith Banister and Andrew Campbell, eds., *The Encyclopedia of Aquatic Life* (New York: Facts on File Publications, 1985), 148-49. Reproduced by permission of Equinox (Oxford) Limited.

25. The main idea of this passage can be summed up best by which of the following statements?

    A. There are many more invertebrates than are known to most of us.
    B. Invertebrates are considerably more diverse than they are similar.
    C. Invertebrates vary greatly in size and place of habitation.
    D. Zoologists have created a classification system to keep track of invertebrates.

26. If a new invertebrate were to be discovered, it would most likely:

    A. have ancestors that could be traced back to the sea.
    B. be a uniramian.
    C. live in the sea.
    D. be microscopic in size.

27. According to this article, the most important factor in classifying animal types is:

    A. DNA.
    B. presence or absence of a backbone.
    C. complexity of the nervous system.
    D. number of cells.

28. Based on the passage, one could assume that:

    A. barnacles are parasites.
    B. some parasites are of commercial significance.
    C. the invertebrates that provide agricultural benefits are not the same ones as those that find hosts in people and animals.
    D. free-living vertebrates are more ecologically beneficial than those that attach themselves to the substrate.

Write two questions with four responses each, based on the passage. Do not base your question on information used in the items above. Use a separate piece of paper.

Feathers, together with adaptations of muscles, heart, bones, and lungs, make birds the most efficient of flying machines. Feathers have many advantages. They are light. They are regularly replaced when worn, lost, or damaged. Each is individually attached to a muscle for greater maneuverability. Feathers enable birds to ride effortlessly on the wind, to travel faster than 100 miles per hour, to hover and fly backwards, to fly more than 48 hours without resting, and to migrate thousands of miles a year. No bird does all of these things, but feathers make them all possible. Swifts, for example, are such accomplished aerialists that they feed, drink, bathe, court, and even mate while flying. In addition to flying at the great speeds (80 miles per hour and faster) that have given them their name, swifts sometimes spend the night on the wing a few thousand feet above the ground.

The shape of the wings and tail tells us at a glance how specialized a bird is for flight. Some of the fastest fliers—falcons and swallows, for example—have long pointed wings and long narrow tails. This streamlined profile creates the least resistance as the bird moves through the air. The Peregrine falcon, diving after prey, has been clocked at 175 miles per hour. The broader wings and tail of slower fliers, such as vultures, eagles, and storks, catch every movement of air so these birds can soar and wheel high in the sky. Birds such as pheasants and grouse, which seldom fly, have short rounded wings that provide quick lift but little sustaining power. Their leg muscles are much more developed than those used in flight. Because the hardest working muscles are nourished by more capillaries and are therefore darker, earthbound birds like chickens and turkeys have "dark meat" in their legs and "white meat" in their breasts. In most birds the breast muscles form the dark meat.

The bird's skeleton, a marvel of flight engineering, fuses lightness with strength. Most birds do not have a bone like the one in humans that separates the nasal cavity from the mouth—one of the many adaptations that keep flying weight to a minimum. Their skulls are usually paper thin. The heads of woodpeckers, however, are specially reinforced to absorb the constant stress of hammering trees. Many powerful fliers are equipped with hollow bones, which are filled with air sacs to increase buoyancy. The skeleton of the frigate bird, a soarer with a seven-foot wingspan, weighs only four ounces—less than its feathers. Hollow bones are stronger than solid bones of the same weight because they bend more easily and the air inside them absorbs shocks. Longer wing bones are reinforced with struts, a device also found in airplanes.

Strong fliers have proportionately larger hearts that pump blood more rapidly than those of nonfliers, weak fliers, and soaring birds. When hovering, a hummingbird beats its wings about 50 times a second, with its heart pulsing 1,200 times a minute. The lungs, aided by air sacs in the bones and other cavities—even the toes—supply oxygen needed for flight. The reproductive system also enhances aerodynamic efficiency; the testes of male birds expand in size and weight only during the brief season they are producing sperm.

Roger F. Pasquier, "The Diversity of Birdlife," in *The Wonder of Birds* (Washington, D.C.: National Geographic Society, 1983), 38–39. Reprinted by permission.

29. According to the passage, one might conclude that the most important point about feathers is that they:

   A. appear to be more important than muscles, heart, bones, and lungs in adaptation for flying.
   B. allow for a great deal of versatility in possible types of flying feats but are not solely responsible for what a bird actually can do.
   C. are responsible for maneuverability.
   D. lessen air resistance.

30. One can infer from the phrase "make birds the most efficient of flying machines" that:

   A. natural features are more efficient than manufactured ones.
   B. airplanes have been structured after birds.
   C. a bird's parts function in a mechanical way.
   D. none of the above.

31. All of the following statements are true EXCEPT:

   A. peregrine falcons probably have long, pointed wings and a long, narrow tail.
   B. a broad tail and wings allow for greater height than a long pointed tail and wings.
   C. length of wings affects endurance.
   D. storks have highly developed leg muscles and wider wings than many other birds.

32. Based on heart size, one could infer which of the following?

   I. A swift would be proportionately larger than a frigate bird.
   II. A hummingbird would be proportionately larger than a swift.
   III. A grouse would be proportionately equal to a turkey.
   A. I only
   B. I and II only
   C. II only
   D. I and III only

33. Based on the information presented on bone structure, one might conclude that:

   I. the bone structure of most birds weighs proportionately less than that of humans.
   II. the bones of peregrine falcons are hollow.
   III. the bones of powerful fliers have air sacs that increase buoyancy and decrease speed.
   A. I only
   B. I and II only
   C. II only
   D. I, II, and III

34. Which of the following facts is/are true?

   A. Hummingbirds have very fast heartbeats compared with many other birds.
   B. Air sacs can be found in the toes of some birds.
   C. A bird's skeleton is compared to flight engineering.
   D. All of the above.

Passage VIII (Questions 35–39)

The tape handling system (of a tape recorder) consists of two hubs that hold the tape supply reel and a take-up reel plus the machinery necessary to pull the tape past the heads. The drive mechanism typically comprises a constant-speed motor coupled by a rubber friction drive wheel to a capstan, which moves the tape. The motor shaft can drive various-size wheels, hereby offering differing tape speeds . . . .

Early tape machines fed tape through the recorder from one reel to a second reel. For the purposes of convenience, tape deck manufacturers developed cartridges to eliminate the need for an independent take-up reel. The first tape cartridge contained a single reel on which the tape was spooled in an endless loop. The tape was fed to the heads from the inside of the reel and back onto the reel from the outside. This caused the tape to slide over itself as the reel turned and thus early cartridges frequently stopped because a layer of tape stuck to the next layer of tape and wound itself too tightly. These problems were lessened by the development of lubricants . . . .

Current cartridges, called cassettes, use two reels but the entire mechanism is encased in a single shell of plastic, eliminating the inconvenience of open reel-to-reel tapes. The costs of the convenience of cartridges are that, in making smaller cartridges, manufacturers are using thinner tape . . . and running the tape at slower speeds, which has implications for frequency response, head construction, quality of the transport mechanism, and quality of recording . . . .

The quality of a tape recorder is a function of the mechanical or electrical design in its construction. In general, electrical devices are less variable in recording and reproduction quality than mechanical devices so that the more expensive the tape machine, the more likely it is to use electrical rather than mechanical components in its design where there is a choice between the two.

In those machines that might be considered for home use or for other less critical applications, the components of operation are entirely mechanical. The capstan is driven by a belt stretched between a stepped motor pulley with several different sizes and a similar stepped motor pulley on the capstan itself. The speed of the tape can be changed by moving the belt from one set of pulleys on the motor and capstan to another set that has a different size ratio and hence a different ratio between motor speed and capstan speed. When the play button is pressed, the pinch roller is moved against the tape by a system of levers to drive the tape. The rewind and fast forward functions are also mechanically controlled by a system of gears and pulleys so that the motor can also drive the take-up and supply reels.

More expensive machines use an electromechanical system. In this case the activation of a push-button energizes devices called solenoids. A solenoid is an electromagnet and an attached rod that can perform mechanical operations by being attracted or repelled by the electromagnet.

The advantage of solenoid operation is twofold. First, the button needs a much lighter touch because no mechanical function is being performed. The electrical system energizes only the solenoid, and the solenoid itself may be adjusted to determine the distance over which some mechanical linkage moves. Second, solenoid operation allows all of the functions of the tape recorder to be remotely controlled; the operator needs only a set of push-buttons that are electrically connected to solenoids that, in turn, control the mechanical movements of the tape parts.

Jack F. Curtis and Martin C. Schultz, *Basic Laboratory Instrumentation for Speech and Hearing* (Boston: Little, Brown and Co., 1986), 150–52. Reprinted by permission.

35. The passage explicitly states that early tape machines:

   A. utilized one reel that fed the tape to the heads from the inside of the reel, and a second reel that received the tape as it fed onto it from the outside.
   B. did not perform as well as cassette models.
   C. used a constant-speed motor, rubber friction drive wheel, and capstan.
   D. none of the above.

36. Based on the information in the passage, one can infer that:

   I. convenience was the driving force for the development of cartridges.
   II. development of the early cartridge solved some problems and created other problems.
   III. people prefer mechanical components over electrical.
   A. I only
   B. I and II only
   C. II and III only
   D. I, II, and III

37. According to the facts presented, which of the following statements is true in a mechanical machine?

   A. The speed of the tape depends on the ratio between motor speed and capstan speed.
   B. When the machine is on play, levers press against the tape and move it along.
   C. Mechanical action is achieved by an electromagnet and attached rod.
   D. The capstan is driven by a single stepped motor pulley.

38. The key difference between an electromechanical system and a mechanical system is that in the electromechanical system:

   A. there is a more expensive solenoid component.
   B. the solenoid allows all functions to be remotely controlled.
   C. mechanical action is achieved by an electromagnet and attached rod.
   D. solenoids eliminate the need for mechanical operations.

39. Based on this passage, one can conclude which of the following?

    A. The best-quality machine is probably beyond the reach of the average person.

    B. The level of quality provided by the most expensive equipment is most likely not needed for typical home use.

    C. There is an inverse relationship between level of technology and cost.

    D. Only A and B are correct.

Passage IX (Questions 40–45)

Paul was diagnosed as having cystic fibrosis at five years of age. As a youngster, he was watched over and guarded by adults who were oriented to the possibility of imminent death. He was usually avoided by peers and potential friends who would "take a step back" upon learning that he had a serious illness. Teachers from grade school through college were reluctant to make demands or encourage long-range tasks which might prove stressful or be abruptly terminated by death.

The attitudes of others toward illness and death were always difficult for him to deal with. Rather than confront people and ask for clarification of their ideas about his situation, he would withdraw. He became hesitant to involve himself with others because of his anxieties about exposing his feelings regarding the implications of his grave medical problems.

Several times in his life, Paul had felt that psychiatric help would be quite useful in learning to cope with his everyday problems of living. He was unsuccessful in pursuing his idea because he was uncertain whether his vague depression and anxieties were appropriate to take to a psychiatrist. Even when seen by a counselor in college, he found it difficult to describe his needs and guide the therapist toward his areas of discomfort. The therapist, in turn, tended to be more concerned about his illness, following the pattern of seeing him primarily as a sick person.

A doctor friend helped Paul change his self-image from a seriously ill person to a man with a serious illness, a shift of attitude which proved successful in all areas of his life. He was able to broaden his horizons and to persevere in looking for a job. He had graduated from college with a business degree, but interviewers had only to hear that he had a chronic illness to refuse his application. With support from his doctor friend, he finally was hired in a managerial capacity with a major distribution and retail firm. His drive to success carried him quite rapidly into additional areas of responsibility. Having given up a death orientation, Paul decided to marry. Although he denies neither the threat of death nor the reality of being alive, his newfound confidence and strength in dealing with himself and others have led to a more productive, rewarding life.

40. Which of the following phrases best describes the central idea of the passage?

    A. Changing one's lifestyle
    B. Coping with mental illness
    C. Adjusting to life's demands
    D. Learning to live with a serious illness

41. The college counselor's primary concern for Paul was:

    A. his future career.
    B. his imminent death.
    C. his physical illness.
    D. his emotional health.

42. Which adjective best describes people's attitude toward Paul during his childhood?

    A. Authoritarian
    B. Compassionate
    C. Hostile
    D. Protective

43. Why didn't Paul seek psychiatric help?

    A. He considered his illness only a physical disorder.
    B. He refused to talk with others about his emotional distress.
    C. He doubted the suitability of psychiatric help for solving his coping problems.
    D. He felt inhibited when talking with medically trained people about his inner feelings.

44. Paul's success in dealing with his illness was due to:

    A. his desire to get well.
    B. his change in mental attitude.
    C. his attainment of a college degree.
    D. his strict adherence to medical treatments.

45. From information in the passage, one can infer that:

    A. cystic fibrosis can be cured.
    B. cystic fibrosis can be inherited.
    C. cystic fibrosis is difficult to diagnose.
    D. cystic fibrosis is an emotionally disabling disease.

Passage X (Questions 46–50)

Senate Joint Resolution One: This Resolution proposes an Amendment to the Constitution of the United States to abolish the antiquated electoral college and undemocratic "unit vote" system and substitute direct popular election of the President and Vice-president. The proposed amendment provides, further, in the unlikely event no candidate receives 40 percent of the popular vote, the President and Vice-president will be elected in a runoff election between two pairs of candidates receiving the highest number of votes.

Senator Smith's Speech: "Under our present electoral system, a member of the losing party carries no long-term liability. Losing neither invites insidious discrimination, nor endangers the security of one's liberty. Among the losers may be a person representing a geographic area or an ethnic, religious, social, or economic group. Most Americans are inclined to forget that they are members of some minority group and this group, potentially, might become a vulnerable minority. The power of minorities comes from the skill with which they are able to join forces with other minorities. Indeed, a minority group which fails to align itself with other minorities finds its political power greatly diminished. One of the chief virtues of the electoral college system is that it not only encourages such alliances, it virtually requires them. It builds moderate majorities, while protecting the interests of all minorities that are willing to compromise."

Senator Brown's Speech: "Perhaps the one aspect of the electoral-college system which carries the greatest burden for ethnic or racial minorities is the 'unit rule.' This system awards all of a state's electoral votes to the candidate who wins a majority of the popular vote. It carries real potential to erase the views of the minority voter, while magnifying the strength of the majority voter. I have considered the argument that a direct election would deprive my constituents of an advantage they now possess under the electoral system. The 'one-man, one-vote' rule has effectively enfranchised black Americans and other minority group members in voting for Congress. In a similar way, the direct election of the President will effectively enfranchise black Americans and other minority and ethnic groups. It will ensure that their vote will count in those states where it is currently ineffectual. It will mean that the people will vote for President as a citizen of the United States rather than merely as a citizen of a state. It will allow the vote of each person, black or white, to carry equal weight."

46. The "unit vote" system is best described in which of the following statements?

   A. All the electoral votes of a state are committed to one candidate.
   B. The Republican votes go to the Republican candidate and the Democratic votes go to the Democratic candidate.
   C. Each candidate receives a "unit" or a proportion of the vote based on the state population.
   D. Only Senate votes count since each state has two senators to encourage fairness.

47. In the event that neither presidential candidate receives 40 percent of the vote under the current system, how would the president and vice president be elected?

   A. By a runoff election between the two pairs of candidates
   B. By popular vote of the people
   C. By naming the president from one party and the vice president from another party
   D. No process stipulated in the passage

48. Senator Smith asserts that the electoral college provides protection for individuals within religious groups. This statement is:

   A. supported by the passage.
   B. contradicted by the passage.
   C. neither supported nor contradicted by the passage.
   D. not discussed in the passage.

49. Senator Brown indicates that election of the President should be similar to the election of state officials. This statement is:

   A. supported by the passage.
   B. contradicted by the passage.
   C. neither supported nor contradicted by the passage.
   D. not discussed in the passage.

50. Each speaker believes his proposal will enfranchise minority and ethnic groups. This statement is:

   A. supported by the passage.
   B. contradicted by the passage.
   C. neither supported nor contradicted by the passage.
   D. not discussed in the passage.

Passage XI (Questions 51–55)

The three components of population growth are births, deaths, and net migration. The birth rate in the United States has varied in importance in the determination of overall population trends in different periods in our nation's history. For the 50 years between the Civil War and World War I, changes in the birth and death rates generally paralleled each other. This produced a rather smooth, declining rate of natural increase (birth rate minus death rate) during this period. As a result, the net growth rate (natural increase plus net migration) was heavily influenced by changes in the rate of net migration rather than by birth or death rates during the late 1800s and early 1900s.

Low migration rates, combined with the influenza epidemic of 1918, resulted in a net growth rate of 10.5 per 1,000 population for the 1915–1920 period. This was the lowest rate of population growth recorded until the "Great Depression" when the net growth rate fell to 7 per 1,000 population during the 1930–1935 period. The Immigration Act of 1924, which established immigration quotas based on national origin, substantially reduced the number of immigrants to about 1 per 1,000 population per year. The fairly constant net migration rate and death rate since the 1920s have made the birth rate the primary factor in the determination of population growth patterns for the last 50 years.

Increases in the birth rate (from 7.0 to 15.6 per 1,000) contributed to the doubling of the net rate of population growth between the 1930–1935 and 1945–1950 periods. However, a decline occurred in the net annual growth rate from 1.7 percent in the 1950–1955 period to less than 1 percent in the 1970–1975 period. This decline was almost entirely due to corresponding declines in the birth rate (from 24.8 to 15.9 per 1,000).

51. Changes in the rate of population increase in the 1930–1935 period and the 1945–1950 period were due to:

    A. declining death rate.
    B. increases in birth rates.
    C. a relaxation of immigration laws.
    D. a declining death rate.

52. What factor most influenced the net population growth in the United States during the late 1800s and early 1900s?

    A. Lower death rates
    B. An epidemic-free period
    C. An increased immigration rate
    D. More accurate recording of births

53. In what historical period was the United States population growth the lowest?

    A. During World War II
    B. During the Depression years
    C. Following the 1918 influenza epidemic
    D. After passage of the Immigration Act

54. If the most recent census count showed that the birth rate had been miscalculated in the country, the most important effect would be:

    A. a higher number of deaths.
    B. a change in the ratio of births to deaths.
    C. the use of the new numbers to determine population growth.
    D. retaking the census count.

55. The main topic of this passage is the:

    A. rationale for demographic studies.
    B. effects of birth declines on population.
    C. population declines in the United States.
    D. net population growth in the United States.

Passage XII (Questions 56–61)

The following comments are from an interview with a recent winner of the Nobel Prize in Physiology/Medicine. His work revealed the overall structure of the antibody molecule.

"Since getting the Nobel Prize, I've been asked to do a lot of talking to nonscientists about research. It's a frustrating thing. Scientists, and certainly I'm included, forget about how abstract what we do is. How getting that structure depends on feeling about Avogadro's number more or less the way I feel about the ends of my fingers. That's because after living with it for ten years, I think I understand it. Maybe that's all understanding is—a terrific familiarity.

"Scientific research proceeds by a process of self-correction and linearization. It falsified the actual events of discovery. Later, it's hard to remember that it really didn't happen that way, that you were blundering around, and something happened. You said 'ah-so!,' and you looked back and regularized it, thereby wiping out the serendipitous nature of the experience.

"We can now see the relationship of one class of antibodies to the other, and the relationship of structure to function. The whole genetic language in immunology emerged as a result of this. It became quite clear in a very nice 'why-didn't-I-think-of-it?' way. The initial impact of such an organizing principle is always astonishing, and then it becomes a habit. We accept it as dogs accept automobiles—they were here forever.

"It's interesting that there is a kind of conviction that leads to any major discovery, but the person who has that conviction hardly knows that the result is going to come out so neatly. What he has is the feeling of 'Well, this is the most important thing.' That's all he has.

"I remember reading a book by Simone de Beauvoir that had to do with growing old. She commented in an anecdotal way about scientists and artists, and how artists, as they grow older, seem to be able—if they are really great—to just churn it out. That just isn't true in science, by and large. And there are deep reasons why. First of all, it's not fair to compare a painting with a long, analytical effort that involves a communal enterprise. Second, that effort to try to remove the arbitrary from what you're doing sure does slow you down! You can have a million, beautiful ideas—if only they would be accepted. With the artist—all due credit to his tradition—they are. So maybe it's that, or maybe it's some other deep factor that we don't understand. If you have an impatient nature, as I think I do, it can be pretty hard to hang in there. And once you have hung in there, and understand that there is no other choice, it takes an awful lot of promise to convince you to take another 15 years of your life to do it.

"I wonder, in fact, whether structure work is the only thing where that's true. It may really be true in some sense about all scientific experimental enterprise. There is a kind of logistic sense, a quartermastering sense, that good scientists will have. They'll tell you 'Well, I don't know how to work it, or make it go, but I can tell you it's going to take five years.'"

56. The main topic of this passage is:
- A. the discovery of the structure of the antibody molecule.
- B. the impact of organizing principles on a science.
- C. the demands of scientific research on a scientist.
- D. the relationship of structure to function in science.

57. According to the author, explaining research to the layperson is frustrating because:
- A. much of science depends on intuition.
- B. it is a very long and time-consuming process.
- C. real comprehension comes only by close contact.
- D. interpretation of the results involves complex numbers and mathematics.

58. According to the passage, all of the following might accompany or characterize a major scientific discovery EXCEPT:
- A. sudden insight.
- B. the ability to see new relationships.
- C. conviction of the importance of the work.
- D. accurate initial perception of the outcome.

59. Which of the following is NOT implied or stated in the passage comparing artists and scientists?
- A. Scientists must prove their ideas.
- B. Artists and scientists have different standards for "greatness."
- C. Some artists continue productively in old age.
- D. Artists and scientists have different traditions of "acceptance."

60. The passage indicates that a good scientist needs:
- A. organization.
- B. a good memory.
- C. language abilities.
- D. a quartermastering sense.

61. The writer perceives scientific research to be all of the following EXCEPT:
- A. anecdotal.
- B. abstract.
- C. analytic.
- D. serendipitous.

Passage I

1. **B**   Statements I and II are in paragraph two. The Museum of London is conducting the dig.

2. **D**   Choice B is not mentioned. Choice A is probably true, but is not the major point of significance. Choice C is incorrect because excavation has not proceeded. The answer is in the last paragraph.

3. **D**   Lambarde wrote of how the Rose and the Theatre were similar, findings that are now being refuted. See paragraph three.

4. **A**   Choices A and C are the closest answers, but the author prioritizes their relationship in the last sentence of paragraph four.

5. **D**   Choices A, B, and C are not indicated by the passage. Choice D is most closely stated in paragraph one.

Passage II

6. **D**   The "new sources" refer to officials in Kennedy's administration as they reveal insights on the international climate that provided the background to Kennedy's decision-making process.

7. **B**   If the Jupiter missiles were found to be defective, Kennedy would have had fewer options, which would weaken the author's argument that he had additional alternatives through the use of missiles.

8. **B**   The passage uses phrases such as "look back and reflect" and "in retrospect." When these phrases are combined with a change in the standard interpretation of the crisis, it would indicate that the officials' views have altered with time. Choices A and D are not indicated by the passage, and Choice C is negated by sentence one in paragraph two.

9. **C**   Choice A is not discussed. Choices B and C are negated by the article. Paragraph three indicates that President Kennedy had more "cushion" than had previously been thought.

Passage III

10. **B**   Choice B is stated in paragraph two.

11. **D**   At various points in the story, he exhibited all three behaviors.

12. **A**   Because he indicates that the "lacteal opacity" is "familiar," we can assume from the context that he is referring to the milky color mentioned earlier.

13. **A**   Because he had failed before, and there was no improvement during this course, the probability is great that he will fail again.

14. **D**   At the end of paragraph one, the author states that the professor adjusted the microscope for his own eyes.

15. **B**   The ending is ironic in that he can finally see an image, but the image is an unexpected one.

Passage IV

16. **A**   The passage indicates that Michelangelo and the Pope had a very stormy relationship; the Pope even hit Michelangelo and threatened to throw him from the scaffold. There is no indication that they were colleagues, religiously similar, or that they libeled each other.

17. **B**   A might be true, but it is not the primary reason. Choice C is incorrect because the sculpture was already completed. Choice D uses an incorrect name for the Pope. The passage indicates that Michelangelo grumbled constantly, asking to be released from painting the Sistine Chapel. By signing "sculptor" under his name, Michelangelo exemplified his bickering with the Pope over art, and this was most likely meant to be provoking or annoying.

18. **B**   This question asks for a difference. Choice B is different in that Michelangelo painted onto fresh plaster, which sealed the color.

19. **C**   Choice A is incorrect because he altered his designs as he worked. Choice B is not discussed. Choice D is backward because the passage indicated that he painted onto fresco. In the first paragraph, Michelangelo sketches and adapts as he designs.

Passage V

20. **A**   The molecules must be fast enough to exceed a speed of 11.3 km/s (paragraph two). These include light as well as heavy gas molecules.

21. **A**   The answer is in paragraphs one and three, because the gases bubbled to the surface.

22. **D**   Statements I, II, and III are correct.

23. **C**   Statements II and III are in paragraph three.

24. **A**   Paragraph one indicates the earth's age is five billion years. If there were enough oxygen to sustain life two billion years ago, the ratio would be $5:2$.

Passage VI

25. **B**   Although choice A is a correct idea, it is too broad and lacks the specific focus of the idea that is developed. The information in choice C is too narrow since diversity other than size and habitation is discussed. Choice D is incorrect because the need for a classification system is a result of the main idea, which is expressed in choice B.

26. **A**   Paragraph two states that virtually all major invertebrate groups have marine representatives, so it would be most likely that a newly discovered invertebrate would also have ancestors that could be traced from the sea. All other choices have an implied lower frequency.

27. **D**   DNA is discussed only relative to the definition of a cell, so choice A is incorrect. Although choices B and C may be factors used in classifying animals, the last paragraph states that organization based on number of cells is the most fundamental factor considered.

28. **C**   Paragraph three states that barnacles attach to the substrate, making choice A incorrect. There is no mention of commercial importance to parasites, negating choice B. Choice D is incorrect because no comparison of value between free living and attached invertebrates is provided. Choice C is the correct answer. The last two sentences in paragraph three indicate that invertebrates that improve the soil and those that are parasites in humans and animals are two separate groups, because one is described in a positive and the other in a negative context.

Passage VII

29. **B**   Choice A is incorrect because sentence one in the first paragraph indicates that all five things are important, and it does not indicate the level of importance of each. Choice C is wrong since the muscle attachments are important in maneuverability. Wing shape affects air resistance, making choice D incorrect. Choice B is supported by the discussion of other factors that play a role in a bird's capabilities, as well as by the statement indicating that not all birds do all things.

30. **A**   No specific comparisons are made to airplanes, leaving no support for choice B. The emphasis is on the natural features of the bird, and no mention is made of functioning in a mechanical way, eliminating choice C. Choice A is correct because sentence one provides a list of natural features and involves an implied comparison with machines.

31. **D**   Choice A is correct based on the fact that long, pointed wings and long, narrow tails (streamlining) are important for speed, and that peregrine falcons have been clocked at 175 miles per hour. Sentence five in paragraph two confirms choice B. Choice C is correct since paragraph two makes reference to the fact that some birds have short, rounded wings, which give them quick lift but limited sustaining power. Choice D is the only statement that is not true, because storks are slower, but soaring fliers, and highly developed leg muscles would indicate that the stork is more of a land bird.

32. **D**   This answer requires putting several pieces of information together. The first sentence of the last paragraph contains information about which type of bird has the larger heart. You must go back to the passage to determine which category each bird fits.

33. **A**   Lightness of bone structure is stressed in paragraph three, and birds do not have the bone separating the nasal cavity from the mouth cavity, as do humans. Peregrine falcons cannot be assumed to have hollow bones since paragraph three says "many" and "not all" powerful fliers have hollow bones. Air sacs are associated with buoyancy in the third paragraph, but there is no mention of effect on speed.

34. **D**   This question tests your attention to detail. Choices A, B, and C are directly stated in the passage, making choice D (all of the above) the correct answer.

Passage VIII

35. **D**   Choice A is wrong because feeding the tape from the inside of one reel to the outside of a second reel refers to the first tape cartridge. Choice B is not explicitly stated. Choice C is wrong because these details refer to tape handling systems now. Choice D is the correct answer.

36. **B**   The second sentence in paragraph two supports statement I. Statement II is supported in that the first cartridges eliminated the need for an independent take-up reel but had the problem of sticking tape. While people buy mechanical equipment for home use because of cost, there is no discussion of preference, so statement III is incorrect.

37. **A**   The answer to this question depends on your understanding of the details, which are presented in paragraph five.

38. **C**   The answer involves identifying the structural difference between the two machines. The information in paragraph six indicates that choice C is the correct answer. According to the passage, electromechanical systems are more expensive, but the cost of parts is not broken down, ruling out choice A. Choice B is cited as a benefit but not as the key difference. Choice D is incorrect since solenoids are responsible for the mechanical operations; they do not eliminate them.

39. **D**   Choice A is a correct statement. This involves considering that the most expensive machines provide the best quality and yet people buy mechanical equipment for the home. If the cost were within the average range, one might assume that more people would opt for better quality. Choice B is also correct because the first sentence of paragraph five implies home use is less critical and mechanical operation provides adequate performance. The opposite is true of choice C.

Passage IX

40. **D**   Choices A, B, and C do not mention the central fact of the passage—Paul's illness.

41. **C**   The last sentence in the third paragraph indicates that the counselor's primary concern was Paul's illness.

42. **D**   The second and fourth sentences in the paragraph state that Paul was "watched over," "guarded," and discouraged from undertaking tasks "which might prove stressful."

43. **C**   This choice is a restatement of the reasons given by Paul in the second sentence in paragraph three.

44. **B**   The first sentence in the fourth paragraph indicates Paul's success was due to a "change in his self-image."

45. **A**   No information is given in the passage to support the conclusion of choices B and C. Although cystic fibrosis may require therapy for emotional issues, the disease may not be "emotionally disabling." The passage supports choice A—that cystic fibrosis is an incurable, terminal illness.

Passage X

46. **A**   "Unit rule" is defined under Senator Brown's speech as awarding all of the state's electoral votes to the candidate with the highest popular vote.

47. **D**   The discussion about how the election would be conducted if neither candidate received a 40 percent vote relates to the proposed amendment. The question, however, focuses on the current system, for which no information is provided.

48. **A**   Senator Smith discusses how the electoral system "virtually requires" that minority groups band together into alliances. These groups encompass persons from various geographic areas as well as various ethnic, religious, social, and economic groups.

49. **B**   Senator Brown discusses how votes will count in states where presently the power of minority votes can be diminished in the "winner take all" approach. He does not compare it with the election procedures for state officials.

50. **A**   The senators present quite different views on how the election of a president should be handled. However, they all believe that their own way is the most advantageous.

Passage XI

51. **B**   The answer to this question is in the first sentence of the last paragraph.

52. **C**   Once you have found the right time period in the passage, the key phrase in

the stem is "most influenced." The last sentence in the first paragraph indicates that migration was the primary influencing factor.

53. **B** To answer this question correctly, you need to read the second sentence of the second paragraph all the way through (otherwise, you might choose D) and rephrase the information found therein. If you'd made notes in the margin indicating growth or decline (perhaps in the form of arrows up or down), you would have found this information more quickly.

54. **C** Choice A is incorrect because births would not affect the number of people dying. There is no support for choice D. Choices B and C are both true answers, but the stem asks for the "most important effect," which would be the impact of the numbers in determining trends.

55. **D** If you look carefully at choices A and B, you will see that they deal with specifics—demographic studies, birth rate, and immigration. Choices C and D are more general—population decline versus population growth. Choosing the correct answer is a matter of deciding between two statements expressing opposite ideas.

Passage XII

56. **C** Only choice C can serve as a thesis or summary of the passage as a whole. Choices A, B, and D apply to single paragraphs, but not to the whole (too narrow). Choice A comes from the introductory or background material (too broad).

57. **C** Although all of the choices may be true about scientific research in general, choice C is a paraphrase of the specific conclusions found in the paragraph regarding talking to nonscientists about research.

58. **D** Choice D in this negative-stemmed question is false. The last sentence in paragraph three and the first sentence in paragraph five indicate that, at the outset, scientists have no clear idea of the results of their research.

59. **B** This is another negative-stemmed question. Choice C is directly stated in paragraph six. Choices A and D are implied in that scientists must "remove the arbitrary" from their work. Choice B is neither stated nor implied, since no comparison is made between scientists and artists on the criteria for "greatness."

60. **D** This fairly easy question is answered in the third sentence of the last paragraph.

61. **A** This is yet another negative-stemmed question. All of these words are found in the passage, but "anecdotal" refers to Simone de Beauvoir's book, not to scientific research.

Bibliography

Atkinson RH, Longman DG: *Reading Enhancement and Development*, St Paul, West Publishing, College and School Division, 1992.

Black H, Black S: *Building Thinking Skills*, 4 volumes, Pacific Grove, California, Midwest Publications, 1984.

Cohen R, et al.: *QUEST: Academic Skills Program*, San Diego, Harcourt Brace Jovanovich, 1973.

Dramer D: *Literary Tales: Inside Stories to Literature for Critical Reading and Thinking*, Providence, Jamestown Publications, 1980.

Flemming LE: *Reading for Results*, Boston, Houghton Mifflin, 1987.

Fry EB: *Reading Faster: A Drill Book*, 10th printing, Cambridge, England, Cambridge University Press, 1983.

Heilman, AW: *Improve Your Reading Ability*, 4th ed., Columbus, Merrill Publishing, 1983.

Hurley P: *A Concise Introduction to Logic*, 4th ed. Belmont, California, Wadsworth Publishing, 1991.

Miller PA: *Managing Your Reading*, Littleton, Colorado, Reading Development Resources, 1987.

Quinn S, Irvings S: *Active Reading in the Arts and Sciences*, Boston, Allyn and Bacon, 1991.

4 Writing Sample

The Importance of Writing Skills

The presence of a writing module in the MCAT is a clear message on the importance of communication in medicine and the need for effective writing. It is a strong reminder that a health professional must not only acquire information but also must consider it critically and then communicate it to patients, medical team members, and professional colleagues. Science majors who have not written much during college may find this a disturbing prospect. However, with practice and with an understanding of some guiding principles, you can learn to write clearly and logically. This chapter can help you improve your writing in general, as well as prepare you for the Writing Sample portion of the MCAT.

What the MCAT Writing Sample Covers

To assess your ability to develop and express ideas in a logical and organized manner, you are asked to write two essays for the MCAT. This portion of the MCAT lasts 60 minutes, with 30 minutes allowed to complete each essay.

The essay topics are statements derived from general interest fields, including history, literature, ethics, business, politics, or art. For each essay, you are given a three-part task. The first task asks you to provide an explanation of what you think the statement means. The second task asks you to demonstrate your understanding of the essay statement by describing an example or a situation that may negate the statement. And finally, the third task requires you to demonstrate your understanding by discussing the topic's broader aspects, which may resolve the conflict between the original statement and the contradictory example that you provided.

The information available from the Association of American Medical Colleges (AAMC) states that you are not expected to have prior specific knowledge on the essay topic. Furthermore, the MCAT essay does not include:

- A demonstration of technical or scientific knowledge
- Topics based on religious issues
- A duplication of the American Medical College Application Service (AMCAS) essay that you submit with your medical school application
- Questions designed to prove your character, morality, or personality
- Topics based on ''social and cultural issues that are not part of most college students' general experience''

According to the AAMC information, you will be evaluated for your skills in:

- Developing a central idea
- Synthesizing concepts and ideas
- Presenting ideas clearly, cohesively, and logically
- Observing the accepted practices of grammar, syntax, punctuation, and spelling (recognizing, of course, that your essay is a timed, first-draft composition)

Sample Essay for Skills Assessment

How well will you do on the Writing Sample Section of the MCAT? The following writing exercise is similar to those on the MCAT. Read the quotation and respond to the directions. Simulate the real test situation by following these five guidelines:

1. Limit yourself to 30 minutes for the planning and writing of your essay.
2. Spend at least 10 minutes of the allotted time considering the essay statement and organizing your ideas.

3. Allow at least 5 minutes at the end of the period to proofread and make corrections. Check the spelling, punctuation, and grammar. You can add a sentence or change a word where necessary.

4. Note that there are three parts to the essay directions: First, you are asked to demonstrate your specific understanding of the given statement. Second, you are asked to move from this specific understanding to an application of the concept. Third, you are asked to discuss the topic in a broader context. (Remember, the Writing Sample is a pen-and-paper exam. Therefore, practice writing your essay on paper, not on a computer with word-processing software.)

5. Write your essay in three parts. Write (1) an introduction (one paragraph), (2) the body (two to four paragraphs), and (3) a conclusion (one paragraph). On the MCAT, the content of each of these parts is evaluated for the depth, clarity, and precision of your argument.

SAMPLE ESSAY TOPIC

Consider the following statement:

"Often the test of courage is not to die but to live." (Alfieri)

Write a unified essay in which you perform the following three tasks:

- Explain what you think the statement means.
- Describe a specific situation in which dying rather than living is a test of courage.
- Discuss what you think determines the qualities of a courageous human.

Now that you have written your essay, evaluate your work using the Writing Sample Analysis Form (Table 4-1). Ask a study partner or an English composition instructor to evaluate your work and discuss it with you. Compare your evaluation with their evaluation to see what improvements may be needed.

Conclude by reviewing the sample essays at the end of this chapter. These sample essays are responses to this essay topic from several students who wrote under MCAT testing conditions. Note the differences in the quality of organization and thought among their responses, and see how your essay stands against their essays.

WRITING SAMPLE ANALYSIS FORM

Evaluate your essay using this form. Variable points are provided for all elements except those covered in the organization section so that you can judge your performance within the range provided. For the organization section, record the total points only if you can identify the item in your essay. Total the points for all the questions and use the score to compare your performance on this essay with other essays you will write as part of your writing preparation. You may want to make copies of this sheet.

APPLYING VERBAL REASONING SKILLS TO YOUR WRITING ANALYSIS

In addition to the specific criteria in Table 4-1, you can also use elements discussed in Chapter 3, Developing Verbal Reasoning Abilities, to analyze your writing performance. You can practice verbal reasoning skills and sharpen your writing skills. Remember that analysis considers structural elements of writing, such as a main idea, supporting evidence, and a summary. You also need to determine whether your premises led to the appropriate conclusions, and you may want to re-evaluate your essay to see whether your argument included any of the following fallacies (see Chapter 3):

Appeal to authority	Equivocation
Appeal to tradition	Hasty generalization
Argument from analogy	Non sequitur
Begging the question	Semantic ambiguity
Either-or	Slippery slope

Developing Your Writing Skills

Like an athlete, you must be in shape before you can exercise your writing skills and perform them well. The following strategies should be part of your long-term plan for developing writing fluency. As you work through the rest of this chapter, pay particular attention to your weak areas on Table 4-1.

GETTING STARTED

Picking up a pen and staring at a blank sheet of paper is enough to give anyone writer's block, regardless of how much one knows about a topic. If this is true for you, then you may need to pressure yourself into writing. If you are intimidated by a blank sheet of paper, there are ways to break your writer's block and begin to develop writing fluency.

For starters, prepare a list of topics so that you will be less likely to put off writing

TABLE 4-1. Writing Sample Analysis Form

Elements of Writing	Points	Essay			
		#1	#2	#3	#4
Preparation Before writing, did you outline the topic either formally by jotting notes or by establishing the purpose?	1 to 5				
Organization Underline the main idea statement and label it MI in the margin.	0 or 5				
Underline the statements of detail that support the main idea and label them by number in margin.	0 or 5				
Underline the topic sentence in the concluding paragraph and label it SS (summary statement).	0 or 5				
Content Judge the effectiveness of the main idea statement. Does it comprehensively cover the supporting details?	1 to 5				
Do the details follow in a logical sequence? Do they have a direct relationship to the main idea?	1 to 5				
Are there statements of transition between the paragraphs?	1 to 5				
Is the evidence persuasive? Is there use of examples, authorities, comparison and contrast, or cause and effect?	1 to 5				
Is there a balance in presenting both sides of the issue before a stance is taken?	1 to 5				
Is there clear differentiation between opinions and statements of fact?	1 to 5				
Is the summary statement directly related to the details presented?	1 to 5				
Does the conclusion go beyond the superficial to show some insight into the topic?	1 to 10				
Vocabulary Is the range of word choice good?	1 to 5				
Mechanics Is the sample free of grammatical errors?	1 to 20				
Spelling Is spelling correct?	1 to 10				
Total	100				

practice for lack of something to write about. To write, you must have something to say. Prepare yourself by reading newspapers, editorials (e.g., the *USA Today* Debate section), and magazines such as *Time* or *Newsweek*. Look for short quotations, philosophical sayings, and proverbs. Read about current issues to find suitable writing topics. Attend seminars and meetings in social sciences to become more aware of current issues.

Writing Topics

Writing is easier if you feel strongly about the subject matter, so you might begin by gathering topics that make you feel uncomfortable. Writing about an intimidating subject makes the subject more approachable, because you probably have an opinion about it. Make a list of topics that fit into this category and use the list to get started.

Although you may not have time to write a reactive essay, spend some time formulating an opinion and synthesizing your thoughts about these topics. Find the time to enrich your perspective by thinking about philosophical and social issues.

WRITING FLUENCY 10-Minute Exercises

After you decide on a topic, write about the topic for no more than 10 minutes. Be sure to time yourself. Even if you become involved in what you are writing, stop at the 10-minute time limit. Your goal in this exercise is to initiate and sustain the active process of writing on a topic for a 10-minute period without stopping. Next time, you can pick up writing where you stopped if the topic still seems compelling. Although you should write in complete sentences, do not worry now about syntax, grammar, spelling, or organization. Instead, work to keep your ideas flowing and your hand moving steadily across the page. Do not spend time pondering word choices: substitute and move on.

This simple 10-minute writing exercise should be done each day. Do not postpone this exercise until a day when you can write for 50 minutes, because this will not accomplish your goal. If you regularly jog 1 mile each day, you would not postpone all of your jogging until Friday to run 5 miles at a stretch. The same is true for this writing exercise.

Your writing skills can always be improved. Even if you can easily write 2 pages in 10 minutes, continue working to improve your writing fluency. Keep in mind that your finished product should not be a list of what you did on a given day, but rather ideas relating to a single event, topic, or issue. Keep pushing yourself to write a little more during each 10-minute period. After 1 week or so, you should see an improvement in your writing fluency and an increase in the amount you can write in 10 minutes.

Writing about your course work provides an additional 10-minute exercise for improving your writing skills daily. Anytime after class (but on the same day), write for 10 minutes about everything you remember from class without looking at your notes. Your studies will benefit from this approach as well, because it will provide timely review and an opportunity to break down the information into its component parts (analyze) and then put them back together again in your own words (synthesize). Unless you can explain something you have learned in your own words, you have not really learned it. Timely review will reinforce learning and increase long-term retention.

WRITING FOR THE MCAT

Remember, each essay should have three parts: an introduction, a body, and a conclusion. The content of each of these three parts will be evaluated for the depth, clarity, and precision of your argument.

The introduction. Do not use factual examples in the introduction. Instead, write your own explanation or interpretation of the given statement. Think of the introduction as an explanation of your understanding of the given statement, a restatement of the main idea with a paraphrase of the given statement, or a declaration of what the given statement means to you.

The body. Use new information for the body of the essay and state whether you agree or disagree with the given statement. Think of the body as providing a concrete example of how you evaluate the contradictions in the given statement and describing a specific situation (real or hypothetical) that illustrates the contradiction in the statement.

The conclusion. Your conclusion should address the conflict in the given statement. Think of concluding your essay in these terms:

- Explain what you think are the determining factors that support either the given statement or the contradiction of the given statement
- Conclude by resolving the conflict inherent in the given statement

WRITING FOR QUALITY

After you have achieved writing fluency, you are ready to address writing for quality. Many people think first about writing "correctly" (i.e., mechanical considerations). However, writing effectively is a more complex task and should be tackled before grammar and punctuation. Writing effectively involves organizing one's thoughts into a clear, cohesive, and logical written form, making these thoughts intelligible to the reader. There are many books available to help students develop effective writing skills. Many of these books are helpful, especially if you are interested in developing more than just basic writing skills. These books offer a systematic approach that builds on a sequence of steps, ranging from brainstorming to writing drafts, revising, and ultimately polishing the finished product.

Writing for the MCAT, however, requires special consideration because you are confined to a limited time period. For each essay you have only 30 minutes to analyze the task, formulate and organize your ideas, and get them down on paper. Because you do not have the time to develop, revise, and refine multiple drafts, it is crucial to achieve a systematic approach for writing your essay in fewer steps. The following suggestions and guidelines will help you achieve this approach.

THE FOUR WRITING STAGES

Creating an MCAT essay consists of four stages: **analysis**, **organization**, **writing**, and **editing**. Once again, practice is required to improve quality.

Analysis	### Rule 1: Understand the Essay Topic

Rule 1: Understand the Essay Topic

Analyze the topic statement carefully to make sure you understand it. Do not rush through the analytical stage—it can result in misdirected efforts based on an initial misunderstanding of the statement.

Rule 2: Interpret the Topic as Serious, not Frivolous

MCAT topics tend to ask questions with broad philosophical implications, meaning that the topics presented are of a serious nature. The comparisons you make and the examples you provide should therefore be serious as well.

Organization

Rule 3: Organize Your Time

Take time to think and organize. Do not be put off by the test-takers around you who start to write furiously the minute after the essay portion of the MCAT begins. In general, thinking and note-taking should take up to 50% of the time allotted for each essay portion, or about 10–15 minutes. Then, you have another 10–15 minutes for actual writing and about 5 minutes to edit and proofread.

Rule 4: Organize Your Ideas

Write ideas down in the margin or on the back of your paper, and do not start writing your essay until you have thought through the essay topic, formulated your thesis, and decided on the supporting information and the organizational structure you are going to use. Group together related ideas and organize them according to the essay's introduction, body, and conclusion. You might construct a key word outline. If you limit your notes to single words or even abbreviations, this process should take only a few minutes. Time invested at this stage will make your actual writing go faster. As you group ideas, eliminate any that seem irrelevant to the development of the topic.

Writing

Rule 5: Respond Directly to the Quotation

Expand your outline into fully developed ideas that relate directly to the quotation. As you elaborate on your ideas, be sure that you are developing and clarifying the main idea and not digressing. Maintain focus by eliminating anything that is irrelevant to the main idea. It is tempting to try to demonstrate everything you know about a topic, but your goal is not to showcase your range of information but to develop those specific aspects of the topic that are requested.

Rule 6: Understand Essay Format

As shown in Figure 4-1, standard essay format consists of an opening paragraph, two or more supporting paragraphs, and a concluding paragraph. Writing in standard format makes your task easier because it frees your energy for thinking through the problem and expressing your thoughts in a coherent manner. It also makes evaluation easier for the essay grader, who has certain expectations.

Rule 7: Focus Your Essay in the Introduction

Begin your essay by restating the main idea of the quote. It will orient the reader and serve as a reminder of the main elements that you need to develop. Also, it gives you an immediate beginning and provides an early feeling of control. Your restatement of the quote should lead to a thesis statement (i.e., the controlling idea). The thesis statement is one of the most important sentences of your essay. A carefully written thesis statement facilitates the writing of the rest of the essay, because it provides the guideline for what you should include in the body of the essay. The thesis statement should be broad enough to cover the theme of the essay but focused enough to delineate the aspect of the topic you will cover or the position you will take.

Rule 8: Use Your Thesis Statement to Guide the Development of the Body of the Essay

With supporting paragraphs using new information, the body of the essay expands on the thesis statement. The body of the essay:

- Provides a concrete example of a specific situation (real or hypothetical) that illustrates a contradiction to the statement
- Describes how you evaluate the contradiction (i.e., where you come down on it and why)

The number of paragraphs in the body of the essay is determined by the number of main ideas needed to fully develop your thesis statement. Each paragraph should develop

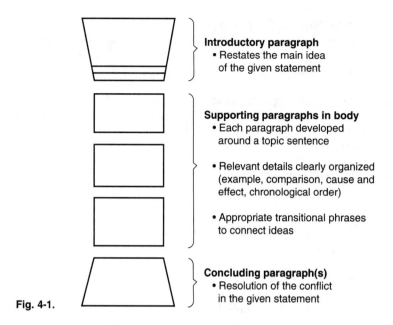

Introductory paragraph
• Restates the main idea of the given statement

Supporting paragraphs in body
• Each paragraph developed around a topic sentence

• Relevant details clearly organized (example, comparison, cause and effect, chronological order)

• Appropriate transitional phrases to connect ideas

Concluding paragraph(s)
• Resolution of the conflict in the given statement

Fig. 4-1.

only one point; therefore, each paragraph should have a main idea statement that tells the reader what the paragraph is about.

Rule 9: Show the Relationships Among Details in the Paragraphs

After you have determined what information to include in a paragraph, present it in an organized form. In Chapter 3, organizational patterns are discussed in terms of the role they play in validating reading comprehension. In writing an essay, your job shifts from *identifying* organizational structure to *constructing* it and providing appropriate examples.

Rule 10: Present Information in a Logical Progression

Information may progress logically in either an ascending or descending order of importance. The order that you choose depends on the kind of effect you want to make. If you want the reader's immediate attention, then begin with your most important point. The less important points that follow are used to add additional confirmation. If you would rather build gradually to a climax to lock in the reader's attention toward the end, save the most important point for last.

Rule 11: Include Good Writing Techniques

Besides presenting information logically, a well-written essay contains the following:

- **Smooth transitions.** To move the reader smoothly from one idea to the next, your essay should have unity. Without transitional words or phrases, some of the meaning is lost. Your reader understands each sentence or paragraph individually, but not the way the ideas are connected. Use transitional words and phrases, such as *moreover, then, however, accordingly, besides, therefore, nevertheless, on the other hand,* and *on the contrary.* Also, use transitional statements: "Although the author's comments resulted from a very specific situation, one can see broader implications and after considering the essence of what this statement means, it is important to examine the potential outcomes that arise from this philosophy."
- **Careful and precise word choice.** *Junction* is a better word than *gap* if you are defining *synapse.*
- **A mix of sentences that vary in length and complexity.** A short, simple sentence at the end of a paragraph provides a powerful, effective finish.
- **Use of active rather than passive voice.** Read old essays and underline every passive form of the verb *to be.* Revise the essays by exchanging what you underlined with an active verb (e.g., "In 1909 the Futurist manifesto was written by the poet Marinetti" becomes "In 1909 the poet Marinetti wrote the Futurist manifesto").

Rule 12: Provide the Reader with a Summary

Your essay should end with a summary paragraph. This paragraph should not include any new information. Instead, the summary should restate the thesis sentence and provide a resolution of the conflict between the original statement and its contradiction.

Editing and Proofreading

Rule 13: Assess the Content of your Essay

After you have completed your essay, reread it to evaluate content. Have you addressed all parts of the question? Is there a well-formulated thesis statement? Does your concluding paragraph relate back to your thesis? Have you changed your mind in the course of writing? If so, it is quicker to modify your thesis than it is to rewrite the body of the paper.

What about the body of the paper? Are your ideas broad enough? Do you support them with adequate, specific details or examples? Are logical connectors provided or clearly implied?

Rule 14: Correct Mechanical Errors

The MCAT evaluators expect you to proofread and correct your essay for mechanical errors (i.e., grammar, spelling, and word choice) after you have finished writing. They do not give you enough time to recopy your essay, and they do not expect you to do so. However, they do expect you to correct mechanical errors. Mark your corrections as neatly and legibly as possible so that the reader can follow your changes; if possible, use an erasable pen.

As you proofread, look for errors that you commonly make. Repeated errors are a sign of careless preparation. (In your practice essays, direct extra effort toward improving these areas.) Proofread for the following:

- **Sentence fragments.** Check for sentences beginning with *and, or,* and *but.*
- **Run-on sentences.** Correct these sentences by changing a comma to a semicolon; or, make two sentences by changing the comma to a period, crossing out any connecting word, and capitalizing the first letter of the new second sentence.
- **Subject-verb agreement.** Watch especially for the third person singular.
- **Verb tense errors.** Avoid beginning a sentence in one tense and shifting to another.
- **Spelling errors.** People tend to repeat spelling errors (e.g., *mathmatics* versus *mathematics, recieve* versus *receive, comparible* versus *comparable, seperate* versus *separate*).
- **Homophones.** These words sound alike but have different spelling and meaning (e.g., *there* versus *their* or *they're, to* versus *too* or *two, here* versus *hear*).
- **Common punctuation errors.** Watch for *its* versus *it's,* and inappropriate use of commas.

Writing for the MCAT—Practice Essays

Practice your writing skills by developing an essay for each of the following essay topics, which typify the ones you will encounter on the MCAT. As you practice, simulate the real MCAT situation by following the guidelines for test simulation (see Sample Essay for Skills Assessment). After you have finished an essay, evaluate it using Table 4-1.

ESSAY TOPICS
Topic 1

"Education is the cheap defense of nations."
(Edmund Burke)

Write a cohesive essay in which you do the following: Explain what you think the statement means. Describe a situation in which education might not prevent more expensive solutions. Discuss whether education is always the solution to problems of national importance.

Topic 2

"Every calling is great when greatly pursued."
(Oliver Wendell Holmes)

Write a cohesive essay in which you do the following: Explain what you think the statement means. Describe a situation in which a calling was greatly pursued but did not result in greatness. Discuss those elements which you think comprise a great calling.

Topic 3

"What we need is not more government in middle America but more middle America in government."
(George Bush)

Write a cohesive essay in which you do the following: Explain what you think the statement means. Describe a situation in which having more middle American involvement would not improve the functioning of government. Discuss what you think is the ideal working relationship between citizens and government.

Topic 4

"Many readers judge the power of a book by the shock it gives their feelings."
(Henry Wadsworth Longfellow)

Write a cohesive essay in which you address the following: Explain what you think the statement means. Describe a book that might have a strong impact on one's feelings but might not be considered a powerful book. Discuss whether impact on one's feelings is the key indicator of a powerful book.

Topic 5

"Fine art is that in which the hand, the head, and the heart of man go together."
(John Rankin)

Write a cohesive essay in which you address the following: Explain what you think the statement means. Describe a piece of art or an art form that you did not feel reflected the unity of hand, head, and heart. Discuss the components that you think are important in defining fine art.

Topic 6

"[In business,] the chairperson of the team should be someone with an easy conversational access to the very top management."
(Philip B. Crosby)

Write a cohesive essay in which you address the following: Explain what you think the statement means. Describe a situation in which a person with easy conversational access to the top management should not be the team leader. Discuss criteria for selecting an effective team leader.

Topic 7

"What is essential is invisible to the eye."
(Antoine de Saint-Exupery)

Write a cohesive essay in which you do the following: Explain what you think the statement means. Describe a situation in which something essential is visible to the eye. Discuss whether essential things are perceived to be invisible or really are invisible.

Essay Topic with Sample Student Essays

'Often the test of courage is not to die but to live."
(Alfieri)

ESSAY TOPIC

Write a unified essay in which you perform the following tasks: Explain what you think the above statement means. Describe a specific situation in which dying rather than living is a test of courage. Discuss what you think determines the qualities of a courageous human.

Sample Key Word Outline For Essay Topic

○	I.	What does it mean:
		one test of courage is not to die but to live
		–Test-indicator
		–Courage-strength
		–Fighting an illness; accident
○	II.	Dying Rather than Living: Test of Courage
		Young men willing to die for abolishment of slavery
	III.	Courageous Human
		–Someone who is strong, fearless, undaunted
○		–will stand if he must stand alone
		–will not cower in the face of iniquity
		–will not yield to temptation
		–inner strength

Sample Sentence Outline For Essay Topic

(This sample is from an actual student's essay notes. The errors intentionally have not been corrected.)

○	Being courageous is associated with the will to live rather than accepting defeat and accept death. A test of courage means that a person wants to fight for their life it means that they realize how precious their time on this earth really is. There are some instances in which a person is courageous by giving up his right to live and accepts death. An example would be the soilders lost during the Vietnam War. These soilders that put themselves in a situation where saving a
○	country from dictatorship was more important then their own life. Soilders are taught to think this way in an effort to benefit another.
	Qualities of a courageous human
	—Accepts what lies ahead and gives his best shot to succeed.
○	—A door to door salesperson takes each new customer as a challenge.
	—Takes one day at a time and cherishes every men of that day.
	—A person with a terminal illness learns the value of life and cherishes. What others might
	consider small and
○	—Letting guards down
	—Emotionally speaking a courageous person is one who will allow themselves to be vulnerable
	espically in a relationship were feeling are concerned.
	—Accepting Defeat as a last resort

Sample Essay 1

(Sample Essays 1, 2, 3, and 4 are actual student essays. These essays contain many errors made by the students. These errors intentionally have not been corrected.)

○	Being courageous is antiquated with the will to live rather then to accept death. A test of courage to live means that a person wants to fight for his life and realizes how precious time is on this earth and how there is so much to live for. All of life's challenges are right at a person's fingertips as long as they are courageous enough to live.
○	There are some instances in which a person is courageous by giving up the right to live and will accept death as his duty to mankind. For example, the brave soldiers that fought in the Vietnam War. Those soldiers fought so that they could defeat communistic views and set a country free from communisim. These soldiers were very brave to place their lives in jeopardy for the sake of principles, that they believed to be right.
○	Qualities of a courageous person are often found in people who have gotten over the hurdles of lifes experiences such as what life holds ahead and determination to see any obstacle through. For instance the salesman that takes each new customer as a new challenge. Or the individual that takes life one day at a time and cherishes every minute. A person with a terminal illness
○	would display this sort of courage. An individual who drops his guard and reveals his emotions might also be described as having courage. A final component of courage is knowing when to

accept defeat and realizing that there will be times like this but that life is full of unexpectancies and as a human learning to deal with defeat is also a brave ordeal.

In conclusion, it is more courageous to deal with the challenges of life then to accept death so willingly.

Sample Essay 2

Often the test of courage is not to die but to live.

A test is a tool which challenge's a persons level of knowledge about a particular subject, skill or a reaction to a situation. Courage is having the ability to take on a task that entails doing something one normally would not do and the task also has a level of risk. When one states, "often the test of courage is not to die but to live, he means that being courageous does not mean to be a show off

Perform tasks that are done without thought and do not unnecessarily place oneself in a situation to die because that's not courageous; that's foolish.

An example of a situation in which dying rather than living is a test of courage is when a seven year old female is about to do die in a week and decides to donate her lungs to an eight year old female is in need of a lung transplant. The aspect which is courageous is that the donor will give up her lungs before her week to die is up. This is extraordinary because although she knows she is going die her time is up. She has decided to leave a place filled with her loved ones, go to a place (Heaven) which she knows nothing about and most importantly, she's giving up her life. Most people try to hold onto life as long as they can because they feel safe and it's familiar therefore, many of them would not have donated their lungs although, they were going to die anyway. This is definitely an example of when dying rather than living is courageous because it will allow someone else to lend a normal & healthy life.

The qualities that exemplify a courageous human being are having the ability to take a stand when others may not agree, be willing to sacrifice for others, take risks that will enhance the other person but not pull the courageous person down and one who desires to help other's by any means but can also recognize when things are out of his control.

Therefore, the test of courage is not to die but to live implies that it's okay to be courageous but don't jump into unnecessary situations or situations that are beyond ones control because that is not courageous; it's foolish.

Sample Essay 3

Alfieri's statement "often the test of courage is not to die but to live" presents the vehicle in which the courage of people, real or fictional can be describe and, to some degree, qualitatively examined. One must also look at examples to the contrary and the factors defining courageousness.

The statement means the true courage is not only to battle against your antagonists, struggling through difficulty, one should survive in the process. People find it easier, at times, to just give up the battle and thus dying. This easy way out does not constitute true courage despite the battle waged before surrender. Alfieri says that to fight and survive defines courage. Suicide and surrender do not find a place in courage; only the continued fight against all enemies constitutes courage.

Alfieri's quotation does leave room, however, for courge through death by qualifying it with "often." Indeed there exist in life and literature examples of dying with courageousness. I feel that one such example can be found in Victorian literature. One novel, A Tale of Two Cities, tells us of courage in death. The courageous man has loved a woman from afar for many years; she refuses his love. He remains in love after her marriage to another man. Her new husband receives the sentence of death by a tribunal of the French revolution, but his life is spared when the courageous man decides to demonstrate his love by dying in the place of his love's husband. The courage and bravery exhibited in his death outweighs any that he could have achieved by living.

Several factors determine courageousness in our society. Among the many factors exist the quality of the challenge, the resolve to fight, and the hope maintained throughout. For courage to manifest itself, a challenge of significant proportion must be faced. Battling and defeating many without real threat to yourself, without risk, may be glamorous but not courageous. Courage can be seen when someone fails to succumb to the challenge of the overwhelming. The courage maintains itself when the resolve to continue to fight does not receive significant damage. The desire to battle further must be present to avoid falling into submission. Finally hope should burn within the courageous. Hope bolsters the resolve to continue; without it, people teeter on the edge of submission.

To fight and live remains the test of courage.

Sample Essay 4

War is a devistating time that effects the entire being. Those who have participated, can tell stories which express the most expliceal, catastrophic scenes possible to man. When self esteem, moral and self identity is low, self confidence and courage is most important. During this time, living means the most to solders. If one was to engage in a particular battle, and return alive, intact and sane, he or she would be glorified for their courage and self commitment. Alfieri's statement would now hold true. The test of courage, during war time, is measured by one's ability to survive, and returns alive and well. This experience confirms that he or she was sucessful, determined and extremely committed.

Though a persons performance during war can be based on his courage of survival, ones will to die can be compared as courage in certain situations. For instance, an individual who has been diagnosed for terminal cancer or one who is on a life support system after a devistating accident. There entire exsistance has been placed at a holt. In these cases, if that individual or his/her family can comes to terms with dying, then that is a courageous choice. When one can be frank with reality and say to one self that "My life is comming to a close and I am brave enough to contend with it" then it is just to say that this person can be placed in the same category as the surviving war hero.

Never the less, courage is a personal discription that can be use to define an array of situations. Though time, one can be inudued in several situations, each with their own unique flavor and quality, and still that person can be called courageous. Courage is when a man can sincerely utilize his mind to come to a honest conclusion. He must use his confidence within self, and weigh and judge the senerio well. If he is successful in his endevers, then he can be classified as being courageous.

Scoring the MCAT Essay

On the MCAT, each of your essays is evaluated by two readers. The evaluators are trained in writing and score your essay using a holistic approach—that is, your essay is evaluated as a total unit rather than scored according to separate components of essay writing. Each evaluator scores your essay on a scale from 1 (lowest) to 6 (highest). If the two readers assign scores that differ by more than one point, a third reader evaluates the essay and assigns a final score. Then the scores from both essays are combined and averaged, and the numerical score is converted to an alphabetic score, ranging from J (lowest) to T (highest).

The following scoring-level descriptions are adapted from the *MCAT Student Manual*, published by the AAMC, which provides six sample essays and discusses their competency levels.

6 Addresses all three tasks; presents a complete exploration of the topic; demonstrates depth and complexity of thought; shows coherent organization; expresses ideas with superior clarity and precision.

5 Addresses all three tasks; presents substantial treatment of the topic, shows adequate organization but not at a 6 level; demonstrates some depth of thought; expresses ideas with clarity and precision.

4 Addresses all three tasks; presents only moderate treatment of the topic; demonstrates clarity of thought but may have some lack of complexity; has coherent organization with possible digressions; expresses most ideas with clarity and precision.

3 Lacks or distorts one or more of the writing tasks; shows some clarity of thought but with possible simplistic treatment; demonstrates problems in organization; has fluency but language may not communicate ideas effectively.

2 Shows serious neglect or distortion of one or more of the tasks; demonstrates problems with organization and analysis; may have recurrent mechanical problems making the essay difficult to read.

1 Fails to address the tasks entirely or demonstrates marked difficulty with mechanics and organization.

Before the MCAT

The main focus of the Writing Sample section of the MCAT is to construct a first-draft essay that completes all three tasks. While practicing writing essays, examine the tasks that you do not address well. Try to divide the 30-minute essay time into three 10-minute segments. Look at sample essays from several books and the MCAT practice tests published by the AAMC so you can determine the position and length of each of the three writing tasks.

Write at least five essays, and note how much time it takes you to start the essay and complete each of the three writing tasks. Be sure to time each task. Evaluate and analyze the quality of each task and if you completed it.

On the Day of the MCAT

On the day of the test, bring at least three newspaper editorials with you from *USA Today* or the *New York Times*. Or, bring a news magazine with you. During your lunch break, put yourself in the shoes of a writer or editor to see if the editorials are complete and how the three writing tasks are completed. During the Writing Sample section of the MCAT, jot down phrases and questions as you mentally prepare to write your essays. Use the back of your page to do preliminary work before you begin writing the essay.

Bibliography

Alvarez JA: *Elements of Composition.* San Diego, Harcourt, Brace & Co., 1985.

Fishman J: *Responding to Prose: A Reader for Writers.* New York, Macmillan, 1982.

Gallo JD, Rink HW: *Shaping College Writing: Paragraph and Essay.* San Diego, Harcourt, Brace & Co., 1979.

Kesselman-Turkel J, Peterson F: *Getting It Down: How to Put Your Ideas on Paper.* Chicago, Contemporary Books.

5

Test-Taking Skills for the MCAT

Test-Taking Skills for Verbal Reasoning and the Science Subtests

This chapter presents techniques for solving passage-based problems as you prepare for the MCAT. Review these test-taking strategies at an early stage of your MCAT preparation to become familiar with the MCAT passage-based test items. An Error Analysis Chart is also included in this chapter to help you identify weaknesses in your test-taking skills and to suggest ways to address them constructively.

Both test-taking and study strategies are covered here, including using principles of logic in passages and test items; remembering definitions of scientific terms and concepts; learning how to work with multiple-choice test items; using error analysis; working at a certain speed without sacrificing accuracy; learning how to cope with stress and anxiety; learning how to eliminate wrong answers and guessing; and remembering things to do before, during, and after the MCAT.

QUESTION FORMAT

There are two question formats used on the MCAT: multiple-choice questions and multiple-multiple-choice questions. The following shows you the two formats:

Multiple-Choice Questions

1. A question appears here.

    A. Response 1
    B. Response 2
    C. Response 3
    D. Response 4

Multiple-Multiple-Choice Questions

    I. Premise 1
    II. Premise 2
    III. Premise 3
1. A premise is placed here to be compared with statements I, II, and/or III above.

    A. Response 1
    B. Response 2
    C. Response 3
    D. Response 4

Strategy 1: Visualize Yourself in the Examination

You want to be comfortable and relaxed when you take the MCAT. The best preparation plan may fall flat if you become anxious, because it will reduce your ability to think logically. Anxiety is often the by-product of worrying about the unknown. By conditioning yourself to the idea of successfully taking the examination, you will better control your anxiety.

You have many reasons to feel positive: you have taken all the prerequisite courses; you have done a systematic review of relevant content areas; and you have worked to develop the test-taking skills that will allow you to be in control. *You are ready.* The typical classroom setting in which you will take the test is familiar to you and should give you some reassurance. Picture yourself receiving your test booklet and opening it—another very familiar experience.

Finally, visualize yourself actually taking the test. You have had a lot of practice taking tests in your courses, and your MCAT preparation has involved working with many test questions. What do you think the MCAT questions will be like? Compare your perceptions with the models and exercises included in this manual. As you visualize yourself taking the test, do not dwell on how difficult the questions might be. Rather, try to keep your thinking in perspective by reminding yourself that there will be a range of difficulty as on any other test. Some questions will be easier, some more challenging but manageable, and only a small percentage will be truly difficult.

Most worries are about the test itself. However, as you try to visualize yourself in the exam, are there any other concerns that come to mind? Do you find yourself worrying about the temperature of the room or getting hungry? If you identify something specific, you can plan ahead to eliminate the problem.

Walk through this scenario frequently until you feel comfortable thinking about the test.

Strategy 2: Understanding Logical Connectors and Logical Reasoning

A central component to good test-taking is the ability to understand and use logic and to recognize logical connectors immediately. We use logical reasoning to understand what we read and to organize our thoughts when we write. In national standardized tests in particular, form and syntax are governed by the rules and language of logic. Logical reasoning governs our understanding of test questions in terms of what is being asked and how to choose an answer.

USING DEDUCTIVE AND INDUCTIVE REASONING

Learn to recognize whether a question requires deductive or inductive reasoning. This will help to clarify the question and assist you in working through the problem. As you read the descriptions below, pay attention to the processing differences involved in the two types of reasoning (see Chapter 3).

Deductive Reasoning

Questions that require a recognition of deductive reasoning involve statements that lead to a particular conclusion. If the reasons are accurate or confirmed by facts, the conclusion must follow. For example, if you were to evaluate the statement "Bacteria contain protoplasm," you would note that (1) protoplasm is found in the cells of all living organisms, (2) bacteria are living organisms, and, therefore, (3) bacteria contain protoplasm.

Your job during the test is to evaluate the accuracy of the supporting evidence for a particular statement. If you can say that the supporting evidence is true, you can accept the conclusion. The bacteria example is a syllogism—a deductive scheme of a formal argument. In this form, it is easy to evaluate. However, in a test, the information is rarely, if ever, given to you in this format. The more common test question format is, for example:

Which of the following statements is false?

A. Bacteria do not contain protoplasm.
B. Bacteria consist of prokaryotic cells.
C. Bacteria cannot be seen with the naked eye.
D. Bacteria do not have circulatory systems.

In this format, it is less clear how deductive logic can help you on the test. However, to evaluate these answer choices, you must reconstruct the supporting evidence in your mind. To determine whether choice A is correct, you would recall that protoplasm is found in the cells of all living organisms and, from what you know about bacteria in general, you know that they are living organisms. Hence, bacteria contain protoplasm. Therefore, the correct answer choice is A. Now you construct the syllogism for choices B, C, and D.

Inductive Reasoning

In inductive reasoning, your task is to evaluate the level of probability under which the conclusion does follow. In written text, you can tell by the syntax whether a sentence is a conclusion suggested or a conclusion confirmed. That is, if the sentence is a conclusion suggested, it will contain the conditional verbs such as *may, seem, can,* and so on, or adverbs such as *probably, primarily, most likely,* and *most nearly.* In logic, these conditional verbs and adverbs signify that you are to read the sentence according to the rules of inductive logic; that is, the conclusion is to be judged according to probability.

This is different from a deductively phrased statement in which you are to judge the information according to logical validity. Remember that logical validity states that if the premises are true, then the conclusion must also be true.

Consider the following example: You ask me to dinner at your house, and I say, "I may come." This is very different from saying, "I will come," which is definite. The first statement is to be read as, "I may" or "I may not," and you have to judge whether I will accept your invitation on the basis of probability.

Many students are uncomfortable with inductively phrased questions and their conclusions because they are based on probability. For everyone, in real life and on the MCAT, probability causes trouble in at least two related ways. First, in an inductively phrased multiple-choice question, there can be more than one possible correct answer, but one will be more probable than the other. Second, probability involves a sliding scale of certainty. Consider, for example, a brown paper bag that contains 10 blue marbles, 3 green marbles, and 4 yellow marbles. If one marble is pulled out at random, what is its most probable color? Blue, of course. But now 5 orange marbles and 8 white marbles are added to the bag. Again, one marble is selected at random. What is the most probable color of this second marble?

The answer is still blue, simply because there are more blue marbles than any other one color, but the probability is less. As different-colored marbles are added, *blue* will remain the correct answer as long as there are more blue marbles than any other color. But the answer *blue* will feel less and less certain to you until only the deliberate application of the rules of probability will help you to answer. As the probability lessens, you will no longer feel as certain about which answer is correct.

Don't make the mistake of looking for the obscure (but possible) answer, rather than choosing the probable answer even if it seems too easy. Remember that the syntax of the question stem tells you that you must select your answer based on probability rather than on possibility or certainty.

Strategy 3: Linking Question Analysis to Passage Analysis

CONVENTIONAL MULTIPLE-CHOICE QUESTIONS

The conventional multiple-choice question is composed of a stem and a set of four answer choices. Multiple-choice items appear to be constructed in much the same way on tests from high school-level SATs right through the National Medical Board Examinations for medical students. The test-maker puts the correct answer in one of the slots, and then adds the trickiest and most difficult *incorrect* answer. This most difficult incorrect answer, called the "almost-right" response or the "most likely" distractor, tends to be very close to the correct answer. The test-maker knows that the closer the "almost-right" response is to the correct answer, the more difficulty you will have distinguishing one from the other. For example, if the question stem says, "All of the following are functions of the liver EXCEPT . . . ," the exception might be a function of the spleen, one that the test-maker knows students tend to relate incorrectly to the liver.

To avoid being misled, try not to leap for a single, correct answer. Under the pressure of the real MCAT, you might be tempted to choose the first answer choice that seems correct, but that answer may turn out to be the most likely distractor. You need to read all the answer choices carefully before making your selection. If you do not see at least two "correct" or "nearly correct" answers, you may be responding too superficially.

The Importance of Strategy for Multiple-Choice Questions

As a five-hour exam, the MCAT is more like running a marathon than a sprint and, like a marathon runner, you need an overall plan and specific, well-practiced strategies for each test section well in advance. You need to practice until the targeted actions for the actual test are deliberate yet automatic.

When you have decided on strategies for answering the multiple-choice questions, you will find that it is beneficial to use these strategies consistently until they become habit. Follow these three basic rules:

1. Read all of the options presented before eliminating any of them.
2. Reject a clearly incorrect answer by putting a slash through the identifying letter.
3. Identify the most likely answer choices and consider them carefully to assure the best possible choice.

A word of warning! Much of a student's classroom training runs counter to the deliberate, careful strategies suggested here for best performance on multiple-choice items. Consider that as early as junior high school, many students are already competing not only to get the correct answers, but also to get them faster than everyone else. This focus on speed encourages students to rely on rote memory and intuition leaps rather than carefully working their way to the correct answer. To benefit from the strategy recommended here, you will need to practice consistently until you can respond automatically. On the day of the test, then, you can concentrate on content and your search for correct answers.

Because answer choices require a certain amount of thought, you may be concerned about how you will be able to find time during the MCAT examination to worry about test-taking strategies. However, effective strategies not only lead to the correct answers but are time-efficient as well.

PASSAGE ANALYSIS

Try to understand the type of science passage presented by quickly skimming the entire subtest. The four types of science passages—information, problem solving, research study, and persuasive argument—should give you a method of attack for the problems following each passage. For example, for a research-study passage, look for hypotheses and conclusions (graphical or in text form); for a problem-solving passage look for data, figures, units, and *only* relevant information. Understanding the type of each passage will help you attack problems with a clear strategy.

QUESTION ANALYSIS STRATEGY

For most readers, recall of information from the passage or problem is usually insufficient to pick the best answer on the MCAT verbal reasoning test section. In using a question analysis strategy, however, you read the question stem first so you know what to look for and then you search the passage for the sentence (usually only one) that gives the answer.

You know when you have found the correct sentence in the passage because of the number of important words (primarily significant nouns) that it has in common with the question. For example, if the question asks, "In what historical period was U.S. population growth the lowest?," you can scan the passage for the words "population growth" and "lowest." The passage sentence that provides the answer might read: "This was the lowest rate of population growth recorded until the Great Depression, when the net growth rate fell to 7 per 1,000 population during the 1930–1935 period."

At first, you may find the question analysis strategy awkward and time-consuming. However, practice will increase your accuracy and ensure that you have enough time to complete this section of the test. To develop your skill using the question analysis strategy, follow these seven steps:

1. Skim the passage, reading only the first and last sentence in each paragraph.
2. Read the question stem first, but do not spend time reading all the answer options.
3. Underline the significant words in the question stem, primarily the nouns and active verbs.
4. Scan the passage, marking as you go and looking for words and sentences that match those you underlined in the stem. Words in the passage may appear in a different order than they appear in the question.
5. Put the number of the question in the margin where you found the information in the passage.
6. Steps 1 through 4 can be learned quickly; but after you narrow your choices, slow down to evaluate them carefully.
7. Answer the questions carefully, working back and forth between passage and question. Pay special attention to the remaining words in the sentence, especially to the precise meaning of conjunctions and qualifiers such as adverbs, adjectives, and restrictive phrases.

Practice this strategy with the passages in Chapter 3. Remember to pick out the significant nouns and verbs in the question stem and passage. Note when you begin to anticipate difficulty in choosing the right answer. Continue practicing until you feel you have developed an effective approach to these questions.

Modified Question Analysis Strategy

Many students, even with continued practice, find the question analysis strategy difficult to use. They find that while they have located specific places to look for designated words and phrases, they do not have a sense of the overall development of the topic. This makes it difficult to work with questions that involve interpretation, inference, or application. If this is your problem, you might want to try modifying the question analysis strategy. Begin working with a passage by doing the following:

1. Skim the text quickly to find the main idea of the passage. The statement containing the main idea is typically located in the first or last sentence of the first paragraph, or at the end of the last paragraph.

2. Skim the remaining paragraphs to determine the main idea of each paragraph. Again, look at the first or last sentence in each paragraph to find the main idea.
3. Watch for key words that indicate the topic's pattern of development. Examples of key words include *but, consequently, only, in addition, similar to.*
4. Return to the question analysis strategy, using the seven steps described above.

Work with both the question analysis strategy and the modified question analysis strategy to determine which is best for you. Evaluate your performance, checking your speed and accuracy for each method. Once you have determined the best approach, do not go back and forth between the two methods.

Strategy 4: Tools to Enhance Your Test-Taking Skills

A good strategist will take at least three diagnostic tests and three practice tests at monthly intervals in preparation for the MCAT. Diagnostic tests will help you evaluate your weaknesses, whereas practice tests will help you calculate your potential MCAT scores to indicate your overall MCAT standing. Use the American Association of Medical Colleges (AAMC) practice tests and items as authentic, field-tested, and valid instruments to score yourself. Remember, diagnostic tests should be used to monitor your MCAT review, not the other way around. Always work around your weaknesses and deficiencies, not around your strengths.

Strategy 5: Using Error Analysis to Improve Test Performance

Learning to analyze error patterns is a key element to improvement in all parts of the MCAT. Because we tend to repeat the same errors, it is essential to know our error patterns to begin developing corrective strategies.

ERROR ANALYSIS PROCEDURE

Error analysis is a very useful part of your MCAT preparation. You can keep track of the types of errors you make by completing the Error Analysis Chart (Table 5-1). By analyzing your errors on a regular basis, you will identify your problems and monitor your progress as well. In evaluating your test-taking performance and filling in the Error Analysis Chart, consider the following:

1. **Familiarity with passage content.** Note whether the content was drawn from the social sciences, natural sciences, humanities, or medicine, according to the topics listed in the *MCAT Student Manual.* Review Chapter 1 in this book to develop familiarity with passage format.
2. **Passage type.** Examine passage types in Chapter 1. In the following list, check those types that give you the most trouble:
   _____ Cause/effect
   _____ Comparison/contrast
   _____ Reasons
   _____ Time order
   _____ Definition
   _____ Classification
   _____ Spatial or graphic orientation
   _____ Process

3. **Pattern of organization.** Determine whether your errors more frequently involve:
   _____ Experimental data
   _____ Experimental procedures and designs
   _____ Basic information understanding
   _____ Analysis
   _____ Research methodologies

4. **Question type.** Note whether the question type was multiple choice or multiple-multiple choice.
5. **Reason for choosing the incorrect answer.** Determine the reason for an error by comparing your answer choice with the correct answer:
   • Was your error due to carelessness in choosing the best answer?
   • Did you have trouble with inductively phrased questions?
   • Did you have difficulty sorting out main ideas from details?

- Did you ignore the negative stem?
- Did you begin to feel pressured for time?
- Did you not study the correct information?
- Did the passage mislead you?
- Did you answer a different question from the one that was asked?

6. **Analyze your errors for patterns.** After recording your experience on the Error Analysis Chart, analyze your performance by searching for error patterns in the data. A tally of the frequency of various errors in each column will suffice. This provides important information to use in trying to eliminate repetitive errors.

COMMON ERROR PATTERNS AND SOLUTIONS

Identify error patterns so you can anticipate problems. This method allows you to deliberately apply strategies to eliminate your usual pitfalls, of which you should be aware. You may have your own pattern of error, but you will want to pay attention to some particularly common errors as you analyze your error patterns.

Remember that student errors will be evenly spread across all the alternate answers in a test-maker's ideal question. This means that each distractor ideally represents typical student errors. To complicate matters, we each tend to have patterns of errors that we repeat over and over unless an intervention strategy is introduced.

When you make an error, note what you say to yourself; example, ''I always have trouble with Boyle's law.'' This kind of admission is usually followed by a rationalization—''It's not that I don't know it, it's just that the test items confuse me.'' We tend to confuse recognition with knowing or understanding. If you cannot explain a concept clearly to someone who knows it well and who thus would know how accurate your reasoning is, you really do not know the concept.

TABLE 5-1. Error Analysis Chart

Question Number	Content Area	Passage Type	Pattern Type	Question Type	Reasoning Process	Item Type	Reason for Error
15.	Social sciences	Description	Cause/Effect	Multiple choice	Inductive	Main idea	Careless and hasty reading
25.	Natural sciences	Argument	Definitions	Multiple choice	Deductive	Detail	Inattention
27.	Humanities	Data interpretation	Comparison/ Contrast	Multiple-multiple choice	Proportional	Inference	Language
37.	Medicine	Information presentation	Classification	Multiple choice	Analogy	Application	Definitions
46.	Biological sciences	Research hypothesis	Reasons	Multiple choice	Comparative	Prediction	Language
51.	Physical sciences	Experimental/ Instrumental	Spatial/Graphic	Multiple choice	Visual	Definition	Definitions

Fill out this chart for each question you answer incorrectly (or create your own chart on a separate piece of paper). The top portion of this chart is an example of how to fill it out. Look for patterns in the types of errors you make and concentrate on improving those areas.

The first step in correcting error patterns is to recognize when they occur. The second step is to develop a mnemonic or memory device. Apply your device every time you see an item in the category you have identified. For example, it may help you to remember Boyle's law by thinking of your car. As you step on the accelerator, the piston goes down; and as the volume decreases, the pressure increases. You can even draw a picture in the margin of the test booklet to remind yourself. But the message here is that if you need a mnemonic, you must apply it every time the difficult topic comes up. Patterns of error tend to be well developed and they do not lend themselves to correction by rote memorization alone. Problems with the passages on the MCAT tend to involve difficulty with basic comprehension, analytical reasoning, question format, and concentration, all of which are associated with integrated pre-med skills. Try to analyze your error patterns based on these problems, for test items that you solved incorrectly.

Basic Comprehension Problems

General Reading Skills

Problem: You continue to make frequent errors because of poor reading comprehension, even though you are practicing to build accuracy.

Solution: Take the time to work on basic reading skills. A speed-reading course will not help, because these courses typically do not concentrate on increasing comprehension. One of the best ways to improve comprehension is to read more. Many students limit their reading to materials related to their course work. Consequently, they feel insecure when asked to read in other topic areas. Although reading your textbooks is important, spend at least 30 minutes or more each day reading for pleasure. This provides you with exposure to a wider range of writing styles and formats and stimulates your reading flexibility and rate.

Careless or Hasty Reading of the Passage

Problem: You are able to identify the sentence in the passage that contains the information needed to answer the question correctly, but you still fail to answer the question correctly. The problem may be due to superficial reading.

Solution: Finding the correct passage sentence is only the first step. Once you have found the sentence, read it critically to be sure that you understand what was stated. The entire passage should be read as evidence, and you, as the reader, are the detective looking for very precise clues.

Inattentive Reading of the Question

Problem: You are making errors because of reading the question carelessly, not because of lacking content comprehension. Typical errors of this type include failing to read the question completely; overlooking important qualifying words, such as *some* or *not*; not paying attention to comparison/contrast factors in the passage and questions; and failing to recognize that a question has more than one proposition.

Solution: Go back to labeling the important parts of the question or proposition when you are doing practice questions, and strive to be more active in the strategies you use.

Language Difficulties

Problem: You have comprehension problems involving synonyms because you classify terms inaccurately. For example, *dog* and *German shepherd* are not synonymous because a German shepherd is only one type of dog.

Solution: The discussion of synonyms is actually a discussion of the relationship between two terms under consideration. Using outlines or Venn diagrams can help you to sort out relationships between words.

Reasoning Problems

Analytical Reading Errors

Problem: You are unaccustomed to the precise, problem-solving approach of reading analytically. You read for facts and fail to apply reasoning strategies to develop a more in-depth understanding of the material.

Solution: Do some additional practice in this area. There are a number of excellent books about the art of problem solving that offer strategies and practice exercises.

Reasoning Pattern Identification

Problem: You have difficulty solving questions that are inductively phrased. You either fail to recognize that you are dealing with probability or you do not apply effective reasoning skills.

Solution: Reread the discussion on inductive reasoning in this chapter. Compare inductively phrased questions with deductively phrased questions. Do you see why they are written inductively? Do you see how inductive phrasing allows for more than one possible answer? Inductive phrasing is a clue that you should choose the best or most likely answer.

Proportional Reasoning
Problem: You have trouble with questions that include the words *increase* or *decrease*, especially when proportional reasoning is required to understand the passage or determine the correct answer.

Solution: Use arrows and make a chart in the margin. This helps you visualize what is happening and facilitates choosing the right answer.

Problems Related to Question Format

Questions with Negative Stems
Problem: You have trouble with negative words (e.g., *not, except, least*) in a question or answer. Because we are unaccustomed to reading for what is *not* true, this type of question may require extra concentration.

Solution: When you see an item with a negative stem, circle the negative word. Consider each answer choice and decide whether it is true or false, putting a *T* or *F* next to choice. If you are unsure, make an educated guess and put down a *T?* or *F?*. After you have evaluated all the information, make your choice. When working with this type of question, be sure to focus on *what is not* rather than *what is.*

Double Questions
Problem: You have trouble with questions that have more than one proposition or answers with more than one variable. You may make errors either because you fail to recognize that more than one proposition is involved or because you do not evaluate all the pieces of information.

Solution: Identify each proposition and number it. Then methodically evaluate each proposition to be sure that it satisfies all of the conditions given.

Variations in Degree of Concentration

Length of the Task
Problem: You find it difficult to concentrate for more than 30 minutes at a time. Given the length of each MCAT subtest, this negatively affects your overall test performance. The MCAT is a long examination, requiring both physical and mental stamina. During the examination you will find that when your mind begins to tire, it takes a break of its own accord; you might begin to think about something else (e.g., washing the car on the weekend) or you might begin to read a single question over and over again.

Solution: Stamina is developed over time. As a first step to improving your concentration, eliminate unconscious breaks when you are studying. Take a deliberate break as soon as you need it. Work with a clock in front of you. Deliberately change what you are doing by standing, stretching, or moving around for 2 to 5 minutes. When you go back to studying, try to concentrate just a little longer before your next break. You build slowly to increase speed for the MCAT. Increase your concentration in the same systematic way. Practice doing this so you will be able to work productively, taking only controlled breaks. If you do this, you will be taking the test rather than letting the test take you. Take full-length practice tests under specific time limits to build endurance.

Anxiety
Problem: You find that a high level of anxiety on a test hampers your ability to concentrate. It is serious enough to affect your performance. How do you respond to pressure? Does the first question make your mind go fuzzy, or does anxiety rise as time passes and you are suddenly aware that you are never going to finish in the allotted time unless you speed up?

Solution: If your anxiety tends to increase as soon as you see the first difficult question, do not answer it. Move on until you find a question you can answer with confidence, carefully marking the correct numbers on the answer sheet. Then go back to the question(s) you skipped. If pacing is a problem, work on it before you take the MCAT. Learn the techniques for keeping track of your pace. If you speed up in a "knee-jerk" fashion because you are anxious and feel pressured, you will probably make more careless errors. On the other hand, consciously speeding up because you are keeping track of the time is a confidence-builder and puts you in control. You do not get extra points just for answering every question on the test. However, you may lose points if you do not attempt to answer. By pacing yourself properly, you will be able to record an answer for each question.

YOUR PERSONAL PROFILE   As you work the various practice exercises in this book, enter your errors on Table 5-1 and analyze the data for continued error patterns. The Error Analysis Chart is designed to help you see the areas where you make repeated errors so you can concentrate on improving these areas. You may find that you develop a different profile across subtest areas that will then guide further preparation efforts. Remember that an important part of improving your performance is developing greater self-awareness of your personal test-taking skills and your ability to appropriately modify them.

Strategy 6: Determining Your MCAT Test-Taking Speed

Being "test-wise" means that you are in charge on the day of the MCAT. You have learned the mechanics of handling test questions, and you know how to pace yourself, how to mark the test booklet as you work, how to keep your place on your answer sheet, and so on. You are comfortable with the MCAT test-item format. You have developed your skills for accuracy even if you are not yet working at MCAT speed. You have reviewed the natural science sections, building your mastery of weak areas while maintaining your mastery of strong areas. You are now able to concentrate for 2-hour segments, including short, structured breaks.

If you have disciplined yourself to prepare for the MCAT, and if your accuracy level is satisfactory on all sections of the MCAT practice tests, you are now ready to develop your test-taking speed. The MCAT lasts 5 hours and 45 minutes.

SCHEDULE FOR TEST DAY: MCAT TIMING REQUIREMENTS BY TASK   Time management for the MCAT includes finishing the following tasks within 5 hours and 45 minutes. Your test-taking speed is a function of these tasks. The time range specified for each task below will give you a goal to aim for:

Task 1: Skimming, reading, and classifying passages. There are a total of 30 passages to cover in 60 to 90 minutes. Speed for task 1 = 2 to 3 minutes per passage.

Task 2: Underlining key words and marking passages. Marking up all 30 passages will take 15 to 25 minutes of your total time.
- The verbal reasoning section will take more time to mark up than either the physical or biological science section because of the amount of reading material. This includes nine verbal reasoning passages to be marked in 5 to 9 minutes. Speed for verbal reasoning task 2 = 30 to 60 seconds per passage.
- The science sections have 20 or 21 shorter passages (most are shorter than verbal reasoning passages) to be marked in 10 to 12 minutes. Speed for physical and biological sciences task 2 = 25 to 35 seconds per passage.

Task 3: Writing essays. This task takes 60 minutes. For details see Chapter 4.

Task 4: Answering independent questions. There is a total of 30 independent questions in the biological and physical sciences. These will take about 20 to 30 minutes, an average of 40 to 60 seconds per question.

Task 5: Answering passage-based questions. There is a total of 189 passage-based questions in the verbal reasoning and physical and biological sciences subtests. You can expect to spend about 189 minutes on this task. Pacing is especially important for this task.

Task 6: Marking your answer sheet. You can avoid marking your answer sheet erroneously if you mark after you have completed the passages and questions. Circle the correct responses in your answer booklet as you work, and then spend about 5 minutes filling in the ovals on the answer sheet. This prevents you from skipping questions and marking the wrong lines. Practice this process to get acquainted with the columns and ovals on the answer sheet. One caution: keep track of your time so you have time to fill in the answer sheet.

You have a total of 345 minutes for the entire test. If you add up the times allotted for tasks 1 through 6, you need from 359 to 414 minutes. Therefore, you need to reduce the time spent by 15% to 20% in the areas where you can best afford it. Learning what areas require the most time will help you meet your goal to complete the test. With practice, you will notice that you can work faster with a constant level of accuracy. Remember, there are no extra points given simply for finishing a subtest. Gauge yourself for the best speed-to-accuracy ratio to achieve the highest score.

Your speed will vary from section to section. You will not spend an equal amount of time on each item within a given subtest, but you will spend less time on those that are "easy," saving time for more difficult items. Because there are no extra points for answering the most difficult questions correctly, you will get every point possible by solving the easiest questions first and finishing with the more difficult.

Because separate scores are given for each section, you need to apply an equal effort for each area. Whether or not you like one science better than another, you must develop a disciplined, effective approach for all of them. The pressure of real testing situations tends to make you revert to past behaviors. Maintain your discipline throughout the test.

SPEED AND ACCURACY RELATIONSHIP

Faulty Pacing

Problem: You misunderstand the relationship between speed and accuracy. Managing time during the MCAT is a complex matter. Figuring out how many minutes per question on average that you have for each section of the test does not help, simply because the test-maker does not expect you to spend the same amount of time on each question.

Solution: The test-maker carefully balances relatively quick-to-answer questions with those that take more time. As a sophisticated test-taker, you need to develop a sense for determining both types so you can appropriately judge your time and set a reasonable pace.

Low Accuracy-to-Speed Ratio

Problem: You work too slowly on tests. In the classroom, this may not affect the final score, but working too slowly or too quickly on the MCAT can lower your score.

Solution: The best way to monitor this problem is to evaluate your pace when working practice tests. You may find that your current rate is appropriate; but if it needs modification, do it early in the preparation process so you have a comfortable accuracy-to-speed rate on the day of the MCAT.

PRACTICAL EXERCISES TO BUILD SPEED

Begin working seriously on your speed approximately 6 weeks before the MCAT. Work with a clock in front of you. Start with a passage or two that each have seven or eight questions. First, work for accuracy, noting how much time it takes to reach an accuracy level that satisfies you. On the next set of practice items, push yourself to work a little faster. If your accuracy level stays the same, work just a little bit faster on the next practice set. At the point where your accuracy level begins to suffer, work at that speed to raise your accuracy level. Increase your speed only when the accuracy level meets your standards. Work in this way on passages from each subtest area.

Look for shortcuts as you build your test-taking speed. For example, don't work too hard on calculating something for an equation in which a quick estimate will allow you to eliminate several wrong answer choices quickly. Continually look for the most efficient way to approach a problem, and don't become overly stubborn about answering a question that simply takes too much time.

Practice answering independent questions frequently. This way you will be ready for them when they appear on the test, and you may gain some more time to answer the more complex passage-based items.

Strategy 7: Using Multiple Resources to Identify a Concept

When studying scientific concepts, consult more than one resource. For example, let us examine the concepts of *osmolarity* and *glycolysis*. Review each concept from at least two, maybe three, books (e.g., a lab book and one or two textbooks). Compare each author's definition of each concept and evaluate the credibility of each resource or book. Try to construct a multiresource definition that you can comprehend, draw on, apply, analyze, and explain to another student. Learn each concept in this way to enhance your long-term understanding. Mastery of a medical concept is best achieved if you can find a journal article, a research application, or a specific clinical use of the concept before you determine that you really know and understand it.

Strategy 8: Using Intuition

Avoid guessing. If an item looks unfamiliar or difficult, rely more on your intuition and less on random guessing. Talk to yourself about what you know about a problem topic, even if it seems only tangentially related. This process can trigger associations that did not immediately come to mind, and it will often give you enough information to answer the question correctly. If you remain uncertain after brainstorming about what you know, use common sense to make your decision. Lean toward the answer that makes the best impression on you at that point. If you cannot entirely avoid guessing, you will at least be in a position to make an educated guess.

Strategy 9: Planning Three Weeks Before the Test

Take the full-length simulated MCAT from the AAMC about three or four Saturdays before the test. The AAMC publishes actual tests and you can purchase these tests from Williams & Wilkins (800-791-8042); use MCAT *Practice Tests I* or *II.* Your score on these tests will enable you to determine your readiness for the MCAT and will guide you in spending your time most profitably during your last few weeks of study. During these last few weeks, practice on the following skills for reinforcement:

1. Try to predict test questions while studying science topics
2. Read test directions carefully
3. Read questions carefully and identify key terms
4. Attempt to define key terms in a question before working through the question
5. Determine the intent of the test item without overinterpreting
6. Evaluate all information before choosing an answer
7. Use a problem-solving strategy rather than guessing
8. Apply consistent logic to all answer choices of a test question
9. Be flexible and follow multiple paths to problem solutions
10. Distinguish between fact and opinion provided in the passage
11. Rely on reasoning rather than personal feelings and/or impressions
12. Determine similarities and differences among concepts and detail
13. Draw diagrams or write equations, when appropriate, to sharpen perception and to clarify ideas
14. Test answers for relevancy to a problem

Try to get fellow premed students to participate in the MCAT simulation with you. Carefully follow the time limits in the MCAT test booklet and make your environment as similar to a real test site as possible.

You will benefit from a careful analysis of your results. Score one point for each correct answer. There is no penalty for incorrect or unanswered items. Total your correct answers to produce your raw score. You may then compute your "percent correct" score by dividing your raw score by the number of items in that subtest. If there are 50 questions and you answered 35 of them correctly, you got 70 percent correct. Next, tabulate your converted or scaled score against our simulated MCAT Scoring Chart (see Chapter 1, Table 1-2). *(This scoring chart should in no case be interpreted as part of the actual AAMC scoring system. The MCAT Scoring Chart was developed for test materials in this book only.)* The scoring chart serves only as a guide to check your performance on a relative basis with past test-takers. Actual tests vary depending on how difficult they are, how well the test conditions are simulated, your personal disposition on the day of the test, and other factors. Use the chart to become familiar with the scoring process and to evaluate the status of your preparation.

Be rigorous in maintaining your daily schedule for MCAT preparation. Use the time limits of a real MCAT testing day as a guide. This includes the time you get up, what you do when you wake up, appropriate diet, and the time you go to sleep. You may not be at your best on a test starting in the morning if you have maintained a night-study schedule up until the test day.

Strategy 10: Planning the Last Week Before the Test

On the Saturday before the actual MCAT, drive to the testing location at the time the MCAT will be given the following week. Pay attention to route, traffic, parking, and so on. Locate the testing room, bathroom, snack bar. Overpreparation is a good antidote to anxiety.

Schedule review sessions that emphasize short-term memory tasks. The rest of your MCAT study time should be spent solving passage-based questions from each section under timed conditions. During these final sessions, simulate real test situations as closely as possible. For example, do not allow yourself to spend too much time solving one problem. In a good simulation, the adrenaline should be flowing just enough so you feel the stress, but not enough to make you anxious.

In these final practice sessions, stick to the strategies you have practiced. Be deliberate. Consider statements carefully and mark the answer clues in the question. Cross out wrong answers. Work with a watch in front of you that you intend to bring with you on the real test day. It should have a large, clear face and a minute hand. Work without calculators, because you are not permitted to use them on the MCAT. You know by now that accuracy and speed are a trade-off. Know beforehand what speed on each subtest gives you the highest level of accuracy.

Strategy 11: Planning for the Test Day

PREPARE IN ADVANCE WHAT YOU WILL TAKE WITH YOU

On the day of the test, take along your watch, three or four well-sharpened pencils with erasers, and snacks. Remember to eat a good breakfast. Research at the Johns Hopkins Medical Center shows that protein at breakfast is particularly important for problem-solving activities. Get up in time to eat your breakfast calmly.

ARRIVING AT THE TESTING ROOM

Get to the testing room in time to settle in. Once the test begins, keep the following points in mind:

1. You may want to note in the margins of your test booklet certain short-term memory items.
2. Remember to stick to your strategies throughout the test. Do not be distracted by what others are doing around you. Periodically, make sure your mark on the answer sheet corresponds to the number of the question you are answering, or follow the previous suggestion to mark your answer sheet from marks you make in the test book.
3. If your mind goes blank on the first item, go on to the next one. Continue until you find one you can answer. Then go back. Once you begin, keep to the pace that allows you the highest level of accuracy.
4. Answer all questions. For those you honestly do not know, fill in your predetermined guess answer. There is no penalty for incorrect answers.
5. During breaks, do not talk to other test-takers. Keep your energies focused on the test.
6. Stay in control of your time and energy. Remember, you are taking the test; do not let the test take you.

SUMMARY OF TEST-TAKING RULES

Read all instructions carefully and make sure you understand them. You do not want to miss a question that you knew because you failed to note a detail in the directions.

Scan the test for question types and plan strategy. Certain types of questions take more time than others. Negative-stemmed questions, questions on particularly complex material, and multiple-multiple choice or double-level questions require a little more thought and processing, so you need to budget your time accordingly. If you are worried about finishing on time, leave these questions for last. Plan to answer all questions. Because all of the questions are equally weighted, it is better to answer more questions than to labor over getting just a few correct.

Read the stem of the question carefully. Be particularly careful to notice qualifying words, such as *almost, usually, characteristically, decrease, except,* and *not,* as well as prefixes that change or determine the meaning of a word such as *un-, dis-, in-, pre-,* and *post-.* If you read the qualifiers but tend to forget them when thinking through the question, underline or circle them. Remember to go back and double-check your answer against the words you have highlighted as being important.

Interpret questions at face value. Test questions, especially professionally constructed ones, are not intended to be trick questions, so do not read an intent into the question that is not stated. Interpret the question as straightforwardly as possible.

Avoid liberal guessing. Do not give up and move into a guess mode as soon as something looks unfamiliar or difficult. Talk to yourself about what you do know, even if it seems only tangentially related. This process often triggers associations and may give you enough information to answer the question. If you cannot avoid guessing, you will at least be in a position to make an educated guess that will increase your chances of answering correctly.

Maintain consistent logic. Make sure that your answer rationale does not contain contradictory information. On questions in which several answers may be correct, evaluate each answer choice individually for accuracy, but then look at whether your combination of information is in agreement. Evaluate each answer separately without bias.

Resolve vagueness or ambiguity. It is very difficult to make a decision when you are uncertain of what a word or phrase means. In this situation, determine exactly which word or phrase is unclear, and try to define it according to what you think it might be. Then use that definition to solve the problem. Although there is always the chance that your definition may not be accurate enough for you to arrive at the correct answer, more often than not you will be able to come close enough to the correct definition to answer the question correctly.

Read all information provided, even when you see an immediate answer. Do not allow yourself to respond solely on the basis of familiarity. This can cause you to read carelessly and to ignore the context in which the words are used. You may find that what you had anticipated to be there was, in fact, not there.

Give thought to what the answer should include before reading the answer choices. If you look at the answer choices immediately after reading the question, you run the risk of narrowing the field of information that you use to solve the problem to what is directly in front of you. It is especially important to work with as much information as you can when you are uncertain about the answer.

Transfer answers in a batch to the answer sheet. Mark your answers on the test booklet as you work with the questions. Periodically stop and transfer a block of answers to the answer sheet. This will save you time and reduce the risk of transfer errors.

Pace yourself to answer all questions. Do not spend long periods of time working on a single question. If you are not sure, pick an answer and move on. Circle the number so that if you have time at the end, you can look at it again. Watch your time. Set interim checkpoints for where you want to be on the test at a given time. Then try to pace yourself accordingly.

Void the test if necessary. If you feel sick during the exam or realize that you are not adequately prepared, you can void your test. If you do this, you will not receive scores (and the proctor will record your decision in your presence) and the unsatisfactory scores will not be recorded against your name.

AFTER THE TEST

When the test is finished, do not compare what you remember answering with what someone else remembers answering. It is unreliable at best and often depressing. Be good to yourself!

Both preparation and luck have a part in any event that is going to occur at a specific time. If you have not performed as well as you should, you may take the test again. Start early on a routine that allows you to analyze weaknesses and get your new preparation program under way.

# Applied Math Concepts Required for Physical and Biological Sciences

The mathematics review that follows is an important reference to sample selectively according to the need for specific material.

The Role of Mathematical Skills for Medical Students and Physicians

Historically, collection of medical data can be traced back to 1854, when Florence Nightingale started keeping records of health care systems. She recognized that reliable data on the incidence of preventable deaths made compelling arguments for reform. She was a pioneer in the uses of social statistics in the medical profession. Today, the medical student also relies increasingly on modern technology in the form of computerized medical instrumentation.

In a wide variety of situations, medical students and physicians must deal effectively with quantitative information. For example, it is necessary to analyze data pertaining to research and development. Such analysis includes "looking" at a quantity of numerals and "extracting" useful or pertinent information for later use. Physicians must be able to evaluate data on new diagnostic instruments or experimental drugs and then interpret such data to determine appropriate applications and correct dosages.

An example of making judgments on the basis of quantitative information is the clinical decision surrounding the use of mammography as a detector of breast cancer relative to patient age. To be able to maximize benefits and minimize risks, physicians must be able somehow to match data on the age-group prevalence of breast cancer against data that show mammography as predisposing its recipients to breast cancer.

The mathematical skills of premedical students are tested in the physical and biological sciences subtests of the MCAT, including the ability to estimate, to calculate quickly and accurately, to recognize and analyze inaccuracies in data and identify possible sources of error in information, to predict numeric outcomes from given facts and figures, and to understand the use of graphs, tables, and related figures.

How Mathematics Concepts and Skills Are Tested on the MCAT

No actual mathematics subtest is included in the MCAT. Instead, the applied knowledge of mathematics is tested indirectly in various subtests. Knowing how to compute is not enough for MCAT preparation. It is important to emphasize approach or method of attack, calculation or quick evaluation, interpretation or critical analysis, and finally, speed or time-wiseness. Remember, no calculators are allowed.

The MCAT is designed to determine the following:

1. Can you perform calculations mentally or manually under pressure of time?
2. Can you reason proportionally when comparing two sets of information?
3. Can you remember and use basic formulas learned in plane geometry (Pythagorean theorem, areas and volumes of common figures and shapes)?
4. Can you convert units from one system to the other using scientific notation? Can you convert percentages to fractions?
5. Can you use definitions of trigonometric functions and their relationships?
6. Can you understand the concepts of exponentials, logarithms, reciprocals, semilog and log-log graphs?
7. Can you calculate the probability of an event?
8. Can you add and subtract vectors?

9. Can you conceptualize arithmetical mean, standard deviation, statistical correlation, and relative error analysis of experimental data?
10. Can you identify, explain, and predict mathematical trends in continuous line graphs?
11. Can you determine the underlying equation or function in a line graph or a mathematical plot?

Mathematical Problems in Physical and Biological Sciences Subtests

Mathematics is an integral part of the ability to solve the problems included in the Physical and Biological Sciences subtests. These problems are designed and structured to evaluate certain skills, such as those that involve the following:

- **Detailed information** (raw data) given in a tabular or a graphic format to be interpreted by the student without a calculator (quick mathematical interpretation)
- **Describing** research methodology, experimental methodology, complex organization of types of information collected from natural sciences, social sciences, and medically related topics (analytical reading and reasoning)
- **Comparing/contrasting** proficiency to recognize similarities and differences between two sets of information, such as "statistical summary" (proportional and logical reasoning)
- Tables of **scrambled data** that need an appropriate format, including sorting with the eye, classification, and interpretation (mathematical interpretation)
- **Multiple image graphs** to study correlations, rates of change, or slope, and to discover and explain inconsistent trends using simple mental/manual arithmetic (perceptive proportional reasoning)
- **Actual data** that may lead to deceptive empiric trends and relationships leading to erroneous conclusions if not well analyzed (predictive reasoning)
- **Detection** of an underlying assumption, finding and filling gaps in information given, and forming valid "information-based" conclusions (analytical reading and reasoning)
- **Testing the reliability** of information for precision, accuracy, and validity over long time spans: predicting values in the future (predictive reasoning)
- **Simple arithmetic skills**, such as quick addition, converting numeric data into percentages or fractions, and approximating to get the right answer (learning how to approximate)
- **Sensitivity testing** of a given equation by changing one variable at a time in relation to another variable
- **Components of graphs, figures, and diagrams** to identify and compare various segments (analytical reasoning)

Familiarize yourself with and concentrate your practice on these topics. Resolve to test yourself by solving each problem that appears difficult to you.

Mathematics Diagnostic Test

For the following test, answer each question as quickly as you can and record your answer. Do not use a calculator. If your test score is less than 75 points, further review and practice are essential. Refer to the High-Speed Math Refresher included in the next section. It will help you to reinforce your calculating skills and make your MCAT preparation more fruitful.

The total amount of time allowed for this test (problems 1–4) is 30 minutes. Score your test carefully when you are finished. Additional space is available in the right-hand margin for calculations.

1. Change each of the following numbers to the percent form:

(a)	0.25	= 25%	(b)	0.333	=	(c)	1.65	=
(d)	0.05	=	(e)	0.005	=	(f)	3	=
(g)	1.065	=	(h)	1.25	=	(i)	$3\frac{1}{2}$	=
(j)	0.16	=	(k)	2.05	=	(l)	0.008	=
(m)	10	=	(n)	0.0036	=	(o)	$1\frac{1}{4}$	=
(p)	0.90	=	(q)	0.005	=	(r)	0.7	=
(s)	0.025	=	(t)	$1\frac{1}{2}$	=			

2. Change each of the following percents to the decimal form:

(a)	2%	= 0.02	(b)	200%	=	(c)	0.5%	=
(d)	$\frac{1}{4}$%	=	(e)	1.6%	=	(f)	1.5%	=

(g) 16% =	(h) 25% =	(i) 300% =
(j) $16\frac{1}{2}$% =	(k) 0.05% =	(l) $32\frac{1}{2}$% =
(m) 9% =	(n) $4\frac{1}{2}$% =	(o) 568% =
(p) $\frac{1}{2}$% =	(q) 23.2% =	(r) 0.56% =
(s) 1.7% =	(t) 115% =	

3. Change each of the following percents to a fraction or a mixed number:

(a) 25% = $\frac{1}{4}$	(b) $16\frac{2}{3}$% =	(c) $12\frac{1}{2}$% =
(d) $11\frac{1}{9}$% =	(e) $108\frac{1}{3}$% =	(f) 20% =
(g) 5% =	(h) $3\frac{1}{2}$% =	(i) 30% =
(j) 125% =	(k) 15% =	(l) $83\frac{1}{3}$% =
(m) 60% =	(n) 17% =	(o) 0.22% =
(p) 6% =	(q) $\frac{2}{5}$% =	(r) 38% =
(s) 46% =	(t) 375% =	

4. Change each of the following fractions or mixed numbers to the percent form:

(a) $\frac{3}{8}$ = 37.5%	(b) $\frac{5}{6}$ =	(c) $\frac{1}{12}$ =
(d) $\frac{3}{9}$ =	(e) $\frac{2}{5}$ =	(f) $\frac{5}{12}$ =
(g) $\frac{1}{30}$ =	(h) $\frac{1}{25}$ =	(i) $\frac{1}{2}$ =
(j) $\frac{3}{4}$ =	(k) $\frac{7}{8}$ =	(l) $3\frac{3}{4}$ =
(m) $\frac{1}{6}$ =	(n) $\frac{2}{3}$ =	(o) $\frac{2}{16}$ =
(p) $\frac{4}{32}$ =	(q) $\frac{12}{5}$ =	(r) $\frac{5}{9}$ =
(s) $1\frac{1}{3}$ =	(t) $20\frac{1}{2}$ =	

Answers

1.	(a) 25%	(b) $33\frac{1}{3}$%	(c) 165%	(d) 5%
	(e) 0.5% or $\frac{1}{2}$%	(f) 300%	(g) 106.5% or $106\frac{1}{2}$%	(h) 125%
	(i) 350%	(j) 16%	(k) 205%	(l) 0.8%
	(m) 1000%	(n) 0.36%	(o) 125%	(p) 90%
	(q) $\frac{1}{2}$%	(r) 70%	(s) $2\frac{1}{2}$% or 2.5%	(t) 150%
2.	(a) 0.02	(b) 2.00	(c) 0.005	(d) 0.0025
	(e) 0.016	(f) 0.015	(g) 0.16	(h) 0.25
	(i) 3.00	(j) 0.165	(k) 0.0005	(l) 0.325
	(m) 0.09	(n) 0.045	(o) 5.68	(p) 0.005
	(q) 0.232	(r) 0.0056	(s) 0.017	(t) 1.15
3.	(a) $\frac{1}{4}$	(b) $\frac{1}{6}$	(c) $\frac{1}{8}$	(d) $\frac{1}{9}$
	(e) $\frac{11}{12}$	(f) $\frac{1}{5}$	(g) $\frac{1}{20}$	(h) $\frac{7}{200}$
	(i) $\frac{3}{10}$	(j) $1\frac{1}{4}$	(k) $\frac{3}{20}$	(l) $\frac{5}{6}$
	(m) $\frac{3}{5}$	(n) $\frac{17}{100}$	(o) $\frac{11}{5000}$	(p) $\frac{3}{50}$
	(q) $\frac{1}{250}$	(r) $\frac{19}{50}$	(s) $\frac{23}{50}$	(t) $3\frac{3}{4}$

4. Answers to Problem 4 (a–t) can be obtained by using a calculator once you have finished the test. Now make up and solve your own problems.

SCORE INTERPRETATION

Each problem has 20 parts (a–t). Assign one point for each correct answer. The highest score possible is 4(20) = 80 points. Determine your score by using the following chart.

Score Obtained	Interpretation
75–80	Excellent
70–74	Good
60–69	Satisfactory

If your score is less than 60, your math skills are poor. To improve both speed and accuracy, structure your practice in mathematics with special emphasis on the High-Speed Math Refresher in the following section. You may have to review this type of material for several weeks until you have mastered it. Practice all problems with a clock in front of you. Remember that the actual MCAT is an instrument that checks your ability to solve problems and to calculate quickly and precisely.

The High-Speed Math Refresher—Time and Precision

Science is mostly knowledge; art, such as moving a paintbrush on canvas, the professional strokes of tennis, golf, and baseball, is a skill. Repeated practice of fundamental skills makes them seem automatic. An example of a fundamental skill of mathematic calculation for a typical MCAT student is knowing how to determine that 67 multiplied by 25 equals 1,675 and being able to do so mentally or manually in about 5 seconds. Without this level of skill, you may not be adept at the art of calculation as it is required for successful completion of the MCAT.

Genuine skill in calculation may be acquired by anyone of average intelligence, regardless of educational background. The following section leads you through easy steps to acquire exceptional calculating ability. The key to success in this learning process is the ability to hold and manipulate figures in your head. It is important to develop an understanding of "number sense," which is the ability to recognize the relationships that exist between numbers considered as quantities in terms of their relationship with each other.

EXAMPLE. Using different methods, solve the multiplication problem: 67×25.

Long Method	Horizontal Algebraic Method
$\begin{array}{r} 67 \\ \times\ 25 \\ \hline 335 \\ +1340 \\ \hline 1{,}675 \end{array}$	$\begin{aligned} 67 \times 25 &= (70 - 3)(20 + 5) \\ &= 1400 - 60 - 15 + 350 \\ &= 1750 - 75 = 1{,}675 \end{aligned}$
Vertical multiplication (10 seconds)	Algebraic multiplication (8 seconds)

If you know the multiplication table for 25, you could solve this problem with double-digit multiplication in 5 seconds.

$$67 \times 25 = \begin{array}{r} 6 \\ \times\ 25 \\ \hline 150 \end{array} \quad \begin{array}{r} 7 \\ \times\ 25 \\ \hline 175 \end{array} \text{[carry over to places shown]}$$

$$\frac{''}{1{,}675} \leftarrow$$

The quickest method sometimes is a combination of these methods.

$$67 \times 25 = (70 - 3)25$$
$$= 1750 - 75 = 1675$$

Study the following mathematics concepts at your own pace and practice using these fundamental skills until you have mastered them.

BASIC ARITHMETIC OPERATIONS

Concept 1: Addition, Subtraction, Multiplication, and Division

Adding by Pairs
Instead of adding one vertical column, learn how to add a pair of digits in a vertical column. Try adding your monthly checking account statement when you receive it from the bank, or adding the items of your grocery receipt. Do all of these additions mentally.

Exercise A: Adding Single Columns by Pairs
Add the following columns of figures. Taking successive double-digit numbers one at a time, add from the top down beginning with 51:

1.	2.	3.	4.	5.	6.	7.	8.
51	42	12	34	12	43	58	74
30	53	73	12	81	61	48	48
96	43	32	97	11	38	62	65
24	79	12	19	39	36	49	74
25	87	81	69	43	37	47	71
75	76	11	94	10	33	92	49
48	92	44	83	85	38	34	47
49	52	84	68	99	87	52	35
93	45	70	38	29	62	98	63
80	38	40	46	14	96	87	67
13	18	92	17	95	95	34	84
58	63	67	57	10	44	84	45
88	22	56	66	74			
86	21	16	64	31			
20	47	37	89	77			
99	91	55	92	74			
59	15	27	60	28			
65	78	54	23	84			
1,059							

9. 87	10. 99	11. 14	12. 39	13. 68	14. 63	15. 84
85	84	12	68	55	62	99
91	96	26	23	52	62	36
76	77	29	37	34	63	73
85	87	24	47	69	89	74
82	96	24	35	56	59	56
69	93	18	98	46	67	82
58	21	37	29	67	92	89
49	69	98	85	53	42	68
74	47	36	91	37	64	53
28	89	29	48	64	97	59
95	53	49	96	59	24	84

Answer and Solution to Problem 1

Add 51 and 30 to get 81, then add 81 to 96 to obtain 177, then add 177 to 24 to obtain 201, then add 201 to 25 to obtain 226, then add 226 to 75 to obtain 301, then add 301 to 48 to obtain 349, then add 349 to 49 to obtain 398, then add 398 to 93 to obtain 491, then add 491 to 80 to obtain 571, then add 571 to 13 to obtain 584, then add 584 to 58 to obtain 642, then add 642 to 88 to obtain 730, then add 730 to 86 to obtain 816, then add 816 to 20 to obtain 836, then add 836 to 99 to obtain 935, then add 935 to 59 to obtain 994, then add 994 to 65 to finally get 1059.

Problems 2 through 15 can be solved in the same way. Each problem should take about 10 seconds.

Answers to Problems 2–15

2) 962	3) 863	4) 1028	5) 896	6) 670	7) 745	8) 722
9) 879	10) 911	11) 396	12) 696	13) 660	14) 784	15) 857

Factors of Common Numbers

Factors of numbers should be reviewed from time to time and used frequently for multiplication problems. Remember that a prime number cannot be divided by any number but itself or the number one. Formally, a prime is an integer greater than one that has exactly two distinct positive integer divisors.

$2 =$ prime	$27 = 3 \times 3 \times 3$
$3 =$ prime	$28 = 2 \times 2 \times 7$
$4 = 2 \times 2$	$29 =$ prime
$5 =$ prime	$30 = 2 \times 3 \times 5$
$6 = 2 \times 3$	$31 =$ prime
$7 =$ prime	$32 = 2 \times 2 \times 2 \times 2 \times 2$
$8 = 2 \times 2 \times 2$	$33 = 3 \times 11$
$9 = 3 \times 3$	$34 = 2 \times 17$
$10 = 2 \times 5$	$35 = 5 \times 7$
$11 =$ prime	$36 = 2 \times 2 \times 3 \times 3$
$12 = 2 \times 3 \times 2$	$37 =$ prime
$13 =$ prime	$38 = 2 \times 19$
$14 = 2 \times 7$	$39 = 3 \times 13$
$15 = 3 \times 5$	$40 = 2 \times 2 \times 2 \times 5$
$16 = 2 \times 2 \times 2 \times 2$	$41 =$ prime
$17 =$ prime	$42 = 2 \times 3 \times 7$
$18 = 2 \times 3 \times 3$	$43 =$ prime
$19 =$ prime	$44 = 2 \times 2 \times 11$
$20 = 2 \times 2 \times 5$	$45 = 3 \times 3 \times 5$
$21 = 3 \times 7$	$46 = 2 \times 23$
$22 = 2 \times 11$	$47 =$ prime
$23 =$ prime	$48 = 2 \times 2 \times 2 \times 2 \times 3$
$24 = 2 \times 2 \times 2 \times 3$	$49 = 7 \times 7$
$25 = 5 \times 5$	$50 = 2 \times 5 \times 5$
$26 = 2 \times 13$	

Continue to expand this list to 1000 by regularly adding new numbers.

$$\text{Factors of } 1000 = 2 \times 500 = 2 \times 2 \times 250$$

$$= 2 \times 2 \times 2 \times 125$$

$$= 2 \times 2 \times 2 \times 5 \times 125$$

$$= 2 \times 2 \times 2 \times 5 \times 5 \times 5$$

Divisibility Rules

These rules and examples will enhance your ability to divide quickly.

A NUMBER IS DIVISIBLE BY:	IF:
2	it ends in 0, 2, 4, 6, or 8
3	the total of its digits is divisible by 3 (see example 1)
4	the number formed by the last two digits is divisible by 4 (see example 2)
5	if it ends in 0 or 5
6	if it is divisible by 2 and 3 (use the rules for both and see example 3)
7	(no simple rule)
8	the number formed by the last three digits is divisible by 8 (see example 4)
9	the total of its digits is divisible by 9 (see example 5)

EXAMPLE 1

Is 126 divisible by 3? Total of digits = 9. Because 9 is divisible by 3, 126 is divisible by 3.

EXAMPLE 2

Is 1,748 divisible by 4? Because 48 is divisible by 4, then 1,748 is divisible by 4.

EXAMPLE 3

Is 186 divisible by 6? Because 186 ends in 6, it is divisible by 2. Total of digits = 15. Because 15 is divisible by 3, 186 is divisible by 3. 186 is divisible by 2 and 3; therefore, it is divisible by 6.

EXAMPLE 4

Is 2,488 divisible by 8? Because 488 is divisible by 8, then 2,488 is divisible by 8.

EXAMPLE 5

Is 2,853 divisible by 9? Total of digits = 18. Because 18 is divisible by 9, then 2,853 is divisible by 9.

Divisibility Problems

PROBLEM 1

4,620 is divisible by which of the following numbers: 2,3,4,5,6,7,8,9?

PROBLEM 2

13,131 is divisible by which of the following numbers: 2,3,4,5,6,7,8,9?

Answers to Problems 1 and 2

1) 2,3,4,5,6,7
   2—the number is even
   3—the digits total 12, which is divisible by 3
   4—the number formed by the last two digits, 20, is divisible by 4
   5—the number ends in 0
   6—the number is divisible by 2 and 3
   7—4,620 divided by 7 equals 660
   8—the number formed by the last three digits, 620, is not divisible by 8
   9—the total of the digits is 12, which is not divisible by 9
2) 3,9
   2—the number is not even
   3—the digits total 9, which is divisible by 3
   4—the number is not even
   5—the number does not end in 0 or 5
   6—the number is not even
   7—division yields a remainder, hence not divisible
   8—the number is not even
   9—the digits total 9, which is divisible by 9

More Mental Multiplication and Division Problems

EXERCISE A: mental multiplication

Mentally multiply the following:

1.	46×71	5.	88×75	9.	56×71	13.	96×75	17.	66×71
2.	58×72	6.	96×76	10.	66×72	14.	36×76	18.	76×72
3.	66×73	7.	36×77	11.	76×73	15.	46×77	19.	86×73
4.	76×74	8.	48×77	12.	86×74	16.	56×76	20.	96×74

EXERCISE B: mental division

Mentally divide the following:

1.	$5338 \div 772$	6.	$1859 \div 263$	11.	$2284 \div 282$	16.	$5887 \div 647$
2.	$5393 \div 883$	7.	$2736 \div 374$	12.	$3183 \div 393$	17.	$7123 \div 758$
3.	$6001 \div 994$	8.	$3606 \div 485$	13.	$3956 \div 444$	18.	$8221 \div 869$
4.	$908 \div 145$	9.	$4518 \div 596$	14.	$4795 \div 555$	19.	$9257 \div 973$
5.	$1576 \div 256$	10.	$4711 \div 637$	15.	$5954 \div 666$	20.	$1721 \div 184$

EXERCISE C: mental multiplication

Mentally multiply the following:

1.	47×79	5.	87×84	9.	57×79	13.	97×84	17.	67×79
2.	57×81	6.	97×85	10.	67×81	14.	37×85	18.	77×81
3.	67×82	7.	37×86	11.	77×82	15.	47×86	19.	87×82
4.	77×83	8.	47×87	12.	87×83	16.	57×87	20.	97×83

Answers to Exercises A–C

(Exercise A)

1) $46 \times 71 = 46 (70 + 1)$

$$= 3220 + 46 = 3266$$

2)	4176	3)	4818	4)	5624	5)	6600	6)	7296
7)	2772	8)	3696	9)	3976	10)	4752	11)	5548
12)	6364	13)	7200	14)	2736	15)	3542	16)	4256
17)	4686	18)	5472	19)	6278	20)	7104		

(Exercise B)

1) $\underline{53}38 \div \underline{7}72$: To divide mentally or manually, first try to divide the first digit of the numerator (5) by the first digit of the denominator (7). It is not possible. Next try to divide 53 by 7. It works, but 772 is closer to 800 than 700 and the answer (5404) is too high. Try again with 6: the answer (4632) leaves a remainder (706) or 706 ÷ 772. For the decimal, 7 goes into 70 ten times, but 772 is nearer to 800, so try one less, which is 9. Manual division yields 6.9 as well.

1) Answer: 6 remainder 706, or 6.9 when done manually.

2)	6r95	3)	6r37	4)	6r38	5)	6r40	6)	7r18
7)	7r118	8)	7r211	9)	7r346	10)	7r252	11)	8r28
12)	8r39	13)	8r404	14)	8r355	15)	8r626	16)	9r64
17)	9r301	18)	9r400	19)	9r500	20)	9r65		

(Exercise C)

1) $47 \times 79 = 47 (80 - 1) = 3760 - 47 = 3713$

2)	4617	3)	5494	4)	6391	5)	7308	6)	8245
7)	3182	8)	4089	9)	4503	10)	5427	11)	6314
12)	7221	13)	8148	14)	3145	15)	4042	16)	4959
17)	5293	18)	6237	19)	7134	20)	8051		

Concept 2: Estimating Square Roots of Common Numbers

The square roots of whole numbers from 1 to 100 are floating-point decimal numbers. In the following table, they are rounded to the nearest hundredth. For example, the table has these entries:

Number	Square Root
17	4.12 (rounded from 4.123106 ...)

$$(4.123)^2 = 16.999, \text{ which is close to } 17$$

When the square root entry has a 0 in the thousandths place, the 0 can be ignored. For example:

$$\sqrt{22} = 4.690 \text{ (or simply } 4.69)$$

When using the table, you can round the square root entries even further. For example:
Round the entry below to the **nearest hundredth**:

$$\sqrt{31} = 5.57 \text{ (from } 5.568)$$

Round the entry below to the **nearest tenth**:

$$\sqrt{95} = 9.7 \text{ (from } 9.74)$$

To find a close approximation to the square roots of decimal numbers from 1 to 100, simply round to the nearest whole number and use its square root from the table. For example:

$$\sqrt{12.8} \text{ is close to } \sqrt{13} \text{ or } 3.61$$

$$\sqrt{84.36} \text{ is close to } \sqrt{84} \text{ or } 9.17$$

Note: When rounding to the nearest whole number, you occasionally get a whole number that is a perfect square. As in the following example, use the whole number (5) as an approximation of the square root of the decimal number (25.33). For example:

$$\sqrt{25.33} \text{ is close to } \sqrt{25} \text{ or } 5$$

Square Roots of Whole Numbers From 1 to 100

Number	Square Root
1	1.00
2	1.41
3	1.73
4	2.00
5	2.24
6	2.45
7	2.65
8	2.83
9	3.00
10	3.16

Note: When you do not remember a square root, guess and check. The square root of 640 must be between 20 and 30; guess 25, $25 \times 25 = 625$ (too small), $26 \times 26 = 676$ (too large), $25.5 \times 25.5 = 650$ (too large), $25.4 \times 25.4 = 645$ (too large), $25.3 \times 25.3 = 640.1$ (close enough). Notice that

$$640 = 6.4 \times 100 \ (\sqrt{640}) = (\sqrt{6.4} \times 10)$$

ALGEBRA CONCEPTS

A basic knowledge of algebra that covers solving simple equations, solving quadratic equations, and manipulating formulas is required for the MCAT.
Some **basic definitions** follow.

- A **variable** is a symbol that, without further definition, can stand for any number or an unknown quantity.
- A **constant** is a symbol (or number) that has a fixed value.
- An **expression** is any combination of variables and constants connected by arithmetic symbols, for example, $3x + 7 - 2/x$.
- An **equation** expresses the equality or balance between different expressions. It is satisfied by certain values of the variables.

Concept 3: Simplifying Algebraic Equations

An **algebraic equation** is an algebraic expression in which one variable usually amounts to the isolation of the unknown quantity or variable on one side of the equation. Any operation, except multiplication or division by zero, can be used to achieve this isolation as long as it is done to both sides of the equation. More generally, the basic rule for solving equations is that whatever is done to one side must be done to the other side so that the equality of the sides is not affected. It is like a weighing scale with two balanced sides or pans.

Order of Operations

Before solving some sample equations, it is important to recall that, when manipulating an expression (whether or not it is part of an equation), the order of operations is as follows:

1. Parentheses
2. Powers or exponents
3. Multiplication and division (whichever comes first from the left)
4. Addition and subtraction (whichever comes first from the left)

EXAMPLE 6

Solve for a: $4a + 5 = 13$

$$4a + 5 - 5 = 13 - 5$$
$$4a = 8$$
$$\frac{4a}{4} = \frac{8}{4}$$
$$a = 2$$

EXAMPLE 7

Solve for m: $\dfrac{10}{m} - 8 = \dfrac{5}{3}$

$$\frac{10}{m}(3m) - 8(3m) = \frac{5}{3}(3m)$$
$$30 - 24m = 5m$$
$$30 = 29m$$
$$m = \frac{30}{29}$$

EXAMPLE 8

Solve for c: $3c^2 = 75d^4$

$$c^2 = 25d^4$$
$$\sqrt{c^2} = \sqrt{25d^4}$$
$$c = \pm 5d^2$$

EXAMPLE 9

Solve for q: $3[(q + 2)^2 - 4q] = 2q^2 + 13$

$$3[(q + 2)(q + 2) - 4q] = 2q^2 + 13$$
$$3[q^2 + 4q + 4 - 4q] = 2q^2 + 13$$
$$3q^2 + 12 = 2q^2 + 13$$
$$q^2 = 1$$
$$q = \pm 1$$

PROBLEM 3

Solve for a: $s(a - p) + q = ta + r^2$

PROBLEM 4

Solve for d: $\dfrac{1}{d - 2} + \dfrac{2}{d + 3} = \dfrac{4}{d - 2}$

PROBLEM 5

Solve for x: $3(4x - 2[1 - (x + 5) + 3]) = 13x + 19$

Solutions to Problems 3–5

3) $a = \dfrac{r^2 + sp - q}{s - t}$; $s(a - p) + q = ta + r^2$

$$sa - sp + q = ta + r^2$$
$$a(s - t) = r^2 + sp - q$$
$$a = \frac{r^2 + sp - q}{s - t}$$

4) $d = -13$; $\dfrac{1}{d - 2} + \dfrac{2}{d + 3} = \dfrac{4}{d - 2}$

[Multiply through by $(d - 2)(d + 3)$]

$$d + 3 + 2(d - 2) = 4(d + 3)$$
$$3d - 1 = 4d + 12$$
$$d = -13$$

5) $x = \dfrac{13}{5}$; $3(4x - 2)[1 - (x + 5) + 3]) = 13x + 19$

$$3[4x - 2(4 - x - 5)] = 13x + 19$$

$$3(4x + 2x + 2) = 13x + 19$$

$$18x + 6 = 13x + 19$$

$$x = \dfrac{13}{5}$$

Concept 4: Proportional Analysis of Algebraic Equations

Some problems can be solved by recognizing that the quantities in question are directly or inversely proportional to each other. Two variables, x and y, are directly proportional if their ratio has a constant value, a (Fig. 6-1):

$$\frac{y}{x} = a \quad \text{or} \quad y = ax$$

Consequently, for any distinct values of x, x_1, and x_2, there are corresponding values of y, y_1, and y_2, such that:

$$\frac{y_1}{x_1} = \frac{y_2}{x_2} \quad \text{(x, y directly proportional)}$$

If you know three of the terms in this proportion, you can determine the fourth term.

EXAMPLE 10

If 2 moles of compound A react with 5 moles of compound B to form 3 moles of compound C, how many moles of A are required to react completely with 7 moles of B?

In a chemical reaction, the quantities of reactants/products are directly proportional. (Why?) Let x_1 = 2 moles of A and y_1 = 5 moles of B. Then, x_2 = number of moles of A and y_2 = 7 moles of B such that:

$$\frac{5}{2} = \frac{7}{x_2}; \; x_2 = 2.8 \text{ moles of A}$$

PROBLEM 6

In example 10, how many moles of C are formed? Two variables, x and y, are inversely proportional if their product has a constant value, b (Fig. 6-2):

$$xy = b \text{ or } y = \frac{b}{x}$$

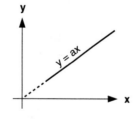

Fig. 6-1. Linear variation.

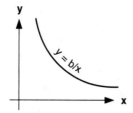

Fig. 6-2. Nonlinear/hyperbolic variation.

Consequently, for any distinct values of x, x_1, and x_2, there are corresponding values of y, y_1, and y_2, such that:

$$x_1 y_1 = x_2 y_2 \text{ or } \frac{y_1}{x_2} = \frac{y_2}{x_1} \quad (x,y \text{ inversely proportional})$$

If you know three of the terms in the equation $x_1 y_1 = x_2 y_2$, you can determine the fourth term.

EXAMPLE 11

A car traveling at x mph takes 5 hours to go from city A to city B. Traveling at $x - 15$ mph, the car makes the return trip in $6\frac{2}{3}$ hours. What was the speed of the car on the return trip? Because displacement = (speed)(time), d = vt, speed and time are inversely proportional for a constant displacement. Let $v_1 = x$ mph and $t_1 = 5$ hours; $v_2 = x - 15$ mph and $t_2 = 6\frac{2}{3}$ hours = $\frac{20}{3}$ hours. Then:

$$5x = (x - 15)\frac{20}{3}$$

$$15x = 20x - 300$$

$$5x = 300$$

$$x = 60; \; v_2 = x - 15 = 45 \text{ mph}$$

PROBLEM 7

Before an engine tune-up, a car with a gas consumption rate of r gallons per mile can go 400 miles on a full tank of gas. After a tune-up, the same car has a gas consumption rate of $r - .01$ gallons/mile and can go 500 miles on a full tank of gas. What was the gas consumption rate of the car before the tune-up?

PROBLEM 8

The ideal-gas law for 1 mole of any gas is PV = RT. Thus, two different macroscopic states of a mole of a particular gas are respectively described by

$$P_1 V_1 = RT_1 \text{ and } P_2 V_2 = RT_2$$

Write an equation that shows the relationship between these two states. According to the equation in problem 8, pressure P is inversely proportional to what quantity?

An important application of proportionality is in finding proportional changes in variables that occur when other related variables change. This application, called sensitivity analysis, is an important part of all subjects tested on the MCAT.

EXAMPLE 12

The equation for the electric field E of a point charge q at a distance r from the point charge is $E = k\,q/r^2$, in which k is a constant. If the charge is doubled and the distance from the charge is halved, how much is the field changed?

It is worth noting that E is directly proportional to q and inversely proportional to r^2 (not r).

1. Define the fields before and after the changes respectively as:

$$E_1 = k\frac{q_1}{r_1^2}, \; E_2 = k\frac{q_2}{r_2^2}$$

2. Consider the ratio E_2/E_1, which is equivalent to determining E_2 in terms of E_1, this being the desired result:

$$\frac{E_2}{E_1} = \frac{k\frac{q_2}{r_2^2}}{k\frac{q_1}{r_1^2}} = \frac{q_2}{q_1} \cdot \frac{r_1^2}{r_2^2}$$

3. Observe that the changes in q and r can be written as:

$$q_2 = 2q_1 \text{ and } r_2 = \frac{r_1}{2}$$

4. Substitute these expressions for q_2 and r_2 into the ratio E_2/E_1 to get the desired result:

$$\frac{E_2}{E_1} = \frac{2q_1}{q_1} \cdot \frac{r_1^2}{\dfrac{r_1^2}{4}} = 8 \text{ or } E_2 = 8E_1$$

The final field E_2 is eight times the original field E_1.

Important Conclusions

- If only the charge is doubled, then the field is doubled.
- If only the distance is halved, then the field is $2(2) = 4$ times the original field.
- If the charge is doubled and the distance is halved, then the field is $2(4) = 8$ times the original value.

The key point to remember is that everything that does not change will cancel out; e.g., in example 12, when considering the ratio of the value of the solved for variable, after any changes in the other variables, to its value before these changes, E_2/E_1.

PROBLEM 9

The force holding an object of mass m on a circular path is

$$F = m\frac{v^2}{r}$$

in which v = its speed and r = the radius of the circular path. How much is the force on this object changed if the radius r is reduced to one third of its original value and its speed v is halved? If the original force was 14 newtons, what is the new force on the object?

Solutions to Problems 6–9

6) $C = \dfrac{21}{5}$ moles.

Let $x_1 = 5$ moles of B and $y_1 = 3$ moles of C; then $x_2 = 7$ moles of B and $y_2 = $ number of moles of C. Because B and C are directly proportional:

$$\frac{y_2}{7} = \frac{3}{5}; y_2 = \frac{21}{5} \text{ moles of C}$$

7) r = 0.05 gallons/mile.

From the problem, $xy = a$, x = gas consumption rate (gallons/mile), y = number of miles that the car can go on a full tank of gas, a = number of gallons in full tank of gas (constant). Thus, x and y are inversely proportional with $x_1 = r$, $y_1 = 400$, $x_2 = r - 0.01$, and $y_2 = 500$

$$r(400) = (r - 0.01)500$$

$$400r = 500r - 5$$

$$r = 0.05 \text{ gallons/mile}$$

8) $\dfrac{P_1V_1}{T_1} = \dfrac{P_2V_2}{T_2}; \dfrac{V}{T}$

$P_1V_1 = RT_1$ and $P_2V_2 = RT_2$ can be rewritten as: $\dfrac{P_1V_1}{T_1} = R$ and $\dfrac{P_2V_2}{T_2} = R$. Therefore, the two states are related by $\dfrac{P_1V_1}{T_1} = \dfrac{P_2V_2}{T_2}$.

From the definition of inversely proportional variables, if P is one of the variables, then the other variable is V/T.

9) $F_2 = \tfrac{3}{4}F_1$; $F_2 = 10.5$ newtons.

$$\text{Let } F_1 = \frac{m(v_1)^2}{r_1}, F_2 = m\frac{(v_2)^2}{r_2}, \text{ then}$$

$$\frac{F_2}{F_1} = \frac{(v_2)^2}{(v_1)^2} \cdot \frac{r_1}{r_2}$$

$$r_2 = \tfrac{1}{3}\, r_1 \text{ and } v_2 = \tfrac{1}{2}\, v_1$$

$$\frac{F_2}{F_1} = \frac{\left(\dfrac{v_1}{2}\right)^2}{(v_1)^2} \frac{r_1}{\dfrac{r_1}{3}} = \frac{\tfrac{1}{4}}{\tfrac{1}{3}} = \tfrac{3}{4}$$

$$\text{or } F_1 = \tfrac{3}{4}\, F_1$$

If $F_1 = 14$ newtons, then $F_2 = \tfrac{3}{4}(14) = 10.5$ newtons.

Concept 5: Percentages Increase or Decrease

A percentage is just another way of representing a fraction or ratio. The statement x is P percent (P%) of y means that:

$$x = \frac{P}{100} \cdot y \text{ or, equivalently, } P = \frac{x}{y} \cdot 100$$

Remember that a percentage is a fraction with a denominator of 100; e.g., a nickel is 5% of one dollar.

EXAMPLE 13

What is the percent increase or decrease in a quantity x when its value is: (a) doubled, (b) halved, (c) reduced by one third, (d) reduced to one third of its original value, and (e) reduced to one fifth of its original value?

(a) $x_2 = 2x_1$; $2x_1 = x_1\left[1 + \dfrac{P}{100}\right]$; $P = 100\%$ increase

(b) $x_2 = \tfrac{1}{2}x_1$; $\tfrac{1}{2}\,x_1 = x_1\left[1 - \dfrac{P}{100}\right]$; $P = 50\%$ decrease

(c) $x_2 = \tfrac{2}{3}x_1$; $\tfrac{2}{3}x_1 = x_1\left[1 - \dfrac{P}{100}\right]$; $P = 33\tfrac{1}{3}\%$ decrease

(d) $x_2 = \tfrac{1}{3}x_1$; $\tfrac{1}{3}x_1 = x_1\left[1 - \dfrac{P}{100}\right]$; $P = 66\tfrac{2}{3}\%$ decrease

(e) $x_2 = \dfrac{1}{5x_1}$; $\dfrac{1}{5x_1} = x_1\left[1 - \dfrac{P}{100}\right]$; $P = 80\%$ decrease

PROBLEM 10

In 1984, a particular item A cost $2,500. In 1986, the price of A rose 20% because of scarcity. In early 1987, the price of A rose 10% over its 1986 price. At the end of 1987, item A was put on sale with a 30% decrease in price. What was the sale price of A?

Solution to Problem 10
Sale price (1987) is $2,310.

$$\text{1984: cost of A} = \$2,500$$

$$\text{1986: cost of A} = \$2,500 + \frac{20}{100} \cdot \$2,500$$

$$= \$3,000$$

$$\text{1987: cost of A} = \$3,000 + \frac{10}{100} \cdot \$3,000$$

$$= \$3,300$$

$$\text{Sale price (1987)} = \$3,300 - \frac{30}{100} \cdot \$3,300$$

$$= \$2,310$$

Concept 6: Exponentials

The simplest use of exponentials is as a shorthand way of symbolizing a repeated multiplication of a number by itself, e.g., $10^3 = 10 \cdot 10 \cdot 10$, in which 10^3 is the exponential expression for this repeated multiplication of 10 by itself. The exponential expression 10^3 is also another way of expressing the number 1,000. In general, for

$$y = x^n = x \cdot x \cdot x \ldots x \leftarrow n \text{ factors of } x$$

in which x^n is defined as an exponential form of y, x as the base, and n as the exponent. In this definition, x can be any number except zero and n is a positive integer.

Rules for Exponentials

The following discussion includes 10 rules for using exponentials. Refer to the chart of rules in exponential algebra at the end of this section when solving problems.

Using the definition for exponentials stated previously, three basic rules for arithmetic operations with exponentials are:

$$1: \quad x^m \cdot x^n = x^{m+n}$$

$$2: \quad \frac{x^m}{x^n} = x^{m-n} \quad m,n \text{ are positive integers; } x \neq 0$$

$$3: \quad (x^m)^n = x^{mn}$$

(Note that the addition/subtraction of exponentials is deferred until the subsequent discussion of scientific notation.) By manipulating these basic exponent rules, we can show:

$$4: \quad x^0 = 1; \; x^0 = x^{n-n} = \frac{x^n}{x^n} = 1$$

$$5: \quad x^{-m} = \frac{1}{x^m}; \; x^{-m} = x^{0-m} = \frac{x^0}{x^m} = \frac{1}{x^m}$$

EXAMPLE 14

Evaluate each expression:

1. $10^2 \cdot \dfrac{10^3}{10^{15}} = 10^{2+3-15} = 10^{-10}$

2. $\left[3^6 \cdot 3^3 \cdot \dfrac{9}{3^0} \cdot 3^{-4} \right]^2 = (3^{6+3+2-0-4})^2 = (3^7)^2 = 3^{7\cdot2} = 3^{14}$

3. $(\frac{1}{4})^{-2} = \dfrac{1}{(\frac{1}{4})^2} = \dfrac{1}{\frac{1}{16}} = 16$

PROBLEM 11

Evaluate each expression:

(a) $4^4 \cdot \dfrac{4^8}{4^5}$

(b) $\left[\dfrac{6^4}{6^2} \right]^3 \cdot 6^{-5}$

(c) $(7^4)^0$

The present discussion of exponentials can be extended to include nonintegral (any real number) exponents. A radical is just a fractional exponent:

$$6: \quad x^{1/n} = \sqrt[n]{x}; \; (\sqrt[n]{x})^n = x \text{ (by definition)}$$

$$(x^m)^n = x \text{ (by letting } x^m = \sqrt[n]{x})$$

$$x^{mn} = x^1$$

$$\text{thus } mn = 1; \; m = \frac{1}{n}$$

It therefore follows in a straightforward manner that:

$$7: \quad x^{m/n} \;=\; (\sqrt[n]{x})^m \;=\; (\sqrt[n]{x^m})$$

$$8: \quad x^{-m/n} \;=\; \left(\frac{1}{x^{m/n}} \;=\; \frac{1}{\sqrt[n]{x^m}}\right) \;=\; \frac{1}{(\sqrt[n]{x})^m}$$

(Note that m and n at this point are still positive integers.)

In these last two exponent rules, an exponent m/n can be any rational number (recall that any rational number can be written as a fraction of two integers). Moreover, because any irrational number can be approximated by a rational number, we can define:

$$y = x^p$$

in which the base x is any number except zero and the exponent p is any real number. If p is not an integer, it represents the combined operations of an integral exponent m and an nth root on the number x where p equals (exactly or approximately if it is irrational) m/n. In other words, the basic exponent rules 1–3 apply for m, n = real numbers, not just positive integers. Finally, observe that:

$$9: \quad (x \cdot y)^n \;=\; x^n \cdot y^n$$

$$10: \quad \left(\frac{x}{y}\right)^n \;=\; \frac{x^n}{y^n}$$

EXAMPLE 15

Find the value of each expression:

1. $8^{4/3} = \sqrt[3]{8^4} = (4{,}096)^{1/3} = 16$

   $\qquad = (\sqrt[3]{8})^4 = 2^4 = 16$

2. $(289x)^{3/2} = (289^3)^{1/2}\, x^{3/2}$

   $\qquad\qquad = (289^{1/2})^3\, x^{3/2} = 17^3 \cdot x^{3/2} = 4913x^{3/2}$

3. $8^6 \cdot 8^3 \cdot \dfrac{\sqrt[3]{8}}{8^{5/3}} \cdot 8^{-7} = 8^{6+3+1/3-5/3-7}$

   $\qquad\qquad\qquad = 8^{2/3} = (8^{1/3})^2 = 2^2 = 4$

PROBLEM 12

Find the value of each expression:

(a) $216^{4/3}$

(b) $256^{3/4}$

(c) $\sqrt{ab} \cdot \dfrac{\sqrt[4]{a^3 \cdot b^3)}}{\sqrt[3]{a^2 \cdot b^2}}$

(d) $\left[\dfrac{3}{5}\right]^{-8} \left[\dfrac{9}{25}\right]^3$

Use the following chart in solving problems.

Rules in Exponential Algebra

1:	$x^m \cdot x^n$	$= x^{m+n}$	$3^2 \cdot 3^3$	$= 3^{2+3} = 243$
2:	$\dfrac{x^m}{x^n}$	$= x^{m-n}$	$\dfrac{3^2}{3^3}$	$= 3^{2-3} = 3^{-1} = \frac{1}{3}$
3:	$(x^m)^n$	$= x^{mn}$	$(3^2)^3$	$= 3^6 = 729$
4:	x^0	$= 1$	3^0	$= 1$

(x is any real positive number)

5:	x^{-m}	$= \dfrac{1}{x^m}$	3^{-2}	$= \dfrac{1}{3^2}$	$= \dfrac{1}{9}$
6:	$x^{1/n}$	$= \sqrt[n]{x}$	$3^{1/2}$	$= \sqrt[2]{3}$	$= \sqrt{3}$

(It is customary to ignore the 2 in $\sqrt[2]{3}$. The figure $\sqrt{3}$ represents the square root of 3.)

7:    $x^{m/n} = (\sqrt[n]{x})^m = \sqrt[n]{x^m}$ $3^{2/3} = (\sqrt[3]{3})^2 = \sqrt[3]{9}$

(The figure $\sqrt[3]{9}$ represents the cube root of 9.)

8:    $x^{-m/n} = \dfrac{1}{x^{m/n}} = \dfrac{1}{\sqrt[n]{x^m}} = \dfrac{1}{(\sqrt[n]{x})m}$

$3^{-2/3} = (\sqrt[3]{3})^{-2} = \sqrt[3]{\dfrac{1}{3^2}} = \sqrt[3]{\dfrac{1}{9}}$

9:    $(x \cdot y)^n = x^n y^n \quad (3 \cdot 4)^3 = 3^3 \cdot 4^3 = 27 \cdot 64 = 1728$

10:    $\left[\dfrac{x}{y}\right]n = \dfrac{x^n}{y^n} \quad (\tfrac{3}{4})^3 = \dfrac{3^3}{4^3} = \dfrac{27}{64}$

Solutions to Problems 11 and 12

11a) $4^4 \cdot \dfrac{4^8}{4^5} = 4^{4+8-5} = 4^7$

b) $\left[\dfrac{6^4}{6^2}\right]^3 \cdot 6^{-5} = (6^2)^3 \cdot 6^{-5} = 6^{6-5} = 6$

c) $(7^4)^0 = 1$; recall $x^0 = 1$

12a) $216^{4/3} = (\sqrt[3]{216^4}) = 6^4 = 1296$

           $= 216^1 \cdot (\sqrt[3]{216}) = 216 \cdot 6 = 1296$

b) $256^{3/4} = (256^{1/4})^3 = 4^3 = 64$

c) $\sqrt{ab} \cdot \dfrac{\sqrt[4]{a^3 b^3}}{\sqrt[3]{a^2 b^2}} = \dfrac{(ab)^{1/2}(ab)^{3/4}}{(ab)^{2/3}}$

           $= (ab)^{1/2+3/4-2/3} = (ab)^{6/12+9/12-8/12} = (ab)^{7/12}$

d) $\left[\dfrac{3}{5}\right]^{-8}\left[\dfrac{9}{25}\right]^3 = \dfrac{3^{-8}}{5^{-8}} \cdot \dfrac{3^6}{5^6} = \dfrac{3^{-2}}{5^{-2}} = \dfrac{5^2}{3^2} = \dfrac{25}{9}$

Concept 7: Scientific Notation

Scientific notation is a convenient method for writing large and small numbers using powers of 10. It is essentially an application of exponentials. A number is said to be in standard scientific notation when it is written in the form:

$$X = a \times 10^m$$

in which a is between 1 and 10 and m is an integral exponent.

EXAMPLE 15a

$$29980000000 \text{ cm/sec} = 2.998 \times 10^{10} \text{ cm/sec}$$

EXAMPLE 15b

$$0.001234 = 1.234 \times 10^3$$

Standard scientific notation does not always have to be used. In examples 15a and b, the numbers could be rewritten as:

EXAMPLE 16a

$$2.998 \times 10^{10} \text{ cm/sec} = 0.2998 \times 10^{11} \text{ cm/sec}$$

$$2.998 \times 10^{10} \text{ cm/sec} = 29.98 \times 10^9 \text{ cm/sec}$$

$$1.234 \times 10^{-3} = 0.1234 \times 10^{-2}$$
$$1.234 \times 10^{-3} = 12.34 \times 10^{-4}$$

Observe that when the decimal point moves one place to the left, the power of 10 increases by 1, and that when the decimal point moves one place to the right, the power of 10 decreases by 1. The arithmetic operations for numbers written in scientific notation are as follows. Recall that to add and subtract numbers in scientific notation, the numbers must be in terms of the same power of 10.

Addition/Subtraction

EXAMPLE **17**

$$3 \times 10^3 + 4 \times 10^3 = 7 \times 10^3$$

EXAMPLE **18**

$$3 \times 10^3 + 4 \times 10^4 = 0.3 \times 10^4 + 4 \times 10^4 = 4.3 \times 10^4$$

Multiplication

$$(a \times 10^m)(b \times 10^n) = (ab) \times 10^{m+n}$$

Division

$$\frac{a \times 10^m}{b \times 10^n} = \left[\frac{a}{b}\right] \times 10^{m-n}$$

Exponents

$$(a \times 10^m)^n = (a^n) \times 10^{mn}$$

EXAMPLE **19**

$$(6.6 \times 10^{12})(1.1 \times 10^{-3}) = (6.6)(1.1) \times 10^{12-3} = 7.26 \times 10^9$$

EXAMPLE **20**

$$\frac{1.8 \times 10^7}{7.2 \times 10^{-10}} = \frac{18 \times 10^6}{7.2 \times 10^{-10}} = \left(\frac{18}{7.2}\right) \times 10^{6-(-10)} = 2.5 \times 10^{16}$$

EXAMPLE **21**

$$(1.2 \times 10^3)^3 = (1.2)^3 \times 10^{3 \cdot 3} = 1.728 \times 10^9$$

PROBLEM **13**
Put in terms of standard scientific notation:

(a)   3430000

(b)   0.000000000824

PROBLEM **14**
Find the value of each expression (in standard scientific notation):

(a) $\dfrac{(4 \times 10^{16})(7 \times 10^{-5})}{(3.455 \times 10^4) - (3.427 \times 10^4)}$

(b) $\dfrac{7 \times 10^7 - 2.8 \times 10^{-6}}{10^{-7} + 1.24 \times 10^{-6} - 1.02 \times 10^{-6}}$

(c) $[(6 \times 10^4)(9 \times 10^3)(4 \times 10^{-1})]^{\frac{1}{3}}$

Solutions to Problems 13 and 14

13a) 3.43×10^6

b) 8.24×10^{10}

14a) $\dfrac{(4 \times 10^{16})(7 \times 10^{-5})}{(3.455 \times 10^4) - (3.427 \times 10^4)} = \dfrac{28 \times 10^{11}}{0.028 \times 10^4} = \dfrac{28 \times 10^{11}}{28 \times 10^1} = 10^{10}$

b) $\dfrac{7 \times 10^7 - 2.8 \times 10^{-6}}{10^{-7} + 1.24 \times 10^{-6} - 1.02 \times 10^{-6}}$

$= \dfrac{70 \times 10^6 - 2.8 \times 10^6}{1 \times 10^{-7} + 12.4 \times 10^{-7} - 10.2 \times 10^{-7}}$

$= \dfrac{67.2 \times 10^6}{3.2 \times 10^{-7}} = \left(\dfrac{67.2}{3.2}\right) \times 10^{6-(-7)} = 21 \times 10^{13}$

$= 2.1 \times 10^{14}$

c) $[(6 \times 10^4)(9 \times 10^3)(4 \times 10^{-1})]^{1/3}$

$= [(6 \times 9 \times 4) \times 10^{4+3-1}]^{1/3}$

$= (216 \times 10^6)^{1/3} = (216)^{1/3} \times 10^{6 \cdot 1/3} = 6 \times 10^2$

Concept 8: Logarithms

Calculators have largely replaced the use of logarithms in solving problems. You cannot use calculators on the MCAT, however, and so learning common logarithms is essential for solving science problems. Conceptually, they are still important for topics such as pH, sound intensity, exponential decay, and growth problems.

In the discussion of exponentials, you learned that:

- $x^m \cdot x^n = x^{m+n}$
- $\dfrac{x^m}{x^n} = x^{m-n}$
- $(x^m)^n = x^{mn}$
- $x^0 = 1$
- $x^{-m} = \dfrac{1}{x^m}$

in which x is any number except zero, and m,n are any real numbers. Logarithms arise when one considers that, by assuming a particular base x, these exponent rules could be rewritten in terms of the exponents only. We define the logarithm of a number M as the power (exponent) m to which a base x must be raised to give the number M; that is, if $M = x^m$, then $m = $ logarithm of M with respect to the base x. This expression is usually written $m = \log_x M$; if $N = x^n$, then $n = \log_x N$, etc.

By definition, logarithms are simply exponents:

$$X^{\log_x M} = M$$

(Take the log (base X) of both sides of this equation.)

EXAMPLE 22

Write each expression in its equivalent logarithmic form.

1. If $8^3 = 512$, then $\log_8 512 = 3$

2. If $10^{4.6990} = 50{,}000$, then $\log_{10} 50{,}000 = 4.6990$

3. If $2^{-2} = \frac{1}{4}$, then $\log_2(\frac{1}{4}) = -2$

EXAMPLE 23

Find the value of x.

1. $\log_2 32 = x \quad \rightarrow 2^x = 32; \ x = 5$

2. $\log_5 1 = x \quad \rightarrow 5^x = 1; \ x = 0$

3. $\log_m (m^{10}) = x \rightarrow m^x = m^{10}; \ x = 10$

4. $2^{\log_2 3} = x \quad \rightarrow \log_2 3 = \log_2 x; \ x = 3$

5. $4^{\log_4 16} = x \quad \rightarrow \log_4 16 = \log_4 x; \ x = 16$

Rules of Logarithms

Using logarithms, five rules for exponentials can now be rewritten as:

Rule 1: $\log_x M + \log_x N = \log_x (MN)$

Rule 2: $\log_x M - \log_x N = \log_x \left[\dfrac{M}{N}\right]$

Rule 3: $\log_x (M^n) = n(\log_x M)$

Rule 4: $\log_x 1 = 0$

Rule 5: $\log_x \left[\dfrac{1}{M}\right] = \log_x (M^{-1}) = -\log_x M$

$(\log_{10} M$ is usually written as $\log M)$

EXAMPLE 24

If $\log 2 = 0.3010$ and $\log 3 = 0.4774$, then:

1. $\log 6 = \log (2 \cdot 3) = \log 2 + \log 3 = 0.3010 + 0.4774 = 0.7784$

2. $\log 5 = \log \left[\dfrac{10}{2}\right] = \log 10 - \log 2 = 1 - 0.3010 = 0.6990$

3. $\log 8 = \log (2^3) = 3(\log 2) = 3(0.3010) = 0.9030$

4. $\log 60 = \log (2 \cdot 3 \cdot 10) = \log 2 + \log 3 + \log 10 = 0.3010 + 0.4774 + 1 = 1.7784$

EXAMPLE 25

Solve for x.

$$2\log x = \log a + \log b - \log c$$

$$\log x^2 = \log \left(\dfrac{ab}{c}\right)$$

$$x^2 = \dfrac{ab}{c}$$

$$x = \sqrt[\pm]{\dfrac{ab}{c}}$$

PROBLEM 15

Express as a single logarithm:

(a) $\log M^2 + 7\log N - \frac{1}{3}\log P$

(b) $\log\sqrt{x^5} - 3\log \sqrt[4]{x} + \log x^3$

PROBLEM 16

Solve for x.

(a) $\log_9 (x + 1) = \frac{1}{2}$

(b) $3\log x = 2\log a + 3\log b + 4\log c - 5\log d$

The two most common bases used for logarithms are 10 (common logarithms) and e (natural logarithms). In a sense, common logarithms are an extension of scientific notation in that the coefficient of the power of 10 (which is between 1 and 10) is also written as a power of 10. Thus, the number in question is written completely as an exponential using the base 10. Consider:

$$y = a \times 10^b \text{ (define } a = 10^c)$$

$$= 10^c \times 10^b = 10^{c+b}$$

$$\log y = c + b$$

in which c is the mantissa and b is the characteristic. The base of natural logarithms, e, is an irrational number that is approximately equal to 2.71828. Natural logarithms and the base e play an important part in many scientific problems, e.g., exponential growth and decay. A basic understanding of logarithms is sufficient for the MCAT. Use the basic principles just presented to work on advanced science problems on your own.

Solutions to Problems 15 and 16

15a) $\log M^2 + 7\log N - \frac{1}{3}\log P$

$$= \log M^2 + \log N^7 - \log\sqrt[3]{P} = \log\left[\frac{M^2N^7}{\sqrt[3]{P}}\right]$$

b) $\log\sqrt{x^5} - 3\log\sqrt[4]{x} + \log x^3$

$$= \log x^{5/2} - \log x^{3/4} + \log x^3$$

$$= \frac{5}{2}\log x - \frac{3}{4}\log x + 3\log x$$

$$= \left(\frac{5}{2} - \frac{3}{4} + 3\right)\log x = \frac{19}{4}\log x = \log x^{19/4}$$

16a) $\log_9(x + 1) = \frac{1}{2} \rightarrow x + 1 = 9^{1/2} = 3$

$$x = 2$$

b) $3\log x = 2\log a + 3\log b + 4\log c - 5\log d$

$$\log x = \frac{1}{3}(\log a^2 + \log b^3 + \log c^4 - \log d^5)$$

$$\log x = \log\left[\frac{a^2b^3c^4}{d^5}\right]^{1/3}$$

$$x = \left(\frac{a^2b^3c^4}{d^5}\right)^{\frac{1}{3}}$$

ANALYTIC GEOMETRY

A working knowledge of analytic geometry is required for successful completion of the MCAT, with a primary focus on the interpretation of information presented in a graphical format, e.g., determining slopes of lines and curves, finding intercepts, and determining equations for experimental curves. The *MCAT Student Manual* states that the premedical student should be able to remember and use important, basic formulas to calculate areas and volumes. Such calculations are used routinely in health science professions, for example, to determine cross-sectional areas of any human artery or vein, volume of blood pumped by the heart, total surface area of the body, area of a cast, and volume of air/oxygen capacity of lungs. Knowledge of the geometry formulas that follow is also useful in the physical and biological sciences subtests.

By memorizing basic formulas, you can:

- facilitate your problem-solving ability and be able to work faster
- improve your mental proportional reasoning ability
- increase your confidence

Plane Geometry

The most commonly used geometric shapes and formulas are provided in Figure 6-3. Learn to apply them to ordinary geometry problems.

Concept 9: Cartesian or Rectangular Coordinate System

The Cartesian coordinate system consists of two perpendicular axes, each representing a variable (Fig. 6-4). The intersection of the two axes in the Cartesian plane is called the origin (O). The origin splits each axis into two segments that respectively represent positive and negative values of that axis's variable. The standard positive (+) and negative (−) segments of each axis are labeled; arrows indicate the directions of positive change for each axis's variable.

Each point in the Cartesian plane is represented by a pair of coordinates (an ordered pair), each of which represents a displacement from the origin along one of the axes [e.g., the point P = (x,y) on the graph above and the origin O = (0,0)]. The first coordinate in the ordered pair is defined as the abscissa or the independent coordinate; the second coordinate is defined as the ordinate or the dependent coordinate.

The abscissa and ordinate are labeled x and y, respectively, unless otherwise specified. With these coordinate labels, the Cartesian plane can be referred to as the xy-plane. Depending on the data or function being graphed, all or part of the xy-plane is used.

Triangle

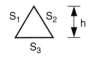

Perimeter = $S_1 + S_2 + S_3$, b = S_3
Area = 1/2 base x height = $(1/2)hS_3$

Square

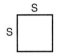

Perimeter = 4S
Area = S x S or S^2

Rectangle

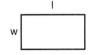

Perimeter = 2(l+w) or 2l + 2w
Area = lw

Fig. 6-3. Common geometric shapes.

Parallelogram

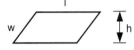

Perimeter = 2(l+w) or 2l + 2w
Area = hl

Trapezoid

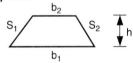

Perimeter = $b_1+b_2+S_1+S_2$

Area = $h\left(\dfrac{b_1+b_2}{2}\right)$

[Hint: draw a diagonal and find the area by summing the areas of the two triangles.]

Circle

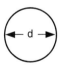

Circumference = $2\pi r$ or πd
Area = πr^2
[Note: r = d/2]

Right triangle (Pythagorean theorem)

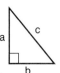

$a^2 + b^2 = c^2$
The sum of the squares of the legs of a right triangle equals the square of the hypotenuse

Cube

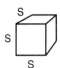

Volume = S x S x S or S^3
Surface area = S x S x 6

Rectangular prism

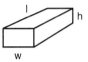

Volume = l x w x h
Surface area = 2(lw) + 2(lb) + 2(wh)

Closed right circular cylinder

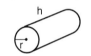

Volume = $\pi r^2 h$
Surface area = $2(\pi r^2) + h(2\pi r)$

Sphere

Volume = 4/3 πr^3
Surface area = $4\pi r^2$

When discussing the relation between two variables, it may be possible or necessary to say that one variable is independent and the other is dependent. When dealing with data, an independent variable is one with values that are predetermined by the experimenter; the dependent variable is then determined for each of the values of the independent variable (it is then dependent on them). When dealing with functions, if y is a function of x, then x is the independent variable on the x-axis and the dependent variable on the y-axis.

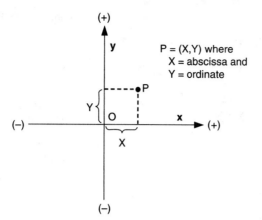

Fig. 6-4. Cartesian coordinate system.

What are Graphs?

Graphs are constructed by plotting values of one variable against the corresponding values of a second variable, i.e., by plotting a set of ordered pairs, as determined by experiments, equations, or some other known relationship between them.

EXAMPLE 26

An experimenter determines the pairs of values for two related variables, x and y (Fig. 6-5). Plotting these points and connecting them by straight line segments generates the graph in Figure 6-6.

x	-2	+3	+4	+5	+6
y	-6	-4	+16	+18	+10

Fig. 6-5.

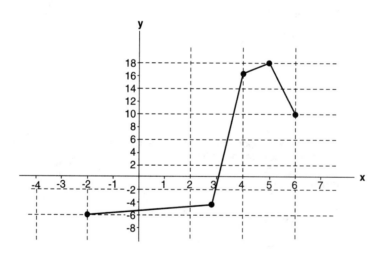

Fig. 6-6.

Concept 10: Graphic Representation of Functions

EXAMPLE 27

Graph $y = \dfrac{a}{1 + x}$ for $x \geq 0$ (reciprocal function). Assume $a > 0$.

Using this function, possible pairs of values for x and y are shown in Figure 6-7. Graphing these points and connecting them by a curve to represent $y = \dfrac{a}{1 + x}$ for $x \geq 0$ generates the graph in Figure 6-8.

EXAMPLE 28

Graph the relationship between two variables, x and y, which are defined in terms of a third variable, t, as: $y = 3t + 1$; $x = 2t$ (three-variable equation).

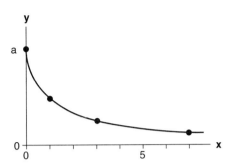

x	0	1	3	7
y	a	$\frac{a}{2}$	$\frac{a}{4}$	$\frac{a}{8}$

Fig. 6-7.

Fig. 6-8.

Using these functions to get ordered pairs for (x,y) (Fig. 6-9) generates the graph shown in Figure 6-10.

Note that this graph can also be represented algebraically:

$$y = \frac{3}{2}x + 1$$

t	-1	0	1	2	3
x	-2	0	2	4	6
y	-2	1	4	7	10

Fig. 6-9.

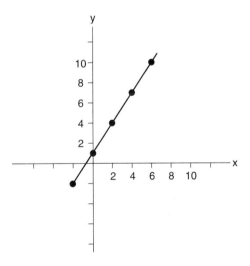

Fig. 6-10.

PROBLEM 17

Graph $y = \frac{5x}{1 + x}$ for $x \geq 0$, after first identifying the ordered pairs for x = 0, 1, 4, 9. As x increases, what value does y approach?

Solution to Problem 17

The ordered pairs requested are: (0,0), (1,5⁄2), (4,4), and (9,4.5). Plotting these four points and drawing a curve through them for $x \geq 0$ yields the graph shown in Figure 6-11.

Applied Math Concepts Required for Physical and Biological Sciences 129

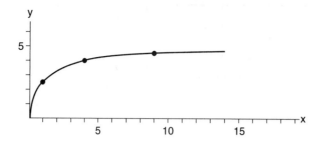

Fig. 6-11.

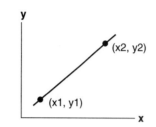

Fig. 6-12.

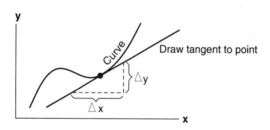

Fig. 6-13. Definition of slope for straight and curved lines.

Measure $\triangle x$, $\triangle y$ for any two points on tangent

Slope $= m = \dfrac{\triangle y}{\triangle x}$ (changes along the curve)

As x gets large, $x \gg 1$, so $y = \dfrac{5x}{1 + x} \cong \dfrac{5x}{x} = 5$. Thus, the value of y approaches 5 as x increases.

Concept 11: Slope or Rate of Change

An important parameter when interpreting the relationship between the two variables in a graph is the slope. The slope of the line segment between two points is defined as the ratio of the change in the ordinate to the change in the abscissa:

$$\text{Slope} = \frac{\text{Change in ordinate}}{\text{Change in abscissa)}} = \frac{\Delta y}{\Delta x}$$

$$= \frac{\text{Rise}}{\text{Run}} = \frac{\text{Change in dependent variable}}{\text{Change in independent variable}}$$

A slope exists at every point on a smooth graph, whether it is a straight line or a curved line. For each point on a graph, the slope is the rate of change (positive or negative) in the ordinate with respect to the change in the abscissa. It may be constant as for straight lines or portions of curves that are straight, or it may be constantly changing as for curved lines. In practice, the slope is calculated for straight (Fig. 6-12) and curved (Fig. 6-13) lines as follows:

For straight lines:

$$\text{Slope} = m = \frac{y_2 - y_1}{x_2 - x_1} = \frac{\Delta y}{\Delta x} = \text{constant}$$

For curved lines:

Measure $\dfrac{\Delta y}{\Delta x}$ for any two points on tangent.

$$\text{Slope} = m = \frac{\Delta y}{\Delta x} \text{ (changes along the curve)}$$

EXAMPLE **29**

Calculate the slope of the line graphed in Figure 6-14.

$$m = \frac{y_2 - y_1}{x_2 - x_1}$$

$$= \frac{8 - 3}{13 - 1}$$

$$= \frac{5}{12}$$

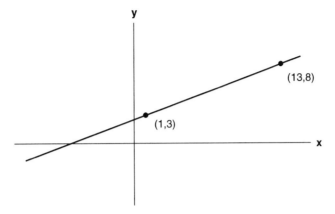

Fig. 6-14.

PROBLEM **18**

Calculate the slope of the line graphed in Figure 6-15 (use the two points indicated).

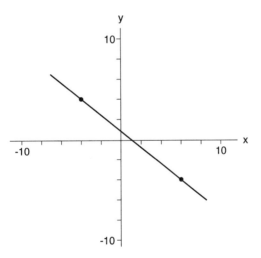

Fig. 6-15.

Large Slope Versus Small Slope

Because vertical lines have slopes $= \pm \infty$ and horizontal lines have slopes $= 0$, the more vertical the line, the larger the magnitude of the slope. In Figure 6-16, the magnitudes of slopes in A and C are greater than those of slopes in B and D, respectively.

Fig. 6-16. Sign convention and magnitude of slope. Magnitudes of slopes in A and C are greater than those of slopes in B and D, respectively.

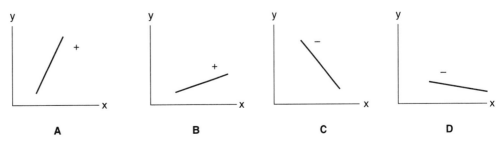

Calculate the slopes of lines 1 and 2 in Figure 6-17. Which line has the slope of greater magnitude?

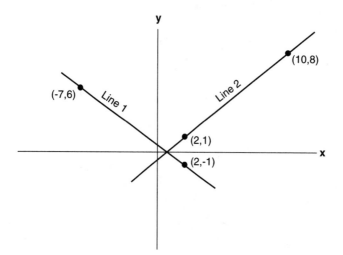

Fig. 6-17.

At which of the three points indicated on the graph in Figure 6-18 is the slope the greatest?

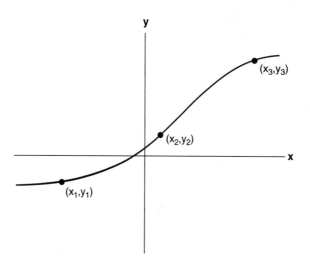

Fig. 6-18.

Maximum and Minimum Points

The relation between two variables often has local maximum point(s) and/or minimum point(s) that appear on graphs, as shown in Figures 6-19 and 6-20.

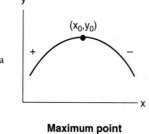

Fig. 6-19. Maximum point on a curve.

Maximum point

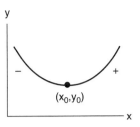

Fig. 6-20. Minimum point on a curve.

(x₀,y₀)

Minimum point

Area Under the Graph

If the quantity represented on the vertical axis is considered to vary as a function of the quantity measured on the horizontal axis, and if the product of these two quantities has meaning [e.g., distance = (speed)(time)], then the area under the graph also represents an important quantity. This area (called A) represents the continuous product of these variables over the interval shown on the horizontal axis.

EXAMPLE **30**

Consider the graph in Figure 6-21. Note that because v is constantly increasing with t, the acceleration is constant; so $v = at$. The area of the triangle for a particular time is $t_0 = \dfrac{(v_0 t_0)}{2} = \dfrac{(at_0^2)}{2}$. The distance formula for uniform acceleration is $s = \dfrac{(at^2)}{2}$. (Recall that $s = vt_0$ holds only when v is constant or an average value over the time between $t = 0$ and $t = t_0$.)

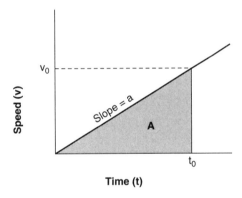

A = (speed) (time)
= distance traveled from time t = 0 to time t = t₀

Fig. 6-21.

The area under the graph, A, and the slope, $\dfrac{\Delta y}{\Delta x}$, are related in the sense that the ordinate in a graph describes how fast A is changing in the same way that the slope describes how fast the ordinate is changing. In example 30, the ordinate v describes how fast s is changing in the same way that the slope = a describes how fast v is changing.

When interpreting the information in a graph, the slope at a particular point on the graph is a more important quantity than the corresponding area under the graph (A). Area A should be kept in mind when analyzing a graph, however, especially when the product of the variables represented on the axes has meaning in terms of representing a third variable.

Solutions to Problems 18–20

18) The two points indicated are $(-4,4)$ and $(6,-4)$. Let $(x_2,y_2) = (6,-4)$ and $(x_1,y_1) = (-4,4)$; then:

$$\text{Slope} = \frac{y_2 - y_1}{x_2 - x_1} = \frac{-4 - 4}{6 - (-4)} = \frac{-8}{10} = \frac{-4}{5}$$

Applied Math Concepts Required for Physical and Biological Sciences   133

19) For line 1, let $(x_2, y_2) = (2, -1)$ and $(x_1, y_1) = (-7, 6)$; then:

$$\text{Slope of line 1} = \frac{y_2 - y_1}{x_2 - x_1} = \frac{-1 - 6}{2 - (-7)} = \frac{-7}{9}$$

$$\text{Magnitude of the slope of line 1} = \frac{7}{9}$$

For line 2, let $(x_2, y_2) = (10, 8)$ and $(x_1, y_1) = (2, 1)$; then:

$$\text{Slope of line 2} = \frac{y_2 - y_1}{x_2 - x_1} = \frac{8 - 1}{10 - 2} = \frac{7}{8};$$

$$\text{Magnitude of the slope of line 2} = \frac{7}{8}$$

Therefore, line 2 has the slope of greater magnitude ($\frac{7}{8} > \frac{7}{9}$).

20) Draw the tangent at each of the three points in Figure 6-22:

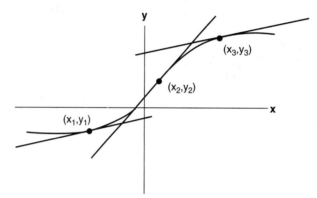

Fig. 6-22.

By inspection, the slope at (x^2, y^2) is the greatest. (See interpretation of sigmoid curve in the discussion of basic graphs.)

Concept 12: Graphic Interpretation of Basic Functions

The interpretation of a second or higher degree function represented by the graph should involve the following steps:

1. Carefully analyze each axis as to:
   a. what variable it represents
   b. the units (scale) used and the range of values on both axes
2. Estimate the overall shape of the graph. Can that lead to classification of linear, hyperbolic, or parabolic functions?
3. Estimate the slope at various points of the function. Is the slope constant or changing? Is the slope the quantity of greatest interest?
4. If the slope is changing, are there any maximum, minimum, or inflection points? If so, is their identification critical to answering the questions asked?
5. Estimate the area under the graph only for specific situations.

The purpose of interpreting a function is to determine whether a mathematical connection or relationship exists between the two variables in it. The graphs in the following review tend to recur in medicine and biology and have well-known functional interpretations of the relations between the variables in them. These commonly encountered graphs are basically examples of interpretation of the quadratic or exponential functions discussed previously.

Linear Functions
The linear (straight line) graph is the simplest type of graph. Any straight line can be described by the equation $y = mx + b$ in which x (usually the abscissa) and y (usually the ordinate) are the two variables, m is the slope of the line, and b is the y-intercept (the value of y when $x = 0$). As observed previously, for any two points (x_1, y_1) and (x_2, y_2) on a straight line:

$$m = \frac{y_2 - y_1}{x_2 - x_1} = \frac{\Delta y}{\Delta x}$$

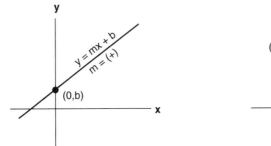
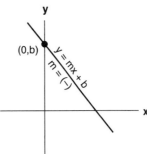

Fig. 6-23. Slope and intercept of straight lines on linear graphs.

Thus, observe that Δy is directly proportional to Δx; observe also that y is directly proportional to x when b = 0. Examples of linear graphs are shown in Figure 6-23.

When the slope is negative, x increases as y decreases and vice versa. Note, however, that y and x are not inversely proportional (see next function considered), in which case they would be related in a nonlinear manner. The basic interpretation for linear functions is that a constant relationship (as given by the slope) exists between x and y.

Hyperbolic Functions

A hyperbolic function results when two variables, x and y, are inversely proportional: xy = a, in which a is a constant. Consider the hyperbolic graphs in Figure 6-24.

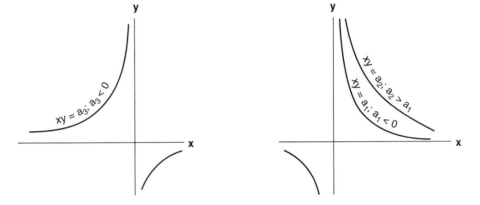

Fig. 6-24. Hyperbolic functions (nonlinear graphs).

Observe that because xy = a is a nonlinear relation for x and y, the slope is different at every point in a hyperbolic graph. Note also that hyperbolic graphs approach but never reach the x- and y-axes; consequently, the x- and y-axes are called the asymptotes in these graphs.

Parabolic Functions

In the xy-plane, a general parabola can usually be described algebraically by $y = ax^2 + bx + c$ or $x = my^2 + ny + p$ in which a, b, c, m, n, and p are constants. Three parabolic functions, with positive values of x and y, are shown in Figure 6-25.

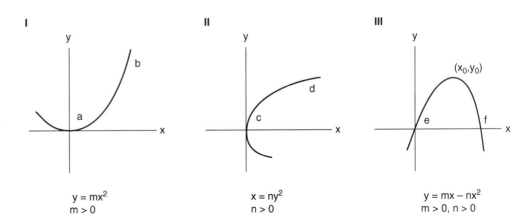

Fig. 6-25. Parabolic functions.

Graph I shows an initially nearly flat slope (region a) that rapidly becomes large (region b). For graph II, the opposite interpretation ensues. A large slope (region c) gives way to a larger region (region d), where the slope is flatter. Graph III shows an initially high positive slope (region e) that decreases to zero at a maximum point (x_0, y_0) and then becomes negative, increasingly so as the x-axis is approached (region f). Note that the slopes at (b), (e), and (f) are not of infinite magnitude and also that the slope at (d) is not zero.

Special Functions in Biologic Sciences

The curve in Figure 6-26 is common in many biochemical situations.

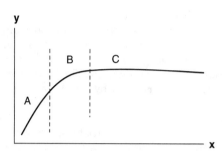

Fig. 6-26. Segmental analysis of slope (three segments).

In this graph, $y = \dfrac{ax}{b + x}$; a, b = positive constants. The limit $x \ll b$ implies that $y = \dfrac{ax}{(b + x)} \approx \dfrac{ax}{b}$ (region A), whereas the limit $x \gg b$ implies that $y = \dfrac{ax}{(b + x)} \cong a$ (region C).

Another graph found in many situations, such as population growth (biology), is the sigmoid or s-shaped curve (Fig. 6-27):

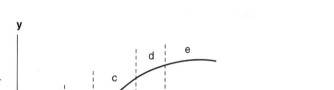

Fig. 6-27. Segmental analysis of slope (five segments),

It can be divided into five phases (or less):

1. An initial latent phase of small positive slope (region a)
2. An accelerative phase of rapidly increasing slope (region b)
3. A phase of fairly constant high positive slope (region c) and note that there is an inflection point where the slope reaches its maximum value in this region
4. A decelerative phase of rapidly decreasing slope (region d)
5. A phase of essentially zero slope (region e)

In general, these curves represent situations in which a latency phase (region a) exists before a phase of rapid changes in y for a given change in x (region c), the latter phase being followed by a phase of saturation of the system with x (region e).

Exponential Functions

Exponential relations between variables are common. In the exponential curves in Figure 6-28, assume $A > 0$.

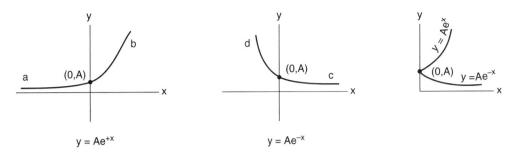

Fig. 6-28. Exponential functions.

$$y = Ae^{+x}$$

$$y = Ae^{-x}$$

Regions a and c approach the x-axis as an asymptote. Regions b and d approach no asymptote, but increase rapidly with ever increasing slopes. Graph I shows exponential growth. Graph II shows exponential decay. Only positive values of x for exponential functions are displayed in graph III. All three graphs have y-intercepts at (0, A). These functions are useful in solving radioactivity decay problems and carbon dating.

PROBLEM 21

A linear graph can be algebraically described by the equation $8x - 6y = 18$. Write it in slope-intercept form and then graph it, labeling the slope and y-intercept.

PROBLEM 22

An experimenter collects data on the pressure (P) versus the volume (V) of 1 mole of ideal gas A at a constant temperature T_1 (sample 1 in Figure 6-29). He repeats the experiment with a 2-mole sample of gas A at a constant temperature T_2 and plots the data (sample 2). What are the relative magnitudes of T_1 and T_2?

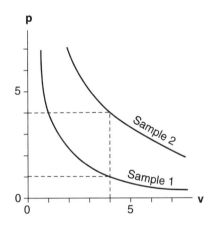

Fig. 6-29.   **p** and **v** axes are scaled with arbitrary units

PROBLEM 23

The relation between variables x and y can be described by the equation

$$y = \frac{ax}{b + x^2}$$

in which a,b = positive constants. Looking at only $x \geq 0$, how does the slope of this curve vary? (Hint: To graph this equation and analyze how its slope varies, split the graph into three regions—$x \ll b$, $x \approx b$, and $x \gg b$ as was done for the graph of $y = \frac{ax}{b + x}$ in Figure 6-26.)

Semi-Log and Log-Log Graphs and Functions

The scales on the axes of the preceding graphs have been linear. For some graphs, alternative scales, such as semi-log and log-log, are useful. A semi-log plot of a graph has

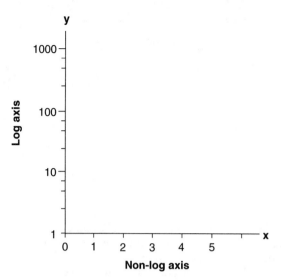

Fig. 6-30. Semi-log axes.

a log scale on one axis (usually the ordinate) and a linear scale on the other axis (usually the abscissa) (Fig. 6-30).

A semi-log scale is particularly useful for plotting exponential graphs, because they become linear on semi-log graph paper. Consider $y = ae^{bx}$, in which a,b = constants. Taking log of both sides:

$$\log_{10}y = \log_{10}ae^{bx} = \log_{10}a + bx \log_{10}e$$

$$= \log_{10}a + 0.4343bx \qquad [\log_{10}e \cong 0.4343]$$

This graph could be used to plot data to verify Newton's law of cooling (temperature difference versus time). Observe that a plot of log y versus x is linear with the y-intercept = log a and the slope = 0.4343b.

As another example, consider:

$$s = s_0 \cdot 10^{kt}$$

$$\log_{10}s = \log_{10}(s_0 \cdot 10^{kt}) = \log_{10} s_0 + kt$$

Observe that a plot of log s versus t is also linear with the y-intercept = log s0 and the slope = k.

When plotting data on semi-log paper, you do not convert the raw data into logs and plot them on the paper. Instead, plot the raw values on the paper, because the scale on the log axis does the conversion. Semi-log plots of exponential graphs are valuable because it is easier to analyze a straight line than it is to analyze a curved line.

EXAMPLE 31

Graph $y = 500(10^{-x/2})$ on both regular and semi-log graph paper (for $x \geq 0$ only). Figure 6-31 demonstrates the regular graph of $y = 500(10^{-x/2})$.

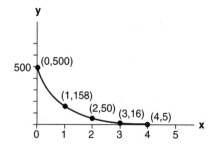

Fig. 6-31.

Figure 6-32 demonstrates the semi-log graph of $y = 500(10^{-x/2}) \rightarrow \log y = \log 500 - \dfrac{x}{2}$.

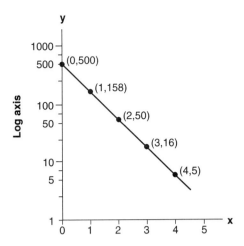

Fig. 6-32.

Two important observations follow:

1. The points on the log axis are not labeled by values of log y but by the corresponding values of y; that is, the point for log 10 = 1 is labeled by 10, not 1; the point for log 100 = 2 is labeled by 100, not 2, etc. This format allows you to read the value of y for a particular value of x directly off the graph. Remember, however, that the slope of a semi-log graphic function, which is $-\frac{1}{2}$, is:

$$\frac{\Delta(\log y)}{\Delta x} \text{, not } \frac{\Delta y}{\Delta x}$$

2. If we had been given experimentally determined values of y for x = 1, 2, 3, 4, and were told that x and y were related by the equation $y = a(10^{kx})$, it would have been easier to determine a and k from the semi-log plot of these points than from their regular plot (these points are indicated in both Figures 6-31 and 6-32), because k = the slope of, and a = the y-intercept extrapolated from, the line drawn through these points.

PROBLEM 24

The relation between two variables, x and y, is described by the equation $y = a(10^{bx})$ in which a,b = constants. Using the data presented in the semi-log graph in Figure 6-33, determine a and b (actual data points are marked with a dot).

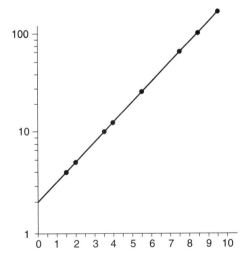

Fig. 6-33.

A log-log plot of a graph, which has log scales on both axes, can be used advantageously when two variables are directly or inversely proportional. When x and y are directly proportional, a log-log plot is especially useful when their values range over several powers of 10. In this graph, a log-log plot of x and y spreads out the data points while preserving linearity:

$$\text{If } y = kx, k > 0$$

$$\text{then } \log y = \log x + \log k$$

In general, if $y = ax^n$ (a,n = constants), then y is directly proportional to x^n and so could be plotted linearly on log-log paper, i.e., $\log y = n\log x + \log a$. A nonlinear graph (for $n \neq 1$) is then transformed into a linear graph of slope n and y-intercept = log a. Again, a linear function is easier to analyze than a nonlinear function.

EXAMPLE **32**

Graph y = x on both linear and log-log paper for $1 \leq x \leq 1000$, identifying the points corresponding to x = 1, 10, 100, 1000.

Figure 6-34 demonstrates the linear graph of y = x (linear scale, both axes). Note that it is hard to show difference on a linear graph.

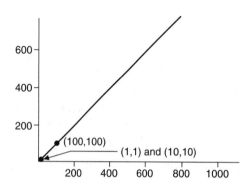

Fig. 6-34.

Figure 6-35 demonstrates the log-log graph of log y = log x. The plotted points in this graph are spread out, compared to the corresponding points in the linear graph, without losing linearity.

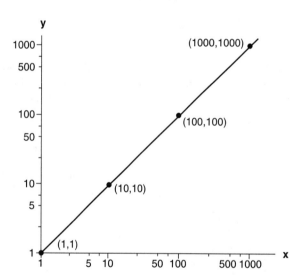

Fig. 6-35.

EXAMPLE **33**

In the discussion of basic graphs, we saw the parabola $y = mx^2$ plotted as a graph with both linear axes. Plot $y = 5x^2$, for $1 \leq x \leq 10$, on log-log paper.

Figure 6-36 shows that the log-log graph is $\log y = 2\log x + \log 5$.

When two variables, x and y, are inversely proportional, a log-log plot converts their hyperbolic function into a linear function.

$$\text{If } y = \frac{k}{x}, k > 0 \text{ (hyperbolic equation)}$$

$$\text{then } \log y = \log k - \log x \text{ (straight line transformation equation)}$$

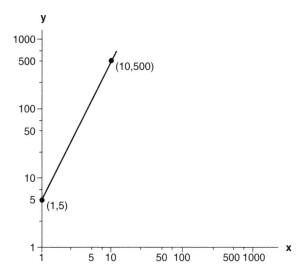

Fig. 6-36.

Actually, $y = \dfrac{k}{x}$ is just a special case of $y = kx^n$ (when $n = -1$).

Solutions to Problems 21–24

21) The slope-intercept form of $8x - 6y = 18$ is: $y = \dfrac{4}{3}x - 3$. It is displayed graphically in Figure 6-37.

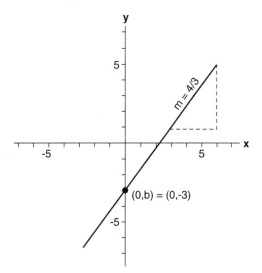

Fig. 6-37.

22) Recall that the ideal gas law is $PV = nRT$. Because n, T = constants for both samples, both P,V graphs are hyperbolic (P and V being inversely proportional). To determine the relative magnitudes of the constant temperatures T_1 and T_2, you must express them in terms of common constant(s) so you can obtain their numeric ratio.

   For sample 1, $PV = RT_1$ ($n = 1$). Because PV = constant, we can select any point on the sample 1 graph to evaluate it numerically. Selecting point $(v,P) = (4,1)$, $(4)(1) = RT_1$, which implies that $T_1 = \dfrac{4}{R}$.

   For sample 2: $PV = 2RT_2$ ($n = 2$). Selecting point $(v,P) = (4,4)$, $(4)(4) = 2RT_2$, which implies that $T_2 = \dfrac{8}{R}$.

$$\frac{T_2}{T_1} = \frac{\dfrac{8}{R}}{\dfrac{4}{R}} = 2; \text{ or, } T_2 = 2T_1$$

23) $y = \dfrac{ax}{b + x^2}$; a,b = positive constants. Splitting the graph (for x ≥ 0) into three regions corresponding to:

(A) $x << b$, $y = \dfrac{ax}{b + x^2} \cong \dfrac{a}{b}x$ (linear)

(B) $x \approx b$, $y = \dfrac{ax}{b + x^2}$ (no approximation)

(C) $x >> b$, $y = \dfrac{ax}{b + x^2} \cong \dfrac{ax}{x^2} = \dfrac{a}{x}$ (hyperbolic)

To graph this equation, use the same three regions (Figure 6-38). For region A, the function looks linear; for region C, the function looks hyperbolic; and, for region B, the two partial graphs are connected by a smooth curve that must have a maximum point and an inflection point.

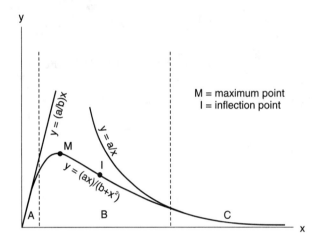

Fig. 6-38.

In the segmental analysis of this compound curve (split into simpler curves), you see that the slope starts off at a finite, nearly constant value (region A). As x increases, it starts to decrease, being zero at the maximum point M and negative thereafter (region B). In the right-hand side of region B, the graph passes through an inflection point (I), where the slope reaches a minimum value and then begins to increase slightly. In region C, the slope approaches zero as the graph asymptotes to the x-axis.

24) $y = 2(10^{x/5})$. For the y-intercept (x = 0), $y = a(10^{b \cdot 0}) = a$. Reading directly from the graph in Figure 6-33, the y-intercept = a = 2. For determining b, consider:

$$y = a(10^{bx}) \rightarrow \log y = bx + \log a$$

The slope of this line $= b = \dfrac{\Delta(\log y)}{\Delta x}$. Selecting two points, $(x_1, y_1) = (3.5, 10)$ and $(x_2, y_2) = (8.5, 100)$, the slope is:

$$b = \log y_2 - \dfrac{\log y_1}{x_2 - x_1} = \dfrac{\log 100 - \log 10}{8.5 - 3.5} = \dfrac{2 - 1}{5} = \dfrac{1}{5}$$

$$y = 2(10^{x/5})$$

Concept 13: Quadratic Equations

Quadratic equations are encountered in the physical sciences, for example, uniformly accelerated motion equations, projectiles, rate law, and reaction order in chemical reactions. Problems related to these topics usually require solution of second order or quadratic equations in one variable. The general quadratic equation is expressed by: $ax^2 + bx + c = 0$, in which a, b, c are constant with $b^2 - 4ac > 0$. For these special values, the general form of solution is represented as:

$$x_1, x_2 = \dfrac{-b \pm \sqrt{b^2 - 4ac}}{2a}$$

in which x_1 and x_2 are the two possible solutions.

Consider a reversible biochemical reaction in which:

$$\text{Reactant} \rightleftharpoons \text{Product 1} + \text{Product 2}$$

The equilibrium constant is

$$K = \frac{[\text{Product 1}][\text{Product 2}]}{[\text{Reactant}]}$$

Assume equimolar amounts of product 1 and product 2 and each is represented by m. Assume we started with a unimolar solution of the reactant.

	Reactant $\rightleftharpoons$	Product 1 +	Product 2
At start,	1	0	0
At equilibrium,	$1 - m$	m	m

$$K = \frac{(m)(m)}{(1 - m)}$$

$$K(1 - m) = m^2$$

$$m^2 + mK - K = 0$$

Comparing this with the quadratic equation $ax^2 + bx + c = 0$, $a = 1$, $b = K$, $c = K$. To obtain the solutions, use the formula:

$$m_1, m_2 = \frac{-K \pm \sqrt{K^2 - 4(1)(K)}}{2(1)}$$

$$\text{Hence, } m_1 = \frac{-K + \sqrt{K^2 + 4K}}{2}$$

$$m_2 = \frac{-K - \sqrt{K^2 + 4K}}{2}$$

Notice that both roots depend on the equilibrium constant. The negative root m_2 is usually hypothetical because equilibrium constants and concentrations cannot be negative. Only one realistic root (m_1) is shown in this solution.

Memorize the fact that, for small numbers, the squares are smaller than the numbers. If $K = 10^{-8}$, then $K^2 = 10^{-16}$, which is negligible for all practical purposes. The interpretation of a quadratic equation will help you save time in solving it. Do not overdo mathematic operations if they do not help you arrive at the correct answers.

Concept 14: Simultaneous Equations

You can solve two equations (linear equations) in two variables. A set of simultaneous equations may be represented as:

$$AX + BY = C \text{ (i)}$$

$$DX + EY = F \text{ (ii)}$$

These equations have two variables (X and Y) and can be solved algebraically or graphically. A, B, C, D, E, and F are real constants.

Algebraic Solution of Simultaneous Equations
Consider the equations:

$$3X + 2Y = 9 \ldots \ldots \text{ (i)}$$

$$4X + 1Y = 11 \ldots \ldots \text{ (ii)}$$

Multiply equation ii by 2 (double both sides):

$$8X + 2Y = 22 \ldots \ldots \text{ (iii)}$$

Subtract equation iii from equation i:

$$3X + 2Y - 8X - 2Y = 9 - 22$$

$$-5X = -13$$

$$X = \frac{13}{5} = 2.6$$

Use X = 2.6 in equation i, ii, or iii to obtain Y.

$$4(2.6) + Y = 11 \text{ yields}$$

$$10.4 + Y = 11 \text{ or } Y = 0.6 = \frac{3}{5}$$

$$\therefore X = \frac{13}{5}, Y = \frac{3}{5} \text{ is the solution set}$$

Graphic Solution of Simultaneous Equations

If you graph both equations, using the techniques discussed in concept 12, you see two straight lines intersecting at a point. Note that the coordinates of that point are the same solution set as obtained using the algebraic solution. On the MCAT, you may be asked to compare two experimental studies to determine if they have a common point. Experiments in chemistry and biology can lead to simultaneous equations to arrive at one solution.

Concept 15: Introduction to Trigonometric Functions

Trigonometry is concerned with the relationships between the angles and sides of triangles. Recall that for similar triangles(Fig. 6-39), i.e., those that have the same angles but are not necessarily the same size, the ratios of the corresponding sides are equal.

$$\frac{X}{x} = \frac{Y}{y} = \frac{Z}{z}$$

$\theta_1, \theta_2, \theta_3$ = angles

Focusing on right triangles(Fig. 6-40), it can be directly deduced that the ratio of any two of the sides of a right triangle is the same for all similar right triangles. In other words, the possible ratios depend only on the angles of the right triangle.

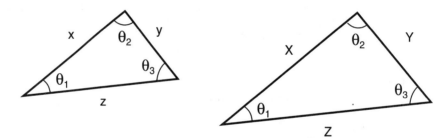

Fig. 6-39. Similar triangles.

X/x = Y/y = Z/z

$\theta_1, \theta_2, \theta_3$ = angles

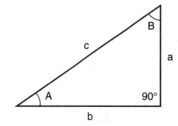

Fig. 6-40. Right triangle. *a* and *b* = legs of the right triangle; *c* = hypotenuse of the right triangle; *A* and *B* = angles.

144   **Applied Math Concepts Required for Physical and Biological Sciences**

The basic trigonometric functions are as follows:

$$\text{Sine of an angle} = \frac{\text{Opposite side}}{\text{Hypotenuse}}$$

$$\sin A = \frac{a}{c}$$

$$\sin B = \frac{b}{c}$$

$$\text{Cosine of an angle} = \frac{\text{Adjacent side}}{\text{Hypotenuse}}$$

$$\cos A = \frac{b}{c}$$

$$\cos B = \frac{a}{c}$$

$$\text{Tangent of an angle} = \frac{\text{Opposite side}}{\text{Adjacent side}}$$

$$\tan A = \frac{a}{b}$$

$$\tan B = \frac{b}{a}$$

Note that definitions are interrelated; for example, observe that $\sin A = \cos B$, $\sin B = \cos A$, and $\frac{\sin A}{\cos A} = \tan A$.

PROBLEM 25

In the triangle in Figure 6-41, find $\sin A$, $\cos A$, and $\tan A$.

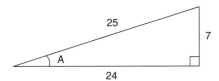

Fig. 6-41.

PROBLEM 26

In the triangle in Figure 6-42, find $\sin B$, $\cos B$, and $\tan B$.

These right triangle definitions of the basic trigonometric functions are restricted to angles between 0° and 90°. Definitions of trigonometric functions can be extended to include all angles.

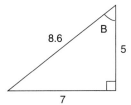

Fig. 6-42.

PROBLEM 27

Using the graphs in Figure 6-43, find $\sin \theta$, $\cos \theta$, and $\tan \theta$ for $\theta = 0°, 90°, 180°,$ and 270°.

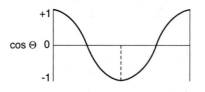

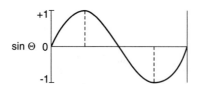

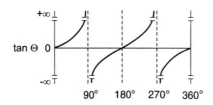

Fig. 6-43. Graphic representation of trigonometric functions.

The trigonometric functions are typically represented graphically for angles between 0° and 360° because they have repeating values; i.e., they are periodic.

If x + angle and n = integer:

$$\sin (x + 360°n) = \sin x$$

$$\cos (x + 360°n) = \cos x$$

$$\tan (x + 180°n) = \tan x$$

Observe and remember two things:

1. Trigonometric functions logically turn up when considering quantities that are periodic in nature, e.g., wave phenomena in physics.
2. Trigonometry should be useful when it is advantageous to represent a quantity as the hypotenuse or a leg of a right triangle, e.g., vectors (see concept 18).

Solutions to Problems 25–27

25) Using the right triangle definitions of the trigonometric functions:

$$\sin A = \frac{7}{25}, \cos A = \frac{24}{25}, \text{ and } \tan A = \frac{7}{24}$$

26) As in the solution to problem 27, using the right triangle definitions:

$$\sin B = \frac{7}{8.6}, \cos B = \frac{5}{8.6}, \text{ and } \tan B = \frac{7}{5}$$

27) Values read directly from the graph are presented in Table 6-1.

TABLE 6-1.

Function	0°	90°	180°	270°
			θ	
$\sin \theta$	0	1	0	−1
$\cos \theta$	1	0	−1	0
$\tan \theta$	0	± ∞ (undefined)	0	± ∞ (undefined)

Concept 16: Characteristics of 30°, 45°, and 60° Right Triangles

The characteristics of a few basic right triangles are shown in Figure 6-44. When preparing for the MCAT, be sure to memorize these characteristics, along with the values of the trigonometric functions for the angles in them.

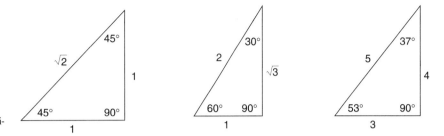

Fig. 6-44. Three special right triangles.

PROBLEM **28**

Using the right triangles in Figure 6-44, find sin θ, cos θ, and tan θ for $\theta = 30°$, 45°, and 60°.

PROBLEM **29**

In Figure 6-45, find x.

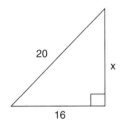

Fig. 6-45.

PROBLEM **30**

In Figure 6-46, find x and y.

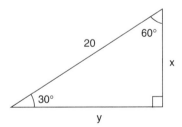

Fig. 6-46.

Up to this point, we have used degrees to measure angles. You should be familiar with an alternative angular measure, which is the radian. Recall that a complete revolution about a point is 360°. The same revolution is alternatively represented by 2π radians (normally it is written as just 2π; the unit of radians is assumed). The 2π to 360° equivalence determines the proportionality of the two angular measures, e.g., $180° = \pi$, $90° = \frac{\pi}{2}$, $720° = 4\pi$, etc. (1 radian = 57.3°).

PROBLEM **31**

What are 30°, 45°, and 60° in radian units?

The Pythagorean theorem (Fig. 6-47) finds many applications in solving problems on the MCAT as well.

$$a^2 + b^2 = c^2$$

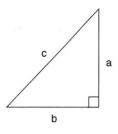

Fig. 6-47. $a^2 + b^2 = c^2$

PROBLEM **32**
In Figure 6-48, find b.

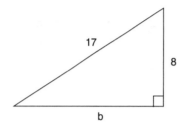

Fig. 6-48.

PROBLEM **33**
In Figure 6-49, evaluate $\sin^2 \theta + \cos^2 \theta$, giving the answer in its simplest form.

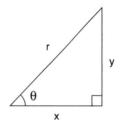

Fig. 6-49.

Solutions to Problems 28–33

28)   Values read from the right triangles in Figure 6-44 are presented in Table 6-2.

TABLE 6-2.

Function	30°	45°	60°
		θ	
$\sin \theta$	$\dfrac{1}{2}$	$\dfrac{\sqrt{2}}{2}$	$\dfrac{\sqrt{3}}{2}$
$\cos \theta$	$\dfrac{\sqrt{3}}{2}$	$\dfrac{\sqrt{2}}{2}$	$\dfrac{1}{2}$
$\tan \theta$	$\dfrac{\sqrt{3}}{3}$	1	$\sqrt{3}$

29)   This 3-4-5 right triangle is recognized by noting some combination of two sides in ratio $3\!:\!4$, $4\!:\!5$, or $3\!:\!5$ corresponding to the positions shown on the standard 3-4-5

triangle; the third is the missing side. The triangle in this problem corresponds to the known triangle in Figure 6-50.

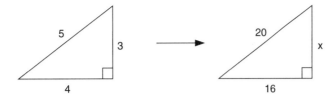

Fig. 6-50.

Because these triangles are similar, the corresponding sides are proportional:

$$\frac{x}{3} = \frac{20}{5} \text{ or } \frac{x}{3} = \frac{16}{4}$$

In either case,

$$x = 12$$

30) $\sin 30° = \dfrac{x}{20}$; $x = 20\sin 30° = 20(\frac{1}{2}) = 10$

$\cos 30° = \dfrac{y}{20}$; $y = 20\cos 30° = 20\left(\dfrac{\sqrt{3}}{2}\right) = 10\sqrt{3}$

31) Using the proportionality based on the equivalence of 360° and 2π:

$$\frac{30°}{360°} = \frac{x}{2\pi} \rightarrow x = \frac{\pi}{6}; \, 30° \rightarrow \frac{\pi}{6}$$

$$\frac{45°}{360°} = \frac{x}{2\pi} \rightarrow x = \frac{\pi}{4}; \, 45° \rightarrow \frac{\pi}{4}$$

$$\frac{60°}{360°} = \frac{x}{2\pi} \rightarrow x = \frac{\pi}{3}; \, 60° \rightarrow \frac{\pi}{3}$$

32) Using the Pythagorean theorem:

$$b^2 + 8^2 = 17^2$$
$$b^2 + 64 = 289$$
$$b^2 = 225$$
$$b = 15$$

33) $\sin \theta = \dfrac{y}{r}$ and $\cos \theta = \dfrac{x}{r}$

$$\sin^2\theta + \cos^2\theta = \frac{y^2}{r^2} + \frac{x^2}{r^2} = \frac{x^2 + y^2}{r^2} = \frac{r^2}{r^2} = 1$$

$(x^2 + y^2 = r^2$ by the Pythagorean theorem)

Concept 17: Inverse Trigonometric Functions

Inverse trigonometric functions are used to determine the angle corresponding to a given value of any trigonometric function.

Find the angle given sine angle = 0.5 or ½. The backward operation of finding the angle from the function is also called inverting the function or finding the inverse of the given function. The angle for which the sine = ½ is 30°.

Inverse trigonometric functions are represented as arcsin, arccos, arctan or $\sin^{-1}$, $\cos^{-1}$, and $\tan^{-1}$. Important values of commonly used inverse trigonometric functions are as follows:

$\sin^{-1} 0 = 0°$ $\cos^{-1} 0 = 90°$

$\sin^{-1} \frac{1}{2} = 30°$ $\cos^{-1} \frac{1}{2} = 60°$

$\sin^{-1} \dfrac{1}{\sqrt{2}} = 45°$ $\cos^{-1} \dfrac{1}{\sqrt{2}} = 45°$

$\sin^{-1} \dfrac{\sqrt{3}}{2} = 60°$ $\cos^{-1} \dfrac{\sqrt{3}}{2} = 30°$

$\sin^{-1} 1 = 90°$ $\cos^{-1} 1 = 0°$

The inverse functions are used when the length of sides of triangles is given. In a right triangle, if the hypotenuse = 11 units and the altitude measures 9 units, then $\sin^{-1} \frac{9}{11}$ = $\sin^{-1} 0.818$. The angle corresponding to $\sin^{-1} 0.818$ will be between 45° and 60° $(\sin^{-1} \frac{1}{\sqrt{2}} = \sin^{-1} 0.707$ and $\sin^{-1} \frac{\sqrt{3}}{2} = \sin^{-1} 0.866)$. These calculations can be used in physical sciences to determine unknown angles from given lengths of various sides of a triangle.

Rules for Inverse Trigonometric Functions

1. For any angle $0 < \theta < 90°$
   (a) $\sin^{-1} (\sin \theta) = \theta$
   (b) $\cos^{-1} (\cos \theta) = \theta$
   (c) $\tan^{-1} (\tan \theta) = \theta$
2. For any $-1 \le A \le 1$,
   (a) $\sin (\sin^{-1} A) = A$
   (b) $\cos (\cos^{-1} A) = A$
3. For any A, $\tan (\tan^{-1} A) = A$
4. If $\theta = \sin^{-1} \left(\frac{y}{r}\right) = \cos^{-1} \left(\frac{x}{r}\right)$ with $x \ne 0$,

   then $\theta = \tan^{-1} \left(\frac{y}{x}\right)$

Concept 18: Vector Operations and Rules

A **vector quantity** is completely specified by a magnitude and a direction. A **scalar quantity** is completely specified by its magnitude, there being no sense of direction. A vector is graphically symbolized by an arrow—the tail is the origin point, the head is the finish point, the length is proportional to its magnitude, and its angle (in relation to a reference) is indicative of its direction (Fig. 6-51).

Right-Hand Rule for Vectors

The right-hand rule is used to determine the sense of the vector that results from the cross-product of two vectors. The torque or rotational moment resulting from the product of the moment arm and the force has a certain sense. Place the vectors (Moment arm = $\vec{r}$ and acting force on the object = $\vec{F}$) $\vec{r}$ and $\vec{F}$ in the same imaginary or fictitious plane. Imagine a line perpendicular to the plane of these two vectors. Call this the axis or line of action of the resulting moment of the force $\vec{F}$. Grasp this axis or action line with your right hand, but be sure to wrap your fingers around this line such that the fingers point as if moving from $\vec{r}$ to $\vec{F}$. The curling of the fingers should point in the same order as the product of $\vec{r}$ and $\vec{F}$. The direction of your thumb point will then indicate the direction of the resulting moment. Figure 6-52 shows how the sense of the resulting vector is determined. Note that $\vec{r}$ and $\vec{F}$ are in the plane of the paper.

Fig. 6-51. Definition sketch for a vector.

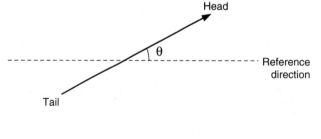

Fig. 6-52. Demonstration of right-hand rule for vectors.

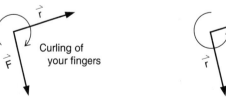

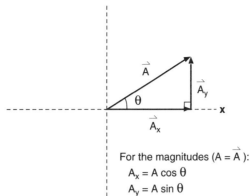

Fig. 6-53. Orthogonal components of a vector. Note: when referring to the magnitude $\vec{A}$, we write A.

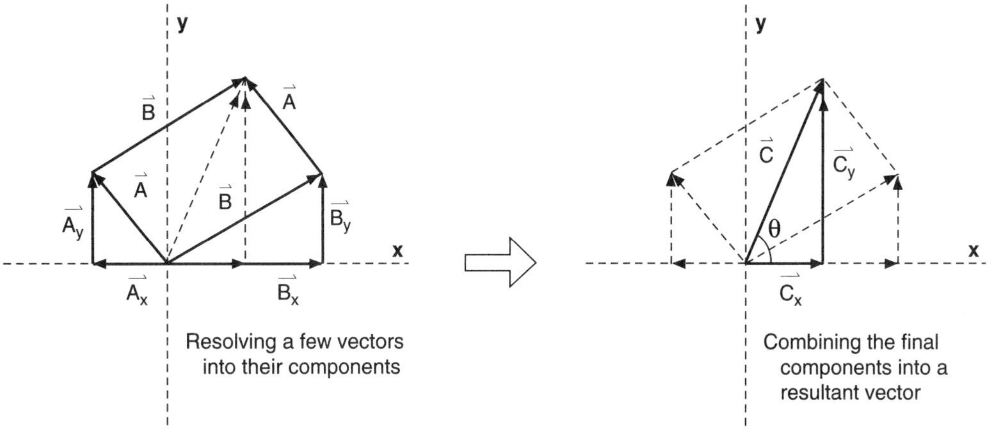

For the magnitudes ($A = \vec{A}$):
$A_x = A \cos \theta$
$A_y = A \sin \theta$
$A^2 = A_x^2 + A_y^2$

Fig. 6-54. Orthogonal components of multiple vectors.

Resolving a few vectors into their components

Combining the final components into a resultant vector

In problem solving, each vector is usually broken down into perpendicular components, identified here as x and y, which added together give the original vector (Fig. 6-53).

In essence, the vector is represented as the hypotenuse of a right triangle in which the legs (i.e., the components of the vector) are chosen to lie parallel to the axes of a convenient Cartesian coordinate system (see Fig. 6-53).

To add (or subtract) two or more vectors, in each reference direction the component of the resulting vector is obtained by adding (subtracting) together all the components of these vectors in that direction. The resulting vector is constructed from its components thus obtained, e.g., for $\vec{A} + \vec{B} = \vec{C}$ (Fig. 6-54).

$$\vec{C}_x = \vec{A}_x + \vec{B}_x, \; C_x = A_x + B_x; \; \vec{C}_y = \vec{A}_y + \vec{B}_y, \; C_y = A_y + B_y$$

$$\vec{C} = \vec{C}_x + \vec{C}_y$$

$$C^2 = C_x^2 + C_y^2; \; \tan \theta = \frac{C_y}{C_x}$$

EXAMPLE 34

Study Figure 6-55. Given $\vec{A} + \vec{B} = \vec{C}$, find C.

$$C_x = A_x + B_x = 12 - 8 = 4; \; C_y = A_y + B_y = 5 - 1 = 4$$

$$C = \sqrt{C_x^2 + C_y^2} = \sqrt{4^2 + 4^2} = 4\sqrt{2}$$

$$\tan \theta = \frac{C_y}{C_x} = \frac{4}{4} = 1 \rightarrow \theta = 45°$$

PROBLEM 34

What is the x-component of the vector $\vec{F}$ in Figure 6-56?

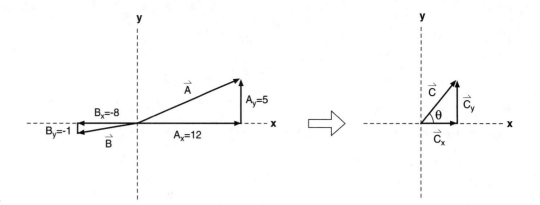

Fig. 6-55.

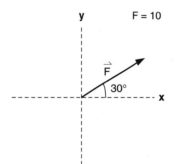

Fig. 6-56.

PROBLEM 35
What is the y-component of the vector $\vec{H}$ in Figure 6-57?

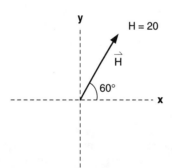

Fig. 6-57.

PROBLEM 36
What are the x- and y-components of $\vec{A} + \vec{B}$ in Figure 6-58?

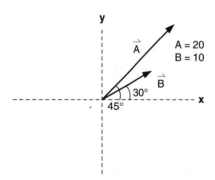

Fig. 6-58.

152   **Applied Math Concepts Required for Physical and Biological Sciences**

Solutions to Problems 34–36

34) Resolving the vector $\vec{F}$ (Fig. 6-59):

$$F_x = F \cos \theta = 10 \cos 30° = 10\left(\frac{\sqrt{3}}{2}\right) = 5\sqrt{3}$$

F = 10

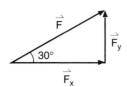

Fig. 6-59.

35) Resolving the vector $\vec{H}$ (Fig. 6-60):

$$H_y = H \sin \theta = 20 \sin 60° = 20\left(\frac{\sqrt{3}}{2}\right) = 10\sqrt{3}$$

H = 20

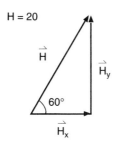

Fig. 6-60.

36) Resolving the vectors $\vec{A} + \vec{B}$ (Fig. 6-61):

$$A_x + B_x = A \cos 45° + B \cos 30° = 20\left(\frac{1}{\sqrt{2}}\right) + 10\left(\frac{\sqrt{3}}{2}\right) = 10\sqrt{2} + 5\sqrt{3}$$

$$A_y + B_y = A \sin 45° + B \sin 30° = 20\left(\frac{1}{\sqrt{2}}\right) + 10\left(\frac{1}{2}\right) = 10\sqrt{2} + 5$$

A = 20   B = 10

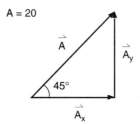   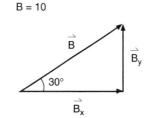

Fig. 6-61.

COMPARATIVE PRINCIPLES

Concept 19: Using Metric and British Unit Systems

Basic Units and Conversions
The **metric system** is based on the decimal system. The three basic units are:

> **length:** meter (m)
>
> **mass:** gram (g)
>
> **volume:** liter (l)

Applied Math Concepts Required for Physical and Biological Sciences   153

All other units of the metric system depend on using the following prefixes:

pico (p) 10^{-12}
nano (n) 10^{-9}
micro (m) 10^{-6}
milli (m) 10^{-3}
centi (c) 10^{-2}
deci (d) 10^{-1}
deca 10^{1}
kilo (k) 10^{3}
mega (M) 10^{6}
giga 10^{9}
tera 10^{12}

Consider the following measurements:

$$\text{kilometer} = 1000 \text{ m}$$

$$\text{centimeter} = \frac{1}{100} \text{ meter}$$

$$\text{kilogram} = 1000 \text{ g}$$

$$\text{milligram} = \frac{1}{1000} \text{ g}$$

$$\text{deciliter} = \frac{1}{10} \text{ liter}$$

The English System has no rational basis. The basic units are:

length: foot (ft)

mass: pound (lb)

volume: gallon (gal)

Multiples of these units are often used:

$$1 \text{ foot (ft)} = 12 \text{ in}$$

$$1 \text{ yard (yd)} = 3 \text{ ft} = 36 \text{ in}$$

$$1 \text{ mile} = 1760 \text{ yd} = 5280 \text{ ft}$$

$$1 \text{ pound (lb)} = 16 \text{ oz}$$

$$1 \text{ ton} = 2000 \text{ lb}$$

$$1 \text{ quart} = 2 \text{ pt}$$

$$1 \text{ gallon (gal)} = 4 \text{ qt}$$

$$1 \text{ pint} = 16 \text{ fluid ounces}$$

The **key conversions** between the metric and English systems are as follows:

length: 2.54 cm = 1 inch

mass: 454 g = 1 pound

volume: 0.95 liter = 1 quart

Converting Units and Balancing Units in Equations

Many MCAT questions require converting units (conversion factors between metric and English systems being provided where needed) and balancing physical units in equations. To convert any unit in the metric system to any corresponding unit in the English system (or vice versa):

1. Write all necessary conversions between units as equations, such as

$$1 \text{ ton} = 2000 \text{ lb}$$

2. Rewrite each equation as either of two ratios, e.g.,

$$1 \text{ ton} = 2000 \text{ lb} \rightarrow \frac{1 \text{ ton}}{2000 \text{ lb}} \text{ or } \frac{2000 \text{ lb}}{1 \text{ ton}}$$

3. Convert between units by multiplying the correct sequence of these ratios so the desired units are obtained and the undesired units cancel out.

EXAMPLE 35

Convert 50 kg to ounces.

$$(50 \text{ kg}) \left(\frac{1000 \text{ g}}{1 \text{ kg}}\right) \left(\frac{1 \text{ lb}}{454 \text{ g}}\right) \left(\frac{16 \text{ oz}}{1 \text{ lb}}\right) = \frac{(50)(1000)(16)}{454} \text{ oz} = 1762 \text{ oz}$$

Observe that kilograms are converted to grams, which are converted to pounds, which are converted to ounces. At each step, the ratio is so chosen as to cancel out the unwanted unit. In this example, all the units except ounces cancel out.

The physical units of the quantities in any equation have to balance. Consequently, in a formula, the units of one quantity can be determined from knowledge of the units of the other quantities. Also, examining to see if the units in a formula balance is a way of checking it for dimensional accuracy.

EXAMPLE 36

The kinetic energy E of a particle of mass m, moving at a speed v, is $E = \frac{1}{2}mv^2$. If E is in units of ergs $\left(\frac{g \cdot cm^2}{sec^2}\right)$ and m is in units of grams, what are the units of speed?

$$E = \frac{1}{2}mv^2$$

$$\frac{g \cdot cm^2}{sec^2} = (g)(\text{units of speed})^2$$

$$(\text{units of speed})^2 = \frac{cm^2}{sec^2}$$

$$\text{units of speed} = \frac{cm}{sec}$$

PROBLEM 37

Convert 20 kg to ounces.

PROBLEM 38

Convert 40 km to miles.

PROBLEM 39

Convert 10 liters to pints.

PROBLEM 40

Because the electric field $E = \frac{F}{q}$, in which F = force = (mass x acceleration) and q = charge, what are the units of E in terms of mass (m), length (l), time (t), and charge (q)?

PROBLEM 41

The equation for the force F of gravity is:

$$F = k \frac{m_1 m_2}{r^2}$$

in which m_1 and m_2 are masses and r is the distance between them. What are the units in terms of mass (m), length (l), and time (t) of the constant k?

Solutions to Problems 37–41

37) $(20 \text{ kg}) \left(\frac{1000 \text{ g}}{1 \text{ kg}}\right) \left(\frac{1 \text{ lb}}{454 \text{ g}}\right) \left(\frac{16 \text{ oz}}{\text{lb}}\right) = \frac{(20)(1000)(16)}{454} \text{ oz} = 705 \text{ oz}$

38) $(40 \text{ km}) \left(\frac{1000 \text{ m}}{1 \text{ km}}\right) \left(\frac{100 \text{ cm}}{1 \text{ m}}\right) \left(\frac{1 \text{ in.}}{2.54 \text{ cm}}\right) \left(\frac{1 \text{ ft}}{12 \text{ in.}}\right) \left(\frac{1 \text{ mi}}{5280 \text{ ft}}\right)$

$$= \frac{(40)(1000)(100)}{(2.54)(12)(5280)} \text{ mi} = 24.9 \text{ mi}$$

39) $(10 \text{ liters})\left(\dfrac{1 \text{ qt}}{0.95 \text{ liter}}\right)\left(\dfrac{2 \text{ pt}}{1 \text{ qt}}\right) = \dfrac{(10)(2)}{(0.95)} \text{ pt} = 21 \text{ pints}$

40) $E = \dfrac{F}{q} = \dfrac{ma}{q} = \left(\dfrac{m\left(\frac{1}{t^2}\right)}{q}\right) = \dfrac{m \cdot 1}{q \cdot t^2}$

41) $F = \dfrac{km_1m_2}{r^2} \rightarrow k = \dfrac{r^2F}{m_1m_2} = \dfrac{r^2(ma)}{m_1m_2}$ for $\dfrac{\text{units}}{\text{calculations}}$

$k = \dfrac{(1^2)(m)\left(\frac{1}{t^2}\right)}{(m)^2} = \dfrac{1^3}{m \cdot t^2}$

Concept 20: Approximation and Estimations

Many MCAT questions involve the ability to estimate an approximate answer quickly. The approximate answer is then compared to the actual answer choices provided. Do not spend too much time finding an exact answer when an approximated answer will give you the information you require.

One part of approximation and estimation is the ability to convert an arithmetic problem into one that can be done quickly in your head. Begin by simplifying the problem. One means of simplification is to recall that multiplication and division may be done in any order.

EXAMPLE **37**

$$\begin{aligned} 40 \times 22 &= (4 \times 10) \times 22 \\ &= (4 \times 22) \times 10 \\ &= 88 \times 10 = 880 \end{aligned}$$

By leaving the 10 until last, you have less to keep in mind for the multiplication steps.

A less obvious, yet useful, simplification is of help when you are required to multiply by 50 or 25 (or by the same numbers with the decimal moved, such as 5, 0.5, 2.5, 0.25, etc.) Remember that 50 is $\frac{100}{2}$ and 25 is $\frac{100}{4}$.

EXAMPLE **38**

$$\begin{aligned} 66 \times 50 &= 66 \times \dfrac{100}{2} \\ &= \dfrac{66}{2} \times 100 \\ &= 33 \times 100 = 3300 \end{aligned}$$

EXAMPLE **39**

$$\begin{aligned} 66 \times 2.5 &= 66 \times \dfrac{10}{4} \\ &= \dfrac{66}{4} \times 10 \\ &= \dfrac{660}{4} = 165 \end{aligned}$$

EXAMPLE **40**

$$\begin{aligned} \dfrac{320}{25} &= \dfrac{320}{\frac{100}{4}} \\ &= 320 \times \dfrac{4}{100} \\ &= \dfrac{320}{100} \times 4 \\ &= 3.2 \times 4 = 12.8 \end{aligned}$$

PROBLEM 42

Mentally multiply the following (simplify the operation as before; then multiply and add or subtract):

(a) 89 × 3

(b) $1.05 × 9

(c) $1.98 × 9

(d) $3.95 × 8

(e) 72 × 30

(f) 44 × 60

PROBLEM 43

Mentally multiply or divide the following:

(a) 36 × 5.0

(b) $\dfrac{440}{50}$

(c) 28 × 25

(d) $\dfrac{120}{25}$

(e) 120 × 0.25

(f) 89 × 33.3

Answers to Problems 42 and 43

42) (a) $89 \times 3 = (90 - 1)\,3$

$= 270 - 3 = 267$

(b) $1.05 \times 9 = 1.05\,(10 - 1)$

$= 10.50 - 1.05 = 9.45$

(c) $1.98 \times 9 = (2.00 - 0.02)\,9$

$= 18.0 - 0.18 = 17.82$

(d) $3.95 \times 8 = (4 - 0.05)\,8$

$= 32 - 0.40 = 31.60$

(e) $72 \times 30 = 72 \times 3 \times 10$

$= 216 \times 10 = 2160$

(f) $44 \times 60 = (40 + 4)\,60$

$= 2400 + 240 = 2640$

43) (a) $36 \times 5.0 = 36 \times \dfrac{10}{2} = \dfrac{36}{2} \times 10 = 18 \times 10 = 180$

(b) $\dfrac{440}{50} = \dfrac{440}{1} \times \dfrac{2}{100} = \dfrac{88}{10} = 8.8$

(c) $28 \times 25 = 28 \times \dfrac{100}{4} = \dfrac{28}{4} \times 100 = 700$

(d) $\dfrac{120}{25} = \dfrac{120}{1} \times \dfrac{4}{100} = \dfrac{480}{100} = 4.8$

(e) $120 \times 0.25 = 120 \times \tfrac{1}{4} = 30$

(f) $89 \times 33.3 = 89 \times \dfrac{100}{3} = \dfrac{89}{3} \times 100 \approx \dfrac{90}{3} \times 100 = 3000$

Approximate Calculations and Percent Errors

Rapid mental calculation to find an approximate answer is a useful skill and one that often involves rounding off to easily handled numbers. In the type of calculation so often encountered in science, however, in which several numbers are to be multiplied and divided, obvious rounding is not always the most useful procedure. Simple rounding off does permit estimation of error type (is the result too large or too small?), and, if necessary, the size of error as a percentage of the answer.

EXAMPLE 41

What is the approximate price of three items that cost $7.98 each? Round off the price to $8. Then 3 × $8 = $24. The actual price is less than that used in the calculation. Therefore, the actual total is less than $24.

To determine not only whether the approximate answer is too large or too small, but also by how much, you can calculate the percent introduced by an approximation. (Usually, an approximate percent is sufficient. Guard against spending more time calculating the percent than you saved by making the rapid approximation.)

Percent error in any calculation is defined by the equation:

$$\text{Percent error} = \frac{\text{Error}}{\text{True value}} \times 100\%$$

The absolute value of error usually is used without any plus or minus signs.

EXAMPLE 42

Calculate the percent error: (a) 14 is rounded down to 10 and (b) 1004 is rounded down to 1000. For each, the error is 4.

(a) % error $= \dfrac{4}{14} \times 100\% = 28.6\%$

(b) % error $= \dfrac{4}{1004} \times 100\% = 0.4\%$

Note that the same size change can result in different percent errors. This calculation should be used to understand proportional reasoning.

PROBLEM 44

Calculate the approximate percent error introduced by the indicated rounding off for each example.
(a) Round 750 to 800
(b) Round 750 to 700
(c) Round 798 to 800
(d) Round 198 to 200
(e) Round 210 to 200

Answers to Problem 44

(a) Error $= 800 - 750 = 50$

$$\text{% error} = \frac{50}{750} \times 100 = \frac{500}{75} = \frac{100}{15} = \frac{20}{3} = 6\tfrac{2}{3}\% \text{ (positive)}$$

(b) Error $= 750 - 700 = 50$

$$\text{% error} = \frac{50}{750} \times 100 = \frac{500}{75} = \frac{100}{15} = \frac{20}{3} = 6\tfrac{2}{3}\% \text{ (negative)}$$

(c) Error $= 800 - 798 = 2$

$$\text{% error} = \frac{2}{798} \times 100 = \frac{200}{798} = 0.25\% \text{ approx.}$$

(d) Error $= 200 - 198 = 2$

$$\text{% error} = \frac{2}{198} \times 100 = \frac{200}{198} = 1\% \text{ approx.}$$

(e) Error $= 220 - 210 = 10$

$$\text{% error} = \frac{10}{210} \times 100 = \frac{1000}{210} = \frac{100}{21} = 5\% \text{ approx. (negative)}$$

EXAMPLE 43

How much solution should you mix to make measurements on eight samples if each requires 110 ml? You will make up more than the minimum required in case of waste, spills, etc., so you do not need to know the precise amount needed. Calculate such that you are sure you are making enough.

Rounding off, approximately 100 ml per sample is needed:

$$8 \text{ samples} \times \frac{100 \text{ ml}}{\text{sample}} = 800 \text{ ml}$$

The number used in calculation, 100, was less than the amount actually needed (110), so the amount calculated is too small. The error is approximately 10%:

$$\frac{10 \text{ ml error}}{110 \text{ ml needed}} \times 100\% \approx 10\%$$

An additional 100 ml will more than make up for the 10% error and 100 ml more to allow for waste would indicate that you should make up at least 1000 ml of solution.

Five rules to remember when rounding off numbers during calculations follow.

Rule 1

In some problems, it is possible to minimize errors caused by rounding off. When you are to multiply two numbers and one is rounded down to a smaller number, try to round the other up to a larger number: $93 \times 69 \approx 90 \times 70$.

EXAMPLE 44

Multiply 2.7×38. The usual way to round off would be to make both numbers larger, but then your answer is too large:

$$2.7 \times 38 \approx 3 \times 40 = 120$$

Rounding 2.7 down to 2 is such a large percentage change that, again, you introduce a large percent error. Consider rounding 2.7 down to 2.5, which in this calculation is a convenient number to use:

$$2.7 \times 38 \approx 2.5 \times 40 = 100$$

The correct answer is $2.7 \times 38 = 103$. Therefore, the second method gives a more nearly correct answer.

Rule 2

In a calculation involving division, it is desirable to round off the numerator and the denominator in the same direction; if the numerator is rounded to a larger number, the denominator should also be rounded to a larger number. This rule is especially important if the rounding off introduces a large percentage change, as in:

$$\frac{68}{47} \approx \frac{70}{50}$$

EXAMPLE 45

Find the approximate quotients:

1. $\dfrac{387}{750}$ 2. $\dfrac{419}{850}$

In each fraction, you can round the denominator up or down equally well. For problem 1, it is also convenient to round the denominator up:

$$\frac{387}{750} \approx \frac{400}{800} = 0.5$$

If the denominator is rounded down to 700, the result is 0.57. Because the correct answer is 0.52, the procedure of rounding numerator and denominator in the same direction gives a more nearly correct answer.

For problem 2, the numerator is rounded down, from 419 to 400. Likewise, the denominator is rounded down:

$$\frac{419}{850} \cong \frac{400}{800} = 0.5$$

The correct answer is 0.49.

Rule 3

When one number is to be divided by another, rounding off can be done in such a way that one number is especially easy to divide by another.

EXAMPLE **46**

$$\frac{298}{2} \times 15 \approx \frac{300}{30} = 10: \text{ means is approximately equal to}$$

$$\frac{685}{702} \approx \frac{700}{700} = 1: \text{ the actual quotient should be less than 1,}$$
$$\text{because the numerator is less than 700}$$

Rule 4

Some combinations cancel well. For example, 9×11 is close to 10×10; 9 is 1 less than 10 and 11 is 1 more than 10. Similarly, 8×12 is also close to 10×10 and, of course, to 9×11.

EXAMPLE **47**

Find the approximate answer.

$$8 \times 6 \times \frac{93}{(7)^2}$$

Because 8×6 is close to 7×7, they can be cancelled.

$$8 \times 6 \times \frac{93}{7 \times 7} \cong 93$$

Rule 5

Some calculations may require cancelling several numbers in order to reach a setup that allows a rapid mental calculation.

EXAMPLE **48**

Find the approximate answer to the following:

$$\frac{273 \times 775 \times 350}{298 \times 760}$$

You can make a gross approximation and consider $273 \cong 298$ so they cancel:

$$\frac{273}{298} \cong 1$$

but your answer will be too large (and 10% error), because you are pretending that 273 is actually a larger number, 298. Cancelling 775 with 760 causes far less error (about 2%), but note that, again, the true answer will be larger than the calculation shows. Similarly, if 273 is cancelled with 298, you know that the true answer will be smaller. The two effects will not entirely counteract each other, because the percent error is not the same.

You could write:

$$\frac{273}{298} \times \frac{775}{760} \times 350 \cong 350$$

Knowing that this answer is too large, you might guess that the correct answer is near 330.

To be more accurate, notice that 273 and 298 are close to 270 and 300, and that they are divisible by 30:

$$\frac{273}{298} \approx \frac{270}{300} = \frac{9}{10} = 0.9 = 1 - 0.1$$

$$\frac{273}{298} \times \frac{775}{760} \times 350 \approx (1 - 0.1) \times 350 = 350 - 35 = 315$$

Knowing that this number is too small (error from $^{775}\!/_{760}$), you might guess the correct answer is about 320.

EXAMPLE **49**

Find the approximate answer:

$$\frac{2(450)}{(0.082)(298)}$$

You can solve this problem using several approaches.

Method 1

In rounding 298 to 300, note that:

$$2 \times 450 = 900, \text{ thus } \frac{900}{(0.082)(300)} = \frac{3}{0.082}$$

To simplify the division, round 0.082 to 0.1, an increase of about 25%:

$$\frac{3}{0.1} = 30$$

For a more accurate answer, consider that 30 is too small, because the denominator used was too big. Estimate that the result should be about 25% larger, or about 37.

Method 2

Round both 450 and 0.082:

$$\frac{2(450)}{0.082(298)} \approx \frac{2(500)}{0.1(300)} = \frac{10}{0.3} = \frac{100}{3} = 33$$

Method 3

Rewrite in exponential notation with slight initial rounding off.

$$\frac{2(450)}{0.082(298)} \approx \frac{2 \times 4.5 \times 10^2}{8 \times 10^{-2} \times 3 \times 10^2}$$

$$= \frac{9 \cdot 10^2}{8 \cdot 3}$$

$$= \frac{3}{8} \times 10^2$$

$$= 0.37 \times 10^2 = 37$$

PROBLEM **45**

Make rapid approximate calculations for each.

(a) $\dfrac{27 \times 720}{59}$

(b) $\dfrac{760 \times 22.4 \times 330}{900 \times 273}$

(c) $\dfrac{9^2 \times 620}{99 \times 0.8}$

Answers to Problem 45

(a) $\dfrac{27 \times 720}{59} \approx \dfrac{30 \times 720}{60} = \dfrac{720}{2} = 360$

$$\text{Correct answer} = 329.5$$

(b) $\dfrac{760 \times 22.4 \times 330}{900 \times 273} \approx \dfrac{760 \times 20 \times 330}{900 \times 270}$

$$= \frac{76 \times 2 \times 33}{9 \times 27} = \frac{152 \times 33}{9 \times 27}$$

$$= \frac{150 \times 50}{10 \times 30} = 20$$

$$\text{Correct answer} = 22.9$$

Applied Math Concepts Required for Physical and Biological Sciences 161

(c) $\dfrac{9^2 \times 620}{99 \times 0.8} \approx \dfrac{81 \times 620}{100 \times 0.8}$

$= \dfrac{80 \times 620}{10 \times 8} = 620$

Correct answer $= 634$

Concept 21: Permutations, Combinations, and Probability

Knowledge of permutations, combinations, and probability is useful in determining the number of logical possibilities of some event without necessarily enumerating each case. Try to memorize the formulas that are included in this section.

Fundamental Principles of Counting

If an event can occur in x different ways, and a second event can occur in y different ways, and a third event can occur in z different ways, then the number of ways the events can occur in the order indicated is $x \cdot y \cdot z$. This multiplication rule of counting is expressed by the formula:

Total number of ways events occur $= x \cdot y \cdot z$

EXAMPLE 50

License plates of a certain state contain three letters followed by three digits, and the first digit cannot be zero. Calculate the number of possible different license plates as follows. Each letter can be selected in 26 different ways, the first digit in 9 ways, and each of the other digits in 10 ways:

Letters	Digits
26 26 26	9 10 10

$26 \cdot 26 \cdot 26 \cdot 9 \cdot 10 \cdot 10 = 15{,}818{,}400$

In other words, about 16 million distinct plates are possible. This principle is particularly useful in understanding genetic codes (see Chapter 7).

Factorial Symbol

The notation n! (read: n factorial) denotes the product of the positive integers from 1 to n, inclusive:

$n! = 1 \cdot 2 \cdot 3 \ldots (n-2)(n-1)n$ (in ascending order)

Equivalently, n! is defined by:

$n! = n \cdot (n-1)!$

It is also convenient to define $0! = 1$, $1! = 1$.

EXAMPLE 51

1. $2! = 1 \cdot 2 = 2$
    $3! = 1 \cdot 2 \cdot 3 = 6$
    $4! = 1 \cdot 2 \cdot 3 \cdot 4 = 24$
    $5! = 5 \cdot 4! = 5 \cdot 24 = 120$
    $6! = 6 \cdot 5! = 6 \cdot 120 = 720$
    $7! = 7 \cdot 6! = 7 \cdot (720) = 5040$

2. $\dfrac{8!}{6!} = 8 \cdot 7 \cdot \dfrac{6!}{6!} = 8 \cdot 7 = 56$

3. $\dfrac{9!}{7!3!} = \dfrac{9 \cdot 8 \cdot 7!}{7! \, 3 \cdot 2 \cdot 1} = 12$

Combination Factorial Symbol

The combination factorial symbol is defined as:

$\binom{n}{r} = n_{C_r} = {}_nC_r$

Read en-see-are, in which r and n are positive integers with $r \leq n$, by:

$$\binom{n}{r} = \frac{n(n-1)(n-2)\ldots(n-r+1)}{1 \cdot 2 \cdot 3 \ldots (r-1)r}$$

$$\binom{n}{r} = \frac{n!}{r!\,(n-r)!}$$

EXAMPLE 52

1. $\binom{8}{3} = \dfrac{8!}{3!5!} = \dfrac{8 \cdot 7 \cdot 6 \cdot 5!}{3 \cdot 2 \cdot 1 \cdot 5!} = 56$

2. $\binom{10}{4} = \dfrac{10!}{4!6!} = \dfrac{10 \cdot 9 \cdot 8 \cdot 7 \cdot 6!}{4 \cdot 3 \cdot 2 \cdot 1 \cdot 6!} = 210$

3. $\binom{12}{1} = \dfrac{12!}{1!11!} = \dfrac{12 \cdot 11!}{11!} = 12$

Permutations

Any arrangement of a set of n objects in a **given order** is called a permutation of the objects (taken all at a time). The arrangement has a **specific** possible order. Any arrangement of any of these objects in a given order is called a permutation of the n objects taken r at a time.

Consider the set of P, Q, R, S.

Permutations of four letters (taken all at a time):

P,Q,R,S	Q,P,R,S	R,P,Q,S	S,P,Q,R
P,Q,S,R	Q,P,S,R	R,P,S,Q	S,P,R,Q
P,S,Q,R	Q,R,S,P	R,S,P,Q	S,R,P,Q
P,S,R,Q	Q,R,P,S	R,S,Q,P	S,R,Q,P
P,R,S,Q	Q,S,P,R	R,Q,S,P	S,Q,P,R
P,R,Q,S	Q,S,R,P	R,Q,P,S	S,Q,R,P

yields 24 permutations in all.

Permutations of four letters (taken three at a time):

P,Q,R	Q,P,S	R,P,S	S,P,Q
P,R,Q	Q,S,P	R,S,P	S,Q,P
P,Q,S	Q,S,R	R,Q,S	S,Q,R
P,S,Q	Q,R,S	R,S,Q	S,R,Q
P,R,S	Q,P,R	R,P,Q	S,P,R
P,S,R	Q,R,P	R,Q,P	S,R,P

yields 24 permutations in all for this case also.

Permutations of four letters (taken two at a time):

P,Q	P,R	P,S
Q,P	R,P	S,P
Q,S	R,Q	S,Q
Q,R	R,S	S,R

yields 12 permutations in all.

The number of permutations of n objects taken r at a time is denoted by:

$$P(n,r) \text{ or } {}_nP_r$$

To find an expression for $P(n,r)$, observe that the first element in an r-permutation of n objects can be chosen in n different ways; the second element in the permutation can be chosen in $n-1$ ways; and the third element in the permutation can be chosen in $n-2$ ways. Continuing in this manner, the rth (last) element in the r-permutation can be chosen in $n-(r-1) = n-r+1$ ways. Thus, by the fundamental principle of counting:

$$P(n,r) = n(n-1)(n-2)\ldots(n-r+1)$$

Formula $P(n,r) = \dfrac{n!}{(n - r)!}$

In the special case in which $r = n$,

$$P(n,n) = n(n - 1)(n - 2) \ldots 3 \cdot 2 \cdot 1 = n!$$

Solve the problem with sets of letters using $P(4,4)$, $P(4,3)$, $P(4,2)$ and check your answers with arrangements shown in the preceding examples with letters P, Q, R, S. (Study this material in conjunction with genetic codes, gene mapping, and other pertinent topics, as outlined in Chapter 8.)

EXAMPLE 53

In how many ways can five people sit in five chairs? In four chairs?

5 people and 5 chairs	Assume all chairs are in a straight row
n = 5 = people	$P(5,5) = \dfrac{5!}{(5 - 5)!)} = \dfrac{5!}{0!} = 5! = 120$ ways
r = 5 = chairs	

5 people, 4 chairs	
n = 5 = people	$P(5,4) = \dfrac{5!}{(5 - 4)!)} = \dfrac{5!}{1!} = 5! = 120$ ways
r = 4 = chairs	

Whether you provide 5 or 4 seats, the number of arrangements does not change. It would be hard to guess at the possible answer without the formula given.

5 chairs	4 chairs
A B C D E	A B C D
A B C E D	A B D C
A B D C E	A B C E
A B E C D	A B E C
and so on	and so on

Compare these permutations with the letter set (P, Q, R, S) permutations.

Combinations

Imagine a collection of n objects. Remember that combinations represent groups, not arrangements. A combination of these n objects taken r at a time is any selection of r of the objects in which order does not count. In other words, an r-combination of a set of n objects is any subset containing r objects. For example, the combinations of the letters a, b, c, d, taken three at a time are:

(a,b,c),(a,b,d),(a,c,d),(b,c,d) or simply abc, abd, acd, bcd

The following combinations are equal:

abc, acb, bca, cab, bac, cba

in that each denotes the same set (a,b,c). The number of combinations of n objects taken r at a time is denoted by $C(n,r)$. The symbols $_nC_r$, C_{nr}, and C_{nr} also appear in various texts. To find the general formula for $C(n,r)$, we note that any combination of n objects taken r at a time determines r! permutations of the object in the combination:

$$P(n,r) = r!\, C(n,r)$$

$$C(n,r) = \frac{P(n,r)}{r!} = \frac{n!}{r!(n - r)!} = \binom{n}{r}$$

EXAMPLE 54

In how many ways can three people sample iced tea, a soft drink, mineral water, and lemonade (1) if each person samples only one drink, and (2) if each person samples only two drinks?

1. Each person must select one of the four drinks, so each has $C(4,1) = \begin{bmatrix}4\\1\end{bmatrix} = \dfrac{4!}{1!3!} = 4$ different possible choices:

    [n = 4 drinks

    r = 1 drink selected]

Because each person makes the selection independently, there are

$$4 \times 4 \times 4 = 64 \text{ possible ways}$$
$$\uparrow \quad \uparrow \quad \uparrow$$

2. Each person must select two of the four drinks (in any order), so each has
C (4,2) = $\binom{4}{2}$ = $\frac{4!}{2!2!}$ = 6 possible two-drink combinations. Because each person selects two drinks independently, there are

$$6 \times 6 \times 6 = 216 \text{ possible ways}$$
$$\uparrow \quad \uparrow \quad \uparrow$$

(Note that this illustration involves combinations rather than permutations, together with the multiplication of choices principle.)

EXAMPLE 55

How many committees of three can be created from nine people? Each committee represents a combination of the nine people taken three at a time. Thus,

$$C(9,3) = \binom{9}{3} = \frac{9!}{3!(9-3)!)} = \frac{9 \times 8 \times 7 \times 6!}{6 \cdot 6!}$$

$$= 84 \text{ different committees can be formed}$$

EXAMPLE 56

A farmer buys three cows, one pig, and four hens from a man who has seven cows, five pigs, and eight hens. How many choices does the farmer have?

The farmer can choose the cows in C(7,3) ways, the pigs in C(5,1) ways, and the hens in C(8,4) ways. Therefore, he can choose the animals in

$$\binom{7}{3}\binom{5}{1}\binom{8}{4} = \frac{7 \cdot 6 \cdot 5}{3 \cdot 2 \cdot 1} \times \frac{5}{1} \times \frac{8 \cdot 7 \cdot 6 \cdot 5}{4 \cdot 3 \cdot 2 \cdot 1} = 12{,}250 \text{ ways}$$

Probability of an Event

It is important to feel confident with the basic concept of probability as applied to genetics (Hardy-Weinberg principle) and physical chemistry (quantum numbers). Probability of something happening is a measure of how likely it is that an event may occur. Probability lies between 0 (impossible) to 1 (certain).

Probability of an event = p(E).

1. p(E) = Number of desired outcomes of E/Number of possible outcomes of E
2. p(success) + p(failure) = 1
3. $0 \le p(E) \le 1$

Note that probability cannot be negative.

EXAMPLE 57

A bag of candy-coated chocolates contains five greens and three yellows. What is the probability of selecting a green candy (1) in one try and (2) on the second try? (After the first try, put the candy back into the bag before you take the second one.)

1. $p(g) = \dfrac{5}{5+3} = \dfrac{5}{8} = \dfrac{\text{Total no. of green candies}}{\text{Total no. of candies}}$

2. During first try: $p(g) = \dfrac{5}{8}$, as shown in part 1

    During second try: $p(g) = \dfrac{5}{8}$ again, because nothing has changed

Observe that under the same given conditions, the probability p(g) does not change for each try. Do not imagine that two trials will double the probability. This is the key to learning the definition of probability and its application. To answer the question, "What is the probability of selecting a green candy after two tries when selection is done with replacement from a bag containing 5 greens and 3 yellows?" you must apply the principle of probabilistic independence (see statistically independent events):

$$p(\text{green in 2 tries}) = 1 - p(\text{no green in 2 tries})$$

$$= 1 - p(\text{no green on 1st try}) \cdot p(\text{no green on 2nd try})$$

$$= 1 - \frac{3}{8} \cdot \frac{3}{8}$$

$$= 1 - \frac{9}{64} = \frac{55}{64}$$

Note: If an identical experiment is repeated under identical conditions in numerous independent trials, the probability for success will remain the same for each individual trial.

A graphic solution is illustrated for students who are using genetics (Punnett squares).

Probability Matrix	
Probability of green on 1st try	$= \dfrac{5}{8}$
Probability of no green on 1st try	$= \dfrac{3}{8}$
Probability of green on 2nd try	$= \dfrac{5}{8}$
Probability of no green on 2nd try	$= \dfrac{3}{8}$

Figure 6-62 is a map showing all (8) possible outcomes. Figure 6-63 displays the possible outcomes for the first and second tries. Using these figures, you can make these assessments:

(i) Probability of 1st candy being green and 2nd candy being green

$$= \left(\frac{5}{8}\right)\left(\frac{5}{8}\right) = \frac{25}{64}$$

(ii) Probability of 1st candy being green and second candy being yellow

$$= \left(\frac{5}{8}\right)\left(\frac{3}{8}\right) = \frac{15}{64}$$

(iii) Probability of 1st candy being yellow and second candy being green

$$= \left(\frac{3}{8}\right)\left(\frac{5}{8}\right) = \frac{15}{64}$$

(iv) Probability of 1st candy being yellow and second candy being yellow

$$= \left(\frac{3}{8}\right)\left(\frac{3}{8}\right) = \frac{9}{64}$$

Fig. 6-62.

Yellow	Green	Green
Yellow	Green	Green
Yellow	Green	

Fig. 6-63. Possible outcomes for first and second tries

		Second try	
		Green	**Yellow**
First try	**Green**	Green, Green	Green, Yellow
	Yellow	Yellow, Green	Yellow, Yellow

Adding i, ii, and iii gives you the probability of getting a piece of green candy in either of two tries:

$$\frac{25}{64} + \frac{15}{64} + \frac{15}{64} = \frac{55}{64}$$

Mutually Exclusive Events

Certain events cannot occur simultaneously; for example, a student cannot attend anthropology and biology classes at the same time. If a college offers 12 classes at 2:30 p.m., the probability that a certain student, known to be in class at that time, will be in anthropology or biology is:

$$p(A \text{ or } B) = p(A) + p(B)$$

$$p(\text{Anthropology or Biology}) = \frac{1}{12} + \frac{1}{12} = \frac{2}{12} = \frac{1}{6}$$

Statistically Independent Events

Events can occur simultaneously, but the first event does not affect the second event. There is a probability that it rains in Miami, Florida, at 4 p.m. and a football game is played at 4 p.m. in Tampa, Florida, on the same day.

$$p(A) = p(\text{rains in Miami}) = \frac{1}{100} \text{ (assume)}$$

$$p(B) = p(\text{game played in Tampa}) = \frac{2}{29} \text{ (assume)}$$

$$p(A \text{ and } B) = p(A) \cdot p(B) = \frac{1}{100} \cdot \frac{2}{29} = \frac{1}{1450}$$

MEMORIZE	
$p(A \textbf{ or } B) = p(A) + p(B)$	Mutually exclusive
$p(A \textbf{ and } B) = p(A) \cdot p(B)$	Statistically independent

Remember that the probability of the union of mutually exclusive events is higher than the probability of either event. On the other hand, the probability of the simultaneous occurrence of statistically independent events is lower than the probability of either event.

EXAMPLE 58

A bag contains five peaches and four plums. Michelle selects one, replaces it, and selects another. What is the probability that both selections are peaches?

These are **independent events.**

$$p(A) = p(\text{peach}) \text{ in first selection} = \frac{5}{5 + 4} = \frac{5}{9}$$

$$p(B) = p(\text{peach}) \text{ in second selection} = \frac{5}{5 + 4} = \frac{5}{9}$$

$$p(A \text{ and } B) = \frac{5}{9} \cdot \frac{5}{9} = \frac{25}{81} \text{ is less than } \frac{5}{9}$$

EXAMPLE 59

Andrew has four nickels, seven pennies, and three dimes in his pocket. He selects one. What is the probability that it is a penny or a dime?

These are **mutually exclusive events** because no coin is both a penny and a dime.

$$p(\text{penny or dime}) = p(\text{penny}) + p(\text{dime}) = \frac{7}{14} + \frac{3}{14} = \frac{5}{7}$$

$\frac{5}{7}$ is more than $\frac{7}{14}$

1. Solve for x: $x^3 = 216a^6b^9$
2. Solve for y: $\dfrac{1}{y-1} + \dfrac{1}{y+2} = \dfrac{1}{5(y-1)}$
3. Solve for b: $6 - 2(3 - 2(5 - 3(b-2) - 4) - 2) - 1 = 50b$
4. The potential of an electric dipole is:

$$V = p\,\frac{\cos\theta}{r^2}$$

   in which p = the strength of the electric dipole, r = the distance from the electric dipole to the point of observation, and θ = the angle between the line to the point of observation and the direction of the dipole. If p is tripled, r is halved, and θ is changed from 0° to 60°, how are the original and final dipole potentials related?

5. The dose of a drug is 5 mg per kilogram of body weight. If a person weighs 70 kg, what amount of drug should be given?
6. The dose of a drug is 5 mg per 40 kg of body weight. If a person weighs 60 kg, what amount of drug should be given?
7. The cost of item A in 1986 was $64. Its cost in 1987 was $89.60. What was the percent increase in the price of item A between 1986 and 1987?
8. Evaluate: $4 \times 10^{-4} + 17 \times 10^{-6}$
9. Evaluate: $(2 \times 10^4)(5 \times 10^{-5})$
10. Solve for x: $x = \left(\dfrac{5 \times 10^3}{25 \times 10^{-5}}\right)^3$
11. Evaluate: $7.15 \times 10^3 + 0.025 \times 10^1$
12. The ideal gas law is PV = nRT. If the absolute temperature T is doubled, the pressure P is decreased by one quarter of its original value, and the number of moles n is unchanged, what is the new volume in relation to the original volume?
13. Find the value of: $\left(\dfrac{2}{3}\right)^{-6}\left(\dfrac{16}{27}\right)^2$
14. Solve for x: $\log(4x) = 2$
15. What is the slope of the line segment connecting the points $(17, -16)$ and $(2, 24)$?
16. The specific heat c (per unit volume) of a metal is described by the formula $= aT + bT^3$, in which T = absolute temperature and a,b = positive constants. If T is doubled, is the new specific heat less than eight times, exactly eight times, or more than eight times greater than the original specific heat?
17. Calculate the slope of the line in Figure 6-64 (use two points indicated).
18. Which slope in Figure 6-65 has the largest magnitude (neglecting signs)?

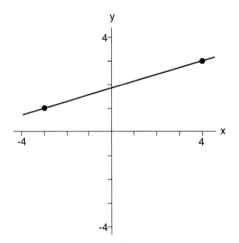

Fig. 6-64.

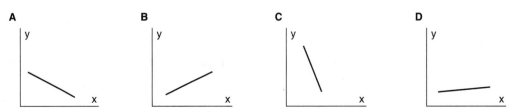

Fig. 6-65.

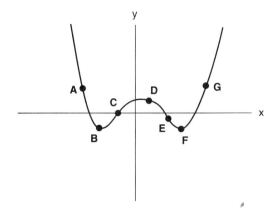

Fig. 6-66.

19. Which points in Figure 6-66, if any, are maximum points? Minimum points?
20. A linear graph can be algebraically described by the equation $2 + 9y = 15x$. What are the slope and y-intercept of this line?
21. The ideal-gas law for 1 mole of an ideal gas is PV = RT. The P,V graph for a constant temperature T is illustrated in Figure 6-67. For constant temperatures T_2 and T_3, such that $T_2 < T_1$ and $T_3 > T_1$, draw possible P,V graphs.

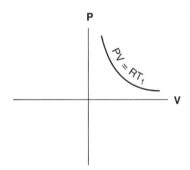

Fig. 6-67.

22. The relation between two variables, C and t, can be described by the equation:

$$C = C_o(1 - e^{-kt})$$

in which C_o, k = positive constants. Looking at $t \geq 0$ only, how does the slope of this curve vary? (Hint: to graph this equation and analyze how its slope varies, split the graph into three regions: $kt \ll 1$—in this region $e^{-kt} \approx 1 - kt$, $kt \approx 1$, and $kt \gg 1$). Plot a segmental graph and explain the connection between various segments.
23. A semi-log plot of $y = a(10)^{bx}$ has a y-intercept = 64 and a slope = 3. What are a and b?
24. In Figure 6-68, find b.

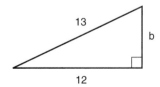

Fig. 6-68.

25. Evaluate: $\sin 30° \cos 60° - \tan 45° \sin 90°$
26. In Figure 6-69, find $\dfrac{\tan A}{\tan(A + B)}$.
27. What are the x- and y-components of A + B in Figure 6-70?
28. Convert 2 tons to grams.
29. Convert 100 ft to centimeters.
30. Convert 128 fluid ounces to milliliters.

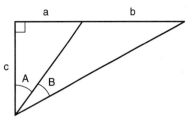

Fig. 6-69.

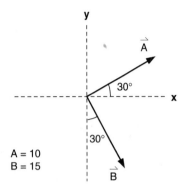

A = 10
B = 15

Fig. 6-70.

31. The electric potential V between two points is given by the formula V = Er, in which E = electric field and r = the distance between the two points. The electric field is given by $E = \dfrac{F}{q}$, in which F = the electrical force and q = charge. The unit of V is the volt. What is the volt equal to in terms of mass (m), length (l), time (t), and charge (q)?

32. Solve for R: $\dfrac{1}{R} = \dfrac{1}{R_1} + \dfrac{1}{R_2}$. Having a formula for R, rewrite the formula explicitly in terms of R_1 and $\left(\dfrac{R_1}{R_2}\right)$. As the value of $\left(\dfrac{R_1}{R_2}\right)$ goes to infinity, what value does R approach?

Solutions to Concepts Test

1) $\quad x^3 = 216a^6b^9$

$\quad \sqrt[3]{x^3} = \sqrt[3]{216a^6b^9} = \sqrt[3]{216}\, a^{6/3}b^{9/3}$

$\quad x = 6a^2b^3$

2) $\qquad \dfrac{1}{y-1} + \dfrac{1}{y+2} = \dfrac{1}{5(y-1)}$

$\quad 5(y+2) + 5(y-1) = y+2$

$\qquad\qquad 10y + 5 = y+2$

$\qquad 9y = -3;\ y = -\tfrac{1}{3}$

3) $\quad 6 - 2(3 - 2(5 - 3(b - 2) - 4) - 2) - 1 = 50b$

$\qquad 5 - 2(3 - 2(1 - 3b + 6) - 2) = 50b$

$\qquad\qquad 5 - 2(1 - 14 + 6b) = 50b$

$\qquad\qquad 5 + 26 - 12b = 50b$

$\qquad\qquad 31 = 62b;\ b = \dfrac{31}{62} = \tfrac{1}{2}$

4) Let $V_1 = p_1\cos\dfrac{\theta_1}{r_1^2}$ and $V_2 = p_2\cos\dfrac{\theta_2}{r_2^2}$, then

$$\frac{V_2}{V_1} = \frac{\dfrac{p_2\cos\theta_2}{r_2^2}}{\dfrac{p_1\cos\theta_1}{r_1^2}} = \frac{p_2}{p_1} \cdot \frac{\cos\theta_2}{\cos\theta_1} \cdot \frac{r_1^2}{r_2^2}$$

$\cos\theta_1 = \cos 0° = 1$, $\cos\theta_2 = \cos 60° = \frac{1}{2}$

$p_2 = 3p_1$ and $r_2 = r_1/2$

$$\frac{V_2}{V_1} = \frac{3p_1}{p_1} \cdot \frac{\frac{1}{2}}{1} \cdot \frac{r_1^2}{(r_1/2)^2} = 3 \cdot (\tfrac{1}{2}) \cdot 4 = 6, \text{ or}$$

$V_2 = 6V_1$

5) The dose of the drug is directly proportional to body weight. The ratio of drug dose to body weight is 5 mg/1 kg. Therefore, if x = the amount of the drug for a person weighing 70 kg, then:

$$\frac{5\text{ mg}}{1\text{ kg}} = \frac{x}{70\text{ kg}} \rightarrow x = 350\text{ mg}$$

6) The dose of the drug is directly proportional to body weight. The ratio of drug dose to body weight is 5 mg/40 kg. Therefore, if x = the amount of the drug for a person weighing 60 kg, then:

$$\frac{5\text{ mg}}{40\text{ kg}} = \frac{x}{60\text{ kg}} \rightarrow x = 7.5\text{ mg}$$

7) The price of A in 1986 = \$64; its price in 1987 = \$89.60. If p = % increase, then:

$$\$89.60 = \$64\left(\frac{1+p}{100}\right) \cdot 1.4 = \frac{1+p}{100} \rightarrow p = 40\%\text{ increase}$$

8) $4 \times 10^{-4} + 17 \times 10^{-6}$

$= 4 \times 10^{-4} + 0.17 \times 10^{-4} = 4.17 \times 10^{-4}$

9) $(2 \times 10^4)(5 \times 10^{-5})$

$= 10 \times 10^{4-5} = 10^1 \times 10^{-1} = 10^{1-1} = 10^0 = 1$

10) $x = \left(\dfrac{5 \times 10^3}{25 \times 10^{-5}}\right)^3 = \left(\dfrac{5}{25} \times 10^{3-(-5)}\right)^3$

$= (0.2 \times 10^8)^3 = (2 \times 10^7)^3 = 8 \times 10^{21}$

11) $7.15 \times 10^3 + 0.025 \times 10^1$

$= 7.15 \times 10^3 + 0.00025 \times 10^3$

$= 7.15025 \times 10^3$

12) Let $V_1 = \dfrac{n_1RT_1}{P_1}$ and $V_2 = \dfrac{n_2RT_2}{P_2}$, then:

$$\frac{V_2}{V_1} = \frac{\dfrac{n_2RT_2}{P_2}}{\dfrac{n_1RT_1}{P_1}} = \frac{n_2}{n_1} \cdot \frac{T_2}{T_1} \cdot \frac{P_1}{P_2}$$

$n_2 = n_1$, $P_2 = \dfrac{3}{4}P_1$, $T_2 = 2T_1$

$$\frac{V_2}{V_1} = \frac{n_2}{n_2} \cdot \frac{2T_1}{T_1} \cdot \frac{P_1}{\frac{3}{4}P_1} = 1 \cdot 2 \cdot \left(\frac{4}{3}\right) = \frac{8}{3}, \text{ or}$$

$V_2 = \dfrac{8}{3}V_1$

13) $\left(\dfrac{2}{3}\right)^{-6}\left(\dfrac{16}{27}\right)^{2} = \left(\dfrac{2}{3}\right)^{-6}\left(\dfrac{2^4}{3^3}\right)^{2} = \left(\dfrac{2^{-6}\cdot 2^8}{3^{-6}\cdot 3^6}\right) = \dfrac{2^2}{3^0} = 4$

14) $\log(4x) = 2$

$\qquad 4x = 10^2 = 100$

$\qquad x = 25$

15) Let $(x_1,y_1) = (17, -16)$ and $(x_2,y_2) = (2,24)$;

$$m = \dfrac{y_2 - y_1}{x_2 - x_1} = \dfrac{24 - (-16)}{2 - 17} = \dfrac{40}{-15} = \dfrac{-8}{3}$$

16) Let $c_1 = aT_1 + bT_1^3$ and $c_2 = aT_2 + bT_2^3$; $T_2 = 2T_1$.

$$\dfrac{c_2}{c_1} = \dfrac{aT_2 + bT_2^3}{aT_1 + bT_1^3} = \dfrac{2aT_1 + 8bT_1^3}{aT_1 + bT_1^3} < \dfrac{8aT_1 + 8bT_1^3}{aT_1 + bT_1^3} = 8$$

Thus $c_2 < 8c_1$

17) The two points on the graph are:

$$(x_1,y_1) = (-3,1) \text{ and } (x_2,y_2) = (4,3)$$

$$m = \dfrac{y_2 - y_1}{x_2 - x_1} = \dfrac{3 - 1}{4 - (-3)} = \dfrac{2}{7}$$

18) By inspection, graph c has the slope of the largest magnitude.

19) Based on the discussion of maximum, minimum, and inflection points in concept 11:
    D is a maximum point
    B, F are minimum points
    C, E are inflection points

20) $2 + 9y = 15x$. Putting this in slope-intercept form:

$$y = \dfrac{5}{3}x - \dfrac{2}{9}$$

Slope, $m = \dfrac{5}{3}$

y-intercept, $b = -\dfrac{2}{9}$

21) $PV = RT$ is a hyperbolic graph when $T = $ constant. If $T^2 < T^1$ and $T^3 > T^1$, possible graphs for $PV = RT^2$ and $PV = RT^3$ are as shown in Figure 6-71.

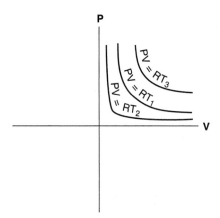

Fig. 6-71.

22) Split the graph (for $t \geq 0$) into three regions corresponding to:
    (A) $kt \ll 1, C = C_o(1 - e^{-kt}) \cong C_o(1 - (1 - kt)) = C_okt$(linear)
    (Note that we used the approximation $e^{-kt} \approx 1 - kt$ for $kt \ll 1$.)
    (B) $kt \approx 1, C = C_o(1 - e^{-kt})$ $\qquad\qquad$ (no approximation)

(C) $kt \gg 1, C = C_o(1 - e^{-kt}) \cong C_o$ (zero slope)
(Note that $e^{-kt} \cong 0$ for $kt \gg 1$.)

To graph this equation, use these three regions. For region A, the graph looks linear; for region C, the graph looks flat (zero slope); and for region B, these two partial graphs are connected by a smooth curve (Fig. 6-72). (Assign different values to kt from 0 to +5 and see if you can join segments I, II, and III with a smooth curve.)

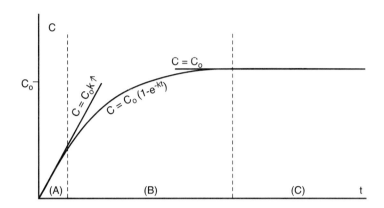

Fig. 6-72.

The slope starts off at a finite ($= C_ok$), nearly constant value (region A). As t increases, the slope decreases (region B) until it becomes zero (region C).

$kt \ll 1$ $C = C_okt$ (segment I)

For region A $0 \leq kt \leq 0.5$

$kt \approx 1$ $C = C_o(1 - e^{-kt})$ (segment II)

For region B $0.5 < kt < 3$

$kt \gg 1$ $C = C_o$ (segment III)

For region C $3 \leq kt < \infty$

23) $y = 64(10)^{3x}$. For the y-intercept ($x = 0$), $y = a(10)^{b \cdot 0} = a = 64$. The slope of the semi-log plot $= b = 3$.

24)   Using the Pythagorean theorem:

$$12^2 + b^2 = 13^2$$

$$b^2 = 13^2 - 12^2 = 169 - 144 = 25$$

$$b = 5$$

25) $\sin 30° \cos 60° - \tan 45° \sin 90°$

$= (\frac{1}{2})(\frac{1}{2}) - (1)(1) = \frac{1}{4} - 1 = -\frac{3}{4}$

26) $\dfrac{\tan A}{\tan(A + B)} = \dfrac{\dfrac{a}{c}}{\dfrac{a + b}{c}} = \dfrac{a}{a + b}$

27)   Recomposing the vectors A and B (Fig. 6-73):

$$A_x + B_x = A \cos 30° + B \sin 30° = 10\left(\frac{\sqrt{3}}{2}\right) + 15(\frac{1}{2}) = 5\sqrt{3} + 7.5$$

$$A_y + B_y = A \sin 30° - B \cos 30° = 10(\frac{1}{2}) - 15\left(\frac{\sqrt{3}}{2}\right) = 5 - \frac{15\sqrt{3}}{2}$$

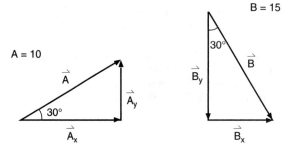

Fig. 6-73.

28) $(2 \text{ tons})\left(\dfrac{2000 \text{ lb}}{1 \text{ ton}}\right)\left(\dfrac{454 \text{ g}}{1 \text{ lb}}\right) = \dfrac{(2)(2000)(454)}{1} \text{ g} = 1,816,000 \text{ g} = 1.816 \times 10^6 \text{ g}$

29) $(100 \text{ ft})\left(\dfrac{12 \text{ in}}{1 \text{ ft}}\right)\left(\dfrac{2.54 \text{ cm}}{1 \text{ in}}\right) = \dfrac{(100)(12)(2.54)}{1} \text{ cm} = 3048 \text{ cm}$

30) $(128 \text{ oz})\left(\dfrac{1 \text{ pt}}{16 \text{ oz}}\right)\left(\dfrac{1 \text{ qt}}{2 \text{ pt}}\right)\left(\dfrac{0.95 \text{ liter}}{1 \text{ qt}}\right)\left(\dfrac{1000 \text{ ml}}{1 \text{ liter}}\right)$

$= \dfrac{(128)(0.95)(1000)}{(16)(2)} \text{ ml} = 3800 \text{ ml}$

31) $\text{volts} = V = Er = \dfrac{Fr}{q} = \dfrac{(ma)r}{q}$ for units analysis

$= \dfrac{(m)\left(\frac{1}{t^2}\right)(1)}{q} = \dfrac{m \cdot 1^2}{q \cdot t^2}$

32) $\dfrac{1}{R} = \dfrac{1}{R_1} + \dfrac{1}{R_2} \rightarrow R_1 R_2 = R(R_1 + R_2)$

$R = \dfrac{R_1 R_2}{R_1 + R_2}$

Alternatively,

$R = \dfrac{R_1}{1 + \left(\dfrac{R_1}{R_2}\right)}$ (as requested)

$\left(\dfrac{R_1}{R_2}\right) \rightarrow \infty, \ R = \dfrac{R_1}{1 + \left(\dfrac{R_1}{R_2}\right)} \rightarrow \dfrac{R_1}{\dfrac{R_1}{R_2}} = R_2$

DATA ANALYSIS IN PHYSICAL/BIOLOGIC SCIENCES

This part of Chapter 6 contains information concerning how to think about the three basic formats of data presentation followed by a brief encyclopedia of data analysis techniques. Read the review of data presentation carefully before you begin to work with data. The information about data analysis techniques should be reviewed quickly and then used for future reference. Most of the material in this section should already be familiar to you.

The new MCAT does not include a separate Quantitative Skills subtest. The data analysis tasks, according to the MCAT Student Manual and the AAMC practice tests, boil down to the following list of questions:

- Are you able to interpret information presented in graphic or tabular format?
- Are you familiar with various types of data, such as graphs, tables, or figures that are presented in passage-based problems?
- What are the basic principles and methods used in the presentation of data?

- Can you explain, identify, or compare the components of graphs, tables, figures, diagrams, and charts?
- Are you able to identify trends and relationships inherent in data?
- Do you always try to understand and determine the background knowledge relevant to a particular interpretation of data?
- Do you know how to select the most appropriate format for representing numeric information?
- Can you perform calculations on a set of numeric data for statistical analysis?
  - (i) Do you know how to determine the arithmetic average, range, and standard deviation?
  - (ii) Do you understand statistical association and correlation as applied to multiple data sets (from various instruments or different experimental investigations)?

Concept 22: Interpretation of Equations

Equations can be complicated. Like graphs, however, they can be broken down into simple parts. Unlike graphs, in which the parts are visually separate, the sections of an equation are often mixed up. There are three basic forms to consider: y may depend on x plus something, x times something, and something divided by x. In the first case, x and y increase at the same rate; in the second case, one variable increases faster than the other; in the third case, one variable increases as the other decreases.

The most important thing to remember about interpreting equations is that they are rules for calculating numbers. They tell you what to do to some numbers to generate a new number. The equation: $y = 8x$ tells you to take a value for x and to multiply it by 8 to generate the value for y. Although glancing at the equation may make you think that the x is bigger than the y, the reverse is in fact the case. Take extra care to avoid this common mistake.

PROBLEM **46**

Test your understanding of how to read equations.

(a) Six out of 10 doctors recommend brand A. Write an equation relating the number of doctors recommending brand A to the number of doctors recommending other brands.

(b) In a large hospital, the number of patients with smallpox (P_{sp}) is related to the number of patients with AIDS (P_a) by the equation $1000\ P_a = P_{sp}$. What is unusual about this situation?

Complicated equations can be understood by holding everything constant except for one pair of variables. If:

$$z = \frac{[a(u + v) - s^2]}{t(w - b)}$$

then z depends linearly on u (or v) and inversely on t (or w). To see this equation more clearly, lump everything together that is not the variable of interest.

$$z = \frac{[a(u + v) - s^2]}{t(w - b)}$$

$$= \left[\frac{au}{t(w - b)}\right] + \frac{(av - s^2)}{t(w - b)}$$

$$= ku + c$$

$$\text{in which } k = \frac{a}{t(w - b)} \text{ and } c = \frac{[av - s^2]}{t(w - b)}$$

With practice, you will learn to make these transformations very quickly in your head so that you can just look at a complicated expression and see how the different variables affect the value of the total expression.

Functions are often written in the form $y = f(x) = x + 2$, instead of $y = x + 2$. For complex expressions, this notation can be useful and you should know what it means and how to use it. The term $f(u,v,w)$ means that the function f depends on the variables u, v, and w and not on others. In the preceding expression for z, it would mean that you should consider u, v, and w as variables and the other letters as constants. In the term $f(s,t)$, u, v, w are constants and only s and t are considered variables.

Tables, graphs, and equations tell the same type of story but each **has its own particular** format. You should know how to relate these three notation systems. **Practice taking** information from one system and expressing it in the other by **using the exercises in** *Beyond Problem Solving and Comprehension* by Whimbey and Lochhead **(see Bibliography).**

Answers to Problem 46

(a) Correct answers are: $4D_A = 6D_X$ or, $\dfrac{D_A}{D_X} = \dfrac{6}{4}$

Common incorrect answers include:

$$6D_A = 4D_X, \quad 6D_A + 4D_X = 10, \quad 6D_A = 10D_X, \quad \dfrac{D_A}{D_X} = \dfrac{6}{10}$$

(b) This equation indicates that there are many more cases of **smallpox than of AIDS:** 1000 people with smallpox for every 1 person with AIDS. **Cases of smallpox are** rare because the disease has been eradicated worldwide. AIDS, **on the other hand, is** increasingly common. The expected ratio would be the reverse **of that indicated** by the equation.

Concept 23: Determining Inherent Trends and Relationships in Data

Usually, when presented with a set of data involving two variables, **say x and y, the data** are plotted as points in an xy-coordinate system in an effort to **identify the relation** between x and y (see previous discussion of graphs based on the **Cartesian coordinate** system, concept 9). Unfortunately, all data so plotted do not always **indicate a clear relation** between x and y. The result of such a plot might be just a **scatter of points or a** graph with no apparent regularity (Fig. 6-74). In these situations, it is **important to avoid** overreading the graphs. It may be necessary to restrict the analysis of **the data to specific** regions of the graph or to make just a general observation (such **as no relationship** between x and y obvious).

Some graphs of data points allow curves to be fitted or approximately **drawn through** them. When eyeballing a curve through points, your approximation **should be reasonably** accurate if there are as many points at (approximately) equal **distances above and below** the eyeballed curve (Fig. 6-75).

Remember that these curve fits are tentative assignments that are **best when you already** have an idea of the relation (linear, hyperbolic, etc.) between x and y. **Curve fitting is** an art and comes with practice and experience. It involves fitting **a simple equation to** a set of data points.

Concept 24: Statistical Data Analysis

In this discussion of quantitative interpretation of a set of data, i.e., **statistics, use the data** from the three sample experiments (A, B, and C) that follow.

Experiment A
In a psychology experiment designed to test the difficulty of a **particular maze, 10 rats** run the maze. The results for their solution times to the nearest 0.1 **second are: 8.3, 7.1,** 8.8, 11.1, 7.0, 13.7, 9.5, 10.3, 10.8, 9.9.

A

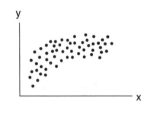

B

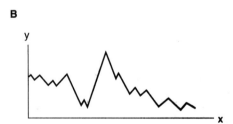

Fig. 6-74. *(A)* Scatter plots for data; *(B)* continuous line graph.

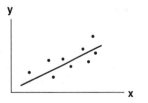

or

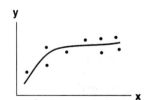

Fig. 6-75. Approximate curve fitting for a scatter plot.

Experiment B

As a physiology experiment, the students in a medical school class have to determine the pulse (number of heartbeats per minute) of 30 patients. The results of one student (which have been frequency grouped instead of recorded individually) to the nearest 5 are:

50: I (1)	65: V (5)	80: III (3)
55: II (2)	70: VII (7)	85: II (2)
60: III (3)	75: VI (6)	90: I (1)

Experiment C

A physiologic study involved measuring the blood cholesterol levels (mg/100 ml) of two groups of 35-year-old subjects, one group of men and one group of women. The data obtained (rounded to the nearest 1 mg/100 ml) are:

Group I (men):   195, 198, 199, 196, 195, 196, 191, 194, 195, 196
Group II (women): 196, 193, 194, 201, 202, 205, 204, 202, 199, 204

Types of Results

It is important to know how to organize and analyze all collected data so they can be interpreted/presented to someone else clearly and meaningfully. The information obtained in the preceding experiments reflects two types of data that are commonly encountered in raw form (as taken during an experiment and not manipulated into graphs, means, ranges, etc.). In experiment A, the data are of a **continuous** nature, because all decimal values of time are possible (e.g., 8.003, 9.1083, etc.) even though they are not recorded. In experiment B, the data are of a discrete, or count nature, because only integer values of pulse rate are possible. As measured, a pulse can be 6 or 7; it cannot be 7.1 or 6.983. The fact that they are count data is particularly evident for categories organized by age or gender in which the number in each group is recorded. The distinction between discrete and continuous data can be important.

PROBLEM 47

Are the data in experiment C count data or continuous data?

Sorting the Data

When presented with a set of data, it is a good idea to make some simple observations. Start by organizing the data in ascending or descending order (or groups). The data from experiment B are already in ascending order; those from experiment A will also be organized into an ascending order: 7.0, 7.1, 8.3, 8.8, 9.5, 9.9, 10.3, 10.8, 11.1, 13.7

Next, look closely at the data in experiments A and B by using the following simple steps.

Experiment A

1. Smallest value = 7.0
2. Largest value = 13.7
3. Range is 7.0 to 13.7: $13.7 - 7.0 = 6.7$
4. Average is about 10: $\dfrac{13.7 + 7.0}{2} \cong 10$

Experiment B

1. Smallest value = 50
2. Largest value = 90
3. Range is $90 - 50 = 40$
4. Most values are around 70, so the average is probably about 70
5. Few values are at the ends of the range (50 and 90), but many are at the middle (65 to 75)

These simple observations, which can be made rapidly, give you some idea about the limits, average value, variability, and distribution of the data over its possible values.

PROBLEM 48

Do the same type of simple analysis on the data for groups I and II in experiment C as was done for experiments A and B.

Suppose you are presented with the data from experiment A. For some reason, you are interested in the percentage of rats with times less than 9.0 seconds. Use the formula:

$$\text{Percent with times} < 9.0 \text{ seconds} = \frac{4}{10} \times 100 = 40\%$$

Now refer to the data from experiment B. An arbitrary definition of bradycardia (slow pulse) is a heart rate that is less than or equal to 60. To determine what proportion of the patients in the sample have bradycardia:

$$\text{Proportion with bradycardia} = \frac{6}{30} = 0.20$$

Observe that it is arbitrary whether you use percentages or proportions. In some cases, a percentage or proportion can be used to calculate a desired result.

EXAMPLE 60

Suppose that you do not know the total number of patients in experiment B. You are told that 12 people have pulse rates of 75 or greater and that this group constitutes 40% of the total number of patients. How many people, N, are included in this study?

$$12 = \frac{40}{100} \text{ N}; \text{ N} = 30 \text{ patients}$$

EXAMPLE 61

You are told that 40% of the rats in experiment A ran the maze in times greater than 10.0 seconds. How many rats, T, ran the maze in times greater than 10.0 seconds?

$$\text{T} = \frac{40}{100} \times 10 = 4$$

PROBLEM 49

What are the respective percentages of subjects in groups I and II in experiment C with blood cholesterol levels of 196 or lower?

Solutions to Problems 47–49

47) The data in experiment C are continuous data.

48) *Group I:* Put the data in ascending order: 191, 194, 195, 195, 195, 196, 196, 196, 198, 199; then:
   1. Smallest value = 191
   2. Largest value = 199
   3. Range is 199 − 191 = 8
   4. Most values are around 195 or 196, so the average is probably about 195 or 196
   5. Few values are at the ends of the range (191 and 199), but many are at the middle (195 to 196)

   Group II: Put the data in ascending order: 193, 194, 196, 199, 201, 202, 202, 204, 204, 205; then:
   1. Smallest value = 193
   2. Largest value = 205
   3. Range is 205 − 193 = 12
   4. Average is about 199: $\frac{193 + 205}{2} = 199$
   5. Values cluster toward the higher end of the range

49) *Group I:* Percentage with blood cholesterol levels of 196 or lower $= \frac{8}{10} \times 100 = 80\%$

   Group II: Percentage with blood cholesterol levels of 196 or lower $= \frac{3}{10} \times 100 = 30\%$

Central Tendency and Variation

Once a set of data is structured in a desired format and preliminary analysis has been done, more formal statistical calculations can be made to describe it. Statistically, the two key features of a set of data are its central tendency and its variation.

The central tendency of a set of data is the value it seems to approach. It is also called the expected value. It is the one value that is taken as representative of the whole set of data. The common measures of central tendency are the mode, median, and average (or mean). The computation of averages is required for the MCAT. The definitions of mode and median are given if needed, but it is best to become familiar with them during your preparative study.

Concept 25: Calculating Expected Value or Average

The **average** takes into account directly the value of each piece of data. It is calculated by adding together each piece of data and then dividing the sum by the total number of pieces of data:

$$\text{Average} = x = \frac{x_1 + x_2 + \ldots + x_n}{n}$$

in which x_1, x_2, . . ., x^n = the individual pieces of data and n = the total number of pieces of data.

In experiment A, the average is:

$$\text{Average} = [7.0 + \ldots + 13.7]/10$$

$$= (9.65) \approx 9.7$$

(Remember that the eyeballed average was about 10.)

In experiment B, the average is:

$$\text{Average} = [1(50) + 2(55) + 3(60) + 5(65) + 7(70) + 6(75) + 3(80)$$

$$+ 2(85) + 1(90)]/30$$

$$= (70.17) \approx 70$$

The **median** is the value in a set of data that is halfway between the lowest and highest values in the set. It is determined by listing all the values in the set of data in ascending order and then identifying the one that is positionally in the middle. For sets of data with an even number of values, the median is calculated by taking the average of the middle two numbers.

In experiment A, the values in ascending order are: 7.0, 7.1, 8.3, 8.8, 9.5, 9.9, 10.3, 10.8, 11.1, 13.7. Because there is an even number of values (10), the two middle values are 9.5 and 9.9. The median is:

$$\text{Median} = \frac{9.5 + 9.9}{2} = 9.7$$

In experiment B, the data are in ascending order as shown in concept 24. Again, given an even number of pieces of data, the median is the average of the two middle values (counting from either end). The median is:

$$\text{Median} = \frac{70 + 70}{2} = 70$$

The **mode** is the most frequent value that appears in a set of data. It exists only if one value occurs more often than any of the other values. In experiment A, no mode exists, because each value occurs only once. In experiment B, the mode = 70, because this value appears seven times.

The question naturally arises as to which measure of central tendency is the best. The answer is that it depends on the distribution of the data. Consider three sets of data, presented graphically in histograms (Fig. 6-76), in which N = the frequency of a particular value of the variable x.

For the data in histogram I, both the mode and the median are good measures of central tendency; the average (mean) is probably not. Whenever the frequency of one value predominates in a set of data, the mode is usually a good measure of central tendency. Unique modes do not exist for the data in histograms II and III.

For the data in histogram II, both the average and the median are good measures of central tendency. When the values of a set of data are distributed fairly evenly over the range of the data, as shown here, the average is sometimes considered better because it takes into account directly the value of each piece of data.

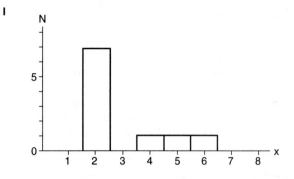

$$\text{Mean} = 2.9 = \frac{7(2)+1(4)+1(5)+1(6)}{7+1+1+1} \approx 3$$

Median = 2
Mode = 2
Data = 2,2,2,2,2,2,2,4,5,6

Fig. 6-76. Histograms showing mean, median, and mode.

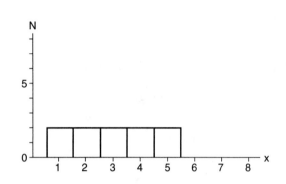

$$\text{Mean} = 3 = \frac{2(1)+2(2)+2(3)+2(4)+2(5)}{2+2+2+2+2}$$

Median = 3
One mode does not exist
Data = 1,1,2,2,3,3,4,4,5,5

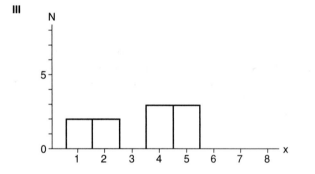

$$\text{Mean} = 3.3 \cong 3 = \frac{2(1)+2(2)+3(4)+3(5)}{2+2+3+3}$$

Median = 4
Two modes = 4,5 (bimodal)
Data = 1,1,2,2,4,4,4,5,5,5

In histogram III, the median is probably better than the average as a measure of central tendency. Typically, the median is preferable to the average when the values in a set of data are clustered toward one end of the range, but not in a way such that the mode would become a good measure of central tendency, as in histogram I.

PROBLEM 50

Calculate the mode, median, and average for each group in experiment C. Identify, if possible, which of the three measures of central tendency is probably best for each group.

SOLUTION

Group I: A unique mode does not exist; both 195 and 196 appear three times. The median is:

$$\text{Median} = \frac{195 + 196}{2} = 195.5 \approx 196$$

The average is:

$$\text{Average} = \frac{191 + 194 + \ldots + 199}{10} = 195.5 \approx 196$$

Both the average and the median are good measures of the central tendency of data in group I.

Group II: A unique mode does not exist; both 202 and 204 appear twice. The median is:

$$\text{Median} = \frac{201 + 202}{2} = 201.5 \approx 202$$

The average is:

$$\text{Average} = \frac{193 + \ldots + 205}{10}$$
$$= 200$$

It is a toss-up as to whether the median or the average is the better measure of central tendency. Qualitatively, the average tends to reflect the spread of data at the lower end of the range more than does the median, whereas the median tends to reflect the cluster of data at the high end of the range more than does the average.

Concept 26: Variation or Dispersion Around Average

Each measure of central tendency discussed in concept 25 gives one value to describe a whole set of data. This one value is inadequate to completely describe the data because it gives no sense of the variation (or the dispersion) of the data about this value. Knowledge of the variation in a set of data is needed to complement our knowledge of its central tendency. The common measures of variation are the range, variance, and standard deviation. Only the computation of the range is required for the MCAT. The definitions of variance and standard deviation are provided if needed, but it is best to become familiar with them during your preparative study.

The **range** is the difference between the highest and lowest values in a set of data. In experiment A, the range is:

$$\text{Range} = 13.7 - 7.0 = 6.7$$

In experiment B, the range is:

$$\text{Range} = 90 - 50 = 40$$

Because the range takes into account only the highest and lowest values in a set of data, it is a rough, and often not a reasonable, measure of variation. When either or both of the extreme values in a set of data are far out of line with the rest of the data, the range is a questionable measure of variation.

Consider the data presented in the histograms in Figure 6-77, in which N = the frequency of a particular value of the variable x. The range of the data in histogram IV gives a good idea of the variability of that data. On the other hand, the range of the data in histogram V does not really give a good idea of the variability of these results.

IV

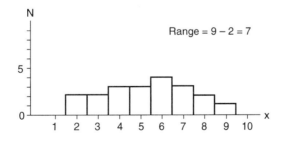

Fig. 6-77. Histograms showing dispersion of data around the mean.

V

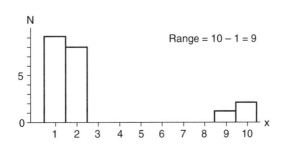

The **variance** (V) and the **standard deviations** (S.D.) are intimately related: S.D. = $\sqrt{V}$. The MCAT requires that you understand these concepts, but you will not have to make calculations. You should review and understand the following material, but you need not memorize it.

The variance, like the mean, takes into account each value in a **set of data**. It is calculated by taking the average value of the squares of the deviation for **each data point** from the mean:

$$\text{Variance} = \frac{(x_1 - \bar{x})^2 + (x_2 - \bar{x})^2 + \ldots + (x_n - \bar{x})^2}{n - 1}$$

in which $x_1, x_2, \ldots, x_n$ = values of individual pieces of data, x = **the mean, and** n = the total number of pieces of data.

The standard deviation is calculated by taking the square root of **the variance so calcu**lated:

$$\text{Standard deviation} = \left(\frac{(x_1 - \bar{x})^2 + (x_2 - \bar{x})^2 + \ldots + (x_n - \bar{x})^2}{n - 1}\right)^{1/2}$$

Calculation of the standard deviation and the variance in **experiments A and B is as** follows:

Experiment A

$$V = \frac{(7.0 - 9.7)^2 + (7.1 - 9.7)^2 + \ldots + (11.1 - 9.7)^2 + (13.7 - 9.7)^2}{10 - 1}$$

$$= 2.714 \approx 2.7$$

$$\text{S.D.} = \sqrt{V} = \sqrt{2.7} = 1.6$$

Experiment B

$$V = \frac{(50 - 70)^2 + 2(55 - 70)^2 + \ldots + 2(85 - 70)^2 + (90 - 70)^2}{30 - 1}$$

$$= 88.793 \approx 89$$

$$\text{S.D.} = \sqrt{V} = \sqrt{89} = 9.43 \approx 9$$

(Recall that these data were rounded off to the nearest 5.)

For a rough estimate of the standard deviation of a set of **data, take its range and** divide by 4:

$$\text{S.D.} \cong \frac{\text{Range}}{4}$$

In experiment A, a rough estimate is:

$$\text{S.D.} \cong \frac{13.7 - 7.0}{4} = 1.675 \cong 1.7$$

In experiment B, a rough estimate is:

$$\text{S.D.} \cong \frac{90 - 50}{4} = 10$$

Comparing these estimates of the standard deviation to the exact **calculations, you can** see that, when the range is a good indicator of the variation in **a set of data, this S.D.** approximation is also good.

PROBLEM 51

Calculate the range, variance, and standard deviation for each **group in experiment C.**

SOLUTION

Group I:

$$\text{Range} = 199 - 191 = 8$$
$$V = [(191 - 196)^2 + (194 - 196)^2 + \ldots + (198 - 196)^2$$
$$+ (199 - 196)^2]/(10 - 1)$$
$$= 5.0 \cong 5$$
$$\text{S.D.} = \sqrt{V} = \sqrt{5} = 2.236 \cong 2$$

Group II:

$$\text{Range} = 205 - 193 = 12$$
$$V = [(193 - 200)^2 + (194 - 200)^2 + \ldots + 2(204 - 200)^2$$
$$+ (205 - 200)^2]/(10 - 1)$$
$$= 18.7 \cong 19$$
$$\text{S.D.} = \sqrt{V} = \sqrt{19} = 4.359 \cong 4$$

Concept 27: Graphic Interpolation

Consider a set of data that relates two variables, x and y. Linear interpolation is a way of approximating the value of one of the variables, e.g., y, for a value of the other variable, e.g., x, which we do not have as a measurement in this set of data. Specifically, if you know that y always increases or always decreases when x increases in the set of data, you can linearly approximate the relation between x and y between any two adjacent data points and thereby calculate an approximate value of y for any value of x between these two points.

Consider the data in Figure 6-78. Suppose you are interested in knowing the value of y when x = 7. You observe (or know for a fact) that as x increases, y increases; thus, linear interpolation is possible. Interpolate the value of y at x = 7 by approximating the relation between x and y as linear between x = 0 and x = 10 (see Figure 6-78). Because y increases by 30 in this interval while x increases by 10, y is taken as increasing by 3 when x increases by 1. Therefore, the interpolated value of y at x = 7 is y = 10 + (7)(3) = 31. Note that when considering the use of interpolation, it is important to verify (or at least be confident) that an increasing/increasing or increasing/decreasing relation exists between the two variables, x and y.

PROBLEM 52

Using the data in Figure 6-78, interpolate the values of y for x = 16, 32, and 48.

SOLUTION

For x = 16: Slope of line segment between x = 10 and x = 20 is $\dfrac{60 - 40}{20 - 10} = 2$, i.e., y increases by 2 when x increases by 1. Thus, at x = 16, y = 40 + 6(2) = 52.

For x = 32: Slope of line segment between x = 30 and x = 40 is $\dfrac{85 - 75}{40 - 30} = 1$, i.e., y increases by 1 when x increases by 1. Thus, at x = 32, y = 75 + 2(1) = 77.

x	y
0	10
10	40
20	60
30	75
40	85
50	90

Fig. 6-78. Graphic interpolation.

Graphically ⟶

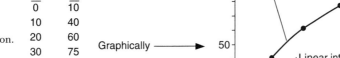

Applied Math Concepts Required for Physical and Biological Sciences 183

For x = 48: Slope of line segment between x = 40 and x = 50 is $\frac{90 - 85}{50 - 40} = \frac{1}{2}$, i.e., y increases by 1 when x increases by 2. Thus, at x = 48, y = 85 + 8($\frac{1}{2}$) = 89.

Concept 28: Problem Solving Using Data Analysis Techniques

1. Take enough time to understand what each number, axis, line, etc., means before trying to answer the questions in a problem. In other words, quickly assess the nature of the information presented, or conquer the given.

2. Read statements/questions carefully. Be sure you are answering the questions being asked, or What is the question? Look for qualifiers, because their presence or absence can determine whether a statement is true/supported or false/contradicted. Examples are:
   a. exactly versus approximately
   b. never versus sometimes (or usually) versus always (or consistently)
   c. greater versus tend to be greater
   d. on the average

3. Select relevant data or information pertinent to the question only. This process may involve simply extracting a particular piece of information from a table or graph. In other instances, you may have to decide which data are pertinent and which are irrelevant or inconclusive, such as when analyzing a set of data for possible correlation between two variables.

   Suppose you are given data relating three variables (A, B, and C). To detect a correlation between the values of A and the values of B (if one exists), you must look at subsets of these data in which C is a constant. Any subset of the data in which C is not constant in value cannot be used to determine a possible correlation between A and B; the only exception is if you already know that no correlation exists between the values of C and the values of A or B. Following the rule of comparison, you can compare only two things at a time.

4. Do not overextend stated facts or assumptions. Consider a composite group C that consists of two subgroups A and B (C = A + B). If you are told that 40% of C falls into a certain category, it is not reasonable to assume that it is true that approximately 40% of A and 40% of B each separately falls into this category. Avoid asking questions that are more detailed than the question itself. Your task is to answer the question before you, not one that you think should have been asked.

5. If the data in a problem are not presented in a good format for answering related questions, reorganize the data. Typically, this step is useful when you are presented with raw data. Suppose the data for experiment B in concept 24 consisted of a list of 30 patients, numbered 1 through 30, with a pulse rate recorded for each (raw format). If you are then asked questions about the distribution of pulse rate values in this set of data, it would be advantageous to reorganize these data into the frequency format as shown in concept 24.

6. Be careful to distinguish between "what" data and "why" data. Consider, as an example, a graph that shows the annual birth rate in the United States for the years between 1935 and 1955. From this graph, you know how the annual birth rate varied during this period, but not why it varied. Thus, the information is insufficient for answering any questions concerning explanations for changes in the birth rate during this period.

7. Be cautious about making value judgments. Although a set of data might show that the smoking of tobacco products predisposes smokers to mouth and lung diseases, you cannot conclude from these data that the sale of tobacco products should be restricted or banned because they are health hazards. Such a conclusion is a value judgment; to say that it is true or false would be to do so using your opinions concerning the regulation of products that are health hazards, not the data presented. You could conclude that doctors ought to warn their patients of the danger.

8. Do not make assumptions about missing information unless explicitly told to do so. Suppose you are given data that show that 4% of men who develop diabetes subsequently suffer blindness, whereas only 3% of women with diabetes are so affected. You are then presented with the statement: More men suffer blindness as a result of being diabetic than do women. It might seem attractive to make the assumption that about as many men develop diabetes as do women and thereby judge this statement as true/supported. This assumption is not justified, however, because you are not told to assume anything. The correct answer is that the information is insufficient to decide whether the statement is true or false.

9. In general, all information needed to answer questions is given in the problem. Nevertheless, general knowledge is to be used to interpret this information, such as in situations in which known relationships exist between the variables. On the other hand, do not use general knowledge to supply missing data or to answer a question on which the problem's data have no bearing.

10. When data are shown graphically, be aware of the slope of the graph as well as the graph itself. When two variables, x and y, are presented, the focus may well be on how the slope varies with x, not in how y varies with x (see discussion of slope in concept 11). Consider a reaction A + B = C. You might be given a graph that plots the amount of C formed versus time. If you are interested in the kinetics of the reaction, your attention will be directed to the rate of change of concentration (which is the slope of the graph) at a time t rather than to the total amount of C formed at the time t.

11. Interpolate values of a variable only when both of the following conditions are met (let the two variables be x and y; you are to interpolate a value of y for a given value of x for which there is not a measured value of y):

   a. A known increasing/increasing or increasing/decreasing relationship exists between x and y.

   b. You are interpolating the value of y for a given value of x that is between two measured data points. Simply, interpolation cannot be done outside the range of the data (see discussion of interpolation in concept 27).

12. Be aware of possibly different information-gathering procedures when comparing two groups of similar data.

13. Be careful when using the range as a measure of variability. Often the best way to make simple comparisons of distributions and relative variabilities of equivalent groups of data is to use frequency representations of them.

Practice Problems in Data Analysis and Reasoning

The problems in the remainder of this chapter are designed to give you practice in data analysis and reasoning to prepare you for the passage-based MCAT. The problems in this section present you with passages in several different forms, primarily written text and graphs or tables. You will need to extract information from all of these sources, which were introduced with exercises in previous sections. These problems are not intended to be exactly like those you will find on the MCAT.

Passage I (Questions 1–10): Physical Sciences Data

A group of introductory physics students were given the task of drawing a variety of graphs for five different situations. The first situation was a coconut on top of a palm tree and the second was a coconut falling from the top of the tree to the ground. The third situation involved a skateboarder, who was actually the professor in the course, coasting across the parking lot; the fourth involved his return hopping with his feet tied together in a bag. The final situation involved the launching of a Sprint missile during the power build-up phase when the missile continues to gain acceleration. Unfortunately, when the coconut dropped, it landed on the head of the student who was keeping track of which graphs referred to which situations. The other students were left with the task of sorting out the graphs representing distance, velocity, acceleration, and time as shown in Figure 6-79.

1. Do the students have at least one graph for each of the five kinds of motion? If not, which kinds of motion have been left out?

2. Which graph represents an object at rest?

3. Which graph represents uniform acceleration?

4. Which graphs represent the same kind of motion?

5. For which of these graphs is a graph of d versus t not a straight line?

6. Over a long time period, which of these motions will have the largest average velocity? (Assume in graph F that d goes as t^2.)
   As additional exercises, draw the following graphs.

7. An a versus t graph that represents the same motion as graph A

8. An a versus t graph that represents the same motion as graph C

9. A v versus t graph that represents the same motion as graph E

10. A v versus t graph that represents the same motion as graph F (assume d goes as t^2 in graph F)

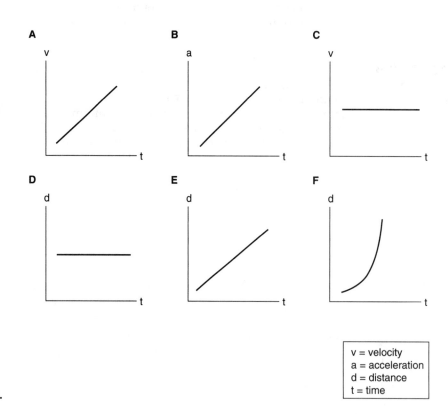

Fig. 6-79.

v = velocity
a = acceleration
d = distance
t = time

Passage II (Questions 11–21): Biologic Sciences Data

Each patient represented in the graph in Figure 6-80 received only one type of treatment. Percentages shown are of total number of patients receiving that treatment. The only dosages actually used are those indicated on the horizontal axis (all integral doses from 1 to 22).

For questions 11 through 16, based on the information given, select:

(A) If the first item is larger than the second

(B) If the second item is larger than the first

(C) If they are equal

(D) If the difference cannot be evaluated on the basis of the information given

11. **1.** Actual dosage of less than 14 units that is closest to the intersection of mitomycin C and Adriamycin lines
    2. Actual dosage of less than 14 units that is closest to the intersection of methotrexate and Adriamycin lines

12. **1.** Number of dosages for which mitomycin C has a higher 5-year survival percentage than methotrexate
    2. Number of dosages for which methotrexate has a higher 5-year survival percentage than mitomycin C

13. **1.** Highest dosage for which mitomycin C has a higher 5-year survival percentage than methotrexate
    2. Highest dosage for which methotrexate has a lower 5-year survival percentage than Adriamycin

14. **1.** Lowest dosage for which mitomycin C is more effective than both methotrexate and Adriamycin
    2. Highest dosage for which mitomycin C is less effective than both methotrexate and Adriamycin

15. **1.** Dosage for which Adriamycin has a higher 5-year survival percentage than mitomycin C and a lower 5-year survival percentage than methotrexate
    2. Half of lowest dosage for which Adriamycin has a higher 5-year survival percentage than methotrexate and a lower 5-year survival percentage than mitomycin C

16. **1.** Range of 5-year survival percentages experienced by groups receiving mitomycin C
    2. Range of 5-year survival percentages experienced by those receiving Adriamycin

17. Can one determine the average 5-year survival percentage of those receiving Adriamycin? If so, what was it? If not, why not?

18. If you are told that each dosage of radiation was received by the same number of patients, can one determine the average 5-year survival percentage of those receiving mitomycin C? If so, what was it? If not, why not?

19. Can one determine the average 5-year survival percentage of those persons receiving 12 units of radiation? If so, what was it? If not, why not?

20. You are also told that the total number of people who received mitomycin C was the same as the respective total numbers of people who received methotrexate and Adriamycin. Can one determine the average 5-year survival percentage of those receiving 12 units of radiation? If so, what was it? If not, why not?

21. You are given the further information that of those receiving 12 units of radiation, the number who received mitomycin C was the same as the respective numbers who received methotrexate and Adriamycin. Can one determine the average 5-year survival percentage of those receiving 12 units of radiation? If so, what was it? If not, why not?

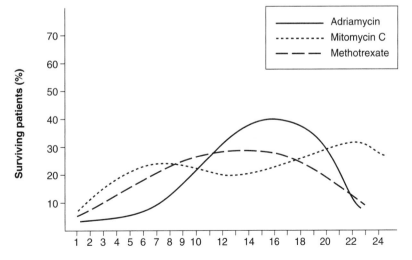

Fig. 6-80. Percentage of lung cancer patients surviving longer than 5 years after receiving 6 weeks of radiation therapy in indicated dosage along with indicated chemotherapeutic agent.

Passage III (Questions 22–26): Biologic Sciences Data

Look at the graph in Figure 6-81.

22. Explain why, at first glance, it seems wrong for these graphs to have a negative slope anywhere.

23. Explain how it is possible for them to have a negative slope.

24. Show where these graphs have a **negative slope.**

25. Which is more closely tied to a **high percentage of people catching measles at a particular age,** a high percentage or a **high positive change in percentage with respect to a change in age?**

26. What quantity indicates change **in percent** with respect to change **in age?**

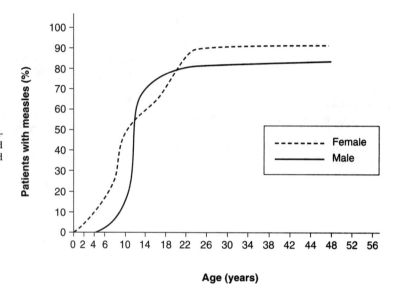

Fig. 6-81. Cumulative percentage of U.S. population that has had 14-day measles by age-group and gender.

Passage IV (Questions 27–32): Biologic Sciences Data

Look at the graph in Figure 6-82. Based only on the information given, select:

(A) If the statement is true or probably true

(B) If the information is not sufficient to indicate any degree of truth or falsity in the statement

(C) If the statement is false or probably false

27. There were more reported cases of whooping cough in country X in 1953 than in any other year studied.

28. More people had whooping cough in 1954 than in any other year.

29. A higher percentage of the population was reported to have fallen ill with smallpox in 1963 than in 1961.

30. If 10% of those reported to have contracted smallpox in 1957 died of it that year, and 3% of those reported to have contracted whooping cough in 1953 died of it in that year, then these figures represent more smallpox deaths than whooping cough deaths.

31. If 2% of the reported new cases of smallpox and 0.1% of the reported new cases of tuberculosis in 1957 died in that year, then more people died of tuberculosis in 1957 than died of smallpox.

32. On average, of the three diseases, whooping cough was the greatest threat to public health in the period between 1950 and 1963.

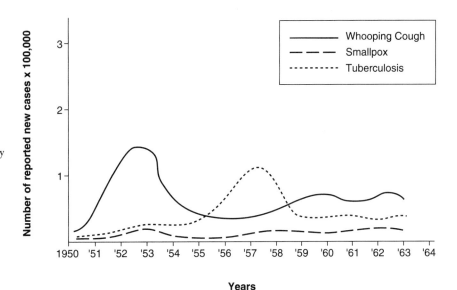

Fig. 6-82. Epidemics in country X between 1950 and 1963.

Passage I

1. **No** Graphs A and F both refer to constant acceleration. Graphs C and E both refer to constant velocity. Thus, only four different kinds of motion are represented. The hopping motion would involve a velocity that cycled up and down and an acceleration that also stepped up and down. The distance versus time graph would look like a staircase.

2. **D** In graph D, d = constant; so the object is at rest.

3. **A** Uniform acceleration = constant acceleration, which means constant change in velocity per unit time. In graph A, v is constantly increasing; so a is constant.

4. **C,E** In graph C, v = constant; so a = 0 (no graph is shown) and d = (constant) × t, as in E.

5. **A,B, or F** Graph of d versus t is a line in D and E. It is also a line if v = constant, as in C. In A, v goes as t, so d goes as t^2. In B, a goes as t, so v goes as t^2 and d goes as t^3. In F, d versus t is obviously not a line.

6. **B** Eventually, the motion in which d goes as t^3 will have the largest d, and hence the largest average velocity. That d goes as t^3 in B was identified in the answer to question 5.

7. Velocity changing constant amount per unit time, as in graph A, is equivalent to a constant acceleration (no graph shown).

8. Constant velocity, as in graph C, is equivalent to a = 0 (no graph shown).

9. Position changing constant amount per unit time, as in graph E, is equivalent to a constant velocity, as in graph C.

10. If d goes as t^2, then v goes as t; so v is constantly increasing, as in graph A.

Passage II

Remember that the real data in the graph for this problem are represented by the distinct points for each of the three chemotherapeutic agents at each of the integral radiation dosages from 1 to 22. The lines drawn through the points of each drug over the range of radiation dosages tend to obscure this fact. These lines clarify the presentation of the data by distinctly separating the data for the three drugs; however, the line segments between any two data points do not themselves represent data to be used in answering the questions for this problem.

11. **B** (1) Actual dosages closest to the intersection of mitomycin C and Adriamycin = 9 units

(2) Actual dosages closest to the intersection of methotrexate and Adriamycin = 10 units

12. **A** (1) Number of dosages for which mitomycin C has a higher 5-year survival percentage than methotrexate = (22 − 15) + (6 − 0) = 13

(2) Number of dosages for which methotrexate has a higher 5-year survival percentage than mitomycin C = 15 − 6 = 9

13. **A** (1) Highest dosage for which mitomycin C has a higher 5-year survival percentage than does methotrexate = 22 units

(2) Highest dosage for which methotrexate has a lower 5-year survival percentage than does Adriamycin = 21 units

14. **B** (1) Lowest dosage for which mitomycin C is more effective than both methotrexate and Adriamycin = 1 unit

(2) Highest dosage for which mitomycin C is less effective than both methotrexate and Adriamycin = 15 units

15. **C** (1) Dosage for which Adriamycin has a higher 5-year survival percentage than mitomycin C and a lower 5-year survival percentage than methotrexate = 10 units

(2) Half of lowest dosage for which Adriamycin has a higher 5-year survival percentage than methotrexate and a lower 5-year survival percentage than mitomycin C = ($\frac{1}{2}$)(20) = 10 units

16. **B** (1) Range of 5-year survival percentages experienced by groups receiving mitomycin C = about (30 − 8) = about 22%

(2) Range of 5-year survival percentages experienced by those receiving Adriamycin = about (43 − 1) = about 42%

Keep in mind when answering questions 17–21 that each experimentally unique group of patients is characterized both by the receipt of one of the three chemotherapeutic agents and by the receipt of a specific dosage of radiation therapy.

17. **No** In addition to the 5-year survival percentage data for Adriamycin shown in the graph, you would also need to know how the total number of patients receiving Adriamycin was distributed over the range of radiation dosages to be able to calculate the average 5-year survival percentage of those receiving Adriamycin. It is not reasonable to assume that the total number of patients receiving Adriamycin was distributed evenly over the range of radiation dosages.

18. **No** To calculate the average 5-year survival percentage of those receiving mitomycin C, it is not sufficient to know that each dosage of radiation was received by the same number of patients. You have not been told how this same number of patients is split among the three chemotherapeutic agents for each dosage of radiation. As in question 17, it is not reasonable to assume that this same number of patients was split among the three chemotherapeutic agents in the same manner for each of the dosages of the radiation.

19. **No** To calculate the average 5-year survival percentage of those receiving 12 units of radiation, you need to know how the total number of patients who received a radiation dosage of 12 units was split among the three groups of patients who received 12 units of radiation and one of the chemotherapeutic agents.

20. **No** The information that the total number of patients who received a particular chemotherapeutic agent was the same for all three drugs does not necessarily mean that the number of patients who received 12 units of radiation and a particular chemotherapeutic agent was the same for all three drugs. Thus, as in question 19, a lack of information about how the total number of patients who received 12 units of radiation was split among the three groups of patients who each received 12 units of radiation and one of the three drugs makes the requested calculation impossible.

21. **Yes, about 25%** The information given allows you to average the survival percentages at 12 units of radiation for the three chemotherapeutic agents shown in the graph to determine the average 5-year survival percentage of those who received 12 units of radiation. Observing that the averages are about 33% for Adriamycin, 26% for methotrexate, and 16% for mitomycin C, the average is about $\frac{(33 + 26 + 16)}{3} = 25\%$.

Passage III

22. You would expect the cumulative percentage of people who have had 14-day measles to increase as occurrences of it in older people became included in this percentage. If this percentage only increases, then the slope can only be positive in this graph (see explanation for question 23).

23. If the relative number of those who have had 14-day measles to those who have not had 14-day measles decreased from one age to the next, then a negative slope would occur. This decrease in the relative number would occur if: (a) those people who have had 14-day measles were removed from the population, or (b) new individuals who have not had 14-day measles were added to the population, such as through immigration.

24. Nowhere. All slopes are positive in this graph.

25. High positive change in percentage with respect to a change in age. The ages at which the change from one age to the next in the cumulative percentage who have had 14-day measles are high can be expected to be those ages at which the chance of catching measles is high. Thus, the slope, the change in cumulative percentage with respect to a change in age, is more closely tied to the chance of catching measles at a particular age than is the cumulative percentage. The cumulative percentage at a particular age is tied to the cumulative chance of catching measles up to that age.

26. Slope. In this graph, the slope indicates the change in cumulative percentage with respect to change in age.

Passage IV

27. **A** A straightforward graph reading shows that about 130,000 new cases of whooping cough were reported in 1953, more than in any other year between 1950 and 1963.

28. **B** The number of people in country X in a particular year who have had whooping cough cannot be calculated from data on the incidence of newly reported cases of it. You need to know such factors as percentage death rate associated with whooping cough over the years before the year in question to be able to determine this number.

29. **B** You must know the size of the population in 1963 relative to that in 1961 in order to compute and then compare the percentage of the given population that contracted smallpox in 1963 to the percentage that contracted it in 1961. It is not reasonable to make any assumptions with respect to the size of the population in 1963 relative to that in 1961.

30. **C** From the graph, approximately 10,000 people contracted smallpox in 1957 and approximately 130,000 people contracted whooping cough in 1953. Then:
Number of smallpox deaths $= (0.10)(10,000) = 1,000$ deaths
Number of whooping cough deaths $= (0.03)(130,000) = 3,900$ deaths
These figures represent fewer smallpox deaths than whooping cough deaths.

31. **B.** Between the information in this statement and that in the graph, you can calculate the respective numbers of reported new cases of tuberculosis and smallpox in 1957 that resulted in death in that same year: 200 for smallpox and just over 100 for tuberculosis. Note, however, that the statement asks for a comparison of the total number of deaths (including those occurring in cases reported before 1957) caused by tuberculosis in 1957 to the total number caused by smallpox in 1957. The respective numbers of deaths caused by tuberculosis and smallpox in 1957 for cases of these diseases reported before 1957 cannot be determined, and so this comparison cannot be accomplished.

32. **B** This type of value judgment cannot be made on the basis of simple incidence data, as are presented in the graph for this problem.

Bibliography

Whimbey A, Lochhead J: Beyond Problem Solving and Comprehension. Hillsdale, NJ, Lawrence Erlbaum Associates, 1984.

Edwards B: Drawing on the Right Side of Your Brain. Los Angeles, Jeremy P. Tarcher, Inc., 1979.

Pauk W: How to Study in College, 4th or later ed. Boston, Houghton Mifflin Co.

Perkins DN (ed): Knowledge as Design. Hillsdale, NJ, Lawrence Erlbaum Associates, 1986.

Novak JD, Gowin DB: Learning to Learn, 2nd or later ed. Boston, Cambridge University Press.

Whimbey A, Lochhead J: Problem Solving and Comprehension, 4th or later ed. Hillsdale NJ, Lawrence Erlbaum Associates.

Hayes JR: The Complete Problem Solver, 2nd or later ed. Hillsdale NJ, Lawrence Erlbaum Associates.

Vitale BM: Unicorns are Real: A Right-Brained Approach to Learning. New York, Warner Books, 1986.

Buzan T: Using Both Sides of Your Brain. New York, Dutton, 1983.

Engel SM: With Good Reason: An Introduction to Informal Fallacies, 3rd or later ed. New York, St. Martin's Press.

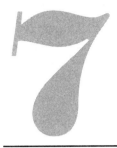

Problem Solving in the Physical Sciences

Introduction

Merely memorizing scientific facts and solving physics and chemistry problems with mathematical calculations are not adequate when preparing for the MCAT. Each section in Chapter 7 should be reviewed to develop a conceptual understanding of scientific facts and their application to medically or health-related situations.

Reading a conceptual section, such as that concerning chemical bonding, involves the use of critical verbal reasoning skills to extract information and precise scientific reasoning, which includes definitions, perception, and association with previous knowledge. Reading this section will help you to read longer passages filled with text, formulas, and equations in association with various sketches and schematic drawings. Apply the concepts you have learned to the review questions at the end of each section.

Chemistry-related physics should be reviewed with an intent to link concepts in physics and chemistry. Medical problem-solving takes aim at solving scientific problems that include a mix of physiology, anatomy, pharmacology, and biochemistry. Before the review questions in each section is a list of experimental and research concepts related to the field of medicine that should be included in your physical sciences review.

Finally, refer to introductory textbooks in anatomy, physiology, and biochemistry, to answer the following questions:

1. How will you relate to information presented in the book?
2. How will you extract basic concepts from the information?
3. How will this information relate to passages in the MCAT?
4. What forms of reasoning will you use to master new information?
5. How will you use this new information to construct questions in the review style of *CompPrep*?
6. Why is it more difficult for you to extract basic concepts from a new book?

Chapters 2, 3, and 6 in this book are designed to provide intellectual tools to help you become a good problem solver. These tools are reasoning, critical thinking, interpretation of graphic information, and acquiring scientific knowledge. The MCAT emphasizes the use and application of these intellectual tools. Look at the following physical science passage and apply your own intellectual skills to it.

"As a scientist, I boil water in a pot and observe the chaotic mixture of water, steam, and bubbles. As I become more curious, but bored with boiling plain water, I choose to boil an egg. I take an egg and carefully lower it with a spoon into the boiling pot. I know that adding sodium chloride or table salt will make it much easier to peel the egg."

To answer specific questions relating to the situation just described, use the following intellectual tools or skills:

1. Reading for scientific information—see Chapters 2 and 6
2. Developing scientific vocabulary—refer to a thesaurus or dictionary
3. Deriving any conclusion (based on supported or unsupported claims)—see Chapter 3
4. Constructing science problems—see Chapters 2 and 5
5. Looking for missing information (including unstated assumptions)—see Chapter 3

READING FOR CAUSE AND EFFECT

The passage explains that boiling water (implied word is "heating" water to a certain temperature) increases its temperature. The heat causes the bubbles of water vapor to expand because the vapor pressure is greater than the external pressure. The heating of the liquid yolk and white inside the porous egg shell causes it to solidify. Why? Remember, heating a cube of ice changes it from a solid to a liquid, which is a physical change. Hence, boiling an egg is a chemical reaction. Studying the chemical composition of egg yolk and egg white would explain how this change occurs. Salt in the water provides salt ions that travel through the egg shell, making it easier to peel. Is that a valid conclusion? Does the salt lower or raise the boiling point? All these questions can be connected to concepts in biology, physics, or chemistry.

READING FOR SCIENTIFIC INFORMATION

This skill builds your knowledge of physics, chemistry, biology, and mathematics. Knowing the definitions of scientific words makes comparative and analogic reasoning easier. Important scientific words in this passage are water, boiling, steam, bubbles (air), egg, sodium chloride, and temperature. Try to define these words and their usage in physics, chemistry, and biology. Learn to integrate definitions and develop concepts, e.g., would sodium chloride create an acidic medium or a basic medium?

DERIVING ANY CONCLUSIONS

The following conclusions are **obvious (direct)**:

1. Heat is required to boil water.
2. Eggs solidify after a certain time if put in boiling water.
3. Peeling an egg shell is easier if salt is added to the water.

The following conclusions are **implied (indirect)**:

1. The scientist is trying to explain a simple, everyday situation in a highly sophisticated scientific and logical way.
2. Egg shells can be hard to peel.
3. Water should be boiling at a certain temperature before eggs are lowered into it.
4. The specific heat of an egg and the specific heat of water are different.
5. Thermodynamic equilibrium is achieved when water boils.
6. Elevation of boiling point by adding salt can be measured by using a thermometer.
7. The egg used in the experiment could be fresh, stale, or rotten.

CONSTRUCTING SCIENCE PROBLEMS

These multiple-choice or mixed-choice questions are based on the scientific situation explained. In this exercise, ask yourself the following questions:

1. What is egg yolk made of?
2. What is the egg shell made of?
3. What is egg white made of?
4. At what temperature does water boil? Why?
5. Are egg molecules biologic molecules?
6. How long does it take to boil an egg? Why?
7. How much water should you boil?
8. How much salt should you add to the water? Why?
9. When should you peel the egg?
10. How should you lower the egg into the water (with what size spoon)?
11. Who is a scientist?
12. Does this experiment represent a scientific situation?
13. Do egg molecules arrange themselves differently when salt is added? If so, why?

Be sure to add "why?" after each question as shown and double check your answers. Feel free to open a chemistry or physics book for basic help.

SOLVING SCIENCE PROBLEMS AND LOOKING FOR MISSING INFORMATION

These last two steps are well covered in Chapter 2. In this passage, an unstated assumption or missing information would be that a raw egg should be lowered carefully to prevent it from breaking or cracking. Review diagramming and reasoning skills carefully before moving ahead in this chapter. Take note of how the simple situation in this example reflects integration of physics, chemistry, reading, reasoning, and some mathematics. MCAT questions, which are much more complicated, focus on the integration of various subject areas. In physical sciences, the focus is on integration of physics concepts and chemistry concepts with reading and reasoning to improve overall performance. Review and integrate various sections or subsections of chapters as you progress in your overall MCAT review; e.g., electronic structure of an atom should be linked with atomic and nuclear structure in physics.

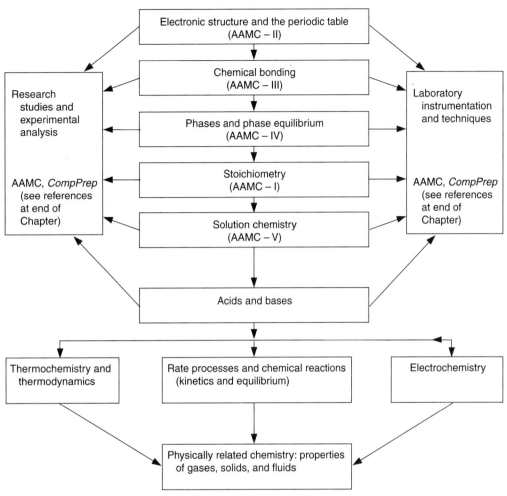

Fig. 7-1. Building blocks for studying general chemistry based on topics listed in the AAMC *MCAT Student Manual.* Roman numerals denote major topics related to the physical sciences.

Logical continuity, conceptual building blocks, and coherent subject matter were important objectives in developing the sequence of this book. See the charts in Figures 7-1 and 7-2 for direction in studying key principles in general chemistry and physics. The coverage of topics and the amount of detail in the background knowledge for these topics has been kept to bare essentials so you can grasp all related concepts. The reordering of sections is beneficial because items are randomly arranged on the MCAT.

Solid and Fluid Properties

Self-Managed Learning Questions

1. How would you classify a candle flame or a fire? As a solid, liquid, or gas? Prepare a persuasive argument with your hypotheses, evidence, and conclusions.
2. How much energy is required to boil and eventually evaporate 1 mole of water?
3. Prove that different liquids at the same temperature have different vapor pressures. Explain the working principles of an indoor humidifier.
4. Is it true that the vapor pressure of every liquid increases as the temperature is raised? Why?
5. Which liquid has stronger intermolecular forces, water or benzene? Why?
6. Is it true that alloys such as steel are solid solutions? Why?
7. Is it true that gem stones such as emeralds, rubies, and sapphires are solid solutions? Why?
8. What is supercritical fluid? (Hint: water at 374.1°C and 218 atm becomes a supercritical fluid.) How is caffeine extracted from coffee using supercritical CO_2? Call

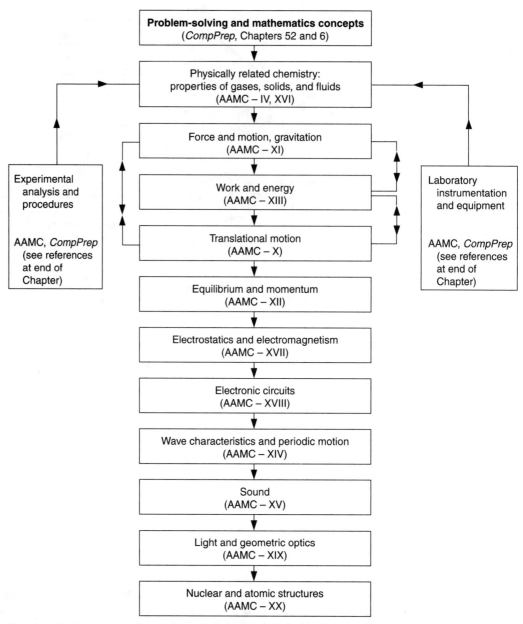

Fig. 7-2. Building blocks for studying physics based on topics listed in the AAMC *MCAT Student Manual.* Roman numerals denote major topics related to the physical sciences.

a coffee production company and learn the equipment, parts, and functions of a supercritical CO_2 extractor.

9. How does surface tension help in an organic separation process called chromatography?

FLUIDS

Density and Specific Gravity

Density is one of the key properties of fluids (liquids or gases); the other is pressure. Pressure (P) is defined as force (F) per unit area (A): $P = F/A$. F is the normal (perpendicular) force. Fluids can only exert P at an enclosed surface or body. Otherwise, fluids will flow under a shearing stress instead of being deformed elastically, as occurs with solids. Pressure is formulated as potential energy per unit volume as follows:

$$P = \frac{F}{A} = \frac{mg}{A} = \left(\frac{mg}{A}\right)\left(\frac{h}{h}\right) = \frac{mgh}{V} = \rho gh$$

in which ρ = density, h = depth below surface, and g = acceleration due to gravity.

Characteristics of force and pressure of fluids are:

1. Forces exerted by fluids are always perpendicular to the container
2. The fluid pressure (hydrostatic) is directly proportional to the depth of the fluid and to its density: $P \propto \rho h$
3. At any particular depth, the fluid pressure is the same in all directions
4. Fluid pressure is independent of the shape or area of its container
5. External pressure applied to an enclosed fluid is transmitted uniformly throughout the volume of the liquid (Pascal's law)
6. An object that is completely or partially submerged in a fluid experiences an upward force equal to the weight of the fluid displaced (Archimedes principle):

$$\text{Buoyant force } (F_B) \text{ is } F = V\rho g = mg$$

Buoyant force is equal to the weight of displaced fluid. An object that floats must displace its own weight (not volume) in fluid.

Buoyancy and Archimedes Principle

In Figure 7-3A, assume that the body is totally immersed in the liquid. Now suppose the fluid inside the surface is removed and replaced by a solid body with exactly the same shape. The pressure at every point will be exactly the same as before, so the force exerted on the body by the surrounding fluid will be unaltered. The fluid exerts on the body an upward force (F_y) that is equal to the weight (mg) of the fluid originally occupying the boundary surface, the line of action of which passes through the original center of gravity. The submerged body, in general, will not be in equilibrium. Its weight may be greater or less than F_y, and if it is not homogeneous, its center of gravity may not be on the line of F_y.

The weight of a dirigible floating in air, or of a submarine floating at some depth below the surface of the water, is just equal to the weight of a volume of air, or water, that is equal to the volume of the dirigible or submarine; that is, the average density of the dirigible equals that of the air, and the average density of the submarine equals the density of the water.

If p1 and p2 are the pressures at elevations y1 and y2 above some reference level and when ρ and g are constant, then:

$$p_2 - p_1 = -\rho g(y_2 - y_1).$$

Hydrostatic Pressure

Apply this equation to a liquid in an open vessel, as shown in Figure 7-3B. Take point 1 at any level and let p represent that pressure at this point. Take point 2 at the top where the pressure is atmospheric pressure, p_a. Then:

$$p - p_a = \rho g(y_2 - y_1),$$

$$p = p_a + \rho g h.$$

Note that the shape of the containing vessel does not affect the pressure, and that the pressure is the same at all points at the same depth.

Concept of Mass Flux

Mass flux is the rate of change of mass of a fluid. It represents mass flow per unit time. This parameter is important when measuring flow of blood from the heart, flow of substances into the kidneys, and flow of air into the lungs. Mass flux is proportional to the rate of flow R mentioned in the next section.

Viscosity

Another important property of fluids, viscosity is analogous to friction between moving solids. It may, therefore, be viewed as the resistance to flow between layers of fluid (as

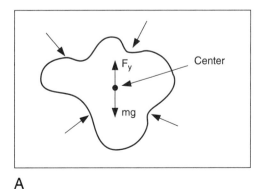

Fig. 7-3. Buoyancy (A) and hydrostatic pressure (B).

A

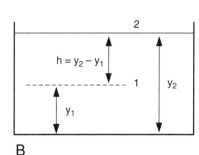

B

in streamline or laminar flow) sliding relative to each other. As friction, viscosity results in dissipation of mechanical energy. As one layer slides over another, its motion is transmitted to the second layer and sets this layer in motion. Because a mass (m) of the second layer is set in motion (v) and some of the energy of the first layer is lost, a transfer of momentum (mv) occurs between the layers. The greater the transfer of this momentum from one layer to another, the more kinetic energy (av^2) is lost and the slower the layers move. The viscosity coefficient (h) is a measure of the efficiency of transfer of this loss of mechanical energy and, consequently, greater loss of velocity. The reverse situation holds of low viscosity coefficients; a high viscosity (coefficient) substance flows slowly (e.g., molasses) and a low viscosity (coefficient) substance flows relatively fast (e.g., water or, especially, helium). Note that the transfer of momentum to adjacent layers is, in essence, the exertion of a force on these layers to set them in motion (Newton's first law; see subsequent section concerning equilibrium and momentum). Whether flow is streamlined (laminar) or turbulent (chaotic loss of layers flowing past each other and their replacement with eddies and whirlpool, etc., with resultant dissipation of more mechanical energy) depends on a combination of factors discussed previously. A convenient measure is Reynolds number (R):

$$R = \frac{vd\rho}{\eta}$$

in which v = velocity of flow, d = diameter of the tube, ρ = density of fluid, and η = viscosity coefficient. In general, if R is < 2000, flow is streamlined; if R is > 2000, flow is turbulent. Note that as v ↑, d ↑, ρ ↑, or η ↓, the flow becomes more turbulent.

Continuity Equation

Fluids in motion are described by two equations, the continuity equation and Bernoulli's equation. Fluids are assumed to have streamlined flow, which means the motion of every particle in the fluid follows the same path as the particle that preceded it. Turbulent flow occurs when one path is not followed, molecules collide, energy is dissipated, and frictional drag is increased. Rate of flow (R) is:

$$R = \text{volume past a point/time} = Avt/t = Av$$

$$\text{Volume} = \text{(cross-sectional area)(length)} = (A)(vt) = Avt$$

$$\text{Length} = \text{distance} = \text{(velocity)(time)} = vt$$

Another way to write this equation is the continuity equation:

$$A_1v_1 = A_2v_2 = \text{constant}$$

in which subscripts 1 and 2 refer to different points in the line of flow. Note that the velocity of the fluid is faster where the cross-sectional area is smaller and vice versa. Also, where the velocity is faster, the pressure (P) exerted is smaller and vice versa.

Bernoulli's Equation

Bernoulli's equation (Fig. 7-4) is an application of the law of conservation of energy:

$$P + \rho gh + \tfrac{1}{2}\rho v^2 = \text{constant}$$

$$\text{Pressure energy} + \text{potential energy} + \text{kinetic energy} = \text{constant}$$

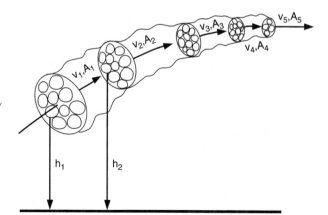

Fig. 7-4. Concept of mass flux/ Bernoulli's equation.

An equivalent expression follows:

$$P_1 + \rho gh_1 + \tfrac{1}{2}\rho v_1^2 = P_2 + \rho gh_2 + \tfrac{1}{2}\rho v_2^2$$

in which the subscripts 1 and 2 refer to different points in the flow. All symbols are as defined in the discussion of the continuity equation.

Turbulence

The Hagen-Poiseuille law for laminar viscous flow of blood through small size tubes is calculated by using the formula:

$$\text{Flow rate} = Q = \frac{\pi R^2 F_v}{8\eta L} = v\pi R^2 \ \text{(from continuity equation)}$$

in which Q = flow rate = m^3/sec, R = radius of flow tube or blood vessel (m), F_v = viscous force causing flow (nt), η = viscosity of blood $\frac{nt \cdot s}{m^2}$, L = length of tube or blood vessel (m), and v = average velocity of blood flow (m/sec). Use proportional reasoning to remember that flow rate is directly proportional to R^2 and pressure difference is inversely proportional to R^2 (Fig. 7-5). To determine viscous force per unit area, divide F_v by the cross-sectional area, which is represented by Δp or pd.

Surface Tension

Molecules of a liquid exert attractive forces toward each other (**cohesive forces**), and exert attractive forces toward surfaces they touch (**adhesive forces**). If a liquid is in a gravity-free space without a surface, it will form a sphere (smallest area relative to volume). If the liquid is lining an object, the liquid surface will contract (because of cohesive forces) to the lowest possible surface area. The forces between the molecules on this surface will create a membrane-like effect. Because of the contraction, a potential energy (PE) will be present in the surface. This PE is directly proportional to the surface area (A). An exact relation is formed as follows:

$$PE = s_t A$$

$$s_t = \text{surface tension} = \frac{PE}{A} = \frac{\text{joules}}{m^2}$$

An alternative formulation for surface tension (s_t) is:

$$s_t = \frac{F}{l}$$

in which F = force of contraction (of surface) and l = length along surface.

Because of the contraction, small objects that would ordinarily sink in the liquid may "float" on the surface membrane.

A liquid will rise or fall on a wall or in a capillary tube if the adhesive forces are greater

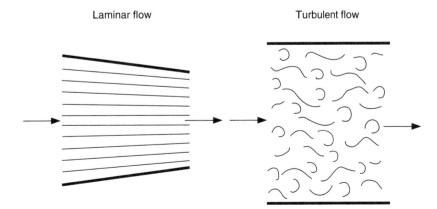

Laminar flow   Turbulent flow

Fig. 7-5. Turbulence.

than cohesive or cohesive are greater than adhesive forces, respectively (Fig. 7-6). The distance the liquid rises or falls in the tube is directly proportional to the s_t and inversely proportional to the liquid density and radius of the tube.

SOLIDS

When a force acts on a solid, the solid is deformed. If the solid returns to its original shape, it is **elastic**. The effect of a force depends on the area over which it acts. Stress is the ratio of the force to the area over which it acts. Strain is the relative change in dimensions or shape of the object caused by the stress. These concepts are embodied in the definition of the modulus of elasticity (ME) as ME = stress/strain.

Density

What is meant by "heavy as lead" and "light as a feather?" Clearly, a grain of lead is light, whereas a mountain of feathers has considerable weight. Such comparisons are based not on a the mass of a body, but on the density of the material from which it is made.

The mass of a unit volume of a body is its **density**. A grain of lead and a massive block of lead have the same density. Density is an **intensive property**, usually expressed as the number of grams (g) per cubic centimeter the body weighs; the symbol g/cm^3 is placed after this number. To determine the density of an object, divide the number of grams by the number of cubic centimeters (the fractional line in the symbol is a reminder).

Certain metals are among the heaviest materials—osmium, the density of which is equal to 22.5 g/cm^3, iridium (22.4), platinum (21.5), tungsten (19.3), and gold (19.3). The density of iron is 7.88, and that of copper is 8.93. Lighter substances include air, with a density of 0.0013 g/cm^3.

Density determinations so far discussed pertain to continuous bodies. If there are pores in a solid, it will be lighter. Frequently used porous bodies include cork, sponge, and steel wool. The density of sponge may be less than 0.5, although the solid matter from which it is made has a higher density. As all other bodies with a density of less than 1, sponge floats superbly on water, unless it is soaked.

The lightest liquid is liquid hydrogen; it can only be obtained at extremely low temperatures. One cubic centimeter of liquid hydrogen has a mass of 0.07 g. Organic liquids, such as alcohol, benzene, and kerosene, do not differ significantly from water in density. Mercury is heavy; it has a density of 13.6 g/cm^3.

Gases fully occupy any given volume. Even though emptied into vessels of different volumes, gas bags with the same mass of gas will fill the volumes uniformly. The density of gases is defined under so-called normal conditions or at STP (temperature of 0°C and pressure of 1 atmosphere, atm). The density of air under normal conditions is equal to 0.00129 g/cm^3; chloride is 0.00322 g/cm^3. Gaseous hydrogen, like the liquid, is the lightest gas, with a density of 0.00009 g/cm^3.

Density represents the packing of material in a certain volume (Fig. 7-7).

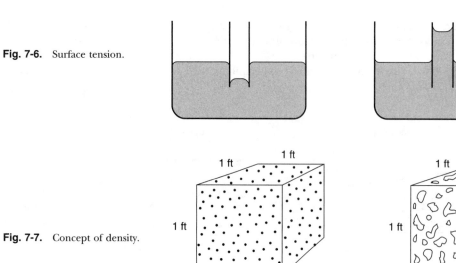

Cohesive > adhesive   Adhesive > cohesive

Fig. 7-6. Surface tension.

Fig. 7-7. Concept of density.

Water	Mercury
62.4 lb/ft³	848.64 lb/ft³

$$\text{Mass density} \qquad \rho = \frac{\text{mass}}{\text{volume}}$$

$$\text{Weight density} \qquad \gamma = \frac{\text{weight}}{\text{volume}}$$

As an example, a human being weighing 150 lb with 90% water is like a container of water about the same weight:

$$150 \times 0.90 = 135 \text{ lb. Weight density of water} = 62.4 \text{ lb./ft}^3$$

$$\text{Using weight density} = \text{weight/volume:} \quad 62.4 = \frac{135}{\text{volume}}$$

The result is the average volume of the human body at 2.16 ft^3. This example shows the fundamental use of the density equation.

Generally, solids are more dense than liquids, which are more dense than gases. The **specific gravity** (SG) is defined as: $SG = \dfrac{\text{Density of a substance}}{\text{Density of water}}$ at a given temperature. The density of water is about 1 g/ml over most common temperatures. So, in most instances, the specific gravity of a substance is the same as its density. Note that the units of density are mass per volume, whereas SG has no units.

Elementary Topics in Elastic Properties

It is important to understand elastic solids. As an example, steel is more elastic than rubber. Rubber is more stretchable, but not more elastic, than steel. Do not confuse the words elastic and stretchable.

Some of the different types of stresses are **tensile stress** (equal and opposite forces directed away from each other), **compressive stress** (equal and opposite forces directed toward each other), and **shearing stress** (equal and opposite forces that do not have the same line of action). Two commonly useful moduli of elasticity follow:

1. Young's Modulus (Y) for compressive or tensile stress (Fig. 7-8):

   $$Y = \text{longitudinal stress/longitudinal strain} = (F/A)/(\Delta l/l)$$

   $$l = \text{original length} = Fl/A\Delta l$$

   $$\Delta l = \text{change in length}$$

   $$A = \text{the area normal (perpendicular) to the force}$$

2. Shear modulus (S) or the modulus of rigidity (Fig. 7-9) is:

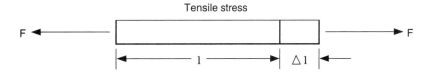

Tensile stress

Fig. 7-8. Tensile stress and compressive stress.

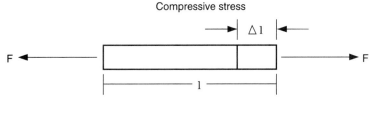

Compressive stress

Fig. 7-9. Shear stress.

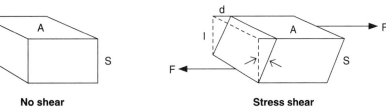

No shear　　　　　　　**Stress shear**

$$S = \text{shearing stress/shearing strain} = (F/A)/\phi = (F/A)/\tan\phi = (F/A)/(d/l) = Fl/dA$$

A = the area tangential to the force; $\phi = \tan\phi$ for small angles

APPLIED CONCEPTS

The fundamental properties of solids and fluids have numerous applications in human physiology. Important basic concepts to learn include the following:

1. External and internal homeostatic balance related to optimal quantities of ions, water, and cellular fluids at optimal pressure and temperature
2. Structural differences between (a) short, long, flat, and irregular bones and (b) compact and spongy bone; mechanical stress and the piezoelectric effect in bones; bone fracture
3. Various types of joints, ligaments, and tendons, as related to movement, including gliding, rotating, hinged, pivotal, ball and socket, etc.
4. Types of contractions in muscles: isotonic, isometric, and treppe
5. Relationships of heart beats to atrial pressure, arterial pressure, atrial systole, ventricular systole and diastole, cardiac output, and stroke volume
6. Working of an artificial heart as a fluid pump
7. Hydrostatic and osmotic pressure related to filtration through capillaries
8. Glomerular filtration rate, renal clearance
9. Operation of an artificial kidney or a hemodialysis machine
10. Physical characteristics of urine and blood, such as volume, color, pH, specific gravity, temperature, and pressure

SOLID AND FLUID PROPERTIES: REVIEW QUESTIONS

1. Mechanical stress, as used in physics, is defined as:
   A. the maximum weight an object can support.
   B. the force per unit length.
   C. the ratio of the force to the area over which it acts.
   D. the relative change in dimensions of an object caused by a force.

2. When an object is deformed by forces acting on an object along the same line of action but in the opposite directions, the resulting stress is called:
   A. tensile stress.
   B. traction stress.
   C. compressive stress.
   D. shearing stress.

3. If D = density, m = mass, and V = volume occupied by that mass, then density is:
   A. $D = (m)(V)$.
   B. $D = 1/(m)(V)$.
   C. $D = m/V$.
   D. $D = V/m$.

4. Pressure may be conceptualized as:
   A. force per unit volume.
   B. work times volume.
   C. potential energy per unit volume.
   D. weight per unit volume.

5. All of the following statements describe characteristics of forces and pressures exerted by fluids EXCEPT:
   A. forces are always perpendicular to the container walls.
   B. pressure is directly proportional to the product of depth and fluid density.
   C. pressure depends on the shape and size of the container.
   D. buoyant force of a submerged object equals the weight of the displaced fluid.

6. Pascal's law (of fluids) states that:
   A. an external pressure applied to an enclosed fluid is transmitted uniformly through the volume of the fluid.
   B. at any depth, the fluid pressure is the same in all directions.
   C. fluid pressure depends on the shape or area of its container.

D. an object completely or partly submerged in a fluid experiences an upward force equal to the weight of the fluid displaced.

7. Bernoulli's equation is an application of:

   A. the second law of thermodynamics.
   B. the law of conservation of momentum.
   C. the law of conservation of mass.
   D. the law of conservation of energy.

8. All of the following statements about viscosity are true EXCEPT:

   A. it is analogous to friction.
   B. no dissipation of mechanical energy is involved.
   C. transfer of momentum occurs between adjacent layers.
   D. as viscosity increases, rate of flow decreases.

9. A certain metal has a mass (m) = 36 g and occupies a volume (V) = 4 ml. What is the density (d) of this metal?

   A. 144 g/ml
   B. 9 g/ml
   C. $\frac{1}{9}$ ml/g
   D. $\frac{1}{444}$ g^{-1} ml^{-1}

10. A substance has a density (d) of 7 g/ml. If 42 g are required, what will be the volume (V) of the substance?

    A. $\frac{1}{6}$ ml
    B. 6 ml
    C. 294 ml
    D. Insufficient information provided

11. A fluid has a density (d) of 5 g/ml and fills a container to a height (h) of 10 cm. What is the pressure (P) on the floor of the container?

    A. 49,000 dynes/cm^2
    B. 50 nts/m^2
    C. 50 V dynes/cm^2, in which V = volume (in ml)
    D. Insufficient data provided

    $P = \rho g h$

12. If an object is moved from a depth of 4 meters to a depth of 8 meters beneath the surface of a large tank of water, the pressure on it will:

    A. remain the same.
    B. quadruple.
    C. halve.
    D. double.

13. At a depth of 10 meters in a large container of water, 3 sheets of glass are placed parallel to the surface. Sheet A is 3 m × 5 m, sheet B is 4 m × 4 m, and sheet C is 2 m × 9 m. Which sheet has the greatest fluid pressure on its surface?

    A. A
    B. B
    C. C
    D. All are equal

14. The buoyant force (F_B) on an object that has a mass of 10 g, a volume of 10 ml, and displaces 2 ml of a liquid with a density of 5 g/ml is:

    A. 10 dynes.
    B. 9800 dynes.
    C. 1000 dynes.
    D. 40 dynes.

    $F = V \rho g$

15. For an object to float in a fluid, it must:

    A. be made of a substance more dense than the fluid.
    B. be made of a substance less dense than the fluid.
    C. displace its own weight in the fluid.
    D. displace its own volume in the fluid.

16. A pipe has a section with a 10-m diameter (A) and another section with a diameter of 5 m (B). Which statement best describes the flow of a given quantity of fluid through this pipe?

    A. It moves at the same speed at A and B.
    B. Flow is faster at A.
    C. Flow is faster at B.
    D. Need to know volume of fluid to evaluate.

17. Fluid is flowing through a pipe. Which point represents the area of highest pressure exerted by the fluid (pipe is filled with fluid at all points)? Points A, B, C, and D are at the same elevation.

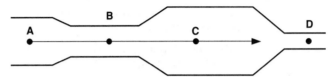

    A. A
    B. B
    C. C
    D. D

18. In this constant diameter pipe, which point represents the area of least pressure exerted by the fluid? Assume all pipes are of constant diameter and points A, B, C and D are not at the same elevation.

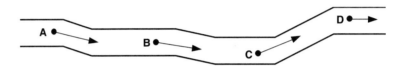

    A. A
    B. B
    C. C
    D. D

19. The relative diameters of the blood vessels of the body and the relative flows are expressed as: arteries > arterioles > capillaries. Which of these vessels is most likely to have turbulent flow?

    A. Artery
    B. Arteriole
    C. Capillary
    D. All equal

1–8. 1-C, 2-A, 3-C, 4-C, 5-C, 6-A, 7-D, 8-B. See text for explanation.

 9. **B** d = m/V = 36 g/4 ml = 9 g/ml

10. **B** d = m/V
        V = m/d = 42 g/7 g per ml = 6 ml

11. **A** P = F/A = ρgh
        P = (5 g/cm^3)(980 cm/sec^2)(10 cm) = 49,000 (g-cm/sec^2)/cm^2
        P = 49,000 dynes/cm^2
        dyne = (g-cm)/sec^2

12. **D** The pressure (P) exerted by the fluid is:

$$P = \rho gh \text{ or } P \propto h$$

in which h = depth under surface. So, P is directly proportional to h, and if h doubles ($\frac{8}{4}$ = 2), then P doubles, OR

$$P_1 = \rho gh_1 = \text{original depth}$$

$$P_2 = \rho gh_2 = \text{final depth}$$

$$P_2/P_1 = \rho gh_2/\rho gh_1 = h_2/h_1 = 8 \text{ m}/4 \text{ m} = 2$$

$$P_2 = 2P_1$$

13. **D** Fluid pressure (P) is independent of the area or shape of its container or objects. The P ∞ ρh in which ρ = density and h = depth. At any particular depth, the pressure is equal in all directions.

14. **B** From Archimedes' principle:

$$F = V\rho g$$

$$V = \text{volume displaced} = 2 \text{ ml}$$

$$\rho = \text{density of fluid} = 5 \text{ g/ml}$$

$$g = 980 \text{ cm/sec}^2$$

$$F = (2)(5)(980) = 9800 \text{ dynes}$$

15. **C** Two factors determine the ability of an object to float: (1) the overall density of the object, not the substance it is made of, and (2) the buoyant force versus the weight of the object.

16. **C** The continuity equation is: $A_{1v1} = A_{2v2}$. Note that the larger the cross section, the smaller the fluid velocity, and vice versa.

17. **C** The velocity (v) is slowest where the cross-sectional area (A) is greatest, from the continuity equation ($A_{1v1} = A_{2v2}$). At faster velocities, the pressure is lower, and at slower velocities, the pressure (P) is higher, from Bernoulli's equation:

$$P + \rho gh + \tfrac{1}{2}\rho v^2 = \text{constant}$$

ρgh does not change if h = constant. Then, $\tfrac{1}{2}\rho v^2$ increases as v increases, and P must decrease because the whole expression is constant. As the fluid moves faster, pressure energy (P) is converted to kinetic energy ($\tfrac{1}{2}\rho v^2$) and the pressure drops.

18. **D** Because the diameter is constant, the velocity of fluid flow is constant by the continuity equation ($A_{1v1} = A_{2v2}$). From Bernoulli's equation:

$$P + \rho gh + \tfrac{1}{2}\rho v^2 = \text{constant}$$

$\tfrac{1}{2}\rho v^2$ does not change; ρ = density and v = velocity. ρgh changes because h (height above some arbitrary reference point) is changing. The larger h means the larger this term; the larger ρgh means the smaller the P term becomes. Thus, the higher the pipe (because of h), the smaller the pressure (P).

19. **A** Turbulence is best estimated using Reynolds number (R) or by remembering the relations from R. The viscosity and density of the fluid (i.e., the blood) is constant. Because diameter (d) and velocity (v) are greatest in the arteries, and turbulence ∞ (v)(d), arteries have the highest turbulence. The velocity is greater in these vessels because the sum total of all cross-sectional areas of the arteries in the human body is less than the total cross-sectional areas of all the capillaries.

Phases and Phase Equilibria

Self-Managed Learning Questions

1. Perform complete information analysis on biologic molecules, e.g., sugar and artificial sweeteners. Review the organic structure of artificial sweeteners, e.g., saccharin, cyclamate, and aspartame, and how they compare to sucrose or sugar. Review the chemical bonds, boiling point, dipole moments, and other characteristics of each compound.

2. Review the melting point and freezing point of clinical solvents and check at least a dozen phase diagrams for biologically relevant substances, e.g., acetic acid, glucose, urine, blood plasma, milk, epinephrine, and norepinephrine.

3. List at least 30 solids, 30 liquids, and 30 gases that are relevant to the study of medicine. Write their chemical structure and where they are used in clinical chemistry.

The physical characteristics of solids, liquids, and gases are summarized in Table 7-1.

TABLE 7-1. Physical Characteristics of Solids, Liquids, and Gases

Solids	Liquids	Gases
1. Solids are rigid.	1. Liquids are fluid.	1. Gases are extremely fluid.
2. Solids have a definite shape.	2. Liquids have no definite shape, but have a well-defined surface.	2. Gases are shapeless; they occupy the entire container.
3. Solids have a definite volume.	3. Liquids have a definite volume.	3. Gases have no definite volume.
4. Solids have a higher density because their molecules are closely packed together.	4. Liquids are lighter than solids in most cases (except water) because molecules are farther apart.	4. Gases are extremely light because their molecules are far apart.
5. Solids are extremely cohesive.	5. Liquids, except for mercury, are less cohesive.	5. Gases have almost no cohesion at all. There is almost no interaction between their molecules.
6. Solids diffuse at an extremely slow rate, e.g., lead and gold diffuse into each other when left for 6 months or more.	6. Liquids exhibit various types of diffusion such as convective, turbulent, and molecular, e.g., preparing coffee or tea in boiling water.	6. Gases diffuse at high speeds, e.g., air freshener in a room.
7. Well-known theories and laws have been established to study solid behavior.	7. As of today, there is a large gap in the study of liquid behavior. No good model exists to represent a liquid.	7. Well-known theories have been established to study behavior of gases.
8. Solids are almost incompressible.	8. Liquids are slightly compressible (do not confuse the slipping of liquid molecules under pressure with compression).	8. Gases are highly compressible, which gives them the property of resiliency.

GAS PHASE

Standard Temperature and Pressure and Standard Molar Volume

Many gas laws and theories are used in both chemistry and physics. Gases have relatively high translational kinetic energies per molecule as compared with liquids. Gases, like liquids, take the shape of the object that contains them. Unlike liquids, however, they completely fill any container. The key characteristics of gases are the pressure (P), the volume (V), the temperature (T), and the quantity (moles = n). Note that 22.414 liters of an ideal gas at S.T.P. (standard temperature and pressure: 273°K and 1 atm pressure) represent 1 mole of that gas.

Ideal Gas Law

Gases are broadly considered ideal or nonideal. An **ideal gas** has no intermolecular forces, and the gas molecules occupy no volume (they are points in space), which means they should have low density (density depends on molecular weight). In general, at high temperatures and low pressures, most gases can be considered ideal. A **nonideal gas** has intermolecular forces, and the molecules do have a finite volume.

When considering laws that pertain to the behavior of ideal gases, recall that metric pressure units are expressed as millimeter of mercury (mm Hg = torr). The English system uses atmospheres (atm). The conversion is 760 torr = 1 atm. (For temperature scales, see the subsequent section concerning thermodynamics and thermochemistry.)

The **ideal gas law** is:

$$PV = nRT$$

in which P = pressure, V = volume, n = moles, T = absolute temperature, R = Ideal gas constant = $0.0821 \, 1-atm/°K\text{-mole}$. Another useful way of writing the ideal gas law is:

$$\frac{PV}{T} = \text{constant or,} \quad \frac{P_1 V_1}{T_1} = \frac{P_2 V_2}{T_2}$$

At constant temperature ($T_1 = T_2$), the above equation reduces to:

$$P_1 V_1 = P_2 V_2$$

This is **Boyle's Law,** which states that pressure and volume are inversely related. Thus, if we double the pressure (i.e. $P_2 = 2 \, P_1$), the resulting volume is:

$$V_2 = \frac{1}{2} V_1$$

Similarly, at constant pressure ($P_1 = P_2$), the equation reduces to:

$$\frac{V_1}{T_1} = \frac{V_2}{T_2}$$

As demonstrated, volume and temperature are directly related—as temperature increases, volume increases, and vice versa. This is **Charles' Law.**

Kinetic Molecular Theory of Gases

The kinetic theory of gases attempts to describe the energy characteristics of gases as a whole by analyzing the motion and mass characteristics (e.g., forces, momentum) of

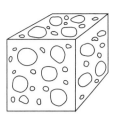

Fig. 7-10. Model of "kinetic molecular theory" and "solubility of molecules." Stirring grains of salt or sugar in water results in a homogenous solution. The salt or sugar molecules do not disappear but occupy the intermolecular spaces in H_2O. The result of this mixing, according to the kinetic molecular theory of liquids and solids, is a solution.

individual molecules. The theory is based on the following basic postulates:

1. All gases consist of small, spherical particles called molecules, which are similar to mini-tennis balls bouncing in a box as shown in Figure 7-10.
2. These molecules are in constant or perpetual motion. They move at high velocities. The size of these molecules is around 2 to 5Å, and they travel in random directions with speeds of about 1000 m/sec (almost 0.5 miles/sec).
3. The distance between individual molecules is great as compared to their diameter. They may be 70Å or more apart.
4. Collisions between molecules are perfectly elastic, on the order of 5 billion collisions per second.

The kinetic theory for gases can also be applied to liquids and solids. The kinetic theory illustrates the concept of solubility. An atom in the bottom of a potential well carries out small thermal oscillations about its equilibrium position.

The kinetic theory of gases has its limitations but its application achieves some important results.

1. Boyle's law, Charles' law, and the ideal gas law are derived from it
2. P and V can be related to the kinetic energy of molecules:

$$PV = \tfrac{2}{3}NE_k \text{ (on a molecular scale)}$$

in which N = the number of molecules and E_k = translational energy/molecule, or

$$E_k = (3/2) RT \text{ (on a mole scale)}$$

Also, at a given temperature, all molecules have the same average E_k.

3. **Graham's law of diffusion** is determined from E_k as follows:

$E_{k1} = E_{k2}$, i.e., the average E_k values are equal (kinetic energies of molecules)

1, 2 = molecules

Also $\tfrac{1}{2} m_1 v_1^2 = \tfrac{1}{2} m_2 v_2^2$

$v_1/v_2 = \sqrt{m_2}/\sqrt{m_1} = \sqrt{m_2/m_1}$

in which v = velocities of diffusion (e.g., ml/min) and m = molecular weights or densities.

4. Values for heat capacities of monoatomic gases are calculated. When C_v = specific heat at constant volume and C_p = specific heat at constant pressure:

$$C_v = \frac{3}{2}R$$

$$C_p = C_v + R$$

$$C_p/C_v = 1.67$$

$$R = 1.99 \text{ cal/mole-}°K = \text{gas constant}$$

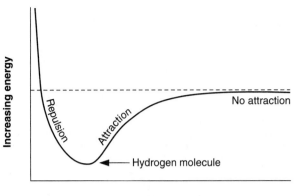

Fig. 7-11. Motion of molecules related to kinetic energy of molecules. The temperature of the medium is a measure of the average kinetic energy of the molecules. The sketch at right shows the energy of molecules as related to internuclear distance between atoms. Note that the curve first goes down, then turns up, forming a "potential well."

Qualitative Aspects of Deviation of Real Gas Behavior from Ideal Gas Law

Movements from left to right in Figure 7-11 represent phase changes from solids to liquids to gases. This diagram illustrates "cohesion" and "adhesion" between molecules, which results in internuclear or van der Waals forces for real gases. One of the simpler equations for nonideal gases, the **van der Waals equation** applies corrections to account for the false assumptions of ideal gases.

$$\left(P + \frac{n^2a}{V^2}\right)(V - nb) = nRT$$

in which a, b are constants; n^2a/V^2 corrects for intermolecular forces = pressure correction; and nb corrects for the volume occupied by gas molecules = volume correction.

Note that if the density is very low, then $V \gg nb$ and $n^2a/V^2 \to 0$, and the ideal gas law results. The effect of the intermolecular forces is to decrease the pressure of the gas. The effect of the volume of molecules is to increase the volume occupied by the gas. The terms just described bring the pressure and volume back to ideal levels.

Partial Pressure and Mole Fraction

The **partial pressure** (P_i) of a gas in a mixture of gases is determined as follows:

$$P_i = X_i P_t$$

P_t = total pressure

X_i = mole fraction of gas in the mixture

$$X_i = \frac{n_i}{n_1 + n_2 + n_3 + \dots} = \frac{n_i}{\Sigma n_i}$$

n_i = moles of a gas

Σn_i = sum of the moles of all gases

Dalton's Law

Dalton's law states that the total pressure (P_t) of a mixture of gases is equal to the sum partial pressures (P_i) of the gases:

$$P_t = P_1 + P_2 + P_3 + \dots$$

LIQUID PHASE

In the liquid phase, a substance has no definite shape but it has a definite volume. Intermolecular forces are the attractive forces between molecules, between ions, or between ions and molecules.

Hydrogen Bonding

Hydrogen bonding takes place when a hydrogen atom covalently bonds intermolecularly with an highly electronegative atom (such as O, N, or F). When a hydrogen atom in a molecule acquires a partially positive charge in the vicinity of a molecule containing an electronegative atom, the resulting interaction between the hydrogen atom and the neighboring electronegative atom draws the hydrogen atom into alignment between the nuclei of electronegative atoms:

$$R-O-H\cdots\overset{\overset{\textstyle H}{|}}{O}\diagdown_R$$

This process is important because many natural materials are chains of amino acids that can interact internally or with a neighboring chain by hydrogen bonding.

Dipole Interactions

Dipole interactions are the intermolecular forces between polar molecules. Details related to the four kinds of dipole interactions are provided in Figure 7-12.

Ion–dipole interactions are not as strong as ionic attractions, and the strength of the attraction depends on three factors:

1. The distance between the ion and the dipole. The closer the ion and the dipole, the stronger their attraction.
2. The charge on the ion. The greater the charge on the ion, the stronger the resulting attraction.
3. The magnitude of the dipole. The greater the magnitude, the stronger the attraction.

In **dipole–dipole interactions**, energy is released when polar molecules interact with each other. Energy is required to separate interacting dipoles. For example, you must cool a gas of polar molecules to convert it into a liquid, and you must heat a polar compound to convert the molecules to the vapor phase.

In **dipole–induced dipole interactions**, polar molecules can induce a dipole in nonpolar molecules by reason of their structure (e.g., H_2O, polar, will dissolve CO_2, nonpolar). **Induced dipole–induced dipole interactions,** sometimes called London or dispersion forces, often are stronger than permanent dipole–permanent dipole interactions. They generally become stronger with increasing mass, which necessitates a higher temperature to overcome these forces and so allow molecules to leave the liquid to go into the vapor phase. Electron clouds around nonpolar atoms or molecules become distorted from the attractions or repulsions between their electrons, leading to intermolecular attraction.

Van der Waals Forces

These weak intermolecular forces do not involve ions.

PHASE EQUILIBRIA (SOLIDS, LIQUIDS, AND GASES)

Phase Changes and Phase Diagrams

The **three phases** of matter are gases, liquids, and solids. Conversions between these states are illustrated in Figure 7-13. As a substance moves from solid to liquid to gas, several changes occur: (1) the molecules become more disordered, (2) the kinetic energy of the molecules increases, (3) the intermolecular forces become weaker, and (4) the molecules become more separated (density decreases).

In general, the heat of vaporization is significantly greater than the heat of fusion for the same compound. In the forward direction, heat must be put into the system and the

Fig. 7-12. Types of intermolecular forces. Ion–dipole forces involve ionic compounds or molecules (e.g., NaCl + H_2O). Dipole–dipole forces involve covalent bonds and no ions are involved (van der Waals forces) or polar molecules (e.g., CO_2 + CO_2). Dipole-induced forces involve polar and nonpolar molecules (e.g., H_2O + Cl_2). Induced dipole–induced dipole forces involve nonpolar molecules (e.g., O_2 + O_2).

Conceptual sketch	Intermolecular forces	Force (kJ/mole)
(+) (- +)	Ion–dipole	50 - 550
(- +) (- +)	Dipole–dipole	5 - 30
(- +) (- +)	Dipole–induced dipole	1 - 10

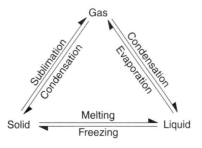

Fig. 7-13.

surroundings become cooler (e.g., vaporization of sweat cools the body). In the reverse direction, heat is given off from the system and the surroundings become warmer (e.g., condensation of water vapor from the air warms the body). **Brownian motion** (e.g., the random motion of a pollen grain that results from collision with the liquid molecules) is evidence for the motion and kinetic energies of liquid molecules.

Molecules have a range of kinetic energies. The number in a given energy range (ΔE) is proportional to $e^{-\Delta E/kT}$ (from the Boltzmann distribution). Molecules above a certain kinetic energy level can escape into the vapor phase (i.e., evaporate). To evaporate, the molecules must have enough energy to overcome the intermolecular forces (the stronger the attractive forces, the more energy required; see subsequent section about chemical bonding for intermolecular forces). The molecules that evaporate become gases and exert **vapor pressure**.

Solids also have a vapor pressure based on a similar argument. Generally, substances with stronger intermolecular attractive forces have lower vapor pressures. Substances with weak intermolecular forces tend to have high vapor pressures. Note: as the temperature increases, the average kinetic energy per molecule increases, and the liquid (or solid) evaporates faster (Fig. 7-14).

Another way of describing the relationships between freezing points and boiling points is the **phase diagram** (Fig. 7-15). This diagram is a plot of **pressure (P) versus temperature (T)**. TP is the **triple point**, which is the value of P and T at which solid, liquid, and gas coexist in equilibrium. **Regions** marked solid, liquid, and gas signify the existence of only that phase. The **lines** represent the coexistence of two phases in equilibrium and the vapor pressures: **AD** = solid and liquid in equilibrium, transition is melting (freezing); **BD** = solid and gas in equilibrium, transition from solid to gas is called sublimation (reverse is condensation); **CD** = liquid and gas in equilibrium, transition is vaporization (condensation); **CD** = vapor pressure of the liquid at different temperatures; and **BD** = vapor pressure of the solid at different temperatures.

Note that all lines in the diagram, with the exception of AD for H_2O, have **positive slopes**, which means that as the pressure is increased on solid H_2O (ice), its melting point decreases and ice can melt at a lower temperature. Observe also that the **location of the 1 atmosphere of pressure relative to the TP** determines if a solid melts at atmospheric pressure or sublimes. If:

1 atm is above the TP, solid → liquid, as for water (see Fig. 7-15A)

1 atm is below the TP, solid → gas (sublimation), as for CO_2 (see Fig. 7-15B)

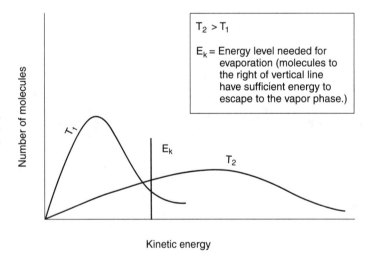

Fig. 7-14. Note that as temperature (T) increases ($T_1 \rightarrow T_2$), more molecules have E_k high enough to evaporate.

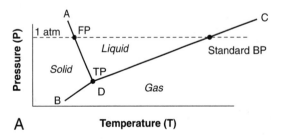

Fig. 7-15.

Freezing Point, Melting Point, and Boiling Point

The **boiling point** (BP) of a liquid is the temperature at which the vapor pressure of the liquid equals the atmospheric (opposing) pressure. For the normal BP, this pressure is taken to be one atmosphere. As the atmospheric pressure decreases, the liquid can boil at lower temperatures. Boiling points depend on intermolecular forces. Remember that nonpolar molecules have weaker forces. Note that symmetric molecules tend to have smaller intermolecular attractive forces. The **freezing point** (FP) of the liquid (or melting point, MP, of the solid) is the temperature at which the vapor pressure of the solid equals the vapor pressure of the liquid.

Molality

Molality is defined as the moles of solute per kilogram of solvent, or

$$m = \frac{\text{mol solute}}{\text{kg solvent}}$$

The extent of freezing-point lowering can be used to determine the molar mass of a nonvolatile solute. For this calculation, solute concentration must be expressed as molality. The molality and molarity of a solution cannot be the same.

Colligative Properties

A solute added to a pure liquid changes some properties of that liquid. The effect of a solute on a pure liquid primarily depends on the relative number of particles present and not on their identity. Properties that are affected by the number of particles present and not by the characteristics of the particles are called colligative properties (boiling point elevation, freezing point depression, vapor pressure, and osmotic pressure). The effect of the number of solute particles (usually nonvolatile, so there is no contribution to the overall vapor pressure) on the boiling point (BP) and freezing point (FP) can be understood by considering their effect on vapor pressure (VP) and using the phase diagram.

When a solute is dissolved in a pure liquid, the solute molecules are bound by liquid molecules. The resultant increase in potential energy must be overcome by kinetic energy if the molecules are to escape. This requirement leads to fewer molecules that have enough kinetic energy to escape into the vapor phase, resulting in a lowering of the VP (Fig. 7-16).

Equations can be derived using thermodynamics to calculate the effect of a solute on the FP or BP of a liquid. A simplified equation for freezing point depression and boiling point elevation follows:

$$\Delta T = +k_b m$$

$$\Delta T = -k_f m$$

ΔT = elevation (for BP) or depression (for FP) of BP or FP, respectively

$$m = \text{molality} = \frac{\text{moles of solute particles}}{\text{kilogram of solvent}}$$

The equation calls for moles of solute particles, which means that if a solute dissociates (e.g., NaCl), the moles of particles are greater than the moles of solute. If the solute dimerizes, there are fewer moles of particles. Taking this fact into account, an alternative way to write the formula is:

$$\Delta T = -ik_f m$$

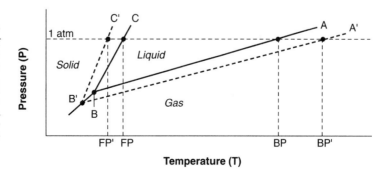

Fig. 7-16. Effect of solutes on BP and FP. AB = original VP line of the liquid, CB = original FP line of the solid, A'B' = lowering of the VP of the liquid by added solute, C'B' = lowering the FP of the solid by the solute, ΔBP = BP' − BP = boiling point elevation, FP = original freezing point, FP' = new FP caused by solute, ΔFP = FP' − FP = freezing point depression.

in which:

$$i = \text{\# of particles the solute dissociates into}$$

$$m = \frac{\text{moles of solute}}{\text{kilogram of solvent}}$$

k_b = boiling point elevation constant depends on the pure liquid used

k_b = 0.51 for H_2O

k_f = freezing point depression constant depends on the pure liquid used

k_f = 1.86 for H_2O

These equations can be used for a variety of purposes:

1. To calculate k, using the formula $k = \dfrac{\Delta T}{m}$

2. To infer the number of actual particles. Make a known m for a liquid with a known k and calculate the expected ΔT. If ΔT (by experiment) is greater than that calculated, then more particles than expected were present and the solute must have dissociated. If ΔT (by experiment) is less than that calculated, then fewer particles than expected were present, and the solute must have aggregated (e.g., dimerized). You can calculate the actual molality of the particles because ΔT (from experiment) and k are known.

3. Most often, to estimate molecular weight = MW (given that corrections are made for dissociation or aggregation). Take a liquid with a known k. Dissolve x grams of solute (MW unknown) in y kg of liquid (solvent). The molality of the solute is determined by measuring ΔT, and employing the formula:

$$m = \frac{\Delta T}{K}$$

Since the (weight of solute)/(kg of solvent) ratio is known, the molecular weight of the solute can be calculated.

Example:

1.02 g of a solid was dissolved in 50.00 g of water. This corresponds to 20.4 g of solute per kg of water. The solution gave a freezing point depression of 0.28°C. Since the molal freezing depression constant of water *k* is 1.86°C, the molal concentration *m* of the solid was:

$$m = \frac{\Delta T}{k}$$

$$m = \frac{\Delta T}{k} = \frac{0.28}{1.86} = \frac{0.15 \text{ mole}}{\text{kg of solvent}}$$

$$MW = \frac{\dfrac{\text{g of solute}}{\text{kg of solvent}}}{m} = \frac{\dfrac{20.4 \text{ g of solute}}{\text{kg of water}}}{\dfrac{0.15 \text{ mole}}{\text{kg of water}}} = \frac{136 \text{ g}}{\text{mole}}$$

4. Definitions:

Suspension: a heterogeneous mixture of solute suspended in solvent, e.g., clay particles suspended in water.

Colloids: solutes that, when mixed with water, do not pass through parchment membranes, e.g., starch, glue. (Substances in solution that do pass through parchment membranes are called crystalloids, e.g., sugar, salt.)

Emulsion: a colloidal suspension of two liquids that are not soluble in each other, e.g., oil and vinegar in a salad dressing.

Foam: a mixture of a gas in a liquid, e.g., aerosol shaving cream.

Gel: colloids that flow at a very slow rate and behave more like solids, e.g., jelly, stick antiperspirant.

APPLIED CONCEPTS

Gas Properties

The premedical student should review applications of the gas theories and laws to the biologic and physical sciences, with particular emphasis on the human respiratory system (inhalation and exhalation). It is necessary to understand the working of a spirometer in order to solve problems as they relate to tidal volume and residual volume in the human lungs. Review the following the gas laws that relate to the physiology of the respiratory system.

Dalton's Law

Definition
Each gas in a mixture of gases in a closed space exerts its own characteristic pressure as if no other gases were present. This pressure is also called partial pressure, or p. Atmospheric pressure is equal to the sum of the partial pressures of all the different gases in the closed space.

Application
Partial pressures are important when studying the movement of gases in the lungs, blood, and tissues. A gas will diffuse from a region where the partial pressure is high to one where the partial pressure is lower. For example, PO_2 is 105 mm Hg in the alveoli and 40 mm Hg in deoxygenated blood. Thus, oxygen will diffuse into the blood to oxygenate it.

Henry's Law

Definition
The volume of a gas that will dissolve in a liquid depends on its partial pressure and its solubility coefficient.

Application
Air gases dissolve in different amounts in the blood. For example, the solubility coefficient of O_2 is 0.024 and of CO is 0.57. Some trauma, such as near-drowning or carbon monoxide poisoning, causes the body to need more O_2 in the blood. Increasing the partial pressure of O_2 in the patient's environment allows more O_2 into the blood. Such a process occurs in a hyperbaric chamber, where the PO_2 is about 3000 mm Hg, thus raising the solubility of O_2 in the blood.

PHASES AND PHASE EQUILIBRIA: REVIEW QUESTIONS

1. Which of the following variables are used to describe gases?

    A. pressure.
    B. volume.
    C. moles.
    D. all of the above.

2. Ideal gases have all of the following characteristics EXCEPT:

    A. absence of intermolecular forces.
    B. nonideal gases may exhibit ideal behavior at high pressure and low temperature.
    C. the molecules occupy no space.
    D. all of the above are correct.

3. Boyle's law states that:

    A. volume varies inversely as temperature at constant pressure.
    B. volume varies directly as temperature at constant pressure.
    C. pressure varies inversely as volume at constant temperature.
    D. pressure varies directly as volume at constant temperature.

4. Charles' law states that:

    A. volume varies inversely as temperature at constant pressure.
    B. volume varies directly as temperature at constant pressure.
    C. pressure varies inversely as volume at constant temperature.
    D. pressure varies directly as volume at constant temperature.

5. All of the following equations are expressions for the ideal gas law EXCEPT:

    A. $PV = nRT$

    B. $\dfrac{PV}{T} = \text{constant}$

    C. $\dfrac{P_1V_1}{T_1} = \dfrac{P_2V_2}{T_2}$

    D. $\left(P + \dfrac{n^2a}{V_2}\right)(V - nb) = nRT$

6. Which of the following characteristics does not describe one mole of an ideal gas at STP?

   A. volume = 1 liter.
   B. temperature = 273°K.
   C. pressure = 1 atmosphere.
   D. all of the above are correct.

7. Each gas in a mixture exerts a partial pressure. The total pressure of all the gases in the container is:

   A. less than the sum of the separate pressures of each gas.
   B. more than the sum of the separate pressures of each gas.
   C. equal to the sum of the separate pressures of each gas.
   D. the sum is variable.

8. What is the correct expression for the partial pressure (P_A) of n_A moles of a gas in a mixture of gases with a total of n_T moles and a total pressure = P_T?

   A. $P_A = (n_A + n_T)P_T$
   B. $P_A = (n_T - n_A)P_T$
   C. $P_A = n_A P_T$
   D. $P_A = (n_A/n_T)P_T$

9. All of the following are conclusions of the kinetic theory of gases EXCEPT:

   A. derivation of the van der Waals equation.
   B. derivation of Boyle's and Charles' law.
   C. relation of average kinetic energy of gases to temperature.
   D. Graham's law of diffusion.

10. In the van der Waals equation for nonideal gases:

$$\left(P + \frac{n^2 a}{V^2}\right)(V - nb) = nRT$$

    which of the following statements is NOT true?

    A. $\frac{n^2 a}{V^2}$ corrects for intermolecular forces.

    B. nb corrects for the volume occupied by gas molecules.
    C. At high densities, the equation reduces to the ideal gas law.
    D. All of the statements are correct.

11. When the pressure on a sample of gas is tripled, the new volume is:

    A. nine times the original volume.
    B. three times the original volume.
    C. one third of the original volume.
    D. one ninth of the original volume.

12. One mole of an ideal gas occupies 3 liters at 37°C. Approximately what pressure, in atmospheres, does the gas exert?

    A. 1.1
    B. 4.2
    C. 8.5
    D. 12.3

    $P = \frac{nRT}{V}$ $R = .082$

13. What approximate volume will 2 liters of a gas at 27°C and 2 atm occupy at STP. (STP = 0°C, 1 atm)?

    A. 3.6 liters
    B. 5.1 liters
    C. 1.1 liters
    D. Cannot be determined

    $\frac{P_2 V_2}{T_2} = \frac{P_1 V_1}{T_1}$

14. If 2 g of a vaporized liquid occupy 0.82 liters at STP, what is the approximate molecular weight of the gas?

    A. 13.5 g
    B. 27 g
    C. 54 g
    D. Cannot be determined

15. A container of pure oxygen has a pool of water at its bottom. The atmospheric pressure is 760 torr and equals the total pressure of the container. If the temperature is 37°C and the vapor pressure of water is 47 torr (torr = mm Hg) at this temperature, what is the pressure of the dry oxygen?

    A. 700 mm Hg
    B. 684 mm Hg
    C. 807 mm Hg
    D. 713 mm Hg

    $P_{tot} = P_{O_2} + P_{H_2O}$

16. A mixture of 2 moles of O_2, 3 moles of N_2, and 5 moles of H_2 exerts a pressure of 700 torr. What is the partial pressure of N_2?

    A. 700 torr
    B. 210 torr
    C. 490 torr
    D. 760 torr

    $\dfrac{3}{2+3+5} \times 700 \text{ torr}$

17. A mixture of 5 moles of O_2, 4 moles of N_2, and 1 mole of CO is collected above water at a temperature of 27°C. The total pressure is 760 torr and the vapor pressure of water at 27°C is 27 torr. What is the partial pressure exerted by O_2?

    A. 76 torr
    B. 100 torr
    C. 367 torr
    D. 380 torr

    $\dfrac{5}{5+4+1}$

    $760 - 27 = 733 \text{ torr}$

18. Oxygen (molecular weight = 32) diffuses at a rate of 10 ml/min. Under the same conditions of temperature and pressure, how fast will hydrogen (molecular weight = 2) diffuse?

    A. 20 ml/min
    B. 40 ml/min
    C. 160 ml/min
    D. Insufficient information provided

    $\dfrac{V_{H_2}}{10} = \sqrt{\dfrac{32}{2}}$

    $= \sqrt{16} = 4$

    $\dfrac{V_{H_2}}{10} = 4$

    $V_{H_2} = 40$

19. As a substance moves from a solid to a liquid, all of the following changes occur EXCEPT:

    A. molecules become more disordered.
    B. kinetic energy of the molecules decreases.
    C. intermolecular forces become weaker.
    D. molecules become farther separated.

20. Vaporization of a liquid from the skin will cause the skin to become:

    A. cooler.
    B. warmer.
    C. extremely hot.
    D. extremely cold.

21. Which of the following forces in liquids result in the highest vapor pressure?

    A. Strong intermolecular forces
    B. Weak intermolecular forces
    C. Tangential viscous forces
    D. Intermolecular forces have no effect on vapor pressure

Questions 22–26
Use the data in the following illustration for this group of questions.

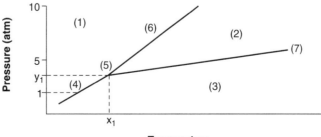

22. Gaseous state is represented by:

    A. 1.
    B. 3.
    C. 4.
    D. 7.

23. What is the triple point?

    A. 1
    B. 4
    C. 5
    D. 7

24. Liquid state can exist only in region:

    A. 1.
    B. 2.
    C. 3.
    D. 5.

25. At atmospheric pressure, the solid phase of this substance will only:

    A. remain a solid.
    B. melt.
    C. freeze.
    D. vaporize.

26. Colligative properties depend on:

    A. the chemical properties of the solute.
    B. the physical properties of the solute.
    C. the chemical properties of the solvent.
    D. the number of solute particles present in solution.

27. Which equation relates the freezing point depression (ΔT) with the freezing point constant (k_f) and the molality (m) of the solution (excluding the minus sign and i)?

    A. $\Delta T = k_f/m$
    B. $\Delta T = m/k_f$
    C. $\Delta T = 1/k_f m$
    D. $\Delta T = k_f m$

Questions 28–30
Five grams of a compound with a molecular weight of 80 is placed in 500 g of a liquid that has a normal freezing point of 58.5°C. The freezing point of the solution is now 57°C. Next, 2 g of an unknown compound is placed in 250 g of the same liquid, and the freezing point is now 58°C.

28. What is the freezing point depression constant (k_f) of the liquid?

    A. 12
    B. 6
    C. 3
    D. 1.5

29. What is the expected molecular weight of the unknown compound by freezing point analysis?

    A. 192
    B. 96
    C. 48
    D. 72

30. A mass spectrograph analysis shows the true molecular weight of the compound is 384. What inference can be made about the compound's behavior in the liquid?

    A. It dissociates.
    B. It forms dimers.
    C. It forms tetramers.
    D. No inference can be made.

1–10. **1-D, 2-B, 3-C, 4-B, 5-D, 6-A, 7-C, 8-D, 9-A, 10-C.** See text for explanation.

11. C This is a direct application of Boyle's law. Volume varies inversely as pressure. So, if pressure is increased by a factor of 3, the volume is decreased by a factor of 3.

12. C This problem deals with one gas under one set of n-P-V-T, and so the equation to use is PV = nRT. Solving for pressure yields:

$$P = \frac{nRT}{V}$$

By knowing the units used, determine R as follows:

$$R = \frac{PV}{nT} = \frac{(1 \text{ atm})(22.4 \text{ liters})}{(1 \text{ mole})(273°K)} = 0.082 \frac{(\text{atm})(\text{liters})}{(\text{mole})(°K)}$$

(Because 1 mole of an ideal gas at STP—273°K, 1 atm—occupies 22.4 liters.) Also, remember that the temperature is the absolute temperature:

$$T = 37° + 273° = 310°K$$

Then:

$$P = \frac{(1)(0.082)(310)}{(3)} \approx 8.2 \text{ atm}$$

$$\frac{310}{3} \approx 100 \text{ and then } (100)(0.082) \approx 8.2$$

Note the approximations made. 8.2 is closest to 8.5 atm.

13. A This problem requires comparing the gas at two different conditions of P-V-T. The best equation to use is:

$$\frac{P_2 V_2}{T_2} = \frac{P_1 V_1}{T_1}$$

$$(\text{STP}) \qquad (\text{Original})$$

Solving for V_2:

$$V_2 = V_1 \left(\frac{T_2}{T_1}\right)\left(\frac{P_1}{P_2}\right) = (2)\left(\frac{273}{300}\right)\left(\frac{2}{1}\right) \approx 3.6$$

$$T_1 = 27 + 273 = 300$$

the approximation is made as follows:

$$\frac{273}{300} \approx \frac{270}{300} \approx \frac{27}{30} \approx \frac{9}{10}$$

$$\text{then, } (2)\left(\frac{9}{10}\right)(2) = \left(\frac{36}{10}\right) = 3.6$$

14. C First determine the number of moles. Because the substance is a gas and there is one set of P-V-T conditions, use:

$$PV = nRT$$

Solving for n:

$$n = \frac{PV}{RT} = \frac{(1)(0.82)}{(0.082)(273)} \approx \frac{1}{27}$$

the approximation for n is:

$$\frac{0.82}{0.082} = 10, \text{ then } \frac{10}{273} \approx \frac{10}{270} \approx \frac{1}{27}$$

The definition of moles (n):

$$\text{moles} = \frac{\text{weight}}{\text{molecular weight}} \text{ or,}$$

$$\text{molecular weight} = \frac{\text{weight}}{\text{moles}} \approx \frac{2}{1/27} \approx (2)\left(\frac{27}{1}\right) \approx 54 \text{ g}$$

Alternatively, because n = wt/mw, PV = (wt/mw)RT; mw = wt(RT/PV).

15. **D** When gases are collected over a liquid (e.g., water), the vapor pressure of that liquid must be subtracted from the total pressure to get the pressure of the gases without the added effect of the liquid's vapor pressure. The vapor pressure varies with temperature. Note that the total pressure of the gases is still the sum of the partial pressures (Dalton's law),

$$p_{tot} = p_{O_2} + p_{H_2O} \text{ vapor}$$

$$p_{O_2} = p_{tot} - p_{H_2O} \text{ vapor} = 760 - 47 = 713$$

16. **B** This problem involves a direct application of Dalton's law of partial pressures. The partial pressure of $N_2 (P_{N2})$ is:

$$p_{N_2} = X_{N_2} p_T$$

$$p_T = 700 \text{ torr}$$

$$X_{N_2} = \frac{nN_2}{nN_2 + nO_2 + nH_2} = \frac{3}{3 + 5 + 2} = \frac{3}{10}$$

$$p_{N_2} = \frac{3}{10}(700) = 210 \text{ torr}$$

17. **C** This problem involves a combination of the principles addressed in questions 15 and 16. First, take into account the effect of the water vapor on the total pressure:

$$P_T(\text{Total pressure of gases}) = \text{total pressure} - \text{water vapor pressure}$$

$$P_T = 760 - 27 = 733 \text{ torr}$$

Then, apply Dalton's law using 733 torr:

$$P_{O_2} = X_{O_2} P_T$$

$$X_{O_2} = \frac{nO_2}{nO_2 + nN_2 + nCO_2} = \frac{5}{5 + 4 + 1} = \frac{5}{10} = \frac{1}{2}$$

$$P_{O_2} = (\tfrac{1}{2})(733) = 367 \text{ torr}$$

18. **B** In general, the lighter gas will diffuse faster. Using the formulation of Graham's law of diffusion:

$$\frac{V_{H_2}}{V_{O_2}} = \sqrt{\frac{MW_{O_2}}{MW_{H_2}}}$$

$$\frac{V_{H_2}}{10} = \sqrt{\frac{32}{2}} = \sqrt{16} = 4$$

$$V_{H_2} = (10)(4) = 40 \text{ ml/min}$$

19–27. 19-B, 20-A, 21-B, 22-B, 23-C, 24-B, 25-D, 26-D, 27-D. See text for explanation.

28. **A** The complete formula is: $k = \Delta T/-im$, in which i = the number of particles into which the substance dissociates, and the negative in the denominator offsets the negative temperature drop. If the absolute value of ΔT is taken, ignore the minus sign. If the molecule does not dissociate, then i = 1 and may be ignored.

$$m = \text{moles/kg of solvent} = (\tfrac{1}{16})/(\tfrac{1}{2}) = (\tfrac{1}{16})(\tfrac{2}{1}) = \tfrac{2}{16} = \tfrac{1}{8}$$

(moles = weight/molecular weight = $\tfrac{5}{80} = \tfrac{1}{16}$
kg = grams of substance/1000 g = $\tfrac{500}{1000} = \tfrac{1}{2}$)

$$\Delta T = 58.5°C - 57°C = 1.5°C = 1\tfrac{1}{2} = \tfrac{3}{2}$$

To use the formula $k = \Delta T/-im$, ΔT must be determined as follows:

$$\Delta T = T_f - T_i = 57 - 58.5 = -1.5°C$$

In which f = final and i = initial.
Finally, $k = (\tfrac{3}{2})/(\tfrac{1}{8}) = (\tfrac{3}{2})(\tfrac{8}{1}) = \tfrac{24}{2} = 12$

29. **A** Use the results from question 28 and the procedure outlined in the text:

(a) $m = \Delta T/k = \tfrac{1}{2}/12 = \tfrac{1}{2} \cdot \tfrac{1}{12} = \tfrac{1}{24}$

$$\Delta T = 58.5 - 58 = 0.5 = \tfrac{1}{2}$$

(b) moles of solute = (m)(y) = $(\frac{1}{24})(\frac{1}{4})$ = $\frac{1}{96}$

y = kg of solute = $\frac{250}{1000}$ = $\frac{1}{4}$

(c) MW = x/moles of solute = $2/(\frac{1}{96})$ = $(2)(\frac{96}{1})$ = 192

x = weight of solute = 2g

30. A The expected freezing point depression using the molecular weight given is:

$$\Delta T = km = (12)(\frac{1}{48}) = \frac{12}{48} = \frac{1}{4} = 0.25°C$$

$$m = \text{moles/kg solvent} = (\frac{2}{384})/(\frac{1}{4}) = (\frac{2}{384})(\frac{4}{1}) = (2)(4)/384 = \frac{1}{48}$$

So, the expected ΔT is 0.25°C. Because the actual is 0.5°C, there must have been more particles present than expected, and the compound must have dissociated, or,

$$i = \Delta T/-km = -(\frac{1}{2})/-(12)(\frac{1}{48}) = (\frac{1}{2})(\frac{48}{12}) = \frac{48}{24} = 2$$

$$= 2 \text{ particles per original molecule}$$

Electronic Structure of the Atom

The **atom** is the smallest unit of an element that retains the characteristic properties of that element. It consists of a very dense nucleus, which contains neutrons and positively charged protons, that is surrounded by a cloud of negatively charged electrons. Their properties are summarized in Table 7-2.

In its ground state, the atom has an equal number of protons and electrons and is therefore electrically neutral. The subatomic particles occupy a minute fraction of the space in an atom. A greatly magnified model of an atom would show the nucleus as a roughly spherical shape one foot in diameter, containing over 99.95% of the total mass, with the electrons orbiting about 10,000 feet away.

The atoms of each element have a specific **atomic number,** which is defined as the number of protons, and a specific **atomic mass number,** which is the sum of the neutrons and protons in the nucleus.

Not all atoms of the same element have the same number of neutrons. Atoms with the same atomic number and different mass number (and therefore a different number of neutrons in the nucleus) are called **isotopes.** For a more detailed discussion of nuclear and atomic structures, see p. 381–384.

Orbital Structures of Atoms

The chemical properties of an element depend on the number of electrons present, which also determine the element's atomic number. Electrons can exhibit both particle and wave characteristics, depending on the measurement that is carried out on them. According to quantum mechanics, electrons can occupy an array of discrete orbits around the nucleus.

An **atomic orbital** describes the probability that an electron will be found at a specific location in the vicinity of the nucleus. Each electron in an orbital has a set of four quantum numbers that uniquely define it. **Pauli's exclusion principle** states that no two electrons in the same atom may have the same set of quantum numbers. The quantum numbers are:

1. Principal quantum number (n). The **principal quantum number** defines the energy and the distance from the nucleus of an electron in an orbital. The values of **n** are positive integers and range from 1 to infinity. As **n** increases, the energy of the electron and its average distance from the nucleus increase. Thus, when **n** = 1, the electron is in the orbital closest to the nucleus. For any given value of **n,** there can be a maxiumum of n^2 orbitals, each containing up to two electrons. The orbitals with the same **principal quantum number** form a **shell.** Thus, for each shell there can be up to $2 n^2$ electrons.

TABLE 7-2. Basic Properties of Subatomic Particles

Name	Charge	Mass at rest (grams)	Symbols
Electron	−1	9.1091×10^{-28}	β, e^-
Proton	+1	1.67252×10^{-24}	p, p^+
Neutron	0	1.67482×10^{-24}	n

Value of n		1	2	3	4
Shell designation		K	L	M	N
Maximum number of electrons in the shell		2	8	18	32

2. Angular momentum quantum number (l). The **angular momentum quantum number** can have a total of n values, from 0 to $(n - 1)$. The angular momentum of the electron will increase with increasing values of l. The value of l determines the subshell of the atomic orbital.

Value of n	1	2	2	3	3	3	4	4	4	4
Value of l	0	0	1	0	1	2	0	1	2	3
Designation of subshell	1s	2s	2p	3s	3p	3d	4s	4p	4d	4f

All **s** orbitals, in which the angular momentum quantum number l equals 0, are spherically symmetrical. The **p** orbitals ($l = 1$) have a dumbell shape, with two regions of high electron density at opposite sides of the nucleus. The **d** and **f** orbitals have more complex shapes (Fig. 7-17). Note that all orbitals have zero amplitude at the nucleus, which means that there is zero probability of finding an electron there. The energy of the electrons increases with increasing principal quantum number **n**; within any given shell the energy increases in the order **s** < **p** < **d** < **f**.

3. Magnetic quantum number (m_l). The **magnetic quantum number** describes the orientation of an electron's magnetic field in an external field. The magnetic quantum number can have any integral value from $-l$ to $+l$; therefore, there are $(2l + 1)$ values of m_l for each value of l. Each value of m_l defines an atomic orbital in the subshell. Thus, when the principal quantum number $n = 3$, the angular momentum quantum number l can have values of 0, 1, and 2. When $l = 0$ (**s** subshell), only one value of m_l, and therefore only one orbital, which can have a maximum of two electrons, is possible. When $l = 1$, m_l can have $(2l + 1) = 3$ values (**p** subshell), and a maximum of three orbitals and six electrons are possible; when $l = 2$ (**d** subshell) a maximum of 5 filled orbitals and 10 electrons are possible.

Value of l	0	1	2	3
Subshell	s	p	d	f
Values of m_l	0	$-1, 0, +1$	$-2, -1, 0, +1, +2$	$-3, -2, -1, 0, +1, +2, +3$
Number of orbitals	1	3	5	7
Maximum number of electrons	2	6	10	14

4. Spin quantum number (m_s). Each orbital can contain up to two electrons, which have identical values for the **n, l,** and **m_s** quantum numbers. These two electrons spin in opposite directions, and are assigned **m_s** values of $+\frac{1}{2}$ and $-\frac{1}{2}$, respectively, depending on the direction of their spin with respect to an external magnetic field.

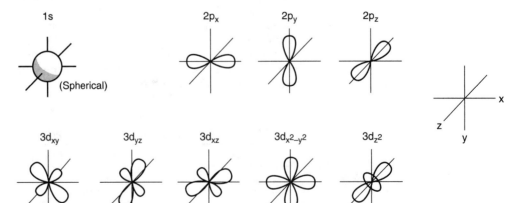

Fig. 7-17. Orbitals.

The electronic configuration of an atom is shown by using the value of each principal quantum number **n,** followed by the letter corresponding to the value of the l quantum numbers (i.e., s = 0, p = 1, d = 2, f = 3). The number of electrons actually present in a subshell is shown as a superscript of the letter. For example, the electronic configuration of aluminum and calcium, whose atomic numbers are 13 and 20, respectively, is shown in the following way:

$$\text{Al:} \quad 1s^2 \quad 2s^2 \quad 2p^6 \quad 3s^2 \quad 3p^1$$

$$\text{Ca:} \quad 1s^2 \quad 2s^2 \quad 2p^6 \quad 3s^2 \quad 3p^6 \quad 4s^2$$

The orbitals are filled in sequence, from the lowest energy to the highest. The filling sequence is shown in Figure 7-18. The actual order is: 1s 2s 2p 3s 3p 4s **3d** 4p 5s **4d** 5p 6s **4f 5d** 6p 7s **5f 6d** 7p. In this sequence, the electrons in the **d** and **f** subshells have higher energies than those in the **s** and **p** subshells with higher principal quantum numbers, and therefore are filled later.

The filling of atomic orbitals of the same shape and energy (i.e., in the same subshell) follows **Hund's rule,** which states that electrons will occupy each orbital with parallel spins until all the orbitals are half filled; only then are electrons paired with opposite spinning electrons in the same orbital (Fig. 7-19).

GROUND STATE AND EXCITED STATE

The **ground state** of the electrons of an atom is when the electrons are in the lowest energy states available to the electrons. For example, the ground state of aluminum is $1s^2 \, 2s^2 \, 2p^6 \, 3s^2 \, 3p^1$.

An **excited state** of the atom occurs when one or more electrons occupy orbitals (energy levels) other than the lowest available to the atom. Input of some energy "excites" the electron to a higher state. As an example, for aluminum:

$$1s^2 \, 2s^2 \, 2p^6 \, 3s^2 \, 3p^1 \xrightarrow{\text{energy}} 1s^2 \, 2s^2 \, 2p^6 \, 3s^0 \, 3p^3$$

Both 3s electrons are in the higher energy level 3p.

For the electrons, the higher the n or l quantum numbers, the higher the energies. When electrons shift between the different orbitals, energy is absorbed or emitted as a frequency of light. When energy is emitted (the electron moves from higher orbitals to lower orbitals, i.e., closer to the nucleus), a bright band appears at that frequency (or wavelength) in a spectrum (the continuum of all frequencies or wavelengths). The results are **emission spectra.** When energy is absorbed by the electron (as must occur in the preceding example), a dark band appears at that frequency because energy is removed from the spectrum. In this instance, the result is **absorption spectra.** Consider the spectrum as a source of light containing all the frequencies (wavelengths) representing different energies. As it passes through a substance, energy may be added (by emission from

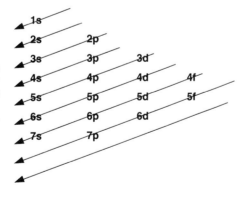

Fig. 7-18. The sequence begins with the orbital on the top arrow (1s) and proceeds to the next arrow, from the right to the left. The sequence is 1s, 2s, 2p, 3s, 3p, 4s, 3d, 4p, 5s, etc.

Fig. 7-19. Hund's rule.

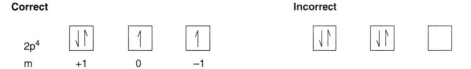

atoms) and certain frequencies become more intense (brighter) or energy may be removed (by absorption by atoms) and certain frequencies become less intense (less bright).

CONVENTIONAL NOTATION FOR ELECTRONIC STRUCTURE

Bohr used the theories and experimental data of Planck, Einstein, and Rutherford to develop his theory of the atom. He proposed that the angular momentum of the electron was in multiples of $\dfrac{h}{2\pi}$ $\left(\text{or } mvr = \dfrac{nh}{2\pi}\right)$ (see the discussion of momentum in the physics section), and that electrons circulated in discrete circular orbits, stabilized by having the centrifugal force on the electron equal the Coulomb force of attraction between the nucleus and the electron. From these inferences, he derived the energy states of the electrons given by:

$$E = -\frac{2\pi^2 mZ^2 e^4}{n^2 h^2}$$

in which n = 1,2,3, ... defines the energy states or levels; m = mass of electron; e = charge on the electron; Z = atomic number (nuclear charge); h = Planck's constant.

Energy transitions occur between states with energy change equal to hv, which could be calculated from above (h = $|E_f - E_i|$). Note that $E \propto \dfrac{1}{n^2}$, and as n becomes larger, the energy levels are closer together. Bohr was able to explain some of the hydrogen spectrum lines with his theory. Another key to his theory was that electrons in any one of the energy states do not radiate energy.

The major flaws in Bohr's theory were the discrete orbits and the determination of exact momentum of the electron concurrently. **Heisenberg's uncertainty principle** states that it is impossible to determine simultaneously the position and momentum of an electron, as in Bohr's theory. This principle led to the probabilistic theory of electronic structure, as derived by Schrodinger.

ELECTRONIC STRUCTURE OF THE ATOM: REVIEW QUESTIONS

1. All of the following were theorized by Bohr in his description of the atom EXCEPT:

   A. angular momentum of electrons is in multiples of $\dfrac{h}{2\pi}$.

   B. electrons circulate in discrete circular orbits.

   C. energy of each electron is inversely proportional to n^2.

   D. electrons radiate energy continuously in a given orbit.

2. The statement, "It is impossible to determine simultaneously the position and momentum of an electron," is attributable to:

   A. Heisenberg.
   B. Einstein.
   C. Planck.
   D. Schrodinger.

3. The following shape represents what type of orbital?

   A. p
   B. s
   C. d
   D. f

4. The letters s, p, d and f are used to represent which quantum numbers?

   A. Angular momentum (l)
   B. Principal (n)
   C. Magnetic (m_l)
   D. Spin (m_s)

5. The magnetic quantum number (QN) has its values limited directly by the value of:

   A. principal QN.
   B. angular momentum QN.

C. spin QN.
D. none of the above.

6. Which statement is consistent with Hund's rule?

 A. Electrons fill orbitals with parallel spins until all the orbitals of the same energy are half filled, then they go into suborbitals with anti-parallel (opposite) spins.
 B. Two electrons in the same atom cannot have the same four quantum numbers.
 C. There is a maximum of two electrons in any orbital.
 D. None of the above.

7. Which statement best summarizes Pauli's exclusion principle?

 A. The position and momentum of an electron cannot be determined simultaneously.
 B. Electrons with the same spin cannot go into the same orbital.
 C. No two electrons in an atom may have the same set of the four quantum numbers.
 D. None of the above.

8. When an atom emits energy as light, bands in the spectrum will appear that are:

 A. brighter.
 B. darker.
 C. colorless.
 D. hard to locate.

9. What is the maximum number of electrons in an orbital with m_l (magnetic quantum number) = 3?

 A. 6
 B. 4
 C. 3
 D. 2

10. What is the maximum number of electrons in a shell with n (principal quantum number) = 3?

 A. 6
 B. 8
 C. 18
 D. 32

$2n^2$

11. What is the maximum number of electrons in an orbital with l (angular momentum quantum number) = 3?

 A. 6
 B. 10
 C. 14
 D. 18

$4l + 2$

12. How many electrons are in the 2p orbitals of an element with an atomic number = 22?

 A. 6
 B. 4
 C. 3
 D. 1

13. The electron configuration of magnesium (Mg) with atomic number 12 is:

 A. $1s^2 \, 2s^2 \, 2p^6 \, 3s^2$.
 B. $1s^2 \, 2s^2 \, 3s^2 \, 3p^6$.
 C. $1s^2 \, 2s^2 \, 2p^2 \, 3s^2 \, 3p^2 \, 3d^2$.
 D. None of the above.

14. Sodium has an atomic number = 11. What is the electron configuration of the sodium ion (Na^{+1})?

 A. $1s^2 \, 2s^2 \, 2p^6 \, 3s^2$
 B. $1s^2 \, 2s^2 \, 2p^5 \, 3s^2$
 C. $1s^2 \, 2s^2 \, 2p^6 \, 3s^1$
 D. $1s^2 \, 2s^2 \, 2p^6$

Questions 15–17

The atomic number of manganese (Mn) is 25.

15. What is the electron configuration of the ground state?

    A. $1s^2 2s^2 2p^6 3s^2 3p^6 3d^7$
    B. $1s^2 2s^2 2p^6 3s^2 3p^6 4s^2 4p^5$
    C. $1s^2 2s^2 2p^6 3s^2 2d^{10} 3p^3$
    D. None of the above

16. An excited state of the atom may be:

    A. $1s^2 2s^2 2p^6 3s^2 3p^6 4s^1 3d^6$.
    B. $1s^2 2s^2 2p^6 3s^2 3p^6 4s^2 3d^5$.
    C. $1s^2 2s^2 2p^6 2d^{10} 3s^2 3p^3$.
    D. None of the above.

17. In going from $1s^2 2s^2 2p^6 3s^2 3p^6 4s^2 3d^5$ to $1s^2 2s^2 2p^6 3s^2 3p^6 4s^1 3d^6$, the atom would _____ energy.

    A. absorb
    B. emit
    C. not change its state of

ANSWERS AND EXPLANATIONS

1–8. **1-D, 2-A, 3-A, 4-A, 5-B, 6-A, 7-C, 8-A.** See text for explanation.

9. D All orbitals contain a maximum of two electrons.

10. C Using the formula provided in the text: $2n^2 = 2(3)^2 = 2(9) = 18$. See the example in the text for an alternative method.

11. C Using the formula provided in the text: $4l + 2 = 4(3) + 2 = 12 + 2 = 14$.

12. A The element has 22 electrons (from AN = 22). The electron configuration is: $1s^2 2s^2 2p^6 3s^2 3p^6 4s^2 3d^2$. It might have been clear that the 2p orbital was filled. So, the answer would be a filled p orbital, which has 6 electrons.

13. A Magnesium has 12 electrons, because AN = 12. The sequence of filling is: 1s 2s 2p 3s 3p 4s 3d. The s orbital has a maximum of 2 electrons, and the p orbital has a maximum of 6 electrons.

14. D Ten electrons are in the sodium ion, whereas 11 are in the neutral atom (from atomic number = 11). Because the ion is positive, one less electron is available.

15. D In the ground state, the electrons are in the lowest energy levels available. The sequence of filling for 25 electrons is: $1s^2 2s^2 2p^6 3s^2 3p^6 4s^2 3d^5$. So, none of the answers is correct.

16. A A 4s electron is excited to a 3d electron. In an excited state, electrons in the ground state orbitals are "excited" to higher energy orbitals.

17. A The 4s electron is being excited to become a 3d electron. Because 3d electrons are of higher energy than 4s (because of the penetrance of this orbital and consequent lowering of its energy), it would require energy to move 4s to 3d levels. Therefore, the atom must absorb this energy.

The Periodic Table

REVIEW OF THE PERIODIC TABLE

The periodic table is an orderly arrangement of elements by their atomic numbers based on the quantum theory of the atom (Fig. 7-20). Mendeleev was the first to arrange elements by their atomic numbers. Rows or **periods** represent the principal quantum number (n) and have values from n = 1 to n = 7. Each period is the sequential filling of the orbitals within a shell. Columns or **groups** represent elements with similar chemical and physical properties and with the same electron configuration in the **outermost shell**. Eight groups of elements are given certain names. The A group of elements are **representative**; these elements have the s and p orbitals as the outermost. The **transition**, or B group, elements have the d or f orbitals as the outermost. Roman numerals (I, II, etc.) identify the number of electrons in the outermost orbitals.

Valence Electrons of the Common Groups

Valence electrons are the outer shell electrons of an atom. Each group has a certain number of valence electrons. Group IA, the alkali metals, have a single s electron, or a valence shell configuration of ns^1. Group IIA, the alkaline earth metals, have a valence shell configuration of ns^2. Group IIIA has a valence shell configuration of ns^2np^1; group IVA, ns^2np^2; group VA, ns^2np^3; group VIA, ns^2np^4; group VIIA, the halogens, ns^2np^5; and group O, the noble gases, ns^2np^6 (an octet). Of group O, the only exception is helium, which is $1s^2$.

    The second period atoms will gain or lose electrons, whichever is easier, to reach the

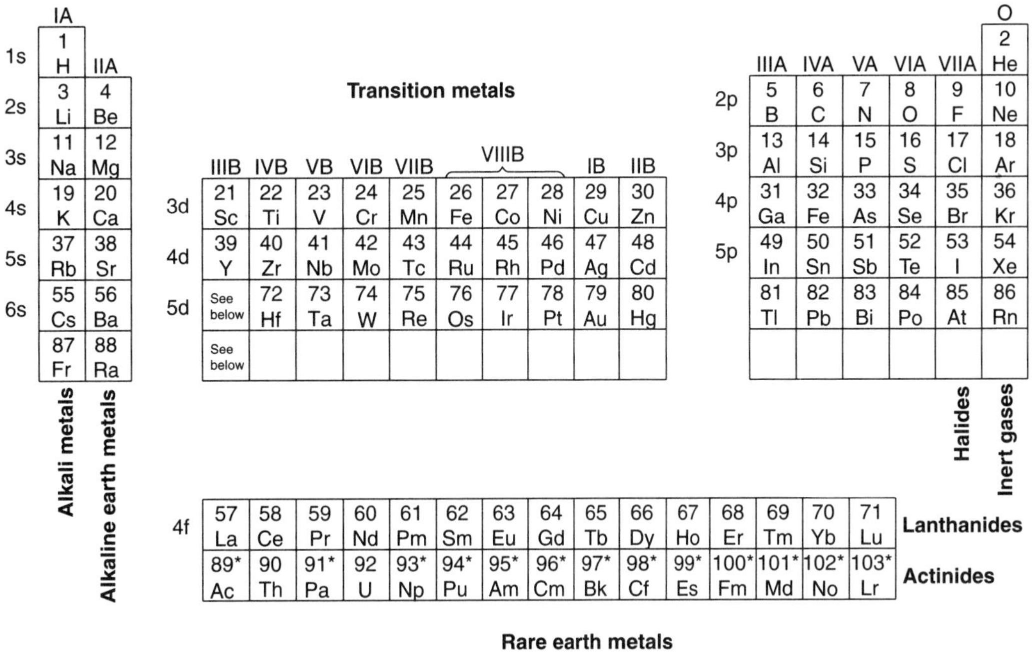

Fig. 7-20. The Periodic Table.

Main group and transition elements:

	IA		IIIB	IVB	VB	VIB	VIIB	VIIIB			IB	IIB	IIIA	IVA	VA	VIA	VIIA	O
1s	1 H	IIA																2 He
2s	3 Li	4 Be											5 B	6 C	7 N	8 O	9 F	10 Ne	(2p)
3s	11 Na	12 Mg											13 Al	14 Si	15 P	16 S	17 Cl	18 Ar	(3p)
4s	19 K	20 Ca	3d 21 Sc	22 Ti	23 V	24 Cr	25 Mn	26 Fe	27 Co	28 Ni	29 Cu	30 Zn	31 Ga	32 Ge	33 As	34 Se	35 Br	36 Kr	(4p)
5s	37 Rb	38 Sr	4d 39 Y	40 Zr	41 Nb	42 Mo	43 Tc	44 Ru	45 Rh	46 Pd	47 Ag	48 Cd	49 In	50 Sn	51 Sb	52 Te	53 I	54 Xe	(5p)
6s	55 Cs	56 Ba	5d (See below)	72 Hf	73 Ta	74 W	75 Re	76 Os	77 Ir	78 Pt	79 Au	80 Hg	81 Tl	82 Pb	83 Bi	84 Po	85 At	86 Rn	
	87 Fr	88 Ra	(See below)																

Transition metals (3d, 4d, 5d block)

Alkali metals (IA) · Alkaline earth metals (IIA) · Halides (VIIA) · Inert gases (O)

Rare earth metals (4f):

4f	Lanthanides	57 La	58 Ce	59 Pr	60 Nd	61 Pm	62 Sm	63 Eu	64 Gd	65 Tb	66 Dy	67 Ho	68 Er	69 Tm	70 Yb	71 Lu
	Actinides	89* Ac	90 Th	91* Pa	92 U	93* Np	94* Pu	95* Am	96* Cm	97* Bk	98* Cf	99* Es	100* Fm	101* Md	102* No	103* Lr

octet state. Remember the mnemonic, "**Asp b**od**y f**ang" for group A-s-p and group b-d-f orbitals.

First and Second Ionization Energies and Trends

Ionization energy (IE) is the energy (or voltage), measured in kilojoules per mole (kJ/mol), required to ionize a gaseous atom, i.e., take the outermost electron away from the atom.

$$\text{Atom(g)} + \text{energy} \rightarrow \text{atom}^+\text{(g)} + e^-$$

$$\Delta E = \text{ionization energy (IE)}$$

Each atom can have a series of ionization energies because more than one electron can be removed. The first ionization energy is the energy needed to remove one electron. The second ionization energy is the energy needed to remove a second electron. The higher the IE, the more difficult it is to remove an electron, which means the nucleus is holding on tighter. IE increases, generally, from left to right in a period, and it decreases from top to bottom in a group. Ionization energy is always positive and the process of ionization is always endothermic.

Electron Affinity

Electron affinity (EA) is the energy released when an electron is moved from infinity into the lowest energy vacant orbital in the gaseous atom.

$$\text{Atom} + e^- \rightarrow \text{anion}^- + \text{energy}$$

The stronger the nuclear attraction for electrons, the higher the EA (absolute value). The EA is subject to configuration variations (Be $2s^2$ < Li $2s^1$ but C > B) and repulsion of electrons in the same energy level (F < Cl but Br < Cl). No overall trend is observed. It may be endothermic or exothermic.

Variation of Properties Within Groups and Rows

The **periodic properties** are properties of the elements that vary in a more or less regular pattern as a function of the atomic numbers, and, hence, electron configuration. To understand the horizontal and vertical structure of the periodic table, consider the following:

1. Reading from left to right in a given period, the nuclear pull on the outermost electrons increases. As a result, the electrons are bound tighter and are closer to the nucleus.
2. Reading down a given column, the outermost electrons are bound less tightly because more electrons are between the nucleus and the outermost electrons. A shell has been completed that effectively shields the outer electrons.

Problem Solving in the Physical Sciences   225

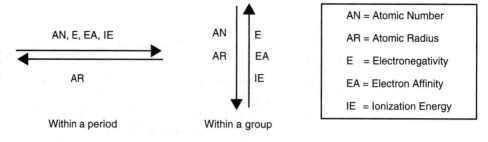

Fig. 7-21. General trends in periodic properties (arrows point toward an increase in the value of a property).

AN, E, EA, IE

AR

Within a period

AN   E
AR   EA
      IE

Within a group

AN = Atomic Number

AR = Atomic Radius

E = Electronegativity

EA = Electron Affinity

IE = Ionization Energy

The gross atomic trends of the periodic properties, illustrated in Figure 7-21, are as follows:

The four major **blocks** (s, p, d, f) of the periodic table (see Fig. 7-20) represent the angular momentum quantum number (l). The number of spaces from left to right in each block is the maximum number of electrons for each quantum number: s has a maximum of 2, p has a maximum of 6, d has a maximum of 10, and f has a maximum of 14. The magnetic quantum number (m_l) and spin quantum number (m_s) are not represented on the table.

Atomic radius (AR) is the distance from the middle of the nucleus to the "outermost limit" of the electrons. The AR is determined by using x-rays on bonded atoms. The AR decreases from left to right in a given period and increases from top to bottom in a given group.

The key feature of a metal is high mobility of electrons, which requires a low IE and/or a low EA. The **metallic character** decreases from left to right in a period but increases from top to bottom in a group. In the periodic chart, the metals are to the left and bottom, and the nonmetals are in the top and right. The semi-metals constitute a region of transition between the metals and nonmetals.

Oxidation state (OS) depends on IE and EA. Low IE elements tend to have positive OS, and high EA elements tend to have negative OS. Metals tend to have positive OS, and nonmetals tend to be negative. Note that the OS of the transition (d orbital) elements tend to be variable but positive and the OS of the inner transition elements (f-orbitals) tend to be + 3.

Chemical activity (CA) depends on the ease of removing an electron (low IE) or the ease of adding an electron (high EA). Either situation leads to high CA. Hence, CA trends are not usually discussed across a period (because the balance of IE and EA changes), but trends are meaningful for groups. On the left side of the table, CA increases as you move down in a given group (because IE decreases). On the right side of the table, CA increases as you move up in a given group (because EA generally increases).

Hydrogen bonding (HB) exists for F, O, N and Cl, but it would theoretically increase as you ascend in a given group.

Substances may be paramagnetic, ferromagnetic or dimagnetic depending on m_s. (Review the section on electrostatics and electromagnetism.)

Electronegativity (E) is a measure of the relative attraction of a bonded atom for the electrons of the other atoms to which it is bonded. In the 1930s, American chemist Linus Pauling was the first to assign numeric electronegativity values to the elements. His theory was that the electronegativity of an element could be determined by measuring the energy needed to break chemical bonds in several of its compounds. Electronegativity is not measured directly, but it can be indirectly obtained from EA, IE and/or bond energies.

The E increases from left to right in a period as atomic size decreases, and decreases from top to bottom in a group as atomic size increases (similar to IE); E increases diagonally upward and to the right in the periodic table. In general, metals have low electronegativities and nonmetals have high electronegativities.

Review these **memory tips**:

1. Ionization energy, electronegativity, and electron affinity follow *similar* trends across groups and periods (with some exceptions)
2. Atomic number and atomic radius follow *similar* trends down a group *but* follow opposite trends across a period (various elements are exceptions)

3. Atomic radii and ionic radii follow *similar* trends across groups and periods. Cations are smaller, whereas anions are larger than the respective parental atoms.

APPLIED CONCEPTS

1. Understand the distribution of calcium and phosphorus in the human body. (All calcium in blood is in the plasma; calcium is absent from red blood cells.) Compare the role of calcium and phosphorus in adults and children. Realize how calcium helps in blood coagulation, regulation of membrane ion transport, and neural impulse transmission. Understand how phosphate provides an important buffer system for urine and blood.
2. Find clinical laboratory procedures and research done on elements such as Ca, P, Mg, Cu, and Fe to determine abnormal levels in the human body. Read how several experimental methods to determine Ca levels have sources of error, e.g., calcium precipitation by oxalate to form CaC_2O_4 may give good Ca excitations because Na and K interfere with the color obtained.

THE PERIODIC TABLE: REVIEW QUESTIONS

1. The periodic table is based on:

    A. atomic weights.
    B. mass number.
    C. neutron number.
    D. atomic number.

2. The periods of the periodic table are _____ and represent the _____ quantum number.

    A. horizontal; principal
    B. horizontal; angular momentum
    C. vertical; principal
    D. vertical; angular momentum

3. Groups of the periodic table:

    A. represent the magnetic quantum number.
    B. represent elements with the same outer electron configuration.
    C. are horizontal.
    D. are all of the above.

4. The transition elements have the _____-orbital as the outermost.

    A. s
    B. p
    C. d
    D. f

5. Which of the following statements about the periodic table is correct?

    A. The nuclear attraction for the outermost electrons decreases from right to left in a given period.
    B. In moving down a given column, the outermost electrons are bound less tightly.
    C. Half-filled or completely filled orbitals have more stability than other incompletely filled orbitals.
    D. All of the statements are correct.

6. The energy required to ionize a gaseous atom is:

    A. ionization energy.
    B. electron affinity.
    C. electronegativity.
    D. none of the above.

7. The relative attraction of the nucleus for the electrons in a chemical bond is:

    A. ionization energy.
    B. electron affinity.
    C. electronegativity.
    D. none of the above.

8. The energy released when an electron is moved from infinity into the vacant orbital (with the lowest energy) is:

    A. electron affinity.
    B. electronegativity.

C. ionization energy.
D. none of the above.

9. Which of the following statements concerning oxidation states (OS) is true?

  A. High ionization energy elements have positive OS.
  B. Metals tend to have negative OS.
  C. Low electron affinity elements tend to have positive OS.
  D. Nonmetals tend to have negative OS.

10. Chemical activity in groups:

  A. increases as ionization energy increases.
  B. decreases as electron affinity decreases.
  C. increases as you read down the left side of the periodic table.
  D. increases as electron affinity decreases.

11. Phosphorus (P) is in group VA. What is the electron configuration of its outermost shell?

  $1s^2\ 2s^2\ 2p^6\ 3s^2\ 3p^3\ 4r\ 3d$

  A. s^2p^3
  B. p^5
  C. d^5
  D. Cannot be determined

12. Bromine (Br) is in group VII A. Which of the following is probably its most common oxidation state (OS)?

  A. $+1$
  B. -1
  C. -2
  D. Cannot be determined

13. The electron configuration of selenium is: $1s^2\ 2s^2\ 2p^6\ 3s^2\ 3p^6\ 4s^2\ 3d^{10}\ 4p^4$. It is probably in what group?

  A. VI A
  B. IV A
  C. VI B
  D. Insufficient information provided

14. The atomic number of chlorine is 17. It is in what group?

  A. VII A
  B. IV A
  C. I A
  D. Cannot be determined by trends

15. Fluorine (F) has an atomic number (AN) = 9 and chlorine (Cl) has an AN = 17. Which has the higher electron affinity?

  A. They are equal
  B. Cl
  C. F
  D. Cannot be determined

16. Sodium (Na) has an atomic number (AN) = 11 and aluminum (Al) has an AN = 13. Which has the higher ionization energy?

  A. They are equal
  B. Na
  C. Al
  D. Cannot be determined

17. Oxygen (O) has an atomic number (AN) = 8 and sulfur (S) has an AN = 16. Which has the greater electronegativity?

  A. S
  B. O

C. They are equal
D. Cannot be determined

18. The atomic number (AN) of magnesium (Mg) is 12, and the AN of sulfur (S) is 16. Which has the larger atomic radius?

    A. Mg
    B. S
    C. They are equal
    D. Cannot be determined

19. Lithium (Li) has an atomic number (AN) = 3 and potassium (K) has an AN = 19. Which has the greater metallic character?

    A. They are equal
    B. Li
    C. K
    D. Cannot be determined

20. Beryllium (Be) has an atomic number (AN) = 4 and strontium (Sr) has an AN = 38. Which has the greater chemical activity?

    A. They are equal
    B. Sr
    C. Be
    D. Cannot be determined

21. Magnesium (Mg) has an atomic number (AN) = 12 and bromine (Br) has an AN = 35. Which has the greater chemical activity?

    A. They are equal
    B. g
    C. Br
    D. Cannot be determined

ANSWERS AND EXPLANATIONS

1–10. **1-D, 2-A, 3-B, 4-C, 5-D, 6-A, 7-C, 8-A, 9-D, 10-C.** See text for explanation

11. A The A means that P is a representative element in the group, and its outermost shell contains s and p orbitals. The V means that P is a fifth group element with 5 outer electrons.

12. B Because Br is in group VII A, the electron configuration of its outermost shell is s2 p5. The closest octet is s2 p6; an extra electron is needed to give it an OS of −1.

13. A Because the outermost incomplete orbitals are s and p (the d orbital is complete), selenium is an A element. The s and p contain $2 + 4 = 6$ electrons.

14. A The electron configuration of chlorine is $1s^2\ 2s^2\ 2p^6\ 3s^2\ 3p^5$. The outermost incomplete orbitals are s and p, which makes it A (representative). With $2 + 5 = 7$ electrons in the s and p orbitals, it is a group VII element.

15. D EA has no overall trend that is useful for predictions.

16. C The electron configuration of Na is $1s^2\ 2s^2\ 2p^2\ 3s^1$ and that of Al is $1s^2\ 2s^2\ 2p^6\ 3s^2\ 3p^1$, which places them in the same period (highest n number is 3 in each). Ionization energy (IE) increases from left to right on the periodic table. Therefore, Al has a higher IE than Na.

17. B The electron configuration of O is $1s^2\ 2s^2\ 2p^4$ and that of sulfur is $1s^2\ 2s^2\ 2p^6\ 3s^2\ 3p^4$, which places both in group VI A. In a group, the electronegativity decreases from top to bottom. Therefore, O has the greater electronegativity.

18. A The electron configuration of Mg is $1s^2\ 2s^2\ 2p^6\ 3s^2$ and that of S is $1s^2\ 2s^2\ 2p^6\ 3s^2\ 3p^4$, which places them in the same period. The atomic radius decreases from left to right in a period. Therefore, Mg is larger than S.

19. C The electron configuration of Li is $1s^2\ 2s^1$ and that of K is $1s^2\ 2s^2\ 2p^6\ 3s^2\ 4s^1$, which places them both in group IA. In a group, the metallic character increases from top to bottom. Therefore, K has more metallic character than Li.

20. B The electron configuration of Be is $1s^2\ 2s^2$ and that of Sr is $1s^2\ 2s^2\ 2p^6\ 3s^2\ 3p^6\ 4s^2\ 3d^{10}\ 4p^6\ 5s^2$, which places them both in group II A. In a group on the left side, the chemical activity increases from top to bottom. Therefore, Sr is more reactive than Be.

21. D The electron configuration of Mg is $1s^2\ 2s^2\ 2p^6\ 3s^2$ and that of Br is $1s^2\ 2s^2\ 2p^6\ 3s^2\ 3p^6\ 4s^2\ 3d^{10}\ 4p^5$. They are in neither the same group nor the same period and therefore cannot be compared by general periodic trends.

1. Understand the limitations of the valence shell electron pair repulsion (VSEPR) theory and draw electron dot structures and predict molecular geometry for H_3O^+, NH_4^+, SO_3, CO_2, and H_2O. (Hints: H_3O^+ is pyramidal, NH_4^+ is tetrahedral, SO_3 is trigonal, CO_2 is linear, and H_2O is angular.)

2. Break and make several molecules using the molecular geometry models (laboratory sticks and balls) and understand several bonds and shapes. Draw all geometric isomers for the PBr_2Cl_3 molecule, with and without dipole moment.

3. Review the dipole moments of common organic compounds and how they correlate with biologic activities of certain molecules, e.g., the three isomers of DDT (para, meta, and ortho) have different dipole moments that cause them to be highly toxic for para DDT compound compared to ortho DDT, which has less toxicity.

4. Understand bond dissociation energy by heterolytic cleavage:

$$H\!-\!H \rightarrow H^+ + H^-:$$

and hemolytic cleavage:

$$H\!-\!H \rightarrow H\cdot + H\cdot$$

THE IONIC BOND

Ionic bonding is the electrostatic attraction between ions of opposite charge. Strong electrostatic forces are evidenced by a high melting point and a high boiling point, and large amounts of energy must be spent to overcome these electrostatic forces. **Ionic forces** are attributable to Coulomb forces (see subsequent discussion of electrostatics and electromagnetism).

The organization of **ionic crystals** is based on the assumption that maximum stability of the crystal is achieved by maximizing the attractive forces between cations (positive) and anions (negative) and minimizing the repulsive forces between ions of the same charge. Hence, anions and cations try to be as close together as possible while minimizing anion-anion repulsion.

Intermolecular forces exist between the molecules of the liquid or solid. These forces depend on the chemical characteristics of the molecules and play a large part in determining the physical behavior (e.g., phase changes, solubility) of the liquid or solid. Several types of forces exist between molecules.

Van der Waals forces are weak attractive forces resulting from the net attraction between the nucleus of one atom and the electrons in another. These forces are effective only over short distances and increase as the molecular weights increase; i.e., as the number of atoms or electrons in a molecule increase. This type of van der Waals force merges with the slightly stronger forces (which may also be considered van der Waals forces) that exist between polar molecules or between molecules that are inducible (i.e., a separation of charge in one molecule can be induced by the presence of a second molecule). **Polar molecules** are made up of elements of different electronegativity:

$$d + d - d + d -$$

$$C\!-\!O, \ C\!-\!Cl$$

and are asymmetric in geometry.

Hydrogen bonds are weak attractive bonds (but stronger than van der Waals) between the hydrogens on chlorine, fluorine, nitrogen, or oxygen, and the nonbonding electrons on these same elements. Hydrogen bonding exists only for these elements. Bonding becomes stronger when the electronegativity of the atoms increases and when the hydrogen bond can have a 180° orientation (Fig. 7-22.).

Hydrophobic bonds are weak attractive bonds between molecules that are nonpolar (no net separation of charges in molecules). These bonds exist because nonpolar molecules (e.g., hydrocarbons, fats, and aromatics) decrease the entropy (see discussion of

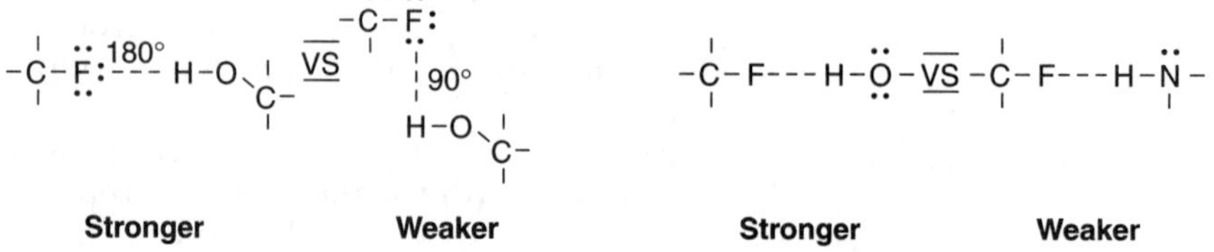

Fig. 7-22. Hydrogen bonding.

Stronger   Weaker   Stronger   Weaker

thermodynamics and thermochemistry) of water when the molecules are apart. When these nonpolar molecules come together and form hydrophobic bonds, the entropy increases, the free energy is lowered, and the bonds become stable.

Although the van der Waals forces, hydrogen bonds, and hydrophobic bonds are weak individually, they are strong when many exist between molecules, as in proteins or nucleic acids. A large part of the stability of these and other polymers is attributable to the multitude of these weak forces. When solids melt or liquids evaporate, it is these collective forces that must be overcome. The greater the number of intermolecular bonds, or the more different types of these bonds present, the greater the stability of the substance and the more difficult it is to melt or evaporate. Temperature increases tend to disrupt these weak intermolecular forces easily, especially when they are few in number.

Note also that molecules of similar type (e.g., hydrophobic or polar or with hydrogen bonding) tend to be soluble in each other because the forces are similar. Conversely, molecules of different types, especially polar versus nonpolar, tend to be insoluble.

When metal (e.g., Na) and nonmetal (e.g., Cl_2) elements are mixed, oppositely charged ions quickly form. Such a compound readily occurs when the atoms involved differ greatly in their attraction for electrons (e.g., a metal of low ionization energy and a nonmetal with a high ionization energy). The resulting ionic compound is more stable (lower in energy) than its elements and owes this stability to the packing of the oppositely charged ions into a lattice.

THE COVALENT BOND

A chemical bond formed by sharing a pair of electrons is a **covalent bond**. Covalent bonds are more prevalent in nonmetallic compounds. Gases such as hydrogen (H_2) or chlorine (Cl_2) are the simplest examples of covalent bonding. Each of the gas molecules depicted in Figure 7-23 shares one pair of electrons.

Organic compounds, many of which are of prime interest in medicine, can have multiple covalent bonds per molecule. The major elements involved in organic compounds are carbon (C), hydrogen (H), oxygen (O), nitrogen (N), and halides (fluorine-F, chlorine-Cl, bromine-Br, and iodine-I). Sulfur (S) and phosphorus (P) are also in many organic compounds. C forms four bonds, N forms three and has one unshared pair of electrons, and O forms two and has two unshared pairs of electrons. H forms one bond, and each halogen forms one bond and has three unshared pairs of electrons—all are assumed to be neutral. The possible bonds are **single bonds** (SB, one shared pair of electrons), **double bonds** (DB, two shared pairs of electrons), and **triple bonds** (TB, three shared pairs of electrons). C and N form all three types, O forms DB and SB, and H and the halides (in organic compounds) form SB only.

The C atom has one s orbital and three p orbitals in its outer bonding electron shells (see previous section on electronic structure of the atom). In organic molecules, these original atomic orbitals are recombined into hybrid orbitals made of part s and part p. Mixing one s and three p results in four hybrid sp^3 orbitals (each consisting of one part s and three parts p) on the C atom. If one s orbital and two p orbitals mix, the result is three sp^2 orbitals and one original p orbital on each C atom. If one s and one p mix, the result is two sp orbitals and two original p orbitals on each C atom.

Lewis Electron Dot Formulas

Electron dot structures are a means of illustrating the valence electrons and how they enter into bond formation. They are used in conjunction with the octet rule stating that a maximum of eight electrons is possible in the outermost shell of atoms. This rule holds only for the second row elements (C, N, O, F). Third row elements (Si, P, S, Cl) can use d orbitals and, hence, can have more. Examples of the use of the electron dot formulas (Fig. 7-24) follow:

1. CO_2 C-4 valence electrons
    O-6 valence electrons
    Combine single electrons (may have to make double or triple bonds)

2. CO_3^{-2} (an example of resonance)

Fig. 7-23.   H·+ ·H ⟶ H:H   :C̈l· + ·C̈l: ⟶ :C̈l:C̈l:

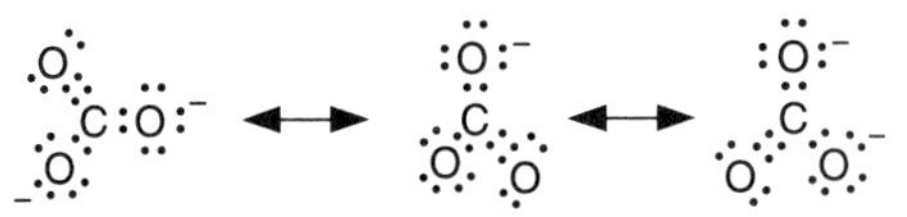

Fig. 7-24.

C-4 valence electrons

O-6 valence electrons

-2 means two extra electrons to place on the atoms

Each element in the final structure counts one half the electrons in a bond as its own and counts all unpaired electrons as its own. The sum of these two numbers should equal the number of valence electrons with which the element began.

Resonance structures are not structures for the actual molecule or ion; they exist only in theory. For example, more than one equivalent Lewis structure can be written for carbonate ion (Fig. 7-25). None of the structures by itself correctly represents the molecule. Rather, the molecule or ion is better represented by a hybrid of the structures.

Formal charge is positive or negative charges assigned to certain atoms in a molecule or ion, the sum of which equals the total charge on the molecule or ion. The formal charge of an atom can be calculated as follows:

Formal charge = (number of valence electrons)

$-$ (number of nonbonding electrons)

$-\frac{1}{2}$(number of bonding electrons)

Another way to calculate the formal charge of an atom is to ask whether the atom has more or fewer electrons in its valence shell than are needed to balance its nuclear charge.

A **Lewis acid** compound is an electron pair acceptor, so it must have a vacant orbital, e.g., HCl, SO_3, BF_3, $AlCl_3$. A Lewis base compound is an electron pair donor, so it usually has a free pair of electrons, e.g., amines, ethers, and carboxylic acid anhydrides (Fig. 7-26).

Consider the reaction:

$$BeF_2 + 2F^- \rightarrow BeF_4^{--}$$

BeF_2 = Lewis acid

F^- = Lewis base

The electron pair geometry of the orbitals and the valence-shell electron pair repulsion models are sp^3-tetrahedral, sp^2-trigonal, and sp-linear (Fig. 7-27). The VSEPR theory, or the valency shell electron pair repulsion theory, explains the different shapes of molecules. The word "valency" or "valence" dictates strength of an atomic bond, or the tendency to bond. Valence electrons are the electrons in the outermost shell or orbit of the atom.

The VSEPR theory states:

1. The geometric or structural arrangement of bonds around an atom (in a molecule) depends on the total number of electron pairs in the valence shell of the atom, including both bonding (shared) pairs and nonbonding (unshared) pairs.
2. Two pairs of electrons have a **linear arrangement**, three pairs of electrons have an **equilateral triangle arrangement**, and four pairs of electrons have a **tetrahedral arrangement**.

Sigma (σ) bonds have electron density between the nuclei. Sigma bonds are formed when hybrid orbitals (sp, sp^2, sp^3) overlap directly. **Pi (π) bonds** have electron density

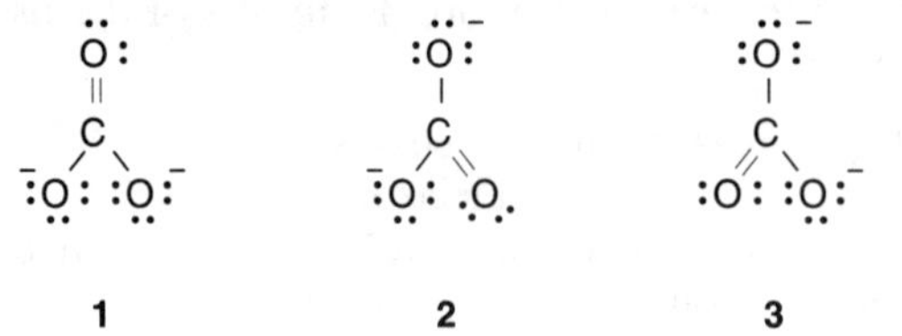

Fig. 7-25.　　1　　　　2　　　　3

Lewis acid	Lewis base
(electron pair)	(electron pair)

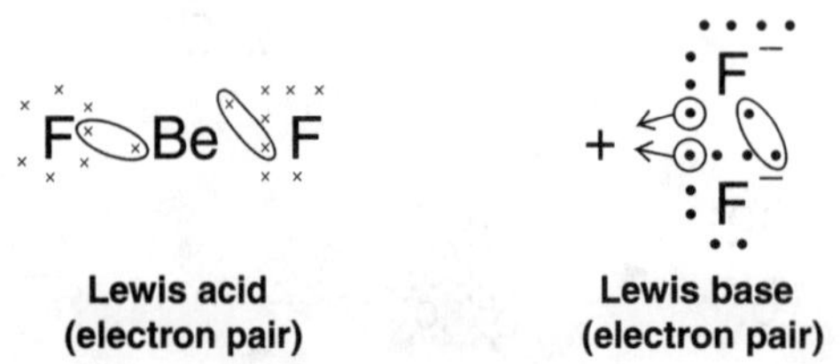

Fig. 7-26.

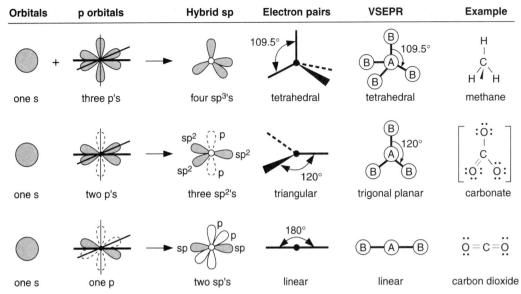

Orbitals	p orbitals	Hybrid sp	Electron pairs	VSEPR	Example

one s / three p's → four sp³'s / tetrahedral (109.5°) / tetrahedral (109.5°) / methane

one s / two p's → three sp²'s (sp², sp², sp², p, p) / triangular (120°) / trigonal planar (120°) / carbonate

one s / one p → two sp's (sp, sp, p, p) / linear (180°) / linear / carbon dioxide

Fig. 7-27. Hybrid bonding orbitals.

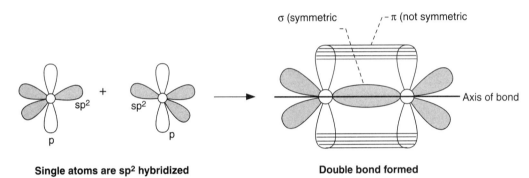

σ (symmetric) — π (not symmetric)

Axis of bond

Single atoms are sp² hybridized → **Double bond formed**

Fig. 7-28. Sigma and pi bonds. Note that the sp² overlap between the nuclei to form the σ bond; the p overlap above and below the axis between the C to form a π bond.

(overlap) above and below the axis (and plane) of the atoms. They are formed by "side-ways" overlap of the p orbitals. **Single bonds** are σ bonds. **Double bonds** are made of one σ bond and one π bond; **triple bonds** include one σ and two π bonds. Note that σ bonds are symmetric about the axis and can rotate freely. Multiple bonds (DB, TB), with π components, are not symmetric about the axis and are not free to rotate about it (Fig. 7-28).

When adjacent atoms are sp² or sp hybridized, there is the possibility of side-to-side overlap of the leftover p orbitals over all of these atoms. This occurrence is called delocalization of the electrons in the π bonds of the molecule. Two ways of depicting these molecules are by the molecular orbital (MO) or the valence bond (resonance) approach. The **MO approach** takes a linear combination of atomic orbitals (LCAO) to form molecular orbitals into which electrons go to form bonds. These molecular orbitals cover the whole molecule, and, hence, the delocalization of electrons is depicted. In the valence bond (resonance) approach, a linear combination of different structures with localized π bonds (and unpaired electrons) depicts the true molecule (the resonance hybrid). No one structure is representative of the molecule (Fig. 7-29).

It is the **valence electrons** (outer shell electrons) that enter into the formation of chemical bonds (see previous sections on electronic structure of the atom and the periodic table).

Partial Ionic Character

When atoms of differing electronegativity form the chemical bond, a situation of charge separation exists. Slight pulling of electron density by the oxygen (the more electronegative) from the carbon (the less electronegative) results in the C—O bond having **partial ionic character**. As shown in Figure 7-30, the separation of charge also sets up an electrical dipole in the direction of the arrow. A dipole has a positive end (C) and a negative end

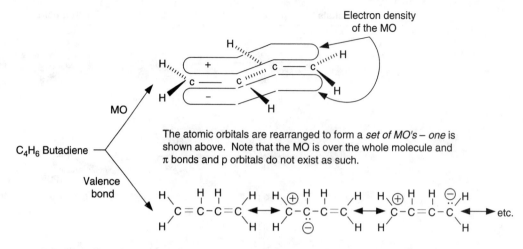

Electron density
of the MO

C_4H_6 Butadiene

The atomic orbitals are rearranged to form a *set of MO's – one* is shown above. Note that the MO is over the whole molecule and π bonds and p orbitals do not exist as such.

Valence
bond

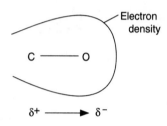

Note that no one structure represents the molecule which is a composite of all of them. The π bonds and p orbitals do exist in each structure above.

Fig. 7-29. Comparison of molecular orbitals (MO) and valence bond approaches.

Electron
density

C ——— O

Fig. 7-30.

$\delta+ \longrightarrow \delta^-$

(O). A dipole will line up in an electric field (see subsequent discussion of electrostatics and electromagnetism). The most electronegative elements are fluorine (4.0) > oxygen (3.5) > nitrogen (3.0) = chlorine (3.0). These elements often are combined with hydrogen (2.1) and carbon (2.5) and, hence, result in bonds with partial ionic character. (The numbers in parentheses show electronegativity of various elements.)

The **dipole moment** is a measure of the charge separation and, hence, the electronegativities of the elements that make up the bond. The larger the dipole moment, the larger the charge separation.

APPLIED CONCEPTS

1. What organic compounds are of prime interest to the field of medicine? Why?
2. What is a "designer drug" and how are the molecules altered to form new compounds?
3. Understand the concept of activators for enzymes. Metal-activated enzymes require the presence of metals, e.g., Mg^{++}, Mu^{++}, Fe^{++}, Ca^{++}, and K^+. Consider some inorganic ions Cl^-, Br^-, NO_3^- in some activator-dependent enzyme reactions.
4. Understand the construction, design, and basic principles behind pH electrode, pCO_2 electrode, or pO_2 electrode. Pay special attention to the maintenance and sources of error for these instruments.
5. Critically examine sigma, pi, and partial ionic bonds as they relate to medical compounds and bioorganic molecules such as proteins, amino acids, carbohydrates, alcohols, enzymes, hormones, and lipids.

CHEMICAL BONDING: REVIEW QUESTIONS

1. Which type of bond has electron density directly between the nuclei?

    A. Pi (π)
    B. Sigma (σ)
    C. Both
    D. Neither

2. Which type of bond is formed by overlap of p orbitals perpendicular to the 2 nuclei?

    A. Pi (π)
    B. Sigma (σ)

C. Both
D. Neither

3. Rotation about the bonding axis can occur with:

    A. pi (π) bonds.
    B. double bonds.
    C. both pi and double bonds.
    D. neither pi nor double bonds.

4. Delocalization of electrons (i.e., resonance) occurs over:

    A. sigma bonds between separated atoms.
    B. sigma bonds on adjacent atoms.
    C. pi bonds on adjacent atoms.
    D. pi bonds between separated atoms.

5. The resonance approach implies that:

    A. one structure cannot be drawn that accurately depicts the electrons in the true molecule.
    B. one structure can be drawn that accurately depicts the electrons in the true molecule.
    C. two structures can be drawn that accurately depict electrons in the true molecule.
    D. none of the above.

6. The octet rule does not have to hold for which of the following elements?

    A. C
    B. O
    C. F
    D. P

7. Select an acceptable resonance form of the ion:

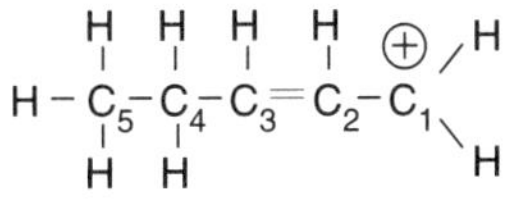

A.

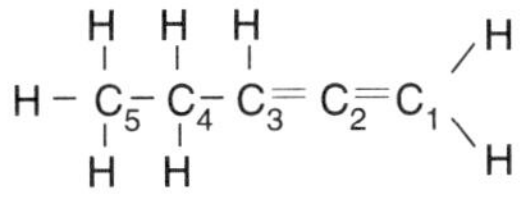

B.

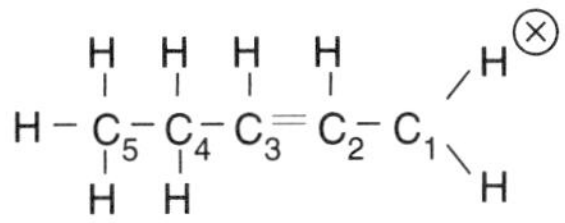

C.

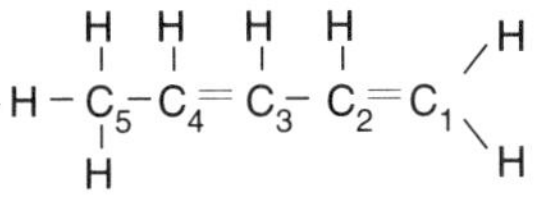

D.

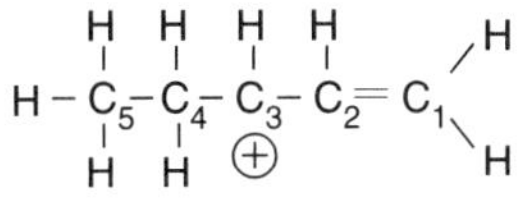

8. Which of the following is NOT an acceptable resonance form of the ion?

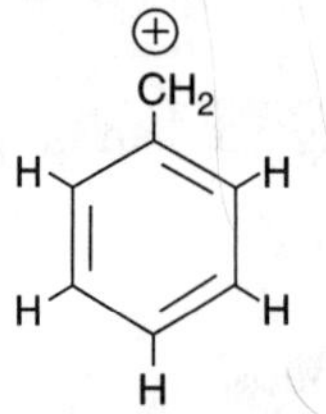

$$\overset{\oplus}{CH_2}$$ attached to a benzene-type ring with H substituents

A. (structure with CH_2 and ring, $\oplus$ on bottom H)

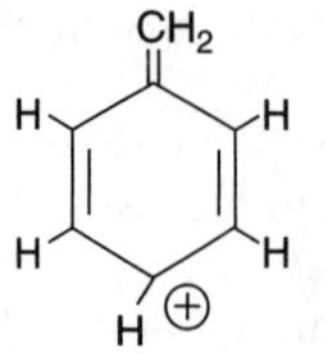

(B.) (structure with CH_2 and ring, $\oplus$H on right)

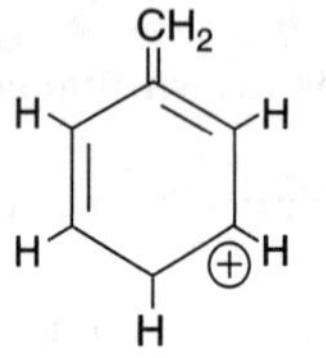

C. (structure with CH_2, $\oplus$ on upper right, ring with H)

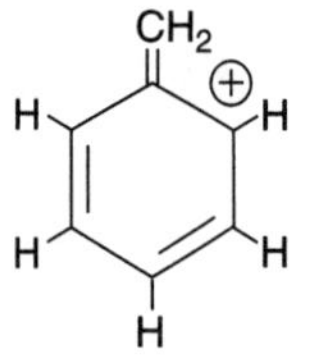

D. (structure with CH_2, $\oplus$ on upper left, ring with H)

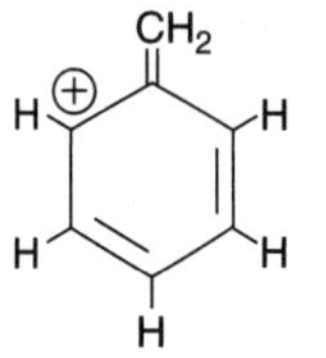

9. What is the electron dot formula for SO_4^{-2}? (Atomic numbers: O = 8, S = 16)

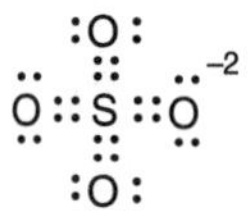

A. $:\!\ddot{S}\!:\!\ddot{O}\!:\!\ddot{O}\!:\!\ddot{O}\!:\!\ddot{O}\!:\!\ddot{O}\!:^{-2}$

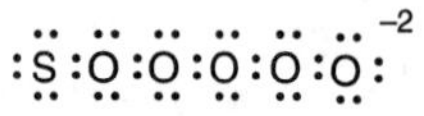

B.
$$
\begin{array}{c}
:\!\ddot{O}\!: \\
\ddot{O}::S::\ddot{O}^{-2} \\
:\!\ddot{O}\!:
\end{array}
$$

C. $:\!\ddot{O}\!:\!\ddot{O}::S::\ddot{O}\!:\!\ddot{O}\!:$

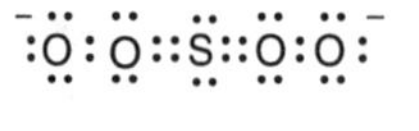

(D.)
$$
\begin{array}{c}
:\!\ddot{O}\!:^{-} \\
\ddot{O}::S::\ddot{O} \\
:\!\ddot{O}\!:^{-}
\end{array}
$$

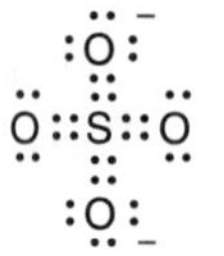

Questions 10 and 11

For these questions, use the electronegativities provided in the text.

10. In which compound does the starred carbon have the largest partial positive charge?

A. 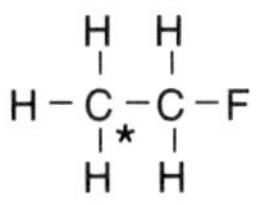
$$H-\underset{\underset{H}{|}}{\overset{\overset{H}{|}}{C}}-\underset{\underset{H}{|}}{\overset{\overset{H}{|}}{C}}-F$$
(star under first C)

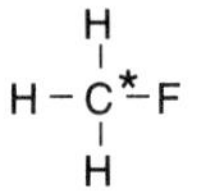

B.
$$H-\underset{\underset{H}{|}}{\overset{\overset{H}{|}}{C}}^{*}-F$$

C.
$$H-\underset{\underset{H}{|}}{\overset{\overset{H}{|}}{C}}-Cl$$
(star)

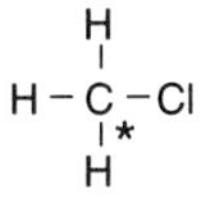

D. 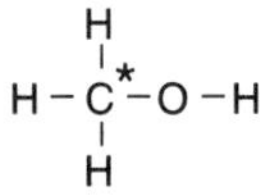
$$H-\underset{\underset{H}{|}}{\overset{\overset{H}{|}}{C}}^{*}-O-H$$

11. Select the compound with the largest dipole moment:

A. CCl_4

B.

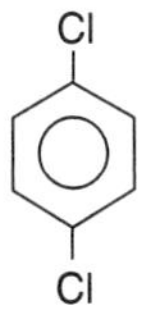

Cl — (benzene ring) — Cl (1,4-dichlorobenzene)

C. 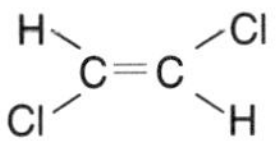
$$\underset{Cl}{\overset{H}{\diagdown}}C=C\overset{\diagup Cl}{\underset{\diagdown H}{}}$$

D. 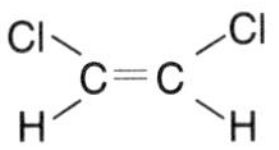
$$\underset{H}{\overset{Cl}{\diagdown}}C=C\overset{\diagup Cl}{\underset{\diagdown H}{}}$$

12. Which of the following is not considered as an intermolecular force between molecules?

A. Covalent bonds
B. Hydrogen bonds
C. Hydrophobic bonds
D. van der Waals forces

13. van der Waals forces depend on:

A. repulsion of the molecules from water.
B. Coulomb attractions between ions.
C. attraction between the nucleus of one atom and the electrons of another.
D. none of the above.

14. The strength of van der Waals forces between molecules is increased by an increase in all of the following factors EXCEPT the:

A. molecular weight of the molecules.
B. number of atoms in the molecule.
C. number of electrons in the molecule.
D. ionic strength of the molecule.

15. The weakest (in strength) of the following intermolecular forces is:

    A. hydrogen bonding.
    B. the typical van der Waals.
    C. forces between polar molecules.
    D. ionic.

16. Hydrogen bonds are possible between all the following elements EXCEPT:

    A. carbon.
    B. nitrogen.
    C. oxygen.
    D. fluorine.

17. The strongest of the forces between molecules is:

    A. van der Waals.
    B. hydrogen bonding.
    C. hydrophobic.
    D. polar.

18. For the three atoms involved in the hydrogen bond (e.g., $^-\!\overset{..}{\underset{..}{A}}\!:$ and $H\!-\!\overset{..}{\underset{..}{B}}\!^-$), the angle that allows the greatest strength (using H as the vertex) is:

    A. less than 90°.
    B. 90°.
    C. 90° to 180°.
    D. 180°.

19. The stability of some polymers may be attributed to:

    A. many of the weak intermolecular forces (bonds).
    B. a few of the weak intermolecular bonds.
    C. factors unrelated to the weak intermolecular bonds.
    D. none of the above.

ANSWERS AND EXPLANATIONS

1–6. **1-B, 2-A, 3-D, 4-C, 5-A, 6-D.** See text for explanation.

7. D A simple "shift" of the bond from C3-C2 to C2-C1 is shown. Pi (π) electrons can be delocalized over charges ($+$ or $-$) and over radicals. So, view the plus charge as if it were an adjacent p orbital ready to overlap. Choices A and C are not acceptable because an atom is displaced (the H); resonance forms are of the same molecule, so no atoms can move. Choice C also places a p orbital on C where none existed. Choice B is incorrect because hydrogen has no p orbitals and can form only one bond. so option (B) is incorrect.

8. B Choices A, C, and D are derived by simple "shifts" of the π bonds around the ring. It is not possible to get the structure in choice B. Also, one carbon has five bonds.

9. D None of the structures accurately depicts the true SO_4^{-2} ion, because resonance is possible with this structure. The electron configurations are:

$$O = 1s^2\, 2s^2\, 2p^4 \quad S = 1s^2\, 2s^2\, 2p^6\, 3s^2\, 3p^4$$

The valence electrons (in the outer shell only) are:

$$O = 6 \text{ and } S = 6 \text{ plus two electrons for charge } (-2)$$

The electron dot formula is:

$$
\begin{array}{c}
:\overset{..}{O}:^{-}\\
:\overset{..}{O}::\overset{..}{S}::\overset{..}{O}:\\
:\overset{..}{O}:^{-}
\end{array}
$$

10. B The element with the highest electronegativity is F, pulling the most electron density away from the C, making it slightly positive. The F is more effective when attached directly to the C, as in choice B, than when another atom (the other carbon) intervenes, as in choice A.

11. D Dipole moments are vectors (directions and magnitude) and are additive as such.

The dipoles for symmetric molecules (choices A, B, and C) cancel because they are opposite and equal.

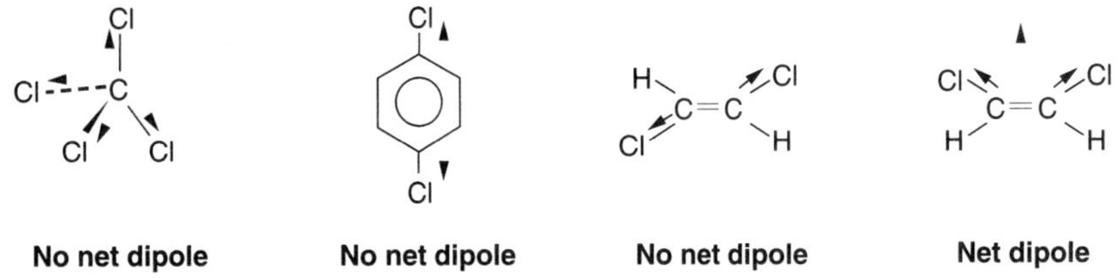

No net dipole   No net dipole   No net dipole   Net dipole

12–19. 12-A, 13-C, 14-D, 15-B, 16-A, 17-D, 18-D, 19-A. See text for explanation.

MOLECULAR WEIGHT

Molecular weight can be determined by adding the atomic weights of all of the atoms in a molecule.

EMPIRICAL FORMULA VERSUS MOLECULAR FORMULA

An **empirical formula** is the simplest formula with the smallest ratio of atoms to each other, but it is not necessarily the actual formula for the molecule or substance. The **molecular formula** is the actual formula of the molecule of the substance. (The empirical formula can be the same as the molecular formula.) The formulas for benzene are shown in Figure 7-31.

It is possible to determine empirical formulas if the percentage composition of the compound is known by following these steps:

1. Assume the given percent of each element as the number of grams of that element (i.e., assume you are given 100 grams = 100% of the compound)
2. Divide the given percentage of each element by its atomic weight to give the moles of each in the compound
3. Divide each of these numbers by the smallest of the numbers obtained from step 2
4. Determine what small number (to multiply the result of step 3), usually 2 to 5, if any, is needed to convert the numbers from step 3 into (approximately) whole numbers. These whole numbers are the ratio of the elements to each other.

This process converts weights (from percent) into moles by step 2. These moles are, themselves, the ratios of elements to each other. Steps 3 and 4 are just simple techniques to obtain whole numbers, because elements are made of atoms and not fractions of atoms.

To determine the molecular formula from the empirical formula, the gram-molecular weight (GMW) must be known from some other source. Then, determine the gram-empirical formula weight (i.e., add up the elements in the empirical formula) and divide the GMW by the gram-empirical formula weight. The resulting number is how many times each element in the empirical formula is to be multiplied to get the molecular formula. For example, a compound of 2.04% H, 32.65% S, and 65.31% O has a GMW = 98 (from other experiments). To determine the empirical formula and molecular formula (H = 1, S = 32, O = 16), follow the steps just outlined:

1. H = 2.04 g; S = 32.5 g; O = 65.31 g

2. H: $\dfrac{2.04}{1}$ = 2.04; S: $\dfrac{32.65}{32}$ = 1.02; O: $\dfrac{65.31}{16}$ = 4.08

3. H: $\dfrac{2.04}{1.02}$ = 2; S: $\dfrac{1.02}{1.02}$ = 1; O: $\dfrac{4.08}{1.02}$ = 4

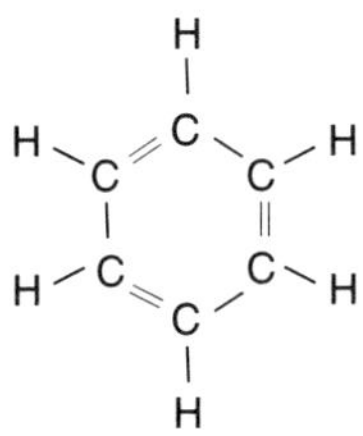

Molecular formula = C_6H_6

Empirical formula = C_1H_1

Fig. 7-31.

4. Not needed because step 3 results in whole numbers.
Empirical formula = H_2SO_4

To calculate the gram-empirical formula weight:

$$2(1) + (32) + 4(16) = 98$$

Divide gram-molecular weight by gram-empirical formula weight: $\frac{98}{98} = 1$

Multiply each element in the empirical formula by the 1 = molecular formula

In this case, the molecular formula and the empirical formula are same.

DESCRIPTION OF COMPOSITION BY PERCENT MASS

The percentage composition by weight of a given element A in a compound with a known formula is calculated as follows:

$$\text{weight \% of A} = \frac{n_A(AW)_A}{\Sigma n_i(AW)_i} \times 100$$

n = number of atoms of an element in the formula
AW = atomic weight of the element
Consider the example of % of oxygen (O) in $KClO_3$ (K = 39, Cl = 36, O = 16)

$$\text{\% of O} = \frac{3(16)}{1(39) + 1(36) + 3(16)} \times 100 = 39\%.$$

The percentages of all components should sum to 100%.

MOLE CONCEPT AND AVOGADRO'S NUMBER

A **mole** of any substance contains 6.02×10^{23} particles (**Avogadro's number**). A mole always contains the same number of atoms or molecules, no matter what the substance. For example, compare a carton of a dozen eggs to a bag of a dozen bagels. Each is a different substance, but they contain the same number of units. For an element, the number of moles present is:

$$\text{Moles} = \frac{\text{weight of sample in grams}}{\text{atomic weight of element in grams (GAW)}}$$

For a compound, the **gram-molecular weight** (GMW) is determined by adding the **gram-atomic weight** (GAW) of all its elements (need the molecular formula). Then, the moles of a compound are determined as follows:

$$\text{Moles} = \frac{\text{weight of sample in grams}}{\text{GMW}}$$

Moles can be calculated in many ways (see subsequent list), all of which are interconvertible via moles. Mole is important because it gives the number of molecules (or atoms) in a given weight of a substance, whereas the weight itself does not. Mole is the key to solving most quantitative mass problems in chemistry.
Methods used to determine the mole of substances are as follows:

1. mole = weight in grams/GMW
2. MV = mole; M = molarity; V = liters (see section on solution chemistry)
3. NV = equivalents; N = normality; V = liters (see section on solution chemistry)
4. mV = mole; m = molality, V = kg of solvent (see section on solution chemistry)
5. Freezing point depression (or boiling point elevation) calculations (see section on phases and phase equilibria) $\Delta T = \kappa m$ where m = molality. First determine κ, then use ΔT to determine mole as in #4
6. One mole of any gas at STP occupies 22.4 liters (see section on phases and phase equilibria)
7. At the same temperature and pressure, equal volumes of ideal gases contain equal numbers of moles (Avogadro's principle)
8. PV = nRT, ideal gas equation
9. $p_1 = X_1 P_T$
p_1 = partial pressure of gas #1, P_T = total pressure, X_1 = mole fraction of gas #1
10. One mole of electrons is one faraday, a faraday is 96,500 coulombs; an ampere (measure of current) is 1 coulomb/sec

11. Law of Dulong and Petit:

$$6.3 \approx (SH)(GAW)$$

Where SH = specific heat in $\dfrac{cal}{gram}$,

GAW = gram-atomic weight of element

Note that the gram-molecular weight can be calculated from moles, and that moles provide a means of conversion between the diverse situations just described.

In the following balanced equation, $N_2(g) + 3H_2(g) \rightarrow 2NH_3(g)$, the numbers in front of the molecules give the smallest ratios of these molecules that will react with each other; that is, they are the number of moles of each that must be present to obtain a complete reaction. With too much (or too little) of a reactant present, that reactant is in excess (or is deficient), and some reactants will remain when the reaction is finished. The reactant and how much of it is left over is calculated from the balanced equation using the ratio of moles. Note that the numbers in the equations reflect ratios of moles and nothing else.

DENSITY AND OXIDATION NUMBER

$$\text{Density} = \frac{mass}{volume} \text{ or } d = \frac{m}{v}$$

Oxidation number is the number assigned to each element in a compound. It is a convenient bookkeeping device for keeping track of the electrons in a reaction. The atoms do not actually possess the charge (when in a molecule) designated by the oxidation state (OS). The following general rules (with exceptions) are useful for determining the oxidation number:

1. All elements have an OS = 0 in the elemental form, e.g., O_2, Fe, Na. (These elements can exist as ions but then they are not in the elemental form.)
2. For ions that have a single atom, the oxidation number equals the charge on the ion.
3. The algebraic sum of the oxidation numbers in a neutral compound equal 0. In a polyatomic ion, the sum equals the ion charge.
4. Hydrogen is $+1$, except when combined with metals as hydrides (-1), and oxygen is -2, except when combined with fluorine (then it is $+2$); in peroxides (-1); or in superoxides $(-\frac{1}{2})$.
5. Fluorine always $= -1$.
6. Group I metals (Li, Na, K, etc.) are $+1$.
7. Group II metals (Mg, Ca, Sr, Ba) are $+2$.
8. Halogens (Cl, Br, I) are -1 unless combined with F or O.
9. Al $= +3$.
10. Charges (not OS) of some common complex ions are as follows:

SO_4^{-2}	sulfate
NO_3^{-1}	nitrate
PO_4^{-3}	phosphate
OH^-	hydroxide
CO_3^{-2}	carbonate
$CH_3CO_2^-$	acetate
ClO_{4-}	perchlorate

Common Oxidizing and Reducing Agents

In an oxidation-reduction reaction, one (or more) atom(s) is always oxidized, and one (or more) atom(s) is always reduced. **Oxidation** is the loss of electrons (or equivalently the loss of hydrogen in organic chemistry), and **reduction** is the gain of electrons (or equivalently the gain of hydrogen in organic chemistry). Remember the mnemonic "OIL RIG," meaning oxidation is loss and reduction is gain of electrons. An **oxidizing agent** is a substance that can take electrons from other atoms and is reduced. A **reducing agent** is a substance that can give electrons to other atoms and is oxidized. As a general rule, metals are reducing agents and halogens act as oxidizing agents.

DESCRIPTION OF REACTIONS BY CHEMICAL EQUATIONS

Chemical equations are concise written descriptions of chemical reactions. They show the reactants and products, their physical states, and the direction in which the reaction proceeds.

Conventions for Writing Chemical Equations

The reactants are shown on the left side of the arrow, and the products are shown on the right side of the arrow. The arrow itself stands for "produce" or "yield." The numbers in front of the formulas are coefficients indicating the smallest number of atoms or other chemical units that are able to take part in the reactions. If no coefficient is present, it is assumed to be 1. Some common symbols that appear in chemical formulas are (s), solid; (g), gas; (l), liquid; and (aq), aqueous solution.

Balancing Equations

Chemical equations should be balanced before attempting stoichiometric calculations. **Balancing** is by trial and error (for non-redox). The goal is to have equal numbers of each element on each side of the equation. A helpful hint is to balance the element(s) that appear in only one compound on each side of the equation and save elements that appear in more than one compound until last.

Practice is the key to balancing equations. An example of a balanced equation is:

$$N_2(g) + 3H_2(g) \rightarrow 2NH_3(g)$$

The numbers in front of the molecules give the smallest ratios of these molecules that will react with each other; that is, they are the number of moles of each that must be present for a complete reaction.

To balance oxidation-reduction equations, follow these few simple steps:

1. Break the process into half-reactions, the oxidation half-reaction and the reduction half-reaction
2. Balance each of the half-reactions separately for mass and for charge
3. Multiply each half-reaction by an appropriate factor so that the reduction half-reaction gives away the number of electrons that the oxidizing half-reaction requires

For example:

$$\text{Overall reaction: } Zn + Cu^{+2} \rightleftharpoons Zn^{+2} + Cu$$

$$\text{Oxidation half-reaction: } Zn \rightleftharpoons Zn^{+2} + 2e^-$$

$$\text{Reduction half-reaction: } Cu^{+2} + 2e^- \rightleftharpoons Cu$$

Note: The e^- (electrons) are on the right side of the arrows in the oxidation (loss) half-reaction and on the left side for the reduction (gain) half-reaction. Also, the sum of the electrons in the balanced half-reactions must cancel out when added (algebraically) to obtain the overall reaction.

Different substances have differing combining powers with each other; that is, one molecule may be two or more times more reactive than another for a specific purpose. A familiar example is H_2SO_4 (a diprotic acid) and HCl (a monoprotic acid) in terms of donation of hydrogen ions (H+). A mole would contain the same number of molecules of H_2SO_4 and HCl, but you do not know their relative strength in giving H+. What is needed is a measure, like mole, that relates the relative or equivalent effectiveness of given weights of substances for specific characteristics. For this reason, the measure called **equivalents** was established. When weights are converted to equivalents, one can be sure, for example, that one equivalent of an acid will be completely neutralized by one equivalent of a base. It cannot be stated, without additional information, that one mole of an acid will react exactly with one mole of a base. Note that in one equivalent of a substance there are 6.02×10^{23} particles of interest (e.g., H+ or OH− for acids and bases).

The formula for calculating equivalents follows:

$$\text{Equivalents} = \frac{\text{weight of sample in grams}}{\text{gram equivalent weight (GEW)}}$$

GEW is calculated as follows:

$$\text{GEW} = \frac{\text{gram molecular weight}}{n}$$

The value of **n** depends on the chemical nature of the compound. For acids, it is the number of hydrogens used in the reaction per molecule. For bases, it is the number of exchangeable OH⁻ used in the reaction per molecule. For oxidation-reduction reactions, n depends on the number of electrons transferred by a given compound in a given reaction.

APPLIED CONCEPTS

1. Try to understand the etiology of hypermagnesemia and hypomagnesemia.
2. Trace the metabolism of copper in the body.
3. Trace the metabolism of iron in the body.
4. What is the effect of protein and pH changes in the interpretation of total calcium values?
5. Analyze and research the effect of calcitonin (32 amino-acid peptide) in bone formation.

REVIEW QUESTIONS

1. Balance the following equation, and determine the coefficient in front of $KClO_3$:
$$4\,KClO_3 \rightarrow KCl + 3\,KClO_4$$

   A. 1
   B. 2
   C. 3
   D. 4

2. What is the coefficient in front of Zn in the equation $Zn + 2\,HCl \rightarrow ZnCl_2 + H_2$?

   A. 1
   B. 2
   C. 3
   D. 4

3. Which reactants or product has the largest coefficient in the following balanced equation?
$$C_{12}H_{22}O_{11} + 12\,O_2 \rightarrow 12\,CO_2 + 11\,H_2O$$

   A. O_2
   B. CO_2
   C. H_2O
   D. O_2 and CO_2

4. What is the coefficient in front of $Ca(OH)_2$ in the following equation when balanced?
$$(NH_4)_2SO_4 + Ca(OH)_2 \rightarrow 2\,NH_3 + H_2O + CaSO_4$$

   A. 1
   B. 2
   C. 3
   D. 4

5. What is the sum of coefficients in the following equation when balanced?
$$3\,CuO + 2\,H_3PO_4 \rightarrow Cu_3(PO_4)_2 + 3\,H_2O$$

   A. 6
   B. 7
   C. 8
   D. 9

6. What is the sum of coefficients in the following equation when balanced?
$$2\,Na_2O_2 + 2\,H_2O \rightarrow 4\,NaOH + O_2$$

   A. 5
   B. 7
   C. 9
   D. 11

7. Consider the following unbalanced equation:
$$2\,N_2H_4(l) + N_2O_4(l) \rightarrow 3\,N_2(g) + 4\,H_2O(l) \quad (H = 1, N = 14, O = 16)$$

   What is the sum of coefficients in the balanced equation?
   A. 4
   B. 6

C. 8
D. 10

8. In the following equation:

$$2FeS(s) + O_2(g) + H_2O(l) \rightarrow Fe_2O_3(s) + H_2SO_4(l)$$

$$(H = 1, O = 16, S = 32, Fe = 56)$$

   what is the sum of the balanced coefficients?

   A. 8
   B. 13
   C. 18
   D. 23

9. Avogadro's number is based on:

   A. the number of liters that make up 1 mole of gas.
   B. 6.023×10^{23} particles per mole.
   C. the number of molecules in a chemical compound.
   D. none of the above.

10. Given that mole = m and the weight = w of a compound with a gram-molecular weight = GMW, which of the following relationships is correct?

   A. $m = (w)(GMW)$
   B. $m = \dfrac{w}{GMW}$
   C. $m = \dfrac{GMW}{w}$
   D. $m = \dfrac{1}{(w)(GMW)}$

11. If equivalents = E, weight of sample = W, and the gram-equivalent weight = GEW, the correct relationship is:

   A. $E = \dfrac{1}{(W)(GEW)}$.
   B. $E = \dfrac{GEW}{W}$.
   C. $E = \dfrac{W}{GEW}$.
   D. $E = (W)(GEW)$.

12. If gram-molecular weight = GMW, gram-equivalent weight = GEW, and the number of groups of interest per molecule = n, the correct relationship is:

   A. $GEW = (n)(GMW)$.
   B. $GEW = \dfrac{1}{(n)(GMW)}$.
   C. $GEW = \dfrac{n}{GMW}$.
   D. $GEW = \dfrac{GMW}{n}$.

13. If the percent composition of element B in a compound = P, the number of atoms of element B in the compound = n, the gram atomic weight of element B = GAW, and the gram-molecular weight of the compound = GMW, the correct relationship is:

   A. $P = \dfrac{(n)(GAW)}{(GMW)} \times 100$.
   B. $P = \dfrac{(n)(GAW)}{(GMW)}$.
   C. $P = (n)(GAW)(GMW)$.
   D. $P = \dfrac{GMW}{(n)(GAW)} \times 100$.

14. Which of the following formulas is NOT correct?

    A. (normality)(volume) = moles
    B. (molality)(kilograms of solvent) = moles
    C. liters of gas at $\dfrac{STP}{22.4}$ = moles
    D. $\dfrac{(Pressure)(volume)}{(ideal\ gas\ constant)(temperature)}$ = moles

15. Moles may be calculated from all of the following types of data EXCEPT:

    A. freezing point depressions.
    B. partial pressures.
    C. electrochemistry (faraday of charge consumed).
    D. valency number of elements.

Questions 16–31
Refer to these atomic weights: H = 1, C = 12, N = 14, O = 16, F = 19, Na = 23, Al = 27, P = 31, S = 32, Cl = 35, K = 39, Ca = 40, Cr = 52, Fe = 56, Cu = 63, Br = 80, Ag = 108, and Pb = 207.

16. What is the gram-molecular weight of $C_6H_{12}O_6$?

    A. 180
    B. 130
    C. 29
    D. None of the above

17. How many moles are 34 g of $AgNO_3$?

    A. 0.20
    B. 0.30
    C. 0.40
    D. None of the above

18. How many grams are in 0.5 mole of NaOH?

    A. 5
    B. 20
    C. 30
    D. None of the above

19. If 5 g of a compound is 0.1 mole of that substance, what is its gram-molecular weight (GMW)?

    A. 25
    B. 100
    C. 150
    D. None of the above

20. What is the approximate gram-equivalent weight (GEW) of HNO_3 when it acts as an acid (donation of H+)?

    A. 21
    B. 63
    C. 126
    D. None of the above

21. What is the approximate gram-equivalent weight of H_3PO_4 when it acts as an acid (donation of H+)?

    A. 33
    B. 49
    C. 98
    D. All of the above

22. In a reaction in which KNO_3 is used, the nitrogen gains 2 electrons. What is the approximate equivalent weight of KNO_3 in terms of its ability to gain electrons?

    A. 21
    B. 32
    C. 63
    D. None of the above

23. In a reaction, the Cr of $K_2Cr_2O_7$ gains 6 electrons. What is the approximate equivalent weight of $K_2Cr_2O_7$ in this reaction in terms of its ability to exchange electrons?

   A. 147
   B. 49
   C. 25
   D. None of the above

24. How many equivalents of base (OH^-) are in 5 g of $Al(OH)_3$ if all OH's react?

   A. 0.10
   B. 0.20
   C. 0.75
   D. None of the above

25. Two equivalents of H + would require what weight of H_2SO_4?

   A. 196
   B. 98
   C. 49
   D. None of the above

26. What is the approximate percentage of H in $(NH_4)_2 SO_4$?

   A. 6
   B. 7
   C. 4
   D. None of the above

27. A compound of carbon and hydrogen contains 92.3% C. The molecular weight (from other experiments) is known to be 52. What is the molecular formula?

   A. C_2H_2
   B. C_4H_4
   C. C_3H_6
   D. None of the above

28. The specific heat of an element is 0.03. What is its gram atomic weight?

   A. 18.9 $0.3 = SH \times GMW$
   B. 210
   C. 189
   D. Insufficient data provided

Questions 29 and 30
Consider the following unbalanced equation:

$$4FeS(s) + 9O_2(g) + 4H_2O(l) \rightarrow 2Fe_2O_3(s) + 4H_2SO_4(l)$$
$$(H = 1, O = 16, S = 32, Fe = 56)$$

29. If 22.4 liters of O are allowed to react with 44 g of FeS, approximately what weight (in grams) of H_2SO_4 is produced (assume reaction run at STP)?

   A. 98
   B. 49
   C. 44
   D. 2

30. If 5 moles of FeS are used in the reaction, what is the maximum number of moles of Fe_2O_3 that can be produced?

   A. 1.0
   B. 2.5
   C. 5.0
   D. 7.5

ANSWERS AND EXPLANATIONS

1. D   O appears in only one compound on each side of the equation, so balance it first. In this type of situation, simply multiply each compound by the number of atoms of the element (i.e., O in this case) in the other compound:

Unbalanced: $KClO_3 \rightarrow KCl + KClO_4$

Balanced O: $4KClO_3 \rightarrow KCl + 3KClO_4$

There is no clear choice between K or Cl, so just pick one to balance. Luckily, both K and Cl are already balanced. Check by counting the total number of each element on each side of the equation:

Check: $4KClO_3 \nrightarrow KCl + 3KClO_4$

K:	4		4
Cl:	4		4
O:	12		12

2. A Select Zn, H, or Cl, because all appear in only one compound on each side. Choose the most complicated, which is H or Cl in this case:

Unbalanced: $Zn + HCl \rightarrow Zn Cl_2 + H_2$

Balanced H: $Zn + 2HCl \rightarrow ZnCl_2 + H_2$

Zn and Cl: both are balanced also

Check: $Zn + 2HCl \nrightarrow ZnCl_2 + H_2$

Zn:	1		1
Cl:	2		2
H:	2		2

3. D

Unbalanced: $C_{12}H_{22}O_{11} + O_2 \rightarrow CO_2 + H_2O$

Balance C: $C_{12}H_{22}O_{11} + O_2 \rightarrow 12CO_2 + H_2O$

Balance H: $C_{12}H_{22}O_{11} + O_2 \rightarrow 12CO_2 + 11H_2O$

Balance O: $C_{12}H_{22}O_{11} + 12O_2 \rightarrow 12CO_2 + 11H_2O$

Check: $C_{12}H_{22}O_{11} + 12O_2 \nrightarrow 12CO_2 + 11H_2O$

C:	12		12
H:	22		22
O:	$11 + 24 = 35$		$24 + 11 = 35$

4. A

Unbalanced: $(NH_4)_2SO_4 + Ca(OH)_2 \rightarrow NH_3 + H_2O + CaSO_4$

Note: Treat SO_4^{-2} as a group in this case

SO_4^{-2} and Ca: Already balanced

Balance N: $(NH_4)_2SO_4 + Ca(OH)_2 \rightarrow 2NH_3 + H_2O + CaSO_4$

Balance O: $(NH_4)_2SO_4 + Ca(OH)_2 \rightarrow 2NH_3 + 2H_2O + CaSO_4$

(note that the O in the SO_4^{-2} balance and do not have to be accounted for in this balancing of the O)

Balance H: Already balanced

Check: $(NH_4)_2SO_4 + Ca(OH)_2 \nrightarrow 2NH_3 + 2H_2O + CaSO_4$

N:	2		2
H:	$8 + 2 = 10$		$6 + 4 = 10$
S:	1		1
O:	$4 + 2 = 6$		$2 + 4 = 6$

5. D

Unbalanced: $CuO + H_3PO_4 \rightarrow Cu_3(PO_4)_2 + H_2O$

Note: the PO_4^{-3} can be treated as a group because it is not changed in the reaction.

Can select Cu, PO_4^{-3}, or H to balance first. The H appear the most complicated so do them first.

Balance H: $CuO + 2H_3PO_4 \rightarrow Cu_3(PO_4)_2 + 3H_2O$

Balance PO_4: Already balanced

Balance Cu: $3CuO \rightarrow 2H_3PO_4 \rightarrow Cu_3(PO_4)_2 + 3H_2O$

Balance O: Already balanced (note again that the O on the PO_4^{-3} were balanced by balancing the PO_4^{-3})

Check: $3CuO + 2H_3PO_4 \not\rightarrow Cu_3(PO_4)_2 + 3H_2O$

Cu:	3		2
O:	3 + 8 = 11		8 + 3 = 11
H:	6		6
P:	2		2

6. **C**

Unbalanced: $Na_2O_2 + H_2O \rightarrow NaOH + O_2$

Balance Na: $Na_2O_2 + H_2O \rightarrow 2NaOH + O_2$

Balance H: Already balanced

Balance O: $Na_2O_2 + H_2O \rightarrow 2NaOH + \frac{1}{2}O_2$

remove fractions by multiplying through by 2:

Check: $2Na_2O_2 + 2H_2O \not\rightarrow 4NaOH + O_2$

Na:	4		4
O:	4 + 2 = 6		4 + 2 = 6
H:	4		4

7. **D**

Unbalanced: $N_2H_4 + N_2O_4 \rightarrow N_2 + H_2O$

Balance O: $N_2H_4 + N_2O_4 \rightarrow N_2 + 4H_2O$

Balance H: $2N_2H_4 + N_2O_4 \rightarrow N_2 + 4H_2O$

Balance N: $2N_2H_4 + N_2O_4 \rightarrow 3N_2 + 4H_2O$

Check: $2N_2H_4 + N_2O_4 \not\rightarrow 3N_2 + 4H_2O$

N:	4 + 2 = 6		6
H:	8		8
O:	4		4

8. **D**

Unbalanced: $FeS + O_2 + H_2O \rightarrow Fe_2O_3 + H_2SO_4$

Balance H, S: Already balanced

Balance Fe: $2FeS + O_2 + H_2O \rightarrow Fe_2O_3 + H_2SO_4$

Rebalance S: $2FeS + O_2 + H_2O \rightarrow Fe_2O_3 + 2H_2SO_4$

Rebalance H: $2FeS + O_2 + 2H_2O \rightarrow Fe_2O_3 + 2H_2SO_4$

Balance O: $2FeS + \frac{9}{2}O_2 + 2H_2O \rightarrow Fe_2O_3 + 2H_2SO_4$

Multiply by 2: $4FeS + 9O_2 + 4H_2O \rightarrow 2Fe_2O_3 + 4H_2SO_4$

Check: $4FeS + 9O_2 + 4H_2O \not\rightarrow 2Fe_2O_3 + 4H_2SO_4$

Fe:	4		4
S:	4		4
O:	18 + 4 = 22		6 + 16 = 22
H:	8		8

9–15. **9-B, 10-B, 11-C, 12-D, 13-A, 14-A, 15-D.** See text for explanation.

16. A GMW = 6C + 12H + 6O = 6(12) + 12(1) + 6(16)

$$= 72 + 12 + 96 = 180$$

17. A $\text{Moles} = \dfrac{\text{weight}}{\text{GMW}} = \dfrac{34}{169} = 0.20$

GMW = Ag + N + 3(O) = 107 + 14 + 3(16)

$$= 21 + 48 = 169$$

18. B weight = (moles)(GMW) = (0.5)(40) = 20 g

GMW = Na + O + H = 23 + 16 + 1 = 40

19. D $\text{GMW} = \dfrac{\text{weight}}{\text{moles}} = \dfrac{5}{0.1} = 50$

20. B $\text{GEW} = \dfrac{\text{GMW}}{n} = \dfrac{63}{1} = 63$

GMW = H + N + 3(O) = 1 + 14 + 3(16)

$$= 15 + 48 = 63$$

n = exchangeable H per molecule = 1

21. D H_3PO_4 can give 1, 2, or 3 protons in a reaction; therefore the reaction must be specified. 3(1) + 31 + 4(16) = 98 = GMW. Then $\frac{98}{1} = 98$, $\frac{98}{2} = 49$, $\frac{98}{3} \approx 33$.

22. D $\text{GEW} = \dfrac{\text{GMW}}{n} = \dfrac{101}{2} \approx 50$

GMW = K + N + 3(O) = 39 + 14 + 3(16)

$$= 53 + 48 = 101$$

n = exchangeable electrons per molecule = 2

23. C $\text{GEW} = \dfrac{\text{GMW}}{n} = \dfrac{294}{12} \approx 25$

GMW = 2(K) + 2(Cr) + 7(O) = 2(39) + 2(52) + 7(16)

$$= 78 + 104 + 112 = 294$$

n = exchangeable electrons per molecule

$$= (2)(6) = 12 \text{ because there are two Cr per molecule}$$

24. B $\text{Equivalents} = \dfrac{\text{weight}}{\text{GEW}} \approx \dfrac{5}{26} \approx 0.20$

$\text{GEW} = \dfrac{\text{GMW}}{n} = \dfrac{78}{3} = 26$

GMW = Al + 3(O) + 3(H) = 27 + 3(16) + 3(1)

$$= 27 + 48 + 3 = 78$$

n = exchangeable OH per molecule = 3

25. B Weight = (GEW)(Equivalents) = (49)(2) = 98

$\text{GEW} = \dfrac{\text{GMW}}{n} = \dfrac{98}{2} = 49$

GMW = 2(H) + S + 4(O) = 2(1) + 32 + 4(16)

$$= 2 + 32 + 64 = 98$$

n = exchangeable H's per molecule = 2

26. A $\%H = \left(\dfrac{\text{weight of H}}{\text{GMW}}\right)(100) = \left(\dfrac{8}{132}\right)(100) \approx 6$

weight of H $= 8(H) = 8(1) = 8$

GMW $= 2(N) + 8(H) + S + 4(O) = 2(14) + 8(1) + 32 + 4(16)$

$= 28 + 8 + 32 + 64 = 132$

27. B Obtain the correct answer by determining the molecular weights of the options. First determine the empirical formula and then the molecular formula from it.

(1) $C = 92.3g$ $H = 100 - 92.3 = 7.7g$

(2) Moles C $= \dfrac{92.3}{12} = 7.7$

Moles H $= \dfrac{7.7}{1} = 7.7$

$C_{7.7}H_{7.7}$

(3) Divide both by 7.7

$$C\ H = C_1H_1 = CH$$
$$\dfrac{7.7}{7.7}\ \dfrac{7.7}{7.7}$$

(4) Not needed

The gram-empirical formula weight is $C + H = 12 + 1 = 13$, which goes into the gram-molecular weight $^{52}\!/_{13} = 4$ times. Therefore, the ratios of elements in the empirical formula must be multiplied by 4, which gives C_4H_4.

28. B This question requires a direct application of the Law of Dulong and Petit (see text for explanation). The approximate GAW is:

$$6.3 = (SH)(GAW)$$

$$GAW = \dfrac{6.3}{SH} = \dfrac{6.3}{0.03} = 210$$

29. C First, convert to moles:

$$\text{Moles of } O_2: \dfrac{x \text{ moles } O_2}{22.4 \text{ liters } O_2} = \dfrac{1 \text{ mole } O_2}{22.4 \text{ liters } O_2}$$

$$\dfrac{x}{22.4} = \dfrac{1}{22.4}$$

$$x = \dfrac{1}{22.4}(22.4) = 1 \text{ mole}$$

Moles of FeS: GMW of FeS $= 56 + 32 = 88$

$$\text{Moles of Fe} = \dfrac{\text{weight}}{\text{GMW}} = \dfrac{44}{88} = \dfrac{1}{2}$$

Then, determine if either reagent is in limiting amounts.
If all the O_2 is used up:

$$\dfrac{x \text{ moles FeS}}{1 \text{ mole } O_2} = \dfrac{4 \text{ moles FeS}}{9 \text{ moles } O_2}$$

$$\dfrac{x}{1} = \dfrac{4}{9}$$

$$x = {}^4\!/_9 \text{ mole of FeS would be required}$$

If all the FeS is used up:

$$\dfrac{x \text{ moles } O_2}{{}^1\!/_2 \text{ mole FeS}} = \dfrac{9 \text{ moles } O_2}{4 \text{ moles FeS}}$$

$$\dfrac{x}{{}^1\!/_2} = \dfrac{9}{4}$$

$$x = \left(\frac{9}{4}\right)\left(\frac{1}{2}\right) = \frac{9}{8} \text{ moles of } O_2 \text{ would be required}$$

So, the O_2 is in limiting amounts because less than $\frac{9}{8}$ mole is available. Note that more than $\frac{4}{9}$ mole of FeS is available to react with the O_2.

Use moles of O_2 to determine how much H_2SO_4 will be produced:

$$\frac{x \text{ moles } H_2SO_4}{1 \text{ mole } O_2} = \frac{4 \text{ moles } H_2SO_4}{9 \text{ moles } O_2}$$

$$\frac{x}{1} = \frac{4}{9}$$

$$x = \frac{4}{9} \text{ moles of } H_2SO_4 \text{ will be produced}$$

$$\text{because moles} = \frac{\text{weight}}{\text{GMW}} \text{ and}$$

$$\text{GMW of } H_2SO_4 = 2(1) + 32 + 4(16) = 2 + 32 + 64 = 98$$

then,

$$\text{Weight of } H_2SO_4 = (\text{moles})(\text{GMW}) = \left(\frac{4}{9}\right)(98) \approx (4)(11) = 44 \text{ g}$$

30. B $\quad \dfrac{x \text{ moles } Fe_2O_3}{5 \text{ moles } FeS} = \dfrac{2 \text{ moles } Fe_2O_3}{4 \text{ moles } FeS}$

$$\frac{x}{5} = \frac{2}{4}$$

$$x = (\frac{2}{4})(5) = \frac{5}{2} = 2\frac{1}{2} \text{ moles of } Fe_2O_3$$

Electrochemistry

Self-Managed Learning Questions

1. Why are cathodes negative and anodes positive?
2. What is electroplating? What are the components of a cell for most efficient electroplating?
3. Are electrons of different elements different? Are copper electrons different from zinc electrons? What substances are electrons made of?
4. What are the medical problems of electrolysis to remove hair from the human body? Are the hair strands oxidized or reduced? Discuss the biochemistry of a hair strand.
5. Is red cabbage juice or red beet juice an electrolyte? Can you find the molarity of either? How?
6. Does the pH of an electrolyte depend on the voltage applied to an electrochemical cell?
7. How would you classify a watch battery—electrochemical or electrolytic? Why?
8. Why is a salt bridge essential in a galvanic cell?

ELECTROLYTIC CELL

Electrolysis

Electrolysis is the process whereby electrons are pushed into a system by an external voltage, and a reaction can be forced to go in a direction it could not go spontaneously. This process is one way by which to recover metals from their salts. Also, gold or silver electroplating is accomplished in this way. The key relations are:

$$1F \text{ (faraday)} = 96,500 \text{ coulombs} = 1 \text{ mole of electrons (Faraday's relation)}$$

$$1 \text{ ampere of current} = \frac{1 \text{ coulomb}}{\text{sec}}$$

These relations are used to determine how much of a metal can be plated out by a given current acting over a certain time, or they can be used to calculate the reverse.

Anode and Cathode/ Oxidation and Reduction at Electrodes

Oxidation and reduction half-reactions may occur at electrodes (substances made of metal or carbon at which electrons may be exchanged). The two types of electrodes are cathode and anode. A **cathode** attracts cations (positively charged ions such as H^+, Ca^{++}, and NH_4^+); it is where reduction occurs. In electrochemical cells (voltaic, galvanic), the reaction is spontaneous, whereas in electrolytic cells, the reaction is nonspontaneous. The cathode is positive in electrochemical cells and is negative in electrolytic cells. An **anode** attracts anions (negatively charged ions such as Cl^-, OH^-, SO_4^-); it is where oxidation occurs. The anode is negative in electrochemical cells and positive in electrolytic cells. Electrons enter the anode by oxidation of a substance and move to the cathode, where they exit by reduction of some substance (Fig. 7-32). A conducting connector (e.g., a wire or a salt bridge) acts as a link between the anode and the cathode (Table 7-3) (Fig. 7-33).

VOLTAIC CELLS AND GALVANIC CELLS

Voltaic cells, which are also called galvanic cells, produce a current and voltage internally by a chemical reaction. Consider, for example, a lead storage battery (Fig. 7-34). The capacity of one substance to give or take electrons from another substance is complex. Suffice it to say, electron affinities, ionization potentials, concentrations, pressures, and temperature are all important. Fortunately, the relative ability of a substance to give or

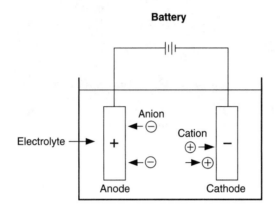

Fig. 7-32.

TABLE 7-3. Electrochemical and Electrolytic Cells

		Contrast			Compare
Electrochemical cells	Voltaic and galvanic	Cathode +	Anode −	Spontaneous	• Oxidation occurs at anode • Reduction occurs at cathode
Electrolytic cells	N/A	Cathode −	Anode +	Nonspontaneous	• Cathode attracts cations in solution • Anode attracts anions in solution

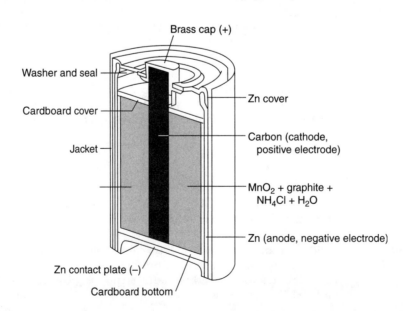

Fig. 7-33.

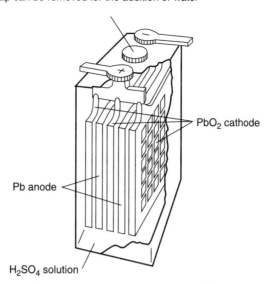

Cap can be removed for the addition of water

PbO$_2$ cathode

Pb anode

Fig. 7-34.

H$_2$SO$_4$ solution

take electrons can be quantified in one number, symbolized by E. E is the potential difference (or voltage, see discussion of electrostatics and electromagnetism) that is generated when two substances are connected. This potential, when standardized, is called the **standard half cell potential** (E°) as follows:

1. A reference half-reaction is established and its E° = 0,

$$2H^+ (1M) + 2e^- \rightarrow H_2(1 \text{ atm})$$

   (atm = atmosphere and M = molar)
2. All other half-reactions are compared to this half-reaction and the E° for each of them is determined
3. To be E°, the following standard conditions must hold:

   • Concentration of all solutes is 1M (one molar)
   • Pressure of all gases is 1 atm
   • Temperature is 25°C (298°K)

The standard half-cell potential (E°) can be written as an oxidation half-reaction:

$$A \rightarrow A^{+n} + ne^-, \text{ or, as a reduction half-reaction } A^{+n} + ne^- \rightarrow A$$

The first is called an **oxidation cell potential**; the second is called a **reduction cell potential**. Usually, the reduction cell potentials are used. Regardless of which one is used, the **interpretation** of E° is the same. The more positive the E°, the more likely the reaction will proceed to the right as written.

It is important to note that if the direction of the equation is reversed, the sign of E° changes to the opposite ($+ \rightarrow -$) or ($- \rightarrow +$). Also, the value of E° is not affected by the stoichiometry of the reaction since conditions are standard.

To determine the standard **potential for a reaction**, call it ΔE°, you must look up the appropriate E° for the half-cell reactions, give it the correct sign, and then add. For example, given the reaction, $2A + B^{+2} \rightarrow 2A^{+1} + B$, the oxidation half-reaction (O) is:

$$(O): 2A \rightarrow 2A^{+1} + 2e^-$$

and the reduction half-reaction (R) is:

$$(R): B^{+2} + 2e^- \rightarrow B$$

If available, a table of standard reduction potentials will include the following:

$$A^{+1} + e^- \rightarrow A \qquad E° = -1.10V$$

$$B^{+2} + 2e^- \rightarrow B \qquad E° = +0.50V$$

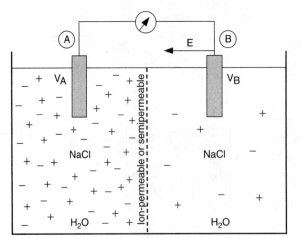

Fig. 7-35. Bioelectric or concentration cell.

Chamber A = higher concentration Chamber B = lower concentration

These half-reactions from the reduction potential table are rewritten as they occur (the direction) in the given reaction:

$$(O): 2A \rightarrow 2A^{+1} + 2e^- \quad E° = -1.10V$$

$$(R): 2e^- + B^{+2} \rightarrow B \quad E° = +0.50V$$

$$\text{overall: } 2A + B^{+2} \rightarrow 2A^{+1} + B \quad \Delta E° = +1.60V$$

Important points to note follow:

1. When balancing the half-reaction, the E° is not affected as for the (O)
2. When reversing the equation as found in the table, the sign of E° (from the table) is reversed as for the (O)
3. If the overall $\Delta E°$ is positive, then the reaction proceeds from left to right as written,
4. If the overall $\Delta E°$ is negative, then the reaction proceeds in the reverse direction and it should be rewritten as such.

The value of E° determines the maximal amount of work the reaction can perform. The relation is:

$$\text{Work (joules)} = (\Delta E)(q) = (\Delta E)(I)(\Delta t)$$

in which ΔE = volts, q = charge in coulombs, I = current in amperes (coulombs/sec), and t = time in seconds. The equation is valid for electrolysis.

Concentration cells can produce a current and voltage by differences in concentrations of the same substance. The larger the concentration difference, the larger the potential produced by the cell (Fig. 7-35). The concentration difference (diffusion) causes ions to flow from higher concentration to lower concentration. The potential of a piece of metal immersed in a solution containing its ions depends on the concentration of the ions. The cell may be set up by deriving its EMF (E volts) from the difference in concentration of solutions of the same electrolyte surrounding the two electrodes. E depends on the concentration differences of A and B.

APPLIED CONCEPTS

1. Understand the chemical structure of dental amalgam (silver, mercury, and tin are usually applied in three layers). When a wrapper (gum or candy) made of aluminum comes in contact with the amalgamated tooth, a small electrical cell is set in operation, leading to minor shock.
2. Understand different types of corrosion of metallic objects, such as statues in museums. Perform an experiment to check the rate of rusting or corroding of iron nails placed in three tubes (one is full of water, one has no water, and one is half empty).
3. Look at several old batteries and understand how they work. Why are rechargeable batteries made of nickel and cadmium?
4. Frogs usually live in fresh water (1–3 M NaCl) and the ECF in a frog's body contains 110 mM NaCl. The frog's environment is hypotonic. Hans Ussing (Danish physiologist) used Ussing chambers to determine the movement of radioactive isotopes of Na^+. Analyze Ussing's experimental techniques to verify active transport of Na^+. Can you support or reject either of the following hypotheses?

I. Energy for active transport of Na+ is provided by the hydrolysis of ATP.
II. The electrical potential generated by active transport of Na+ ions provides energy for Cl⁻ absorption.

ELECTROCHEMISTY: REVIEW QUESTIONS

1. When the oxidation and reduction half-reactions are added, the sum of the electrons is:

    A. positive.
    B. negative.
    C. zero.
    D. any of the above.

2. Where does oxidation of the solution (or solute) occur?

    A. Anode
    B. Cathode
    C. Neither anode nor cathode
    D. Anode and cathode

3. "Positive" substances are attracted to:

    A. the anode.
    B. the cathode.
    C. neither cathode nor anode.
    D. anode and cathode.

4. The direction of electron flow is:

    A. from anode to cathode.
    B. from cathode to anode.
    C. either way.
    D. not determinable.

5. All of the half-cell potentials ($E°$) use the _____ as the reference.

    A. hydrogen (H_2) half-cell
    B. oxygen (O_2) half-cell
    C. carbon (C) half-cell
    D. arbitrarily set zero point

6. On which of the following variables does the ΔE depend?

    A. temperature.
    B. concentrations.
    C. pressures of gases.
    D. all of the above.

7. Half-cell potentials are usually written as:

    A. oxidation half-reactions.
    B. reduction half-reactions.
    C. reactant half-reactions.
    D. product half-reactions.

8. The more negative the value of $E°$:

    A. the more likely the reaction is to proceed left to right.
    B. the more likely the reaction is to proceed right to left.
    C. the less likely the reaction is to proceed left to right.
    D. the less likely the reaction is to proceed right to left.

9. If the coefficients in a half-reaction are doubled, the $E°$ is:

    A. doubled.
    B. halved.
    C. not affected.
    D. tripled.

10. If the potential created by a chemical reaction is used to move a current, what is the type of cell that is created?

    A. Concentration
    B. Galvanic

C. Electrolytic
D. Mixed

11. One faraday corresponds to:

    A. one volt of cell potential.
    B. 96,487 amperes.
    (C.) one mole of electrons.
    D. all of the above.

12. Which of the following would be considered a reduction half-reaction?

    (A.) $A^{+2} + 2e^- \rightarrow A$
    B. $A \rightarrow A^{+2} + 2e^-$
    C. Both
    D. Neither

13. Which of the following is the reduction half-reaction of $A^{+2} + 2B \rightarrow A + 2B^{+1}$?

    A. $2B \rightarrow 2B^{+1} + 2e^-$
    B. $A \rightarrow A^{+2} + 2e^-$
    (C.) $A^{+2} + 2e^- \rightarrow A$
    D. $2B^{+1} + 2e^- \rightarrow 2B$

14. Suppose A and B^{+2} are placed in the same solution. Will there be a spontaneous reaction? If so, what is the balanced equation? The pertinent reduction potentials follow:

$$A^{+1} + e^- \rightarrow A \qquad E^\circ = -1.50V$$

$$B^{+2} + 2e^- \rightarrow B \qquad E^\circ = -1.00V$$

    A. No, because the E° of the reaction is negative
    B. Yes, $A + B^{+2} \rightarrow A^{+1} + B$
    (C.) Yes, $2A + B^{+2} \rightarrow 2A^{+1} + B$
    D. Yes, $2A + B \rightarrow 2A^{+1} + B^{+2}$

Questions 15–17

15. What is the sum of all the coefficients in the following equation when balanced (the solution is **acidic** and **aqueous**)?

$$Ag + NO_3^- \rightarrow Ag^+ + NO$$

    A. 9
    B. 14
    C. 15
    D. 18

16. What is the sum of all the coefficients in the following equation when balanced (solution is **basic** and **aqueous**)?

$$N_2H_4 + Cu(OH)_2 \rightarrow N_2 + Cu$$

    A. 8
    (B.) 10
    C. 12
    D. 14

17. What is the sum of all the coefficients in the following equation when balanced (solution is **basic** and **aqueous**)?

$$ClO_2 + OH^- \rightarrow ClO_2^- + ClO_3^-$$

    A. 5
    B. 7
    C. 9
    D. 10

Questions 18–26
Refer to the following illustration and data to answer the following questions.

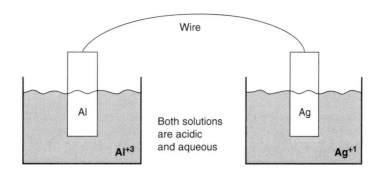

Both solutions are acidic and aqueous

Standard Reduction Potentials at 25°C in Aqueous Solutions

Half-Reaction	E° (volts)
$Ca^{+2} + 2e^- \rightarrow Ca$	-2.9
$Na^+ + e^- \rightarrow Na$	-2.7
$Al^{+3} + 3e^- \rightarrow Al$	-1.7
$Mn^{+2} + 2e^- \rightarrow Mn$	-1.2
$Zn^{+2} + 2e^- \rightarrow Zn$	-0.8
$Cu^{+2} + 2e^- \rightarrow Cu$	$+0.3$
$I_2(s) + 2e^- \rightarrow 2I^-$	$+0.5$
$PtCl_4^{-2} + 2e^- \rightarrow Pt + 4Cl^-$	$+0.7$
$Ag^+ + e^- \rightarrow Ag$	$+0.8$
$O_2 + 4H^+ + 4e^- \rightarrow 2H_2O(l)$	$+1.23$
$Cr_2O_7^{-2} + 6e^- \rightarrow Cr^{+3}$	$\vert\,1.33$
$Cl_2 + 2e^- \rightarrow 2Cl^-$	$+1.36$
$M_nO_4^- + 5e^- \rightarrow Mn^{+2}$	$+1.51$

Equations:

$$\Delta E = \Delta E° - \frac{0.059}{n} \log \frac{[C]^c[D]^d}{[A]^a[B]^b} = \Delta E° - \frac{0.059}{n} \log K \text{ at } 25°C$$

$$= \Delta E° - \frac{RT}{nF} \log K$$

(the Nernst Equation) $\Delta E = 0$ for $aA + bB \rightarrow cC + dD$

$\Delta E°$ = standard cell potential
ΔE = cell potential at new set of concentrations
n = number of electrons exchanged in the reaction as written
K = equilibrium constant
$\Delta G° = -nFE°$ or $\Delta G = -nFE$
F = faraday = 23,000 cal/volts (= 96,500 coulombs)
n = number of electrons exchanged in reaction as written
E = cell potential
ΔG = free energy of reaction = cal
RT = (8.3145)(298) M-K-S units

18. Which substances are the reactants in this cell, assuming concentrations are all standard (1 M)?

    A. Al + Ag
    B. $Al^{+3} + Ag^+$
    C. $Al + Ag^+$
    D. $Ag + Al^{+3}$

19. Write the balanced oxidation half-reaction of this cell.

    A. $Ag^+ + e^- \rightarrow Ag$
    B. $Al^{+3} + 3e^- \rightarrow Al$
    C. $Ag \rightarrow Ag^+ + e^-$
    D. $Al \rightarrow Al^{+3} + 3e^-$

20. At which electrode is reduction of the solution occurring?

    A. Al
    B. Ag
    C. Neither
    D. Both

21. The Al electrode is ——————— and is called the ———————.

    A. positive, anode
    B. positive, cathode
    C. negative, anode
    D. negative, cathode

22. The flow of electrons in the electronic circuit is from the ——————— electrode to the ——————— electrode.

    A. Al, Ag
    B. Ag, Al

23. The sum of coefficients in the balanced equation for the reaction is:

    A. 4
    B. 6
    C. 8
    D. 10

24. The **standard cell potential** ($\Delta E°$) for the reaction is ——————— volts.

    A. -0.9
    B. 0.9
    C. 2.5
    D. 4.1

25. Using the Nernst equation, what is the cell potential (ΔE), in volts, of this reaction? Note: At 25°C, the electrolyte concentrations are $[Al^{+3}] = 0.1$ M and $[Ag^+] = 0.1$ M).

    A. -1.14
    B. 1.14
    C. 2.46
    D. 2.10

26. This type of cell may be best considered a(n):

    A. concentration cell.
    B. galvanic cell.
    C. electrolytic cell.
    D. none of the above.

ANSWERS AND EXPLANATIONS

1–11. 1-C, 2-A, 3-B, 4-A, 5-A, 6-D, 7-B, 8-B, 9-C, 10-B, 11-C. See text for explanation.

12. A A reduction half-reaction has the electrons on the left side.

13. C In the reaction as written, the A^{+2} is being reduced to A: i.e., $A^{+2} \to A$ is a change to a more negative (less positive) oxidation state, which is reduction.

14. C The half-reactions would be:

$$A \to A^{+1} + e^-; E° = +1.50V \text{ (because reversed)}$$

$$B^{+2} + 2e^- \to B; E° = -1.00V$$

because A and B^{+2} are the reactants given. Balance electrons by multiplying half-reactions as necessary so they sum to zero:

$$2A \to 2A^{+1} + 2e^-; E° = +1.50V \text{ (note E° does not change)}$$

$$B^{+2} + 2e^- \to B; E° = -1.0V$$

$$\text{Sum: } 2A + B^{+2} \to 2A^{+1} + B \ \Delta E° = +0.50V$$

Because the $\Delta E°$ is positive, the reaction will occur spontaneously as written.

15. B Follow these steps (see text for explanation)
    1. Ag is oxidized; the N in NO_3^- is reduced

$$Ag + NO_3^- \rightarrow Ag^+ + NO$$

Oxidation states: $0 + 5, -2 + 1 + 2, -2$

2. (a) Oxidation half-reaction

$$Ag \rightarrow Ag^+ + e^-$$

   (b) Reduction half-reaction

$$3e^- + NO_3^- \rightarrow NO$$

3. (a) $Ag \rightarrow Ag^+ + e^-$; already balanced

   (b) $NO_3^- + 3e^- \qquad \rightarrow NO$: N's are balanced

$$4H^+ + NO_3^- + 3e^- \rightarrow NO; \text{ add } H^+ \text{ to left to balance}$$

charge on **both** sides

$$4H^+ + NO_3^- + 3e^- \rightarrow NO + 2H_2O; \text{ add } H_2O \text{ to right to}$$

balance H and O

4. $3\,Ag \rightarrow 3\,Ag^+\; 3e^-$

$$\frac{4H^+ + NO_3^- + 3e^- \rightarrow NO + 2H_2O}{4H^+ + 3Ag + NO_3^- \rightarrow 3Ag^+ + NO + 2H_2O}$$

Sum of coefficients $= 4 + 3 + 1 + 3 + 1 + 2 = 14$

5. Everything checks

Note that for acidic or basic solutions, the H^+ or OH^-, respectively, are usually on the left side of the equation. Also, the balancing of charge does not have to make the overall charge neutral but must make the net charge on one side equal to the net charge on the other.

16. B Follow the steps in question 15:

1. N is oxidized, Cu is reduced

$$N_2H_4 + Cu(OH)_2 \rightarrow N_2 + Cu$$

Oxidation states: $-2, + 1 + 2, -2, + 1\,0\,0$

2. (a) Oxidation half-reaction

$$N_2H_4 \rightarrow N_2 + 4e^-; \text{ (each N loses two electrons)}$$

   (b) Reduction half-reaction

$$2e^- + Cu(OH)_2 \rightarrow Cu$$

3. Balance each half-reaction

$$N_2H_4 \qquad \rightarrow N_2 + 4e^-; \text{ N are already balanced}$$

   (a) $4OH^- + N_2H_4 \rightarrow N_2 + 4e^-$; add OH^- to left to balance charge

$$4OH- + N_2H_4 \rightarrow N_2 + 4e- + 4\,H_2O$$

Add H_2O to right to balance the O (and H)

   (b) $2e^- + Cu(OH)_2 \rightarrow Cu$: Cu are balanced

$$2e^- + Cu(OH)_2 \rightarrow Cu + 2OH^-; \text{ balance charge by adding } OH^-$$

to the right side, H and O are then balanced

4. $4OH^- + N_2H_4 \rightarrow N_2 + 4H_2O + 4e^-$

$$\frac{4e^- + 2Cu(OH)_2 \rightarrow 2Cu + 4OH^-}{N_2H_4 + 2Cu(OH)_2 \rightarrow N_2 + 2Cu + 4H_2O} \text{ (multiply by 2)}$$

Sum of coefficients $= 1 + 2 + 1 + 2 + 4 = 10$

5. Everything checks out

17. B Follow the steps in question 15:

1. Cl is oxidized, Cl is reduced

$$ClO_2 + OH^- \rightarrow ClO_2^- + ClO_3^-$$

Oxidation states: $+4, -2 - 2, +1 + 3, -2 + 5, -2$

2. (a) Oxidation half-reaction

$$ClO_2 \rightarrow ClO_3^- + e^-$$

   (b) Reduction half-reaction

$$e^- + ClO_2 \rightarrow ClO_2^-$$

3. Balance each half-reaction

(a) $ClO_2 \rightarrow ClO_3^- + e^-$; Cl already balanced, add OH^- to left

to balance charge

$2OH^- + ClO_2 \rightarrow ClO_3^- + e^-$

$2OH^- + ClO_2 \rightarrow ClO_3^- + H_2O + e^-$; add H_2O to right to

balance O and H

(b) $e^- + ClO_2 \rightarrow ClO_2^-$; Cl, O and charge are already balanced

4. $2OH^- + ClO_2 \rightarrow ClO_3 + H_2O + e^-$

$$\frac{e^- + ClO_2 \rightarrow ClO_2^-}{2OH^- + 2ClO_2 \rightarrow ClO_2^- + ClO_3^- + H_2O}$$

Sum of coefficients $= 2 + 2 + 1 + 1 + 1 = 7$

18. C Of four possible substances for reactants Al, Al^{+3}, Ag, and Ag^+, only two can be reactants. One will be oxidized and one will be reduced. The candidates for oxidation are Al and Ag; the candidates for reduction are Al^{+3} and Ag^{+1}. Because the ΔE° for $Al \rightarrow Al^{+3} + 3e^-$ (+1.7) is larger than the ΔE° for $Ag^+ + e^- \rightarrow$ Ag (+0.8), which is larger than the ΔE° for $Al^{+3} + 3e^- \rightarrow Al$ (−1.7), the Al must be oxidized and the Ag+ reduced.

19. D From question 18, the Al is oxidized to obtain: $Al \rightarrow Al^{+3} + 3e^-$.

20. B From question 18, the Ag+ is being reduced, causing reduction at the Ag electrode.

21. C Oxidation occurs at the Al electrode (from question 20). Oxidation occurs at the anode, which is negative.

22. A The Al electrode is losing electrons ($Al \rightarrow Al^{+3} + 3e^-$), which travel through the wire to the Ag electrode, where they are used ($Ag^+ + e^- \rightarrow Ag$).

23. C Balance the equation as follows:

1. Al is oxidized, Ag^+ is reduced

$Al + Ag^+ \rightarrow Al^{+3} + Ag$

Oxidation states: 0 +1 +3 0

2. (a) Oxidation half-reaction: $Al \rightarrow Al^{+3} + 3e^-$

(b) Reduction half-reaction: $e^- + Ag^+ \rightarrow Ag$

3. Both are already balanced

4. $Al \rightarrow Al^{+3} + 3e^-$

$$\frac{3e^- + 3Ag^+ \rightarrow 3Ag}{Al + 3Ag^+ \rightarrow Al^{+3} + 3Ag}$$ (multiplied by 3)

Sum of coefficients $= 1 + 3 + 1 + 3 = 8$

5. Everything checks

24. C Using the balanced half-reactions from question 23 and the E° from the table:

$Al \rightarrow Al^{+3} + 3e^-$ $E^\circ = +1.7$ (sign reversed)

$$\text{Sum: } \frac{3e^- + 3Ag^+ \rightarrow 3Ag}{Al + 3Ag^+ \rightarrow Al^{+3} + Ag} \quad E^\circ = +0.8$$

$\Delta E^\circ = +2.5$ volts

25. C The Nernst equation for the balanced reaction is:

$$\Delta E = \Delta E^\circ - \frac{0.059}{n} \log \frac{[Al^{+3}]}{[Ag^+]^3} \approx 2.5 - \frac{0.06}{3} \log \frac{0.1}{(0.1)^3}$$

$$\approx 2.5 - 0.02 \log \frac{10^{-1}}{(10^{-1})^3}$$

$$\approx 2.5 - 0.02 \log \frac{10^{-1}}{10^{-3}} \approx 2.5 - 0.02 \log 10^2$$

$$\approx 2.5 - 0.02(2) \approx 2.5 - 0.04 \approx 2.46 \text{ volts}$$

26. B The voltage in this cell is generated by a chemical reaction. The difference in concentrations reflect that the conditions are not standard. The classic concentration cell would have either Al^{+3}/Al or Ag^+/Ag in both beakers but in different concentrations in each.

Solution Chemistry

Self-Managed Learning Questions

1. What are osmolarity and osmolality? How would you determine osmolality of the following compounds given molarity?
   a. NaCl
   b. $CaSO_4$
   c. C_6H_6
   d. C_2H_5OH
   e. $C_6H_{12}O_6$
   f. $MgCl_2$
2. What organic compounds or molecules are hydrophobic and hydrophilic? Cite some examples of clinical importance.
3. How would the common-ion effect apply to the fluid and electrolyte balance in the human body? (Hint: Lactic acid titrations.)
4. How can solutions change from saturated to supersaturated? Give a kitchen example to demonstrate the concept.
5. What experiment is carried out to determine blood-urea-nitrogen, or BUN? Is a BUN value of 10 mg/dl acceptable for an adult? A child?

IONS IN SOLUTION

Electrolytes are substances that dissociate into positive and negative ions when dissolved in a solvent. An **ion** is an atom, or a group of atoms, that has an electric charge by losing or gaining one electron. The ions are positive (**cations**) and negative (**anions**) and are surrounded by solvent molecules in solution (a process called solvation; when the solvent is H_2O, this process is hydration). In this discussion, we will refer to water as a solvent.

Some substances are only partially soluble in water. The **ion product** is a means of quantifying the solubility:

$$M_mA_a + H_2O \rightarrow mM^{+a}(aq) + aA^{-m}(aq)$$

in which (aq) = dissolved in water; ion product = $[M^{+a}]^m[A^{-m}]^a$; and [ ] = concentration in moles/liter, i.e., molarity. As an example:

For $Ca_3(PO_4)_2$, m = 3, a = 2

Ion product = $[Ca^{+2}]^3[PO_4^{-3}]^2$

The common names, formulas, and charges for familiar cations and anions are listed in Table 7-4.

SOLUBILITY

Solubility is the concentration attained when a designated quantity of liquid has dissolved all the solid it can hold at equilibrium at a given temperature. When the ionic solid is added to water, the water molecules orient around the ions with their positive ends pointing inward toward a negative ion, and vice versa.

Units of Concentration

A **liquid solution** is a homogenous, liquid mixture of variable composition over a limited range consisting of two or more components. Note that a solution may also be gaseous or solid. Given a two component solution, the **solvent** is the component in greater amount (herein, usually a pure liquid), and the **solute** is the component in lesser amount (herein, usually a solid or second liquid). Note that solids, gases, or other liquids can be dissolved in a given pure liquid to make a solution.

Common ways of **measuring the composition of solutions** are outlined as follows:

1. **Percent composition** can be weight/volume, weight/weight, volume/volume, etc. It must be designated as to the type and the units of mass and volume used:

$$\% = \frac{\text{amt solute}}{\text{total amt solution}} \times 100 \text{ (usual form)}$$

2. **Density** (ρ), $\rho = \dfrac{\text{mass of solution}}{\text{total volume of solution}}$

3. **Mole fraction (X)**,

$$x_1 = \frac{\text{moles of one component}}{\text{total moles of all components}} = \frac{n_i}{\sum\limits_{i=1}^{m} n_i}$$

in which n_1 = moles of component #1, for I = 1; I = 1, 2, 3 . . . . . ,

TABLE 7-4. Common Names, Formulas, and Charges for Familiar Ions

Cations

Aluminum, Al^{3+}	Iron(III), ferric Fe^+
Ammonium, NH_4^+	Lead, Pb^{2+}
Barium, Ba^{2+}	Lithium, Li^+
Calcium, Ca^{2+}	Magnesium, Mg_2^+
Chromium(II), chromous, Cr^{2+}	Mercury(I), mercurous, Hg_2^{2+}
Chromium(III), chromic, Cr^{3+}	Mercury(II), mercuric, Hg^{2+}
Cobalt, Co^{2+}	Potassium, K^+
Copper(I), cuprous, Cu^+	Silver, Ag^+
Copper(II), cupric, Cu^{2+}	Tin(II), stannous, Sn^{+2}
Hydrogen, hydronium, H^+, H_3O^+	Tin(IV), stannic, Sn^{4+}
Iron(II), ferrous, Fe^{2+}	Zinc, Zn^{2+}

Anions

Acetate, CH_3COO^-	Nitrite NO_2^-
Bromide, Br^-	Oxalate, $C_2O_4^{2-}$
Carbonate, CO_3^{2-}	Hydrogen oxalate ion, bioxalate, $HC_2O_4^-$
Hydrogen carbonate ion, bicarbonate, HCO_3^-	Oxide, O^{2-}
Chlorate, ClO_3^-	Perchlorate, ClO_4^-
Chloride, Cl^-	Permanganate, MnO_4^-
Chlorite, ClO_2^-	Phosphate, PO_4^{3-}
Chromate, CrO_4^{2-}	Monohydrogen phosphate, HPO_4^{2-}
Dichromate, $Cr_2O_7^{2-}$	Dihydrogen phosphate, $H_2PO_4^-$
Fluoride, F^-	Sulfate, SO_4^{2-}
Hydroxide, OH^-	Hydrogen sulfate ion, bisulfate, HSO_4^-
Hypochlorite, ClO^-	Sulfide, S^{2-}
Iodide, I^-	Hydrogen sulfide ion, bisulfide, HS^-
Nitrate, NO_3^-	Hydrogen sulfite ion, bisulfite, HSO_3^-

m = component number; $\sum n_i$ = sum over moles of all m components. For component #1, if m = 3:

$$X_i = \frac{n_1}{n_1 + n_2 + n_3}$$

This calculation is useful when emphasizing the relation between concentration-dependent properties of solutions and the relative amounts of the components (see subsequent discussion).

4. **Molarity (M)**, $M = \dfrac{\text{moles solute}}{\text{liter solution}}$

Varies with the temperature. ("formality" rather than "molarity" may be used in some texts.)

5. **Molality (m)**, $m = \dfrac{\text{moles solute}}{\text{kilogram solvent}}$

Does not vary with temperature. Note that the molality and molarity of a given solution cannot be the same. (For dilute solutions, however, molality and molarity are almost the same.)

6. **Normality (N)**, $N = \dfrac{\text{equivalents solute}}{\text{liter solution}}$

N = nM relates normality and molarity. The formula is used to calculate the gram-formula weight (e.g., NaCl is the formula for table salt with an equivalent or formula weight of 58.5).

n = number of protons (H^+) or (OH^-) ions.

7. **Mass conservation**. This concept is important for solving problems dealing with solutions and concentrations. Concentration of mass means:

given: C = concentration unit = $\dfrac{\text{amt solute}}{\text{volume solution}}$

(all of the above are similar, except for molality; just substitute kilograms for volume and solvent for solution)

V = volume of solution

then: $(C)(V)$ = amount of solute

amount—grams, moles, equivalents, etc., depending on the concentration unit (C) used.

then: this amount of solute is conserved.

As solutions are diluted:

$$C_1V_1 = C_2V_2 = \text{amount}$$

$$\text{e.g., } M_1V_1 = M_2V_2 = \text{moles}$$

$$(\%_1)(V_1) = (\%_2)(V_2) = \text{grams if \% is } \left(\frac{W}{V}\right)$$

As solutions are made from solids and liquids:

$$CV = \text{amount of solute used to make the solution, e.g.,}$$

$$(M)(V) = \text{moles} = \frac{\text{weight}}{\text{gram-molecular weight}}$$

$$(\%)(V) = \text{grams}\left(\% \text{ is } \frac{W}{V} \text{ here}\right)$$

The correct combination of formulas is chosen depending on the problem.

The Equilibrium Expression

The ion product can be calculated for any solution. The **solubility product** (K_{sp}) is the ion product for a saturated solution (as much as possible of the solute has been dissolved at a given temperature):

$$K_{sp} = [M^{+a}]^m[A^{-m}]^a$$

for a saturated solution. The smaller the K_{sp}, the less soluble a solid. The K_{sp} is larger than the ion product except at saturation, where they are equal. As long as the ion product is less than the **Ksp**, more solute can be dissolved.

APPLIED CONCEPTS

1. Understand calcium methodology for calcium assays. Compare and contrast total calcium methodology versus ionized calcium methodology and analyze sources of error in each procedure. What is the principle controlling chelation with EDTA and Flame photometry for calcium?
2. Read the methods used to detect inorganic phosphorus and wine phosphorus (Hint: read more in Fiske method or Molybdate method). What are clinical values of Ca^{++} and PO_4^{3-} in blood that are normal?
3. Review magnesium methodology from heparinized plasma and compare the dye-complexing method and the atomic absorption method. Define and describe effects of hypomagnesemia and hypermagnesemia.

SOLUTION CHEMISTRY: REVIEW QUESTIONS

1. Fifty grams of sugar are dissolved in enough water (approximately 168 ml) to make 200 ml of solution. What is the composition of sugar in solution in terms of grams per milliliter (g/ml)?

    $\frac{50}{200} \times 100 = 25\%$

    A. 40%
    B. 0.25%
    C. 2.5%
    D. 25%

2. What is the density of the sugar solution (g/ml) in question 1 (assume water weighs 1 g/ml)?

    A. 0.8
    B. 1.00
    C. 1.05
    D. 1.09

3. What weight of salt is in 50 ml of solution with a density of 1.05 g/ml? Assume the volume is mostly water and water weighs 1 g/ml.

    A. 1.05
    B. 2.5
    C. 3.25
    D. 5.0

4. A gas mixture contains 84 g of N_2 ($N = 14$), 64 g of O_2 ($O = 16$), and 10 g of H_2 ($H = 1$). What is the mole fraction of O_2 in this mixture?

    A. 0.4
    B. 0.3
    C. 0.2
    D. Insufficient information provided

5. A solution is made by dissolving 23 g of ethyl alcohol (C_2H_5OH; $C = 12$, $O = 16$, $H = 1$) in 500 ml of water. Water has a density of 1 g/ml. What is the molality of ethyl alcohol?

    A. 0.25
    B. 0.5
    C. 1.0
    D. None of the above

6. Seventy-five grams of Na_2CO_3 ($Na = 23$, $C = 12$, $O = 16$) are dissolved in enough water to make 1 liter of solution. What is the molarity of the solution?

    A. 1.1
    B. 1.0
    C. 0.71
    D. None of the above

7. One-hundred milliliters of a 2 M solution of H_2SO_4 contain how many moles of H_2SO_4?

    A. 0.2
    B. 2
    C. 200
    D. None of the above

8. How many equivalents of H_3PO_4 are in 500 ml of a 3 M solution of H_3PO_4 (all H reacts?)

    A. 1
    B. 2
    C. 6
    D. None of the above

9. What weight of NaCl ($Na = 23$, $Cl = 35$) would be required to make 2 liters of a 1.5 F solution?

    A. 174
    B. 116
    C. 58
    D. None of the above

10. How many milliliters must be added to 500 ml of a 1.5 M solution to make a 1.0 M solution?

    A. 100
    B. 250
    C. 5000
    D. None of the above

$$M_2 V_2 = M_1 V_1$$
$$V_2 = \frac{M_1 V_1}{M_2} = \frac{(1.5)(500)}{1.} \quad 750$$

11. Given the following data:

Ion	Radius (A)	Charge
Li	0.68	+1
K	1.33	+1
Cs	1.67	+1

which ion would most likely have the largest hydration shell in solution?

    A. Li^+
    B. K^+
    C. Cs^+
    D. Cannot be predicted

Consider the following information (numbers are K_{sp} values)

$BaSO_4$ .... 1×10^{-10}
PbS .... 7×10^{-29}
$PbCO_3$ .... 2×10^{-13}
Ag_2S .... 1×10^{-51}
HgS .... 3×10^{-53}
BaF_2 .... 2×10^{-6}
$PbSO_4$ .... 1×10^{-8}
$AgCl$ .... 3×10^{-10}
FeS .... 1×10^{-19}

12. If a saturated solution of $Cu(OH)_2$ contains $[Cu^{+2}] = 3.4 \times 10^{-7}$ and $[OH^-] = 6.8 \times 10^{-7}$, what is the K_{sp}?

    A. 8.2×10^{-21}
    B. 1.6×10^{-19}
    C. 4.6×10^{-13}
    D. None of the above

13. A saturated solution of $Cu(IO_3)_2$ is 3.0×10^{-3} moles/liter (M). What is the K_{sp}?

    A. 6×10^{-6}
    B. 2.7×10^{-8}
    C. 9×10^{-9}
    D. None of the above

14. A saturated solution of $BaSO_4$ contains what concentration of Ba^{+2}?

    A. 2×10^{-10}
    B. 1×10^{-5}
    C. 0.5×10^{-10}
    D. None of the above

15. If enough Na_2SO_4 is added to a saturated solution of $PbSO_4$ to make the total $[SO_4^{-2}] = 2 \times 10^{-2}$ M, how much $[Pb^{+2}]$ is in solution?

    A. 2×10^{-16}
    B. 1×10^{-4}
    C. 5×10^{-7}
    D. None of the above

ANSWERS AND EXPLANATIONS

1. **D** $\% \dfrac{\text{weight of solute}}{\text{volume of solution}} \times 100 = \dfrac{50}{200} \times 100 = \dfrac{50}{2} = 25\%$

2. **D** $\text{Density} = \dfrac{\text{total mass solution}}{\text{total volume solution}} = \dfrac{\text{weight of sugar} + \text{weight of water}}{\text{total volume solution}}$

    $= \dfrac{50 + 168}{200} = \dfrac{218}{200} = \dfrac{25}{20} = \dfrac{5}{4} = 1.09 \text{ g/ml}$

3. **B** $\text{Density} (\rho) = \dfrac{\text{total weight (w)}}{\text{total volume (v)}}$

    $\rho = \dfrac{2}{v}$

    $w = (v)(\rho) = (50 \text{ ml})(1.05 \text{ g/ml}) = 52.5 \text{ g total}$

    $w = \text{total weight} = \text{weight of salt} + \text{weight of water}$

    $\text{Weight of water} = (1 \text{ g/ml})(50 \text{ ml}) = 50 \text{ g}$

    $52.5 = \text{weight of salt} + 50$

    $\text{Weight of salt} = 2.5 \text{ g}$

4. **C** $n_{O_2} = \dfrac{\text{weight}}{\text{GMW}} = \dfrac{64}{32} = 2; = n_{H_2} \dfrac{10}{2} = 5; n_{N_2} = \dfrac{84}{28} = 3$

$$X_{O_2} = \frac{n_{O_2}}{n_{O_2} + n_{N_2} + n_{H_2}} = \frac{2}{2 + 3 + 5} = \frac{2}{10} = 0.2$$

5. C $GMW = C_2H_5OH = 2(12) + 5(1) + 16 + 1 = 24 + 5 + 17 = 46$

Moles of $C_2H_5OH = \dfrac{\text{weight}}{GMW} = \dfrac{23}{46} = \frac{1}{2}$

kg of water $= (500\,ml)\left(\dfrac{1\,g}{1\,ml}\right)\left(\dfrac{1\,kg}{1000\,g}\right) = \dfrac{500}{1000}\,kg = \frac{1}{2}\,kg$

$m = \dfrac{\text{moles solute}}{\text{kg solvent}} = \dfrac{\frac{1}{2}}{\frac{1}{2}} = 1.0$

6. C GMW of $Na_2CO_3 = 2(23) + 12 + 3(16) = 58 + 48 = 106$

Moles of $Na_2CO_3 = \dfrac{\text{weight}}{GMW} = \dfrac{75}{106} = .71$

$M = \dfrac{\text{moles solvent}}{\text{liters solution}} = \dfrac{.71}{1} = 0.71$

7. A $V = (100\,ml)\left(\dfrac{1\,liter}{1000\,ml}\right) = \dfrac{100}{1000} = \dfrac{1}{10} = 0.1$

Moles $= (M)(V) = (2)(0.1) = 0.2$

8. D H_3PO_4 has three hydrogen protons; therefore $n = 3$.

$N = nM = (3)(3) = 9$

$V = (500\,ml)\left(\dfrac{1\,liter}{1000\,ml}\right) = \frac{1}{2}\,liter$

No. of equivalents $= (N)(V) = (9)(\frac{1}{2}) = 4.5$

9. A Find the number of moles that are required, and then find the weight.
Moles $= (F)(V) = (1.5)(2) = 3$
since moles $= \dfrac{\text{weight}}{GMW}$, then:
Weight $= (GMW)(\text{moles}) = (58)(3) = 174$
GMW of $NaCl = 23 + 35 = 58$.

10. B $M_2V_2 = M_1V_1$

$V_2 = \dfrac{M_1V_1}{M_2} = \dfrac{(1.5)(500)}{1.0} = 750\,ml$ total volume

Then, $750 - 500 = 250\,ml$ for the added volume (e.g., pure water)

11. A In general, the ion with the highest charge-to-volume (or radius) ratio will be the most hydrated. Because all the charges are the same, the ion with the smallest radius will be the most densely charged and have the greatest hydration.

12. B $Cu(OH)_2 \rightleftharpoons Cu^{+2} + 2OH^-$

$K_{sp} = [Cu^{+2}][OH^-]^2 = (3.4 \times 10^{-7})(6.8 \times 10^{-7})^2$

$\approx (3 \times 10^{-7})(7 \times 10^{-7})^2 \approx (3 \times 10^{-7})(49 \times 10^{-14})$

$\approx (3 \times 10^{-7})(50 \times 10^{-14}) \approx 150 \times 10^{-21} \approx 1.5 \times 10^{-19}$

Note that estimation works well.

13. D $Cu(IO_3)_2 \rightleftharpoons Cu^{+2}\ 2IO_3^-$

$K_{sp} = [Cu^{+2}][IO_3^-]^2$

$[Cu^{+2}] = $ amt dissolved $= 3 \times 10^{-3}$

$[IO_3^-] = $ twice the amount dissolved $= 2(3 \times 10^{-3}) = 6 \times 10^{-3}$

$K_{sp} = (3 \times 10^{-3})(6 \times 10^{-3})^2 = (3 \times 10^{-3})(36 \times 10^{-6}) = 108 \times 10^{-9}$

$= 1.08 \times 10^{-7}$

Note that when the options are nearly equal, estimation should not be used.

14. B $BaSO_4 \rightleftharpoons Ba^{+2} + SO_4^{-2}$

$$K_{sp} = [Ba^{+2}][SO_4^{-2}]$$

$$[Ba^{+2}] = [SO_4^{-2}]$$

$$K_{sp} = 1 \times 10^{-10} = [Ba^{+2}][Ba^{+2}] = [Ba^{+2}]^2$$

$$[Ba^{+2}] = (1 \times 10^{-10})^{1/2} = 1 \times 10^{-5}$$

15. C $PbSO_4 \rightleftharpoons Pb^{+2} + SO_4^{-2}$

$$K_{sp} = [Pb^{+2}][SO_4^{-2}] = 1 \times 10^{-8}$$

$$[Pb^{+2}][2 \times 10^{-2}] = 1 \times 10^{-8}$$

$$[Pb^{+2}] = \frac{1 \times 10^{-8}}{2 \times 10^{-2}} = 0.5 \times 10^{-6} = 5 \times 10^{-7}$$

Because each $PbSO_4$ gives only one Pb^{+2} per molecule, the $[Pb^{+2}]$ in solution is the same as the amount of $PbSO^4$ that dissolves in the solution—an example of the common ion effect.

Acids and Bases

Self-Managed Learning Questions

1. What are amphiprotic substances? List an example.
2. What are antacid tablets? What chemical reactions do they have with gastric juice?
3. Explain why a solution of a strong base and its salt cannot act as a buffer solution? (HCl + NaOH)
4. How do you find the percentage ionization of an acid or base in the laboratory?

ACID/BASE EQUILIBRIA

Bronsted Definition of Acid and Base

Certain acids or bases fall under one classification; others may fall under more than one. According to the **Brønsted-Lowry definition,** an acid is a substance that can donate H^+ and a base is a substance that can accept H^+. The Brønsted-Lowry concept differs from the Arrhenius definition of acids and bases (substances that can dissociate into H^+ are acids and substances that dissociate into OH^- are bases) in that it does not restrict acids and bases to aqueous solutions. Also, a base need only be able to accept a proton from a donor; it does not have to produce hydroxide ions.

Ionization of Water

K_w is an equilibrium constant that relates hydroxide ion and hydronium ion concentrations in a aqueous solution:

$$K_w = \text{water ionization constant} = [H_3O^+][OH^-]$$

$$K_w = 1.008 \times 10^{-14} \text{ at } 25°C$$

pH is defined as follows:

$$pH = -\log[H+] = \log\left(\frac{1}{[H+]}\right)$$

$[H^+]$ = hydrogen ion concentration in moles/liter as molarity or normality (both are the same in this case).

The pK_A and pOH are similarly defined. The pH of water solutions at 25°C range from pH = 1 to pH = 14. The neutral pH of pure water is 7; a pH < 7 is acid and a pH > 7 is basic. The dissociation of water is:

$$H_2O \rightleftharpoons H^+ + OH^-$$

$$K_w = [H^+][OH^-] = 10^{-14}$$

Note that K_w is not the equilibrium constant. In this relationship:

$$pH + pOH = 14$$

Conjugate Acids and Bases

If an acid is strong, its conjugate base is weak and vice versa. The same is true for bases and their conjugate acids. This terminology is illustrated as follows:

HA	+	B	$\rightleftharpoons$	A$^-$	+	HB$^+$
acid$_1$		base$_2$		conjugate base$_1$		conjugate acid$_2$

Strong Acids and Bases

The strength of an acid (protic, esp.) is determined by its ability to donate protons (H^+). Strength refers to the extent of acid ionization (strong acids ionize 100%), and not to the concentration of an acid in a solution. The strength of a base is determined by its ability to accept protons. This strength is measured by the acid (or base) dissociation constant:

Acid:

$$HA \rightleftharpoons H^+ + A^- \text{ (neglecting solvent, } H^+ (H_2O) \text{ or } H_3O^+ \text{ is more realistic)}$$

$$K_A = \frac{[H^+][A^-]}{[HA]} \text{ at equilibrium}$$

Base:

$$MOH \rightleftharpoons M^+ + OH^- \text{ (for hydroxy bases)}$$

$$K_B = \frac{[M^+][OH^-]}{[MOH]} \text{ at equilibrium}$$

The larger the $K_A(K_B)$, the stronger the acid (base). The smaller the pK_A (pK_B), the stronger the acid (base). Common examples of strong acids are H_2SO_4 (sulfuric acid), HCl (hydrochloric acid), HNO_3 (nitric acid), HI (hydroiodic acid), HBr (hydrobromic acid) and $HClO_4$ (perchloric acid). Examples of strong bases are NaOH, KOH, LiOH and $Ca(OH)_2$. The H^+ of a strong acid or the OH^- of a strong base can be calculated from the normality of the acid or base. Common strong bases include hydroxides or oxides of group IA or IIA metals, the most common of which are NaOH and KOH.

Weak Acids and Bases

Examples of weak acids are H_3PO_4 (phosphoric acid), H_3BO_3 (boric acid), H_2CO_3 (carbonic acid), H_2SO_3 (sulfurous acid), and CH_3CO_2H (acetic acid). Common weak bases include NH_3 (ammonia), CO_3^- (carbonate ion), CH^- (cyanide ion), $(C_2H_5)_3N$ (triethylamine), and $(CH_3)_3N$ (trimethylamine). The important weak base is NH_3 or NH_4OH. Organic acids and some phenols usually are weak acids. The organic bases are amines and are weak. The **H^+ (OH^-) from a weak acid (base)** cannot be calculated from the normality of the acid (base), because they are only partially dissociated. These problems are rigorously solved by using the following equations.

$$K_A = \frac{[H^+][A^-]}{[HA]}$$

$$K_w = [H^+][OH^-]$$

The first equation can be simplified if $K_A \ll [HA]_0$ (original concentration of acid). Then:

$$[H^+] \approx \sqrt{K_A[HA]_0}$$

It is also possible to determine [H+] as follows:

$$HA \rightleftharpoons H^+ + A^-$$

Concentration

At start:	$[H]_0$	0	0
At equilibrium:	$[HA]_0 - x$	x	x (assume negligible H^+ from water)

Then: $K_A = \dfrac{[H^+][A^-]}{[HA]} = \dfrac{(x)(x)}{[HA]_0 - x}$

$$x = \text{amount of HA that dissociates in } \frac{\text{moles}}{\text{liter}} = [H^+]$$

To solve the equation using the quadratic formula, or if the x is small relative to $[HA]_0$, neglect x in the expression $[HA]_0 - x$, and solve for $[H^+] \approx R(KA[HA])_0$ as before.

Dissociation occurs when an acid or base either dissolves in water or breaks up into its ions. A strong acid dissociates completely. A weak acid dissociates incompletely. The conjugate base (acid) of a weak acid (base) is strong.

Hydrolysis occurs when molecules of water are split apart. A general concept is that if a salt is composed of cations from a strong base and anions from a weak acid, the salt will form a basic solution when it is dissolved in water. Strong acids react with strong bases to produce neutral solutions. Strong acids and weak bases produce acidic salts, whereas strong bases and weak acids produce basic salts. Because they hydrolyze in water (the process in hydrolysis): **a salt of a weak acid is basic**

CH_3CO_2H (acetic acid) is a weak acid

$CH_3CO_2^- \, Na^+$ (sodium acetate) is the salt

$CH_3CO_2^- \, Na^+ + HOH \rightleftharpoons CH_3CO_2H + Na^+ + OH^-$ solution is basic

and **a salt of a weak base is acidic**:

NH_4OH is a weak base

NH_4Cl is the salt

$NH_4Cl + HOH \rightleftharpoons NH_4OH + H^+ + Cl^-$ solution is acidic

Equilibrium Constants K_a and K_b and pK_a and pK_b

K_a is the equilibrium constant for a weak acid and K_b is the equilibrium constant for a weak base. The smaller the value of K_a or K_b, the weaker the acid or base.

Buffers

A buffer solution resists changes in pH. For biologic substances, buffers make the pH values rather stable, holding the pH of a solution relatively constant when an acid or base is added. The pH of blood is about 7.4. Carbonate, bicarbonate, and phosphate ions act as buffers for blood. The multiple acid-base groups in biologic molecules, such as proteins and lipids, act as buffers in the human body. Buffers are mixtures of weak acids or bases and their salts. For example:

1. Acetic acid, sodium acetate
   CH_3CO_2H, $CH_3CO_2^-$, Na^+
2. Carbonic acid, sodium bicarbonate
   H_2CO_3, $NaHCO_3$
3. Ammonium hydroxide, ammonium chloride
   NH_4OH, NH_4Cl

Most strong acids or bases and their salts do not make good buffers because they cannot hold the pH constant. A buffer works by having an acid component to neutralize added bases and a basic component to neutralize added acids. It is best to use weak acids or bases and their salts. For example, for acetic acid-acetate buffer:

CH_3CO_2H combines with added base

$CH_3CO_2H + OH^- \rightleftharpoons CH_3CO_2^- + H_2O$

$CH_3CO_2^-$ combines with added acid

$CH_3CO_2^- + H^+ \rightleftharpoons CH_3CO_2H$

Hence, the pH that depends on free H^+ or OH^- is held nearly constant. Clearly, it is the ratio of salt and weak acid or base that is important.

The **Henderson-Hasselbalch relation** points out the importance of the ratio:

$$HA + H_2O \xrightarrow{K_A} H_3O^+ + A^-$$

$$K_A = \frac{[H_3O^+][A^-]}{[HA]}, \text{ for } H_2O$$

(HA = acid and A^- = salt of the acid)

solving for $[H_3O^+]$:

$$[H_3O^+] = \left(\frac{[HA]}{[A^-]}\right)(K_A) \text{ or}$$

$$pH = pK_A + \log\frac{[A^-]}{[HA]}, \text{ which are equivalent expressions}$$

The **effectiveness of a buffer** can be understood in terms of this relation. Buffers are most effective when (1) the desired pH (of the solution) is near the pK_A, and (2) when ratios ($[A^-]/[HA]$) are in the range of 0.1 to 10; the ratio changes slowly and, thus, the pH changes slowly when the ratio = 1 (i.e., $[A^-] = [HA]$).

Important buffers in the human body are: (1) phosphates, inorganic and organic (least important); (2) carbonic acid—bicarbonate (most important); and (3) proteins (moderate importance).

Suppose you are asked to calculate the ratio of $[HCO_3^-]$ to $[H_2CO_3]$ required to maintain a pH of 7.2 in the bloodstream of a mammal. The value of $K_A = 8 \times 10^{-7}$ for H_2CO_3 in blood. The reaction equation is:

$$HCO_3^- + H^+ \rightarrow H_2CO_3$$

Follow these steps to find the solution:

$$pH = -\log [H+]$$

$$7.2 = -\log [H+]$$

$$\log[H+] = -8.0 + 0.8 \text{ (refer to Math Concept 1)}$$

From definition of log (refer to Math Concept 8):

$$[H^+] = 10^{-8} \times 10^{0.8}$$

$$10^{0.8} = 6.31$$

$$[H^+] = 6.31 \times 10^{-8}$$

$$8 \times 10^{-7} = K_A = \frac{[H^+][HCO_3^-]}{[H_2CO_3]} = (6.31)(10^{-8}) \frac{[HCO_3^-]}{[H_2CO_3]}$$

$$\frac{[HCO_3^-]}{[H_2CO_3]} = \frac{8(10^{-7})}{(6.31)(10^{-8})} = 12.7 \approx 13$$

The required ratio is 13.

When the concentration of $H_2CO_3 - HCO_3'$ buffer system deviates from normal, physiologic mechanisms initiate actions to restore the ratio to normal. Blood pH = 7.4 for $\frac{HCO_3^-}{H_2CO_3}$ ratio of concentration of 20:1. The kidneys and lungs tend to change concentration with a disturbance from 20:1.

ACID/BASE TITRATIONS

Titration is the procedure for accurate analysis of the amount of acid or base in a given sample. A titration may be done as follows:

Indicators

$$f = \text{fraction of acid neutralized} = \text{equivalents of base} \frac{\text{added}}{n_o}$$

n_o = original equivalents of acid

V = original volume of acid

v = volume of base added

$[H^+]$ (from acid and water) = $[OH^-]$ at the equivalence point
then,

$$[H^+] = \frac{(n_o)(1 - f)}{(V + v)} + \text{contribution from the } H_2O \text{ (usually negligible)}$$

= acid concentration at any given point during the titration up to

neutralization by base (f = 1.0)

Note that $\frac{(n_o)(1 - f)}{(V + v)}$ = amount of acid not neutralized by

added base

An **acid-base indicator** is a substance that is used to indicate the end point of a titration by some physical property (e.g., a substance that has one color in an acid solution and a different color in a basic solution).

Neutralization

Neutralization reactions are solved using the following equation:

$$N_A V_A = N_B V_B$$

in which N = normality, V = volume in liters, A = acid, and B = base. A neutralization reaction is one in which the number of equivalents of acid is exactly neutralized by an equal number of equivalents of base.

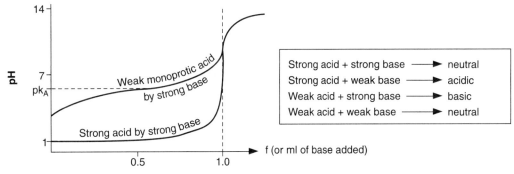

Fig. 7-36. Titration curves.

Strong acid + strong base	→ neutral
Strong acid + weak base	→ acidic
Weak acid + strong base	→ basic
Weak acid + weak base	→ neutral

Interpretation of Titration Curves

Titration curves can be used to calculate the normality of unknown acid (base) solutions, the equivalent weight of an unknown base or acid, or pK_A (pK_B) values. The point in a titration at which the acid has been exactly neutralized by addition of a base is the equivalence point. Examples of titration curves are provided in Figure 7-36. Note that the curve differs for strong and weak acids, and that the pK_A = pH where the acid is half neutralized.

APPLIED CONCEPTS

1. Review the $Na^+ - H^+$ exchange in the kidneys.
2. Review urinary buffer systems that are controlled by the phosphate buffer system, the ammonia buffer system, and the carbonic acid buffer system.
3. Review hypoventilation in which CO_2 is retained, increasing pCO_2 in the lungs.
4. Analyze acid-base disturbances by ionic equations to illustrate metabolic acidosis, metabolic alkalosis, respiratory acidosis, and respiratory alkalosis.

ACIDS AND BASES: REVIEW QUESTIONS

1. An acid is a substance that can donate hydrogen ion (H+). This definition of acids was given by:

   A. Lewis.
   B. Arrhenius.
   C. Brønsted-Lowry.
   D. none of the above.

2. A base is an electron pair donor. This definition of bases was given by:

   A. Arrhenius.
   B. Brønsted-Lowry.
   C. Lewis.
   D. none of the above.

3. The conjugate base of a weak acid (one that dissociates incompletely) is:

   A. weak.
   B. strong.
   C. highly alkaline.
   D. highly acidic.

4. Given the reaction of acid (HA) and base (B):

   $$HA + B \rightleftharpoons A^- + HB^+$$

   which of the following statements is correct?

   A. A^- is the conjugate of acid of HA.
   B. A^- is the conjugate base of B.
   C. HB^+ is the conjugate acid of B.
   D. HB^+ is the conjugate base of HA.

5. The salt of a strong acid and a strong base is:

   A. basic.
   B. neutral.
   C. acidic.
   D. none of the above.

6. The salt of a weak acid and a strong base is:

   A. basic.
   B. neutral.
   C. acidic.
   D. none of the above.

7. The salt of a weak base and a strong acid is:

   A. basic.
   B. neutral.
   C. acidic.
   D. none of the above.

8. Select the weakest acid:

   A. HCl
   B. HNO_3
   C. H_2SO_4
   D. CH_3CO_2H

9. Select the strongest acid:

   A. CH_3CO_2H
   B. H_3PO_4
   C. H_2CO_3
   D. H_2SO_4

10. Select the weakest base:

    A. NaOH
    B. KOH
    C. NH_3
    D. $Ca(OH)_2$

11. All of the following are important buffer systems of the body EXCEPT:

    A. carbonic acid-bicarbonate.
    B. phosphates.
    C. proteins.
    D. nucleic acids.

12. A buffer solution is most effective when:

    A. a strong acid or base and its salt are used.
    B. the desired pH is near the pK of the acid or base.
    C. the ratio of salt to acid (base) is less than $\frac{1}{10}$ or greater than 10.
    D. a strong acid is mixed with a weak acid.

13. A buffer solution is made of:

    A. strong acids and their salts.
    B. strong bases and their salts.
    C. weak bases or weak acid and their salts.
    D. weak acid.

14. Consider the structure for borane:

    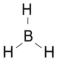

    Given that boron has an atomic number of five, and B-H bonds are relatively strong covalent bonds, borane is a(n):

    A. acid, according to Brønsted-Lowry.
    B. acid, according to Lewis.
    C. acid, according to Arrhenius.
    D. base, according to Lewis.

15. Ammonia is a(n):

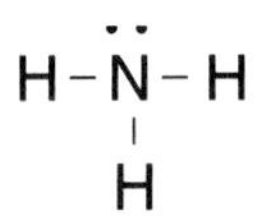

$$H-\overset{\cdot\cdot}{\underset{|}{N}}-H$$
$$H$$

    A. acid, according to Brønsted-Lowry.
    B. base, according to Brønsted-Lowry.
    C. base, according to Lewis.
    (D.) base, according to both Brønsted-Lowry and Lewis.

16. Pyruvic acid is a weak acid. Sodium hydroxide is a strong base. When combined, they form water and sodium pyruvate (a salt). If this salt is placed in water, the solution will be:

    (A.) basic.
    B. neutral.
    C. acidic.
    D. slightly basic.

17. Given the acid HA that dissociates into H^+ and A^-, what is the acid dissociation constant (K_A)?

    (A.) $K_A = \dfrac{[H^+][A^-]}{[HA]}$

    B. $K_A = \dfrac{[HA]}{[HA^+][A^-]}$

    C. $K_A = [HA][HA^+][A^-]$

    D. $K_A = \dfrac{[HA][HA^+]}{[A^-]}$

18. Acid 1 has an acid dissociation constant (K_{A1}) of 5×10^{-5}. Acid 2 has a $K_{A2} = 9 \times 10^{-7}$. Which of the following statements is true?

    A. Acid 1 is a weaker acid than acid 2.
    (B.) The conjugate base of acid 1 is a weaker base than the conjugate base of acid 2.
    C. Both are true.
    D. Neither are true.

19. How many milliequivalents of acid are in 50 ml of a 2 M solution of HCl?

    (A.) 100
    B. 10
    C. 1
    D. 0.1

20. What approximate volume (ml) of a 0.1 M acid would be required to neutralize 50 ml of a 0.3 M base?

    $M_A V_A = M_B V_B$

    A. 17
    (B.) 150
    C. 300
    D. 450

21. If 100 ml of a 2 M solution of acid neutralizes 25 ml of a solution of base, what is the molarity of the base?

    A. 0.5
    B. 2
    C. 4
    (D.) 8

22. Select the incorrect expression for pH ($[H+]$ = hydrogen ion concentration):

    A. $pH = -\log[H^+]$
    B. $pH = \log[H^+]^{-1}$
    (C.) $pH = 1/\log[H^+]$
    D. $pH = \log(1/[H^+])$

23. A solution has a hydroxide ion concentration of 10^{-8}. What is the pH?

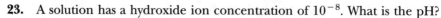

$K_w = [H][OH] = 10^{14}$

A. 0
B. 1
C. 6
D. 8

24. A solution has a hydrogen ion concentration $[H^+]$ of 2×10^{-6}. If $\log 2 = 0.30$, what is the pH?

A. 4.3
B. 5.7
C. 6.3
D. 12.3

$pH = -\log [H^+]$

25. A solution has a pH = 9.3. What is the hydrogen ion concentration (antilog 0.30 = 2, antilog 0.70 = 5)?

A. 5×10^{-9}
B. 2×10^{-9}
C. 5×10^{-10}
D. 2×10^{-10}

26. A solution has a pOH = 9. What is the hydrogen ion concentration?

A. 10^{-9}
B. 10^9
C. 10^5
D. 10^{-5}

$pH + pOH = 14$

27. What is the pH of a 0.01 M solution of HCl (strong acid)?

A. 1
B. 2
C. -1
D. Cannot be determined

28. Calculate the pH of a 0.001 M solution of NaOH (strong base):

A. 11
B. 4
C. 1
D. 3

29. A 0.10 M solution of monoprotic weak acid is 10% ionized. Calculate the pH:

A. 0.01
B. 0.1
C. 1
D. 2

30. If the KA is less than the original concentration, HA_o, of a weak acid in solution, and H^+ = hydrogen ion concentration, then:

A. $K_A \approx [H^+] + [HA]_o$

B. $[H^+] \approx \sqrt{K_A[HA]_o}$

C. $K_A \approx \dfrac{[H^+]}{[HA]_o}$

D. $[H^+] \approx \sqrt{\dfrac{K_A}{[HA]_o}}$

31. The acid dissociation constant (K_A) of a weak monoprotic acid is 4×10^{-5}. What is the $[H^+]$ of a 0.1 M solution?

A. 4×10^{-6}
B. 4×10^{-5}
C. 2×10^{-4}
D. 2×10^{-3}

32. The following graph shows the titration of a weak monoprotic acid by a base. Which point (or line) represents the pK_A of the acid?

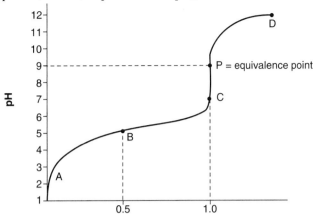

Fraction of acid neutralized (f)

   A. A
   B. B
   C. C
   D. D

33. All of the following acids or bases may be used to make a buffer solution EXCEPT:

   A. H_2CO_3.
   B. H_2SO_4.
   C. NH_4OH.
   D. CH_3CO_2H.

34. Which of the following calculation results indicates the pH of a buffer solution, made of 0.1 M acid (with a $pK_A = 5$), and its salt, which is 1.0 M?

   A. 5.1
   B. 6
   C. 6.1
   D. 7

35. A buffer solution with a pH = 3.3 is desired. An acid (with a $pK_A = 4.3$) and its salt are available. What ratio of salt to acid is required?

   A. 10
   B. 1
   C. $\frac{1}{10}$
   D. $\frac{1}{100}$

ANSWERS AND EXPLANATIONS

1–13. 1-C, 2-C, 3-B, 4-C, 5-B, 6-A, 7-C, 8-D, 9-D, 10-C, 11-D, 12-B, 13-C. See text for explanation.

14. B Because the atomic number is five, the electron configuration is $1s^2\, 2s^2\, 2p^1$. With only 3 bonding electrons ($2s^2\, 2p^1$) to fill the four possible bonding orbitals (2s, $2p_x$, $2p_y$, $2p_z$), there is one vacant orbital that can accept an electron pair. Lewis' definition of an acid is an electron pair acceptor. The information about the covalent bond is to suggest that the H do not dissociate, and, therefore, the Arrhenius and Brønsted-Lowry definitions do not hold.

15. D Ammonia is a base by Brønsted-Lowry because it is a proton acceptor. It is also a base by Lewis, because it is an electron pair donor.

16. A The reaction is:

$$\text{Pyruvic acid} + NaOH \rightarrow H_2O + Na\ \text{pyruvate}$$

$$Na\ \text{pyruvate} + HOH \rightleftharpoons \text{pyruvic acid} + Na^+\ OH^-$$

It is the free OH^- in solution that makes the solution basic. Undissociated acid (e.g., pyruvic acid) has no effect on the acidic or basic nature of the solution.

17. A The K_A is defined as the equilibrium constant of this reaction:

$$HA \rightleftharpoons H^+ + A^- \text{ at equilibrium}$$

which is given as:

$$K_A = \frac{[H^+][A^-]}{[HA]}$$

18. B The larger the K_A, the stronger the acid. Also, stronger acids have weaker conjugate bases (see text for terminology). Note that $10^{-5} > 10^{-7}$, which means acid 1 is stronger than acid 2 and its conjugate base is weaker.

19. A MV = moles if V = liters, M = moles/liter
MV = millimoles (mm) if V = ml, M = mm/ml
(2 mm/ml)(50 ml) = 100 mm

20. B $M_A V_A = M_B V_B$

$$V_A = \frac{M_B V_B}{M_A} = \frac{(0.3)(50)}{(0.1)} = (3)(50) = 150 \text{ ml}$$

21. D $M_A V_A = M_B V_B$

$$M_B = \frac{M_A V_A}{V_B} = \frac{(2)(100)}{(25)} = (2)(4) = 8 \text{ M}$$

22. C Recall that: $-\log x = \log x^{-1} = \log\left(\frac{1}{x}\right)$

23. C Because: $K_w = [H^+][OH^-] = 10^{-14}$

$$[H^+] = \frac{10^{-14}}{[OH^-]} = \frac{10^{-14}}{10^{-8}} = 10^{-6}$$

then: $pH = -\log[H^+] = -\log 10^{-6} = -(-6) = +6$

or: $pOH = -\log[OH^-] = -\log 10^{-8} = -(-8) = 8$

$$pH + pOH = 14$$
$$pH = 14 - pOH = 14 - 8 = 6$$

24. B $pH = -\log[H^+] = -\log 2 \times 10^{-6} = -(\log 2 + \log 10^{-6})$
$= -(0.30 - 6) = -(-5.7) = 5.7$

25. C $pH = -\log[H^+]$
$9.3 = -\log H^+$
$\log[H^+] = -9.3 = 0.7 - 10$
$[H^+] = 10^{0.7} \times 10^{-10}$
$[H^+] = 5 \times 10^{-10}$

Study these steps carefully. Several important log relationships are shown as discussed in Chapter 6.

26. D First method:

Step (a): $pH + pOH = 14$
$pH = 14 - pOH = 14 - 9 = 5$

Step (b): $pH = -\log[H^+]$
$5 = -\log[H^+]$
$-5 = \log[H^+]$
$10^{-5} = [H^+]$

Second method:

$$\text{Step (a): pOH} = -\log [OH^-]$$

$$9 = -\log [OH^-]$$

$$-9 = \log [OH^-]$$

$$10^{-9} = [OH^-]$$

$$\text{Step (b): } [H^+][OH^-] = 10^{-14}$$

$$[H+] = \frac{10^{-14}}{[OH^-]} = \frac{10^{-14}}{10^{-9}} = 10^{-5}$$

27. B The $[H^+]$ of a strong acid is the normality of the acid. For HCl (a monoprotic acid), the molarity and normality are equal.

$$[H^+] = 0.01 = 1 \times 10^{-2}$$

$$pH = -\log [H^+] = -\log(10^{-2}) = -(-2) = 2$$

28. A The hydroxide concentration of a strong base is its normality. The molarity (M) is the same as normality (N) for NaOH. Then:

$$[OH^-] = 0.001 = 1 \times 10^{-3} = 10^{-3}$$

$$[H^+][OH^-] = 10^{-14}$$

$$[H^+] = 10^{-14} [OH^-] = \frac{10^{-14}}{10^{-3}} = 10^{-11}$$

$$pH = -\log [H^+] = -\log 10^{-11} = -(-11) = 11$$

Or,

$$pOH = -\log [OH^-] = -\log (10^{-3}) = -(-3) = 3$$

$$pH + pOH = 14$$

$$pH = 14 - pOH = 14 - 3 = 11$$

29. D For the reaction given:
$$HA \leftrightharpoons H^+ + A^-$$
The concentration of HA is 0.10 M at start; at equilibrium it is 10% ionized.

Then: $[H^+] = (10\%)(0.1) = 0.01 = 10^{-2}$

Then: $pH = -\log [H^+] = -\log(10^{-2}) = -(-2) = 2$

30. B This answer illustrates a formula to determine K_A for weak acids.

31. D The $[H^+]$ of a weak acid must be calculated from K_A. Because 0.1 AF 4×10^{-5}, use the formula:

$$[H^+] = \sqrt{K_A[HA]_o} = \sqrt{(4 \times 10^{-5})(10^{-1})} = \sqrt{4 \times 10^{-6}}$$

$$= \sqrt{4} \times \sqrt{10^{-6}} = \sqrt{2 \times 10^{-3}}$$

and:

$$2 \times 10^{-3} \ll 10^{-1}(0.002 \ll 0.1) \text{ so the assumption is correct.}$$

Another way to solve the problem is:

$$HA \rightleftharpoons H^+ + A^-$$

Concentration

At start: 0.1   0   0

At equilibrium: 0.1 − x   x   x

$$K_A = \frac{[H^+][A^-]}{[HA]} = \frac{[x][x]}{[0.1 - x]} = \frac{x^2}{0.1 - x} = \frac{x^2}{0.1} \text{ (assume x} \ll 0.1)$$

$$4 \times 10^{-5} = \frac{x^2}{10^{-1}}$$

$$x^2 = (10^{-1})(4 \times 10^{-5}) = 4 \times 10^{-6}$$

$$x = \sqrt{4 \times 10^{-6}} = \sqrt{4} \times \sqrt{10^{-6}} = 2 \times 10^{-3}$$

32. **B** Review the discussion of titration curves. The pK_A of an acid is the pH at which it can be half neutralized or $f = 0.5$.

33. **B** H_2SO_4 is a strong acid. Strong acids or bases do not make good buffers.

34. **B** Use the Henderson-Hasselbalch relation.

$$pH = pK_A + \log \frac{[A^-]}{[HA]} = 5 + \log \frac{1.0}{0.1} = 5 + \log 10 = 5 + 1 = 6$$

35. **C** Use the Henderson-Hasselbalch relation.

$$pH = pK_A + \log \frac{[A^-]}{[HA]}$$

$$3.3 = 4.3 + \log \frac{[A^-]}{[HA]}$$

$$-1 = \log \frac{[A^-]}{[HA]}$$

$$10^{-1} = \frac{[A^-]}{[HA]}$$

$$\frac{1}{10} = \frac{[A^-]}{[HA]}$$

Thermochemistry and Thermodynamics

Self-Managed Learning Questions

1. Why does iodine sublime from solid to gaseous state?
2. Why is it better to wear several layers of clothes than to wear one thick jacket when it is cold?
3. What is the function of a catalyst in a chemical reaction? $KClO_3$ is used in the laboratory to produce O_2. If you add MnO_2 (a catalyst), the reaction speeds up. Why?
4. Is it reasonable to say as a thermochemist, "A flame is heat and light energy" when you burn a candle? What evidence would you propose to support or oppose this claim?
5. Are combustion and respiration physically the same? Are they biologically similar? Are they chemically similar? Cite as many examples as possible to explain the similarities.
6. Poikilotherms are animals whose body temperature more or less parallels ambient temperature, such as reptiles, fish, and amphibians. Does temperature affect the ventilation rate of a frog? How would you design an experiment to prove and determine the basic principle behind it?
7. How would you go about verifying the following hypothesis: "Within certain limits, the rates of physiologic processes involved in obtaining oxygen and delivering it to the tissue increase as the temperature of a system increases." Design a complete laboratory with clinical instruments or equipment to verify the hypothesis. What alterations or modifications to the hypothesis would you propose should you fail to support it?
8. Compare and contrast the high pressure (60,000 atmospheres) process to produce artificial diamonds versus the chemical vapor deposition. Read arguments before forming your opinions on both sides of the issue of producing artificial diamonds.

Thermodynamics deals with the physical laws that determine transfer and flow of heat, whereas **thermochemistry** deals with the heat absorbed or given out during chemical reactions.

Equivalence of Mechanical, Chemical, and Thermal Energy Units

All forms of energy—mechanical, chemical, and thermal—can be converted into heat, and all three types have units in common. One unit is the calorie, which can be defined as the amount of heat needed to raise the temperature of 1 g of pure water by 1°C, from 14.5°C to 15.5°C. A kilocalorie is equivalent to 1000 calories. You may know the kilocalorie as the Calorie (with a capital "C"), which is used in nutrition and dieting.

Temperature Scales

Temperature is considered a measure of the average thermal energy of a body; it is also a measure of the amount of energy absorbed or emitted as heat by a body. Thus, when temperature rises, the average kinetic energy per molecule rises, and the object absorbs more energy as heat, and vice versa.

$$\text{Temperature of molecules} = \text{Constant} \times mv^2 \text{ (average)}$$

Measurement of temperature is accomplished by thermometers. A thermometer has (1) a thermometric property (e.g., pressure, density, linear expansion, and resistance), which varies directly as temperature; (2) a lower fixed point (e.g., freezing point (FP) of water); (3) a higher fixed point (e.g., boiling point (BP) of water); and (4) a scale calibrated between these two points and extrapolated beyond them. Relative temperature scales are the **Celsius** or **Centigrade** (FP of water = 0°C, BP of water = 100°C) and the **Fahrenheit** (FP of water = 32°F, BP of water = 212°F). Absolute scales (the zero point of the scale is the true absolute zero) are the **Rankine** (°R) calibrated in °F units and the **Kelvin** (°K) calibrated in °C units. Interconversions of the scales are as follows:

$$°C = \tfrac{5}{9}\,(°F - 32) \text{ or } °F = (\tfrac{9}{5})\,°C + 32 \text{ and 5 units Celsius} = 9 \text{ units Fahrenheit}$$

$$°K = °C + 273, °R = °F + 460$$

The Celsius and Fahrenheit scales are equal at $-40°$.

Remember:

$$\text{Change in temperature } (\Delta T), \text{ heat capacity} = \frac{\text{heat gained}}{\text{temperature change}} = \frac{q}{\Delta T}$$

Measurement of Heat Changes (Calorimetry)

Specific heat capacity (C) is the heat capacity per unit mass per degree Celsius of substance:

$$C = \frac{\left(\dfrac{q}{\Delta T}\right)}{m} = \frac{q}{m\Delta T}$$

This formula can be rearranged to determine the amount of heat exchanged (gained or lost) by a substance:

$$q = (C)(m)(\Delta T)$$

The units of heat most commonly used are calories (or joules). A calorie is the amount of heat required to raise the temperature of 1 gram of water one degree Celsius. A kilocalorie is 1000 calories. Because heat is the transfer of energy, its units must be equivalent to the unit of other energies (kinetic or potential) or work, which is the joule (or other similar units). It is important to know the **interconversion of calories and joules**:

$$4.184 \text{ joules} = 1 \text{ calorie}$$

$$4.2 \text{ joules} \approx 1 \text{ calorie}$$

The **specific heat of water** is then:

$$1\left(\frac{\text{calorie}}{g \times °C}\right)$$

It is in the understanding of **phase transitions** that specific heat, heat of fusion, and heat of vaporization have particular value (see previous sections concerning chemical bonding and phase equilibria). Important features of phase transitions are summarized in Table 7-5. Note that $H_V > H_f$ because usually more kinetic energy per molecule is required to separate liquid molecules to become gaseous than to separate solid molecules

TABLE 7-5. Phase Transitions

Phase Transition	Conditions	Heat Associated
Solid $\underset{\text{freeze}}{\overset{\text{melt}}{\rightleftharpoons}}$ liquid	Solid and liquid vapor pressure in equilibrium Temperature called melting (or freezing) point (MP or FP)	Heat of fusion (H_f) $H_f = q/m$ at MP or $q = m\,H_f$ $q = $ heat transferred $m = $ mass
Liquid $\underset{\text{condense}}{\overset{\text{evaporate (boil)}}{\rightleftharpoons}}$ gas	Gas and liquid vapor pressure in equilibrium Temperature called the boiling point (BP).	Heat of evaporation (H_v) $H_v = q/m$ at BP or $q = H_v\,m$

TABLE 7-6. Changes Associated with Substances Gaining Heat

Phases and Temperatures	Solid Below MP	Solid (1) at → MP	Liquid (2) at → MP	Liquid (3) at → BP	Gas (4) at → BP	Gas (5) Above → BP
Heat changes	(1) Heat is absorbed to raise the temperature as the specific heat of the solid.	(2) Heat is absorbed as heat of fusion to cause solid to melt to the liquid. Note that the temperature does not change.	(3) Heat is absorbed as the specific heat of the liquid to raise its temperature.	(4) Heat is absorbed as heat of vaporization to cause the liquid to be converted to gas. The temperature does not change.	(5) Heat is absorbed as the specific heat of the gas to raise its temperature.	
	$q = C_s\, m\Delta T$	$q = H_f\, m$	$q = C_l\, m\Delta T$	$q = H_v\, m$	$q = C_g\, m\Delta T$	

Note: C_s, C_l, and C_g represent specific heat constants for a material in its solid, liquid, or gaseous phases, respectively.

to become liquid. As a substance gains or loses energy as heat, it passes through the various phases. A scheme for substances gaining heat is outlined in Table 7-6.

The reverse steps would hold if the substance was losing energy as heat. To summarize, heat is used to change the phase or the temperature of a substance. When two objects are in contact and at different temperatures, heat flows from the one with the higher temperature to the one with the lower temperature until the temperatures are equal. It is possible to calculate heat flows and temperatures by using:

Heat flow law: heat loss = heat gain

an equation that is important to memorize.

As an illustration, study the following example and how it relates to the heat flow law. You are preparing a small pot of chicken soup in the kitchen. The pot is made of a special alloy with a specific heat of 0.10. The specific heat of chicken soup is 0.83. Suddenly, you drop a large gold bracelet in the soup. The bracelet has a mass of 75 g. The pot has a mass of 500 g and it contains about 1000 g of chicken soup. The bracelet you were wearing had a temperature of 50°F. The specific heat of the bracelet is 0.032. The temperature of the pot and the soup inside it is 88°C. Find the final temperature of the bracelet.

Solution: Heat lost by hot substances = heat gained by cold substances.

The problem shows that chicken soup and the pot are hot, whereas the bracelet is cold. Convert the temperature of the bracelet to °C, using,

$$\frac{F - 32}{9} = \frac{C}{5}, \quad \frac{50 - 32}{9} = \frac{C}{5}$$

which shows the temperature of the bracelet is 10°C. Next, consider:

Heat lost by pot + heat lost by chicken soup = Heat gained by gold bracelet

Using the following subscripts: s = chicken soup, b = gold bracelet, and p = cooking pot:

$$C_p\,(m_p)(T_p - T_f) + C_s\,(m_s)(T_s - T_f) = C_b(m_b)(T_f - T_b)$$

t_f = Final temperature of bracelet and resulting mixture.

$$0.1\,(500)(88 - T_f) + 0.83\,(1000)(88 - T_f) = 0.032\,(75)(T_f - 10)$$

In other words, the bracelet's temperature is almost the same as the chicken soup, but it rose rapidly from 10°C to 87.8°C.

You could have approximated the answer to this problem by looking at the relative **masses** of various objects. This problem illustrates the use of the heat flow equation. When substances gain (or lose) heat, they usually undergo **expansion** (or **contraction**).

THERMOCHEMISTRY

Thermodynamic System and State Function

Thermodynamics is concerned with physical laws governing the energy states of molecules and chemical reactions. A system consists of a large number of molecules, the so-called "object" under study. It is the reference point. When the system gains energy, the (energy) change is positive. The environment is everything outside the system. Systems exchange energy by the processes of work or heat exchange. Systems do not contain work or heat. Work or heat exchange depends upon the path from the initial to the final state.

In contrast, state functions are independent of the path taken but depend on the initial and final states only. Important state functions are: pressure (P), volume (V), temperature (T), internal energy (E), entropy (S), enthalpy (H), and free energy (G).

Conservation of Energy

When conservation of energy occurs, all energy that is transferred between an object and its surroundings must be conserved, or accounted for, by the heat and work that is transferred between the object and its surroundings. For example, if a croquet ball strikes another croquet ball, the amount of energy that is lost by the first ball is equal to the amount of energy that is gained by the second ball. By transferring energy from one ball to the other, it is conserved.

$$\text{Reactants} \rightarrow \text{Products} + \text{Energy}$$

$$\text{Energy} + \text{Reactants} \rightarrow \text{Products}$$

Some reactions give off energy when products are formed and some reactions require energy to form products. Chemical energy is a form of potential energy. In a closed system or biochemical reaction, the addition of all forms of energy yields the total energy that is mostly conserved.

Endothermic/Exothermic Reactions

Exothermic reactions proceed with a negative ΔH, and endothermic reactions proceed with a positive ΔH:

$$\text{Exothermic: reactants} \rightarrow \text{products} + \text{heat}$$

$$\text{Endothermic: heat} + \text{reactants} \rightarrow \text{products}$$

Enthalpy (ΔH) is the energy change (in terms of heat content) in a chemical reaction that occurs at constant pressure. The natural tendency of systems is toward minimum energy: the lower the energy of the system, the more stable the system. Therefore, a reaction that occurs with loss of energy (or negative energy) is a favorable reaction. The standard enthalpy of formation (ΔH_f°) is the enthalpy change when one mole of a compound is formed from its elements at 298°k. An example is:

$$C + \tfrac{1}{2} O_2\,(g) \rightarrow CO(g) \quad \Delta H_f^\circ\,(CO) = -26.4\ \text{kcal}$$

The standard enthalpy change of a reaction (ΔH°) is:

$$\Delta H_f^\circ = \sum \Delta H_f^\circ\,(\text{products}) - \sum \Delta H_f^\circ\,(\text{reactants})$$

in which the ΔH_f° of all the products are added together and the ΔH_f° of all the reactants are subtracted from them. Note: the enthalpy of elements as they exist at 298°K is zero.

Hess's law of constant heat summation states that the ΔH° of the reactions can be added algebraically to derive the overall ΔH° for the overall reaction. Note that when the direction of a reaction is reversed, the sign of the ΔH° changes (from + to −, or from − to +). Also, if the reaction as written is multiplied (or divided) by a number, the ΔH° must also be multiplied (or divided) by the same number.

Try this sample problem:

Find the enthalpy of formation (ΔH_f°) of $Ca(OH)_2(s)$ given the following:

$$2H_2(g) + O_2(g) \rightarrow 2H_2O(l)$$

$$CaO(s) + H_2O(l) \rightarrow Ca(OH)_2(s)$$

$$2CaO(s) \rightarrow 2Ca(s) + O_2(g)$$

Answer: ΔH_f° of $Ca(OH)_2$ means its formation from $Ca(s)$, $H_2(g)$, and $O_2(g)$. Using the preceding principles:

$$\tfrac{1}{2}[2H_2(g) + O_2(g) \rightarrow 2H_2O(l)] \qquad \Delta H = \tfrac{1}{2}(-136.6\ \text{kcal})$$

$$CaO(s) + H_2O(l) \rightarrow Ca(OH)_2(s) \qquad \Delta H = -15.3\ \text{kcal}$$

$$\tfrac{1}{2}[2Ca(s) + O_2(g) \rightarrow 2CaO(s)] \qquad \Delta H = \tfrac{1}{2}(-303.6\ \text{kcal})$$

Rewriting the above:

$$H_2(g) + \tfrac{1}{2}O_2(g) \rightarrow H_2O(l) \qquad \Delta H = -68.3\ \text{kcal}$$

$$CaO(s) + H_2O(l) \rightarrow Ca(OH)_2(s) \qquad \Delta H = -15.3\ \text{kcal}$$

$$Ca(s) + \tfrac{1}{2}O_2(g) \rightarrow CaO(s) \qquad \Delta H = -151.8\ \text{kcal}$$

Net:

$$Ca(s) + H_2(g) + O_2(g) \rightarrow Ca(OH)_2(s) \quad \Delta H = -235.4 \text{ kcal}$$

(Note: the $CaO(s)$ and $H_2O(l)$ cancel because they are on opposite sides of the equation.)

Bond Dissociation Energy as Related to Heats of Formation

Bonded molecules have lower energy than separate atoms; therefore, when atoms combine to form molecules, they lose energy (when spontaneous). The **bond dissociation energy** (D) is the enthalpy change of the reaction in which a specific bond in a gaseous molecule is broken. The D is positive (i.e., it requires input of energy to break a bond). The **average bond energy** (E) is the approximate energy required to break a bond of a particular type (e.g., C—H) in any compound in which it may be found. Note that each C—H in CH_4 has a different D, but the E would be the average of all four of these bonds. The larger the numeric value (all are positive by definition) of the bond energy, the stronger the bond.

THERMODYNAMICS

Heat is the transfer of energy. Bodies do not contain heat; they either emit or absorb energy as heat. When a body absorbs or emits energy, all of the energy need not be in the form of heat. For example, a body emitting energy may emit some as heat and some as light energy. A body contains **thermal energy** (or internal energy), which is the sum of the potential and kinetic energies associated with the position or motion, respectively, of the molecules (see previous discussion of kinetic theory of gases in the section concerning phases and phase equilibria).

Thermal equilibrium results when the average kinetic energies per molecule of two bodies are equal, when the heat flow between the bodies is zero, and when the temperatures of the two bodies are equal.

First Law of Thermodynamics

Energy is a property of a system and not a process (like heat or work). Specifically, the internal energy change (ΔE) of a system depends on the work done and heat exchanged as follows:

$$\Delta E = q - w \text{ First Law of Thermodynamics}$$

$$q = + \text{ if heat is added to the system}$$

$$q = - \text{ if heat is lost from the system}$$

$$w = + p\Delta V \text{ if work is done by the system}$$

$$(p = \text{external pressure})$$

$\Delta V = V_f - V_i$ change in volume of the system
Note: this gives the sign to the work done by the system

The internal energy depends on the kinetic energies of the molecules, on the potential energies of forces between molecules, and the kinetic and potential energies of the electrons and nuclei. The first law of thermodynamics is a restatement of the law of conservation of energy. The ΔE of a reaction is determined by running the reaction at constant volume and measuring the amount of heat exchanged:

$$\Delta E = q - w = q - p\Delta V = q_v$$

$$\Delta V = 0$$

$$q_v = \text{heat at constant volume}$$

A reversible process is one that occurs in such small increments that it can be reversed at any point. An irreversible process is one that cannot be easily reversed. As an example, if you walked down a flight of stairs one step at a time, it would be fairly easy to reverse your direction at any step. If, however, you jumped out of a window, equivalent to going down a flight of stairs, you could not reverse yourself. For reversible (rev) and irreversible (irrev) processes, the following are true:

$$w_{rev} > w_{irrev}$$

$$q_{rev} > q_{irrev}$$

SECOND LAW OF THERMODYNAMICS

These concepts lead into entropy (S) and the second law of thermodynamics, which is:

$$\Delta S = \left(\frac{q_{rev}}{T}\right) \text{ for a reversible path} = \text{change in entropy}$$

Entropy (S) is a measure of the disorder of a thermodynamic system. It represents that part of the energy that has become unavailable for further work. **Free energy (G)** is the amount of energy that is available to carry out work.

These two quantities are both state functions—their values depend exclusively on the absolute state of the system, rather than the path that was taken to arrive at that state.

The thermodynamic changes that take place during a chemical reaction are expressed by the following equation:

$$\Delta G = \Delta H - T\Delta S$$

in which ΔH is the change in enthalpy of the system and T is the absolute temperature in degrees Kelvin.

Two important points to note:

1. ΔS system is still independent of a particular reversible path
2. ΔS universe is increasing for an irreversible path

For chemical reactions, the following conditions hold. If:

$\Delta G = 0$, then the reaction is at equilibrium
$\Delta G < 0$, then a spontaneous reaction (no change in external conditions) is possible
$\Delta G > 0$, then no spontaneous reaction is possible

The system tends toward a minimal value of ΔG, which is the maximal stability.

The more negative ΔG, the more probable the reaction will go as written. In summary, the ΔG represents the useful energy the system has to do work. As with ΔH:

$$\Delta G^\circ = \sum \Delta G_f^\circ \text{ (products)} - \sum \Delta G_f^\circ \text{ (reactants)}$$

Spontaneous Reactions and ΔG°

When a chemical reaction is spontaneous, it will go to equilibrium if given enough time and will have an equilibrium constant greater than 1. Gibbs equation for spontaneity of a chemical reaction is:

$$\Delta G^\circ_{reaction} = \sum m\Delta G_f^\circ(\text{products}) - \sum n\Delta G_f^\circ(\text{reactants})$$

On the basis of this equation, three rules of thumb about **spontaneity** can be determined: (1) if ΔG has a negative value, the chemical reaction is spontaneous; (2) if ΔG has a positive value, the chemical reaction is not spontaneous, and (3) if ΔG equals 0, the chemical reaction is at equilibrium.

Heat Transfer

Heat flows between substances by conduction, convection, and radiation. **Conduction** is a process in which heat energy is transferred by adjacent molecular collisions throughout a material medium, that is, the medium does not move. The heat energy is carried off by the motion of the electrons. Good electrical conductors, therefore, are usually good heat conductors. The rate of heat transfer (H) by conduction is illustrated in Figure 7-37. Note that the rate (H) is directly proportional to A and Δt and inversely proportional to L. The thermal conductivity, k, is a property of the substance.

Convection is a process in which heat energy is transferred by the actual mass motion of a fluid (gas or liquid). Convection currents are set up that may be natural (caused by density differences, e.g., wind) or forced (as in a house ventilation system). The rate of energy transfer (H) is: $H = Q/T = hA\Delta t$ (note the relations shown). The convection coefficient h is not a property of the substance.

Radiation is a process in which heat energy is transferred by electromagnetic waves absorbed or emitted at the atomic level. All substances radiate heat regardless of the temperature. In general, as the absolute temperature (T) increases, the wavelength of the emitted heat decreases. The rate of radiation (heat) emitted per unit area (R) is:

$$R = e\delta T^4 \text{ (Stefan-Boltzmann law)}$$

in which T = absolute temperature, e = emissivity = the ability to absorb or emit thermal radiation, and δ = Stefan-Boltzmann's constant.

The **key relation** is that R is proportional to the fourth power of the absolute tempera-

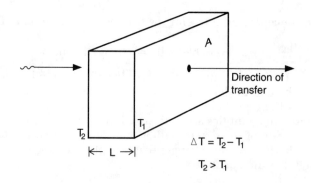

Fig. 7-37.

$$H = \frac{Q}{t} = kA\,(\Delta T/L)$$

Q = heat exchanged
t = time elapsed
A = cross-sectional area
L = length over which transfer occurs
ΔT = temperature difference
H = rate of energy transfer

ture. A body at the same temperature as its surroundings will radiate and absorb heat at the same rate. If not at the same temperature, the net rate of radiation is:

Net rate of radiation = rate of energy emission − rate of energy absorption

$$R = e\delta\, T_1^4 - e\delta\, T_2^4 = e\delta(T_1^4 - T_2^4)$$

in which T1 = temperature of body and T2 = temperature of surroundings.

The **coefficient of expansion** measures the rate at which objects expand for increase in temperature. The **linear expansion coefficient** follows:

$$\alpha = \frac{L_f - L_i}{(T_f - T_i)L_i}$$

$$= \frac{\text{final length} - \text{initial length}}{L_i\,(\text{Final temperature} - \text{initial temperature})}$$

$$L_f - L_i = L_i\alpha\,(T_f - T_i) = a(\Delta T)L_i$$

$$L_f - L_i - L_i\alpha\Delta T$$

$$L_f - L_i\,(1 - \alpha\,\Delta t)$$

The units of a are $(°C)^{-1}$ or $(°F)^{-1}$. The concept of linear expansion can also be applied to areas and volumes (Fig. 7-38).

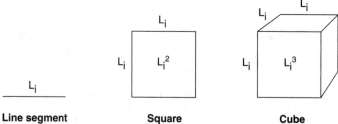

Fig. 7-38.   Line segment   Square   Cube

The **coefficient of expansion for surfaces** follows:

$$\beta = \frac{A_f - A_i}{A_i\,(T_f - T_i)}$$

in which A_f, A_i = initial and final areas.

The **coefficient of expansion** for volumes follows:

$$\gamma = \frac{V_f - V_i}{V_i(T_f - T_i)}$$

in which V_f, V_i = final and initial volumes.

If you know $A_f = A_i(1 + \beta\Delta T)$ and $V_f = V_i(1 + \gamma\Delta T)$ and $L_f = L_i(1 + \alpha\Delta T)$, you can determine (using polynomial approximations) that $\gamma = 3\alpha$, $\beta = 2a$.

As shown in Table 7-7, expansion (contraction) can be by linear dimensions, area, or volume.

Heats of Fusion and Vaporization

Heat of fusion is the energy needed to convert a solid to a liquid. The formula for heat of fusion follows:

$$\text{Heat} = \text{molar enthalpy of fusion} = \Delta H_{fusion} \text{ (J/mol)}$$

The enthalpy of vaporization is the amount of heat needed for a molecule to break free of intermolecular forces and move from the liquid state to the gas state. A low enthalpy of fusion means that a solid melts at a low temperature, and a high enthalpy of fusion means a solid melts at a high temperature.

To change water at $0°C$ to ice at $0°C$ requires 80 cal, and to change water at $100°C$ to steam at $100°C$ requires about 536 cal. It takes energy to form ice from water and to form steam from water. Some substances change directly from solid to gaseous state (try I_2 in the laboratory), where heat of sublimation becomes another heat of vaporization.

APPLIED CONCEPTS

Thermodynamics and thermochemistry have numerous applications to the physiology and biochemical processes in the human body. Consider these topics:

1. Thermal regulation and internal/external homeostasis leading to optimal temperature in the average human; concepts relating input and output of heat energy changes in the body, e.g., hot temperatures lead to sweating to regulate body temperature
2. Heat productivity by skeletal muscles
3. Basal metabolic rate; loss of heat from the body by conduction, convection, and radiation; control of body temperature by the hypothalamus
4. Sunstroke, fever, and hypothermia analysis
5. Biochemical reactions
6. Laboratory instrumentation used for measurements related to temperature, energy, pressure, work, etc.

THERMOCHEMISTRY AND THERMODYNAMICS: REVIEW QUESTIONS

1. The more stable systems with regard to H are systems that have:
   A. zero ΔH.
   B. maximum ΔH.
   C. minimum ΔH.
   D. none of the above.

TABLE 7-7. Concepts of Expansion and Contraction

Type	Final	Original	Change Caused by Heat
(1) Linear	L	L_o	$\alpha\Delta T L_o$
$L = L_o + \alpha\Delta T L_o = L_o(1 + \alpha\Delta T)$			
α = coefficient of linear thermal expansion, ΔT = change in temp			
(2) Area	A	A_o	$\beta\Delta T A_o$
$A = A_o + \beta\Delta T A_o = A_o(1 + \beta\Delta T)$			
β = coefficient of area thermal expansion = 2α			
(3) Volume	V	V_o	$\gamma\Delta T V_o$
$V = V_o + \gamma\Delta T V_o = V_o(1 + \gamma\Delta T)$			
γ = coefficient of volume thermal expansion = 3α			

2. The more stable systems with regard to entropy are systems that have:

    A. minimum ΔS.
    B. maximum ΔS.
    C. zero ΔS.
    D. none of the above.

3. Which of the following equations expresses the relationship between free energy (ΔG), enthalpy (ΔH), entropy (ΔS) and absolute temperature (T)?

    A. $\Delta G = \Delta H + \Delta S$
    B. $\Delta G = \Delta H + T\Delta S$
    C. $\Delta G = \Delta H - T\Delta S$
    D. $\Delta G = T\Delta H - \Delta S$

Questions 4–22
Use the following information for these questions.

Enthalpies of Formation, $\Delta H(^{\circ},f)$ (kcals/mole) at 298°K

$H_2O(g)$	−58	$NO_2(g)$	8	$Ca(OH)_2$	−236	$CH_3CH_2OH(l)$	−66
$H_2O(l)$	−68	$NH_3(g)$	−11	$CaCO_3(s)$	−288	$C_2H_4(g)$	13
$SO_3(g)$	−94	$CO_2(g)$	−94	$C_2H_6(g)$	−20	$C_4H_{10}(g)$	−30
$NO(g)$	19	$CaO(s)$	−152	$CH_3OH(l)$	−57		

Bond Energies (ΔH in kcals/mole)

H-H 104	O-H	111	N = N	226	C-Cl 79	H-Cl	103
O = O	118	C-C 83		C-N	70	C = O 170	C-H 99
Cl-Cl	58	C-O 84		C = C	147		

4. Calculate the ΔH_f° of $H_2SO_4(l)$ given the following equation:

$$H_2O(l) + SO_3(g) \rightarrow H_2SO_4(l) \quad \Delta H^{\circ} = -32 \text{ kcal}$$

    A. −6
    B. −58
    C. −162
    D. −194

5. Calculate the heat (ΔH°) of a reaction for the combustion of n-butane (C_4H_{10})

$$C_4H_{10}(g) + O_2(g) \rightarrow CO_2(g) + H_2O(l) \quad \text{(unbalanced)}$$

    A. −132
    B. −192
    C. −310
    D. −686

6. Which of the following steps releases the most energy?

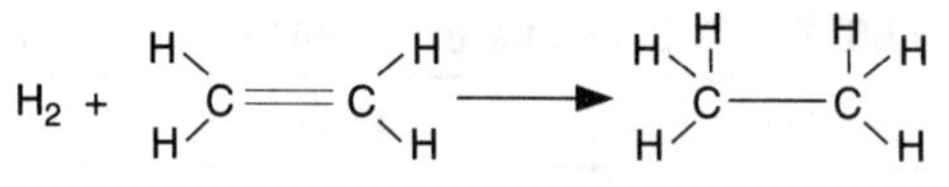

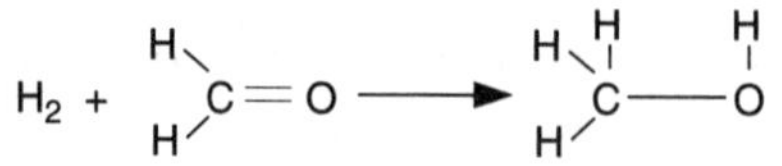

    A. I
    B. II
    C. Neither releases energy
    D. I and II release same amount of energy

7. If C = specific heat capacity, ΔT = change in temperature, and m = mass, then the amount of heat (Q) exchanged is:

A. $q = C/m\Delta t$.
B. $q = C\,m\Delta t$.
C. $q = Cm/\Delta t$.
D. $q = C\Delta t/m$.

8. Heat of fusion refers to the phase change between:

   A. gas and solid.
   B. liquid and gas.
   C. liquid and solid.
   D. all phases.

9. Heat flows between substances by all the following processes EXCEPT:

   A. conjugation.
   B. conduction.
   C. convection.
   D. radiation.

10. What is the process whereby heat is transferred by adjacent molecular collisions throughout a medium?

    A. Convection
    B. Conduction
    C. Radiation
    D. Momentum

11. In heat transfer in a substance (e.g., a heat-conducting rod), the rate of heat transfer is:

    A. directly proportional to the length of the conductor.
    B. indirectly proportional to the temperature difference.
    C. directly proportional to the cross-sectional area of the conductor.
    D. independent of the nature of the substance.

12. The process of transferring heat energy in a moving fluid mass is called:

    A. bulk flow.
    B. radiation.
    C. conduction.
    D. convection.

13. As the absolute temperature increases, the wavelength of radiation emitted by a substance tends to:

    A. increase.
    B. decrease.
    C. remain the same.
    D. change periodically.

14. Which of the following is a statement of the first law of thermodynamics?

    A. $\Delta S = q_{rev}/T$
    B. $\Delta G = \Delta H - T\Delta S$
    C. $\Delta E = q - w$
    D. None of the above

15. The second law of thermodynamics involves the term:

    A. internal energy.
    B. enthalpy.
    C. entropy.
    D. free energy.

16. During the conversion of a liquid to a gas, the heat is used to:

    A. overcome intermolecular forces between liquid molecules and convert them to gaseous molecules.
    B. raise the temperature of the gas.
    C. raise the temperature of the liquid.
    D. do all of the above.

17. The conversion of 10 g of a solid to 10 g of its liquid at the freezing point (25°C) requires 100 cal of heat. What is the heat of fusion of this substance?

   A. 0.40 cal/g · °C
   B. 40 cal · g/°C
   C. 10 cal/g
   D. 250 cal · °C/g

18. A substance weighing 5 g has its temperature raised from 25°C to 75°C without a phase change while absorbing 45 calories of heat. What is the specific heat capacity of this substance?

   A. 1250 cal/g · °C
   B. 450 cal/g · °C
   C. 0.18 cal/g · °C
   D. 4.50 cal/g · °C

19. The amount of heat required to convert 10 g of water (solid) at 0°C to water (liquid) at 50°C (specific heat of solid water is 0.5 cal/g · °C; specific heat of liquid water is 1.0 cal/g · °C; heat of fusion of water is 80 cal/g) is:

   A. 1300 kcal.
   B. 350 cal.
   C. 1300 cal.
   D. 1500 cal.

20. If a heating coil is supplying 50 cal/min to a tank containing water (ice) at 0°C, what amount of water (as a liquid) can be formed in 10 minutes (use specific heat and heat of fusion from question 19)?

   A. 3.5 g
   B. 6.25 g
   C. 420 g
   D. 500 g

21. A temperature of 50°C (Celsius) corresponds to what temperature Fahrenheit (F)?

   A. 122°F $F = \frac{9}{5}c + 32$
   B. 90°F
   C. 82°F
   D. 27.8°F $C =$

22. The coefficient of linear expansion (α) of a substance is $2 \times 10^{-5}\ °C^{-1}$. What would be the coefficient of volume expansion (g)?

   A. $6 \times 10^{-5}\ °C^{-1}$ $y = 3\alpha$
   B. $8 \times 10^{-5}\ °C^{-1}$
   C. $2 \times 10^{-15}\ °C^{-3}$ $= 3(2 \times 10^{-5})$
   D. $9 \times 10^{-5}\ °C^{-1}$

ANSWERS AND EXPLANATIONS

1–3. **1-C, 2-B, 3-C.** See text for explanation.

4. **D** The ΔH_f° is the formation of one mole of the $H_2SO_4(l)$ from its elements: $H_2(g) + S(s) + 2O_2(g) \rightarrow H_2SO_4(l)$, $\Delta H_f^\circ = ?$ Using the information given, a set of equations must be put together that adds up to this net equation:

   (1) $H_2(g) + \frac{1}{2}O_2(g) \rightarrow H_2O(l)$, $\Delta H_f^\circ = -68$

   (2) $S(s) + \frac{3}{2}O_2(g) \rightarrow SO_3(g)$, $\Delta H_f^\circ = -94$

   Rearranged to show how they add up to the desired equation:

   $$H_2(g) + \frac{1}{2}O_2(g) \rightarrow H_2O(l), \Delta H_f^\circ = -68 \text{ kcals}$$

   $$S(s) + \frac{3}{2}O_2(g) \rightarrow SO_3(g), \Delta H_f^\circ = -94 \text{ kcals}$$

   $$H_2O(l) + SO_3(g) \rightarrow H_2SO_4(l), \Delta H_f^\circ = -32 \text{ kcals}$$

   $$\text{Sum: } H_2(g) + 2O_2(g) + S(s) \rightarrow H_2SO_4(l), \Delta H_f^\circ = -194 \text{ kcals}$$

Or, an alternative method:

$$\Delta H^\circ \text{ (product)} - \Delta H^\circ \text{ (reactant)} = \Delta H^\circ \text{ reaction}$$

$$\Delta H^\circ_f \ H_2SO_4 - \{\Delta H^\circ_f \ H_2O(l) + \Delta H^\circ_f \ SO_3(g)\} = -32 \text{ kcal}$$

$$\Delta H^\circ_f \ H_2SO_4 - (-68 \text{ kcal} - 94 \text{ kcal}) = -32 \text{ kcal}$$

$$\Delta H^\circ_f \ H_2SO_4 = -194 \text{ kcal}$$

5. D First balance the equation:
Unbalanced: $C_4H_{10} + O_2 \rightarrow CO_2 + H_2O$
Balance H: $C_4H_{10} + O_2 \rightarrow CO_2 + 5H_2O$
Balance C: $C_4H_{10} + O_2 \rightarrow 4CO_2 + 5H_2O$

Balance O: $C_4H_{10} + \dfrac{13}{2} O_2 \rightarrow 4CO_2 + 5H_2O$ (leave as 1 mole C_4H_{10} because ΔH°

based on one mole of the substance)

Check: C: 4 |4

     H: 10 |10

     O: $\dfrac{13}{2(2)} = 13$ |13

Now apply Hess' law:

$$\sum \Delta H^\circ_f \text{ (products)} = 4 \ \Delta H^\circ_f \text{ of } CO_2(g) + 5\Delta H^\circ_f \text{ of } H_2O(l)$$

$$= 4 \ (-94) + 5(-68) = -376 - 340 = -716$$

$$\sum \Delta H^\circ_f \text{ (reactants)} = \Delta H^\circ_f \text{ of } C_4H_{10} + \dfrac{13}{2\Delta H^\circ_f} \text{ of } O_2(g)$$

$$= -30 + \dfrac{13}{2(0)} = -30$$

and,

$$\sum \Delta H^\circ = \Delta H^\circ_f \text{ (products)} - \Delta H^\circ_f \text{ (reactants)}$$

$$= -716 - (-30) = -716 + 30 = -686 \text{ kcal}$$

6. A Apply Hess' law to each by adding all bond energies in products and reactants:

		ΔH
I	$H_2 + H_2C = CH_2 \rightarrow H_3C - CH_3$	
Reactants:	$H - H + 4(C - H) + C = C$	
	$104 + 4(99) + 147$	647 kcal
Product:	$6(CH) + C - C$	
	$6(99) + 83$	677 kcal
	$\Delta H^\circ = 647 - 677$	-30 kcal
II	$H_2 + H_2C = O \rightarrow H_3C - O - H$	
Reactants:	$H - H + 2(C - H) + C = O$	
	$104 + 2(99) + 170$	472 kcal
Product:	$3(C - H) + C - O + O - H$	
	$3(99) + 84 + 111$	492 kcal
	$\Delta H^\circ = 472 - 492$	-20 kcal

7–15. 7-B, 8-C, 9-A, 10-B, 11-C, 12-D, 13-B, 14-C, 15-C. See text for explanation.

16. A During a phase conversion step, energy is used to break intermolecular bonds and is not used to increase the average kinetic energy of the molecules (raise the temperature).

17. C Heat of fusion $= \dfrac{\text{calories required for phase change}}{\text{mass undergoing phase change}}$

$$= \frac{100 \text{ cal}}{10 \text{ g}} = \frac{10 \text{ cal}}{\text{g}}$$

18. C $C = \dfrac{Q}{m\Delta T} = \dfrac{45 \text{ cal}}{(5 \text{ g})(75 - 25°\text{C})} = \dfrac{9}{50} = 0.18 \text{ (cal/g} \cdot °\text{C)}$

19. C The scheme is:

$$(1) \hspace{5cm} (2)$$

Water (solid) at 0°C → water (liquid) at 0°C → water (liquid) at 50°C
(1) heat of fusion (H_f) of water for phase change
    cals $= (H_f)(\text{mass}) = (80 \text{ cal/g})(10 \text{ g}) = 800 \text{ cal}$
(2) SH of water (liq) to raise temperature
    cals $= (\text{SH})(\text{mass})(\text{temp change}) = C \, m\Delta t$
    $= (1.0)(10)(50 - 0) = (10)(50) = 500 \text{ cal}$
Total: (1) + (2) = 800 + 500 = 1300 cal

20. B Total heat delivered in 10 minutes:

$$\text{Cal} = \left(\frac{50 \text{ cal}}{\text{min}}\right)(10 \text{ min}) = 500 \text{ cal}$$

The scheme for water changes is:
$$(1)$$

Water (solid) at 0°C → water (liquid) at 0°C

(1) Heat of fusion (H_f) of water for phase change
    $H_f = \text{heat change/mass} = Q/m$
    $m = Q/H_f = 500 \text{ cal}/(80 \text{ cal/g}) = 6.25 \text{ g}$

21. A Use ratio and proportion and known facts about temperature scales:

$$\frac{(50 - 0)}{(100 - 0)} = \frac{(F - 32)}{(212 - 32)} = \frac{(F - 32)}{180}$$

$$\frac{(50)(180)}{100} = F - 32$$

$$90 = F - 32$$

$$122 = F$$

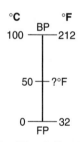

22. A The following relationship holds:

$$\gamma = 3\alpha = (3)(2 \times 10^{-5}°\text{C}^{-1}) = 6 \times 10^{-5}°\text{C}^{-1}$$

Rate Processes in Chemical Reactions— Kinetics and Equilibrium

Self-Managed Learning Questions

1. If a rubber band is stretched and released, then stretched again and released, and the process is repeated many times, the band gets warm. Why? Explain the chemical bonds and the organic chemistry reactions that have taken place. Is this a physical or chemical illustration of kinetics or equilibrium?
2. Why are K_f and K_b (forward and backward) reaction rates called velocities of the chemical reaction if the reaction proceeds faster by adding a catalyst?
3. Are there chemical substances that become more ordered as the temperature increases? (Hint: Biomolecular elastic polymers become more ordered with tem-

perature increase because parts of the polymer chain are hydrophobic and parts are hydrophilic.)
4. Examine the following statements:
   - The total energy of the universe is a constant.
   - The total entropy of the universe is always increasing.
   - The entropy of every pure, perfect substance at absolute zero is zero.

   Can these statements be classified as laws? Why? What evidence exists to support these laws inside and outside a laboratory? Are these statements always valid? (Hint: These statements are the three laws of thermodynamics.)

REACTION RATE

The rates of reactions are affected by four factors: (1) concentration of reagents, (2) energy of activation, (3) temperature, and (4) spatial effects related to the sizes and shapes of colliding molecules that determine which orientations of collisions lead to reactions. The rates of reactions are quantified in terms of **rate expressions**, which relate the change in concentration of one reactant (or product) with time to the concentration of other reactants (or products): for: $aA + bB \rightarrow cC + dD$ (overall reaction), the rate expression might be:

$$\text{Rate} = \frac{\Delta[A]}{\Delta t} = -k[A]^m[B]^n$$

in which the minus sign $(-)$ is present because $[A]$ is decreasing with time, k = rate constant for the reaction, and $[\ ]$ = concentration in moles/liter (molarity). Note that the exponents of $A^{(m)}$ and $B^{(n)}$ do not, in general, equal the coefficients of $A(a)$ and $B(b)$. This point illustrates that rate expressions cannot be determined from stoichiometric equations; they must be determined by experiment. The rate of reaction, and hence, the rate expression, varies during the course of the reaction, because the net reaction rate is as follows:

$$\text{Net rate} = \text{forward rate} - \text{reverse rate}$$

$$\text{Forward rate} = k_f[A]^m[B]^n$$

$$\text{Reverse rate} = k_r[C]^x[D]^y$$

Reactants Concentration

The **forward rate** depends on the concentration of the reactants, and the **reverse rate** depends on the concentration of the products. Early (initially) in the reaction, more reactants are present and the forward rate dominates. As reactants are converted to products, more products accumulate and the reverse rate increases until it equals the forward rate. This point is equilibrium (Fig. 7-39).

Rate Law

For the reason just stated, most rate expressions are for initial rates (reactants present but no products) and, hence, are forward rates, taking the form:

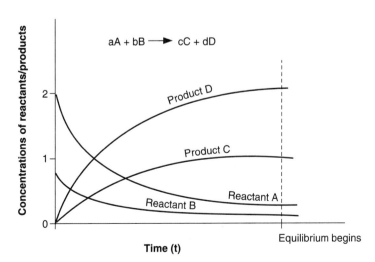

Fig. 7-39. Course of a reaction.

Rate is $\Delta c/\Delta t$ = slope, and this changes going from 5=0 to equilibrium.

$$\text{Rate} = k[A]^m[B]^n$$

Determining the values of m and n is then accomplished by varying the concentration of one reactant while holding other reactants constant and noting how the rate is affected.

Rate Constant

First order kinetics means the first order is one, second order is two, etc. The rate constant can be calculated once you know the orders in each reactant:

$$k = \frac{\text{rate}}{[A]^2[B]^{1/2}}$$

From the collision theory of gaseous reactions, the following equation is derived:

$$k = Ae^{\frac{-E_A}{RT}}$$

in which k = rate constant, A = a constant that includes collision, orientation, and molecular factors, e = base of natural logs, EA = activation energy, R = 1.99 cal/mole − °K, and T = absolute temperature. The EA can be calculated by determining the rate constant at a number of different temperatures and making this plot (Fig. 7-40):

$$\ln k = \ln A - \frac{EA}{R} \cdot \frac{1}{T}$$

Comparing with the slope-intercept form of a straight line equation (y = b + mx), Intercept, b = ln A

$$\text{Slope, m} = -\frac{E^A}{R}$$

$$y = \ln k$$

$$x = \frac{1}{T}$$

Reaction Order

Most reactions proceed as a series of steps that are exemplified by chain reactions. **Chain reactions** are exemplified by radical reactions, such as halogenation. The steps are as follows:

1. **Initiation**: the production of radicals

    $$Cl_2 \rightarrow 2Cl\cdot$$

2. **Propagation**: the production of radicals by reaction with radicals, which keeps the reaction going:

    $$Cl\cdot + R_3CH \rightarrow R_3C\cdot + HCl$$

    $$R_3C\cdot + Cl_2 \rightarrow R_3CCl + Cl\cdot$$

3. **Termination**: the destruction of radicals by the reactions of two radicals with each other, or by the reactions of radicals with the walls of the container:

    $$Cl\cdot + R_3C\cdot \rightarrow R_3CCl$$

    $$R_3C\cdot + R_3C\cdot \rightarrow R_3C - CR_3$$

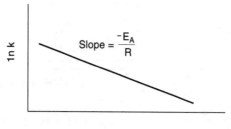

Fig. 7-40.

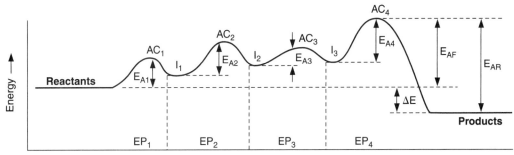

$$\text{Reactants} \rightleftharpoons I_1 \rightleftharpoons I_2 \rightleftharpoons I_3 \rightleftharpoons \text{Products}$$

Fig. 7-41. One of many reaction coordinates that may be taken by reactants being converted to products. EP = elementary process; AC = activated complex, a transient species that may be converted to products or reactants, cannot be isolated; also called the transition state complex; I = intermediates, transient species that may be isolated in some instances; note they are like ''rest points'' between the EP; EA = activation energies; EAF = overall EA for forward reaction; EAR = overall EA for reverse reaction; ΔE = energy of the reaction = EAR − EAF.

Rate-Determining Step

Reactants being converted to products take many possible overall paths (reaction coordinates). If a reaction takes place in a series of steps, and if the first step is slower than the following steps, the reaction rate will essentially be the same as the slowest step. This slowest step is called the rate-determining step. If one molecule is involved in an elementary process, it is said to be **unimolecular**. If two molecules are involved, it is said to be **bimolecular**, if three, then **trimolecular**, and so on. Given an overall path (with its composite elementary processes), the principle of microscopic reversibility states that the elementary processes of the reverse reaction are the same as the forward reaction (Fig. 7-41).

The order of the reaction (contrasted with molecularity) is the sum of the exponents in the experimentally derived rate expression. For example:

given: Rate $= k[A]^2[B]$

then: Order of reaction $= 2 + 1 = 3$

Order of reactant in A $= 2$

Order of reactant in B $= 1$

First order kinetics means the order is one, second order is two, etc.

Temperature and Activation Energy

Temperature can play an important role in determining reaction rate. For many reactions that take place at room temperature, a 10°C increase in temperature can cause the reaction rate to double. The higher the temperature, the higher the number of collisions between reactants, which together have enough energy to surmount the barrier at the higher temperature.

For a chemical reaction to occur:

1. The molecules must **collide** (make contact). The more they collide, the greater the chance of a reaction.
2. The molecules must have enough **energy** to react once they have collided. Remember that molecules have a distribution of kinetic energies (Boltzmann distribution), and only some of the molecules have enough energy to react. Note: Kinetic energy is proportional to the average temperature of the molecules.
3. Given a collision and sufficient energy, a molecule may not react unless the **orientation** is correct. The energy requirements and orientation are related in that some orientations require less energy for reaction to occur.

These factors help to determine the **activation energy** (EA). The EA is the energy barrier that must be overcome for a reaction to occur. The higher the EA, the slower the reaction.

ACTIVATED COMPLEX OR TRANSITION STATE

The **transition state** is an intermediate state lying between the reactants and the products. The transition state is unstable and is the highest energy structure involved in a reaction. There are two kinds of reactions: **exergonic**, which is a reaction with a negative free energy, and **endergonic**, which is a reaction with a positive free energy. If covalent bonds in a reaction are broken, the reactants must first go up an energy hill before they can

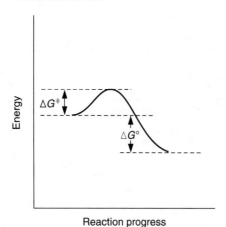

A. Fast exothermic

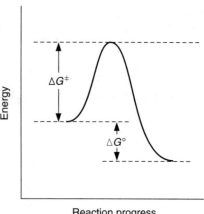

B. Slow exothermic

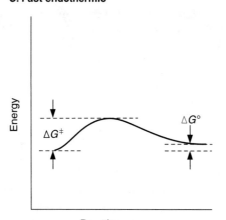

C. Fast endothermic

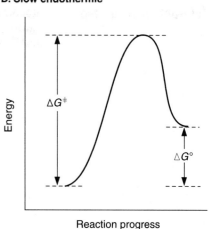

D. Slow endothermic

Fig. 7-42.

go downhill, even if the reaction is exergonic. The top of the hill is the transition state. The difference in free energy between the reactants and the transition state is the free energy of activation, or ΔG (Fig. 7-42).

The energy profile of this reaction:

$$CH_3Cl \qquad + \ OH^- \rightarrow \qquad CH_3OH \qquad + \ Cl^-$$

(chloromethane)   hydroxide ion   methanol   chloride ion

explains the energy relationships between the reactants, the transition state, and the products (Fig. 7-43). The transition state is a high-energy state because energy has been put into the molecule to partially break the carbon-chlorine bond. E^R, E^P, and ΔG^R represent energy levels at each state. The quantity of free energy of activation must be determined experimentally for each reaction (it cannot be predicted).

KINETIC VERSUS THERMODYNAMIC CONTROL OF A REACTION

Kinetics deals with the rates (how fast) of chemical reactions. Therefore, it relates to the activation energy rather than the ΔH (enthalpy change) of a reaction as in thermodynamics (see previous discussion of thermochemistry and thermodynamics).

In an irreversible reaction, there is not enough energy to lift a product out of its deep potential energy valley. Such a reaction is under **kinetic control**, or rate control. At higher temperatures, the intermediate ions in a reaction have enough energy to lift a product out of its potential energy valley to cross over barriers with ease. Both reactions are reversible, and are said to be under **thermodynamic control**, or equilibrium control. The concept of thermodynamic control versus kinetic control is summarized in Figure 7-44.

CATALYSTS

A catalyst (a substance not used up or changed in a reaction) speeds up reactions by lowering the EA. **Enzymes** work in this way. These proteins catalyze chemical reactions.

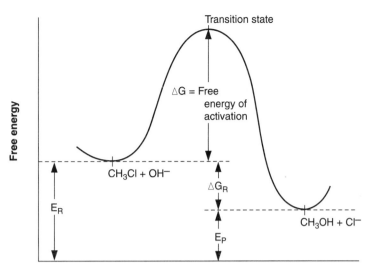

Fig. 7-43.

Free energy

Transition state

ΔG = Free energy of activation

$CH_3Cl + OH^-$

ΔG_R

E_R

$CH_3OH + Cl^-$

E_P

Reaction coordinate

B ⇌ A ⇌ C   Thermodynamic control

Fig. 7-44.   B ⟵ A ⟶ C   Kinetic control

They are highly specific in that each catalyzes only a single reaction or set of closely related reactions. Nearly every biologic reaction is catalyzed by an enzyme. A **substrate** is a reactant that forms a tight complex with the enzyme at the active site on the enzyme. It is the specificity of this enzyme–substrate binding that is largely responsible for the specificity of enzyme catalysis.

EQUILIBRIUM IN REVERSIBLE CHEMICAL REACTIONS

All chemical reactions proceed toward an equilibrium state. The **equilibrium state** exists when the forward rate equals the reverse rate: hence, no change occurs in the components of the reaction. Equilibrium is a dynamic state; i.e., the reactions have not ceased in that reactants are being converted to products and products are being converted to reactants. At equilibrium, ΔG (free energy) is zero, ΔH (enthalpy) is a minimum, and ΔS (entropy) is maximum (see previous discussion of thermochemistry and thermodynamics), or, to summarize, there is minimum energy and maximum randomness in a system at equilibrium. However, these may not be true if ΔH and ΔS drive reactions in different directions.

Law of Mass Action

In reversible chemical reactions, the equilibrium constant is based on the equilibrium concentrations of reactants and products at a certain temperature. The **law of mass action** defines the rate at which a chemical reaction proceeds in relation to its (active mass) concentration of reactants, and the velocity of the reaction is proportional to the products of the concentration of the reactants.

Equilibrium Constant

The equilibrium constant (K) is a quantitative way of describing the interrelationships of the concentrations of components at equilibrium. Given the reaction:

$$aA + bB \underset{k_2}{\overset{k_1}{\rightleftharpoons}} cC + dD$$

Forward rate = $k_1[A]^a[B]^b$ = forward velocity

Backward rate = $k_2[C]^c[D]^d$ = backward velocity

the equilibrium constant is:

Forward rate = backward rate

$$k_1[A]^a[B]^b = k_2[C]^c[D]^d$$

$$K = \frac{k_1}{k_2} = \frac{[C]^c[D]^d}{[A]^a[B]^b} \text{ depends only on temperature}$$

in which [ ] = concentration in moles/liter (molarity), [gases] = atmospheres, and [pure solids] = constant.

The constant K is a measure of the capacity of reactants to be converted to products. Large K values indicate more reactants will be converted to products. The expression:

$$\frac{[C]^c[D]^d}{[A]^a[B]^b}$$

can be determined at points other than equilibrium. The direction the reaction must proceed to get to equilibrium can be determined by comparing the values of the expression with the K. If

$$\text{if } \frac{[C]^c[D]^d}{[A]^a[B]^b} < K$$

then the reaction proceeds to equilibrium from left to right as written (the numerator, products, must increase and/or the denominator, reactants, must decrease for the expression to equal K). If:

$$\frac{[C]^c[D]^d}{[A]^a[B]^b} > K$$

then the reaction proceeds to equilibrium from right to left as written. Several important points to note and memorize:

- The equilibrium constant for the reverse (K_R) of a given reaction (K) is:

$$K_R = \frac{1}{K}$$

- The overall equilibrium constant (K) for a series of reactions is the product of the individual equilibrium constants:

$$K = K_1K_2K_3 \ldots \ldots$$

- When a reaction is exothermic (ΔH is negative), K actually decreases as the temperature increases. The reverse is true for an endothermic reaction.

LeChatelier's Principle

Le Chatelier's principle is a good way to determine how a change in condition (e.g., concentration) will affect the relative concentrations of reactants/products and other factors (e.g., heat, volume) in a reaction. The principle states, "Any perturbation (change) to a system initially at equilibrium will cause that system (if left alone) to adjust in such a way as to offset that perturbation." In essence, the system will go toward a new equilibrium but with concentrations and other factors appropriately adjusted.

A practical way of using this principle follows:

1. Write all the components and conditions of the reaction on the appropriate side of the equation, including all reactants, products, heat, and volume. The heat is the heat of the reaction. If positive, it is a reactant; if negative, it is a product (see previous discussion of thermochemistry and thermodynamics). Remember that an increase in temperature is like increasing the energy (heat) and vice versa.

   The volume can be related to the moles (in the balanced equation) of gases in the reaction. Put the volume on the side with the fewer moles of gas ("balances" out the volume). Remember that as pressure increases, the volume decreases, and vice versa.

2. Apply these rules (from Le Chatelier's) to determine how the equilibrium will shift.
   - If a component or condition increases, the reaction is shifted to the opposite side; i.e., components/conditions on the other side will increase and those on the same side will decrease.
   - If a component/condition decreases, the reaction is shifted to its side, the other

components/conditions on that side increase, and the components/conditions on the opposite decrease.

As an example, consider the reaction:

$$M_2(g) + 3E_2(g) \rightleftharpoons 2ME_3(g), \Delta H = +10 \text{ kcal}$$

Rewrite using the rules just outlined:

$$\text{Heat} + M_2(g) + 3E_2(g) \rightleftharpoons 2ME_3(g) + \text{volume}$$

Examples of effects of perturbations are as follows:

If ↑ M_2, reaction shifts to right
If ↓ E_2, reaction shifts to left
If ↑ pressure, volume decreases and reaction shifts to right
If ↓ temperature, same as decreasing heat and decreasing volume, reaction shift is indeterminate
If add a catalyst, no shift in equilibrium; catalyst only affects rate of reaction

RELATIONSHIP OF THE EQUILIBRIUM CONSTANT AND Δg°

The **equilibrium constant** for a reaction is related to the change in standard free energy by the equation: $\Delta G° = -2.303RT \log K_{eq}$. If $\Delta G°$ decreases during a reaction (it is negative), the equilibrium constant is greater than 1. In this case, the reaction proceeds so that more products than reactants are present at equilibrium. If $\Delta G°$ increases, the reverse reaction is true.

$\Delta G°$ has two components: change in enthalpy (ΔH), the heat of the reaction, and change in entropy (ΔS), the measure of disorder or randomness in the system. The relationship among these components is expressed as: $\Delta G = \Delta H - T\Delta S$.

BIOCHEMICAL REACTIONS IN THE HUMAN BODY

These reactions depend on rate processes in chemical reactions—both kinetics and equilibrium. The study of biochemistry requires a good background in activation energy and metabolic processes applied to the average human body. Carefully review the following basic concepts and terms:

- Maximum catalytic rates of enzymes; fundamentals of enzyme kinetics in relation to Michaelis-Menten equations and graphs; analysis of kinetic tabular data and enzyme inhibitors
- The relation of pH to rate of enzymatic reactions
- Metabolic pathways—catabolism and anabolism, including experimental techniques to study metabolic inhibitors; use of isotopes and autoradiography
- Glycogen metabolism related to blood glucose levels; graphing enzyme activity versus glucose concentration
- Kinetics of mediated transport
- Physiology of protein, carbohydrate, lipid metabolism in the human body

An understanding of the physical and chemical concepts related to biochemical reactions is necessary before you begin your review of the biologic sciences in Chapter 8. Kinetics and equilibrium concepts are directly linked to many basic and more advanced biologic concepts that are essential for the study of medicine.

APPLIED CONCEPTS

1. Biochemists are interested in understanding detailed reaction mechanisms and they study the effect of pH, substrate modification, and inhibitors on reaction rates.

2. Molecular biologists are interested in the regulation of enzyme synthesis or activity and will measure the amount of enzyme activity of a specific enzyme as a function of biologic parameters.

3. Enzymes can be used as laboratory tools to hydrolyze unwanted substances and prepare chemical compounds.

Given these facts:
4. How would rate processes be important to the field of medicine?
5. Why are enzymes important to medicine and research?
6. What kinds of instruments are used? How are they used?
7. Why would a doctor care about how enzymes work and how they are useful?

1. All of the following conditions must be met in order for a chemical reaction to occur EXCEPT:

   A. collisions.
   B. sufficient energy per molecule to react.
   C. appropriate orientation of colliding molecules.
   D. homeostasis.

2. The energy that must be overcome for a chemical reaction to occur is called the:

   A. enthalpy.
   B. activation energy.
   C. entropy.
   D. free energy.

3. Which of the following actions is NOT a step in a chain reaction?

   A. Initiation
   B. Propagation
   C. Acceleration
   D. Termination

4. The step in which radicals already present are used to generate new radicals is called:

   A. initiation.
   B. propagation.
   C. acceleration.
   D. extermination.

Questions 5–7
Use the following diagram to answer this group of questions.

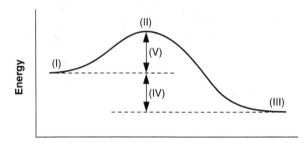

Reaction coordinate

5. The activation energy of the forward reaction is given by:

   A. II.
   B. III.
   C. IV.
   D. V.

6. The heat of the reaction is given by:

   A. II.
   B. III.
   C. IV.
   D. V.

7. The activated complex would be located at:

   A. I.
   B. II.
   C. III.
   D. None of the above

8. The rate-determining step of a reaction with a series of steps is characterized by:

   A. the lowest energy of activation.
   B. the highest energy of activation.
   C. the highest enthalpy.
   D. none of the above.

9. Which of the following statements best defines the role of a catalyst?

   A. It shifts the equilibrium of the reaction in favor of the products.
   B. It speeds up the reaction by raising the activation energy.
   C. It speeds up the reaction by lowering the activation energy.
   D. It shifts the equilibrium of the reaction in favor of the reactants.

10. Which of the following statements relating to the equilibrium state are true?

    A. The forward reaction continues.
    B. The reverse reaction continues.
    C. There is minimum energy and maximum randomness.
    D. All of these statements are true.

11. As the value of K (the equilibrium constant) becomes larger:

    A. more products will be present at equilibrium.
    B. less products will be present at equilibrium.
    C. the faster the reaction will proceed.
    D. the slower the reaction will proceed.

12. Given the reaction:

$$A \rightleftharpoons B$$

if $[B]/[A] = 2 \times 10^{-5}$ and it is known that $K = 5 \times 10^{-4}$ from other experiments, in what direction must the reaction proceed to reach equilibrium?

    A. [B] must increase and/or [A] decrease
    B. [B] must decrease and/or [A] decrease
    C. [B] and [A] should be equal to start the reaction
    D. Cannot be determined from the information given

13. For the reaction:

$$A + 2B \rightleftharpoons 2C,$$

the concentration, in moles/liter, of the components at equilibrium are: $[A] = 1 \times 10^{-2}$ M, $[B] = 2 \times 10^{-3}$ M, and $[C] = 5 \times 10^{-6}$ M. What is the equilibrium constant (K) of the reaction?

    A. 6.25×10^{-4}
    B. 0.225
    C. 25
    D. None of the above

Questions 14–17
Use the following equation to answer this group of questions.

$$C_2H_5OH(l) + 3O_2(g) \rightleftharpoons 2CO_2(g) + 3H_2O(l) \quad \Delta H° = -327 \text{ kcal}$$

14. If the temperature is increased, the equilibrium:

    A. shifts to the left.
    B. shifts to the right.
    C. is unchanged.
    D. can never be achieved.

15. If the pressure is increased, the equilibrium:

    A. shifts to the left.
    B. shifts to the right.
    C. is unchanged.
    D. depends on volume.

16. If $O_2(g)$ is added, the equilibrium:

    A. shifts to the left.
    B. shifts to the right.
    C. is unchanged.
    D. can never be achieved.

17. The addition of a chemical that absorbs CO_2 (g) will cause the equilibrium to:

    A. shift to the left.
    B. shift to the right.

C. remain unchanged.
D. be independent of any catalysts.

Questions 18–21
Use the following equation to answer this group of questions.

$$CH_4(g) + H_2O(l) \rightleftharpoons CH_3OH(l) + H_2(g) \quad \Delta H = +29 \text{ kcal}$$

18. If the H_2 (g) formed is allowed to escape from the reaction, the equilibrium will:

A. shift to the left.
B. shift to the right.
C. remain unchanged.
D. be unattainable in 30 seconds or less.

19. If the pressure is doubled, the equilibrium:

A. shifts to the left.
B. shifts to the right.
C. is unchanged.
D. is acquired within 2 minutes.

20. Suppose CO_2 catalyzes this reaction. If CO_2 is added, the equilibrium:

A. shifts to the left.
B. shifts to the right.
C. is unchanged.
D. cannot be achieved.

21. If the temperature is decreased, the equilibrium:

A. shifts to the left.
B. shifts to the right.
C. is unchanged.
D. is unchanged forever.

ANSWERS AND EXPLANATIONS

1–11. 1-D, 2-B, 3-C, 4-B, 5-D, 6-C, 7-B, 8-B, 9-C, 10-D, 11-A. See text for explanation.
12. A [B]/[A] < K because $2 \times 10^{-5} < 5 \times 10^{-4}$. Then, for [B]/[A] to become equal to K, the [B] must increase and the [A] must decrease.
13. A The equilibrium constant (K) is,

$$K = \frac{[C]^2}{[A][B]^2} = \frac{[5 \times 10^{-6}]^2}{[1 \times 10^{-2}][2 \times 10^{-3}]^2} = \frac{25 \times 10^{-12}}{(10^{-2})(4 \times 10^{-6})}$$

$$K = \frac{25 \times 10^{-12}}{4 \times 10^{-8}} = \frac{25}{4} \times 10^{-12+8} = 6.25 \times 10^{-4}$$

14. A The complete equation is:

$$C_2H_5OH(l) + 3O_2(g) \rightleftharpoons 2CO_2(g) + 3H_2O(l) + vol + heat$$

Volume goes on the right side because fewer moles of gas are on that side. Heat goes on the right because the reaction is exothermic, i.e., heat is a product. An increase in temperature therefore causes an increase in heat, which shifts the reaction to the opposite side (the left).
15. B An increase in pressure causes a decrease in volume. A decrease in volume pulls a reaction to its side (the right).
16. B The added O_2 shifts the reaction to the opposite side (the right).
17. B The CO_2 (g) decreases, which pulls the reaction to its side (the right).
18. B The overall equation is:

$$Heat + CH_4(g) + H_2O(l) \rightleftharpoons CH_3OH(l) + H_2(g)$$

The heat is on the left side because the reaction is endothermic, which means heat is used as a reactant. There is no volume factor because the number of moles of gases on one side is equal to that on the other side. Because the H_2 is being removed, the reaction is pulled to its side (the right).
19. C See the answer to question 18. There is no volume factor, so the pressure has no effect.
20. C Catalysts do not affect the equilibrium of a reaction.

21. A A decrease in temperature is like decreasing the heat, which shifts the reaction to that side (the left).

Translational Motion

Self-Managed Learning Questions

1. Conceptualize a vector and list at least 10 physical quantities that are vectors. Also, list 10 scalars. An example of a vector is the weight of an object, and an example of a scalar is the mass of an object. Learn how to draw scalars and vectors.
2. Understand the equations for translational motion by experimentally understanding quantities such as final velocity, acceleration, initial velocity. Use a stopwatch and a tape measurer to calculate these quantities and verify them against the equations. Plot the calculated quantities versus observed quantities, e.g., acceleration on a graph. Is it a straight line? Why or why not?
3. Understand the definitions of translational motion, rotational motion, and curvilinear motion by drawing actual diagrams from actual real-life examples, e.g., an electric drill is an example of rotational motion. Expand the definitions to surfaces with and without friction when dealing with kinetics (forces, momentum, and included).

UNITS AND DIMENSIONS

The **units** of distance and displacement are lengths, such as feet (ft), meters (m), miles, and kilometers (km). The units of speed and velocity are length divided by time, such as feet/sec (fps), miles/hour, or meters/sec. Acceleration has the units of length/time/time (length/time^2), such as feet/sec^2, meters/sec^2, and miles/hour^2.

VECTORS

Displacement, velocity, and acceleration are added (or subtracted) by vector addition. Speed, time, and distance are **scalars**, whereas velocity, acceleration, and displacement are **vectors**. Review the section on vectors in Chapter 6, making sure to understand how to resolve a vector into its components.

Look at the graph in Figure 7-45. Let the magnitudes of the vectors in Figure 7-45 be $v_1 = 64$ fps, $v_2 = 83$ fps, $v_3 = 31$ fps, and $v_4 = 47$ fps. To find the resultant of vectors v_1, v_2, v_3, v_4, you can use the **quick graphic method,** which involves drawing the vectors tip-to-tail, taking care to preserve lengths and angles.

To start, select any vector. For this example problem, select v_3 as the starting vector. Remember each vector has a **tip** (the arrowhead) and a **tail** (where it is attached to the origin). Start by drawing the vector v_3, making sure of the measurements of **direction** and **length of vector** are fairly accurate. Now select any other vector, such as v_1, and draw it so that the tail of v_1 coincides with the tip of v_3. Proceed to vector v_2 and draw it so that the tail of v_2 coincides with the tip of v_1. You are now left with vector v_4. Using the sequential procedure just outlined, draw v_4 attached to v_2 so that the tail of v_4 coincides with the tip of v_2. The vector diagram is now complete. The vector sum is given by the vector drawn from the origin to the tip of v_4. The resultant vector, $v_R = AB$ (vector sum)

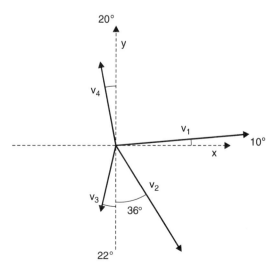

Fig. 7-45.

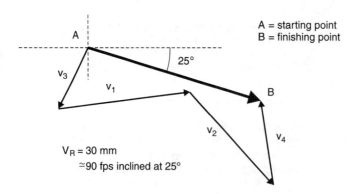

A = starting point
B = finishing point

V_R = 30 mm
≅90 fps inclined at 25°

Fig. 7-46.

has the direction and length shown in Figure 7-46. The direction is inclined from the horizontal by 25° and has length roughly three times the length of v_3 so that $v_R \cong 90$.

This method is also called the "tip-tail method," and it takes about 1 or 2 minutes. You are not able to use a protractor or ruler during the MCAT, so use your answer sheet or the test booklet and your pencil to **measure** as you would with a ruler and a protractor. Your sense of direction and orientation will guide you. Draw the x-axis and y-axis to improve your "angle sense." With practice, this method can be used to obtain approximate solutions to problems with greater confidence.

SPEED, VELOCITY, AND ACCELERATION

Distance depends on the path taken, has no fixed direction, and has magnitude only. **Speed** is the distance traveled divided by the change in time. Both speed and distance are scalar quantities (have magnitude but no fixed direction, and have positive values only). **Displacement** is independent of the path taken (i.e., depends only on initial and final positions of the object). **Velocity** is the displacement divided by the change in time. Both velocity and displacement are vector quantities (i.e., have direction and magnitude). **Acceleration** is the change in velocity divided by the change in time, and it is a vector (Fig. 7-47.) In this section the terms displacement, velocity, and acceleration will refer to **average** quantities, not the instantaneous rate of change, which requires calculus for its characterization.

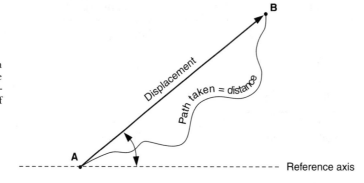

Fig. 7-47. Translational motion parameters. Note that there are many paths from A to B but displacement is the same regardless of the path taken.

The translational motion parameters may be expressed as follows:

$$\text{Speed} = \frac{\Delta \text{distance}}{\Delta \text{time}} = \frac{d_f - d_i}{t_f - t_i}$$

$$\text{Velocity} = \frac{\text{displacement}}{\Delta \text{time}}$$

$$\text{Acceleration} = \frac{\Delta \text{velocity}}{\Delta \text{time}} = \frac{v_f - v_i}{t_f - t_i}$$

where Δ(delta) = change, f = final, i = initial.

Displacement is the "net" area under the velocity-time graph, where area above the t-axis is counted as positive and area below this axis is counted as negative. To compute the total distance traveled, compute the "total" area between the velocity–time graph, where areas above and below the t-axis are both counted as positive.

Note that for systems involving motion in a straight line, the **sign** (+ or −) of displacement, velocity, or acceleration depends on the coordinate system under study. The concept of $+$ or $-$ direction does not apply to motion that is not in a straight line. In this case vector quantities have two components and the components can be described as having $+$ or $-$ directions. A displacement is negative if it is opposite to the direction designated as positive. Velocity is negative if the displacement is becoming more negative. Acceleration is negative if velocity is decreasing in magnitude. **Instantaneous** velocity or acceleration represents a given point in time. Instantaneous velocity is the slope of the graph of distance versus time at the given time. The **average** velocity for straight-line motion is defined for a period of time, and is expressed as $v = \dfrac{v_f + v_i}{2}$ if acceleration is constant.

UNIFORMLY ACCELERATED MOTION

Force is defined as the action of one particle on another, such as pushing a book with your hand. Forces (see subsequent discussion of force and motion and gravitation) act on objects to cause an acceleration. If a constant force is acting, there is a constant (unchanging) acceleration. The motion produced in this situation is **uniform accelerated motion**. If a particle has initial velocity (v_i) and is subjected to a uniform acceleration (a) for a time period (t) then its motion is described by the equation:

$$v_f = v_i + at.$$

For example,

If $a = -10 \text{ m/sec}^2$, 5 seconds elapse, and the final velocity $= 0$, then:

$$v_f = v_i + at \text{ gives } 0 = v_i - (10)(5), \text{ hence } v_i = +50 \text{ m/sec}$$

The acceleration and velocity are both causing a change in displacement (d)—the directions of acceleration, velocity, and displacement are all the same. If

$$d_{vo} = v_o t \text{ displacement because of the initial velocity } (v_o) \text{ at time} = t,$$

$$d_a = \tfrac{1}{2} at^2 \text{ displacement because of the acceleration at time} = t,$$

$$d_o = \text{ initial displacement (if any) from a reference position,}$$

then the total displacement (d) in a time (t) for uniform accelerated motion (**equation for uniform accelerated motion**) is:

$$d = d_o + v_o t + \tfrac{1}{2} at^2$$

or, final displacement (d) $=$ initial displacement from a reference point (d_o) $+$ change in displacement because of initial velocity ($v_o t$) $+$ change in displacement because of acceleration:

$$d = d_o + d_{vo} + d_a$$

These equations illustrate uniform accelerated motion along a straight line. **Translational motion** is the movement of an object in a straight line.

FREELY FALLING BODIES

Free fall motion is vertical motion (in reference to the earth), that is, upward or downward in a straight line. It is always uniformly accelerated motion with the acceleration equal to g. The magnitude of g is 32 ft/sec^2 ($=980 \text{ cm/sec}^2 = 9.8 \text{ m/sec}^2$) and its direction is toward the center of the earth. If a coordinate system takes an upward direction as positive, then g will be -32 ft/sec^2; it is important to keep in mind the direction designated as positive.

The equations for uniform linear motion are applicable when g is substituted for a:

$$y = y_o + v_o t + \frac{1}{2} at^2$$

$$v = v_{y0} + at$$

where $a = \pm g$ depending on the choice of coordinate system.

As an example, in $g = 32 \text{ ft/sec}^2$, g means that for every second an object is falling under the influence of gravity (neglecting air resistance), the velocity is increasing by 32 ft/sec. For an object thrown straight up, its speed is decreasing by 32 ft/sec for every second.

In the free fall of actual objects, the value of g is modified by buoyancy of air and resistance of air. What results is drag force, and depends on the location on earth; the weight, shape, and size of the object; and the velocity of the object (as free fall velocity

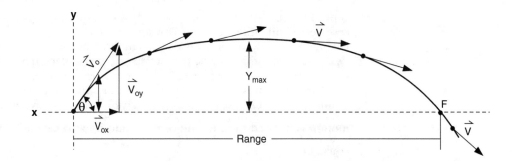

Fig. 7-48. Projectile motion.

increases, the drag force increases). When the drag force reaches the force of gravity, the object reaches a final or terminal velocity, and continues to fall at that velocity.

PROJECTILES

Projectile motion is mathematically represented by two types of translational motion: vertical (affected by g) and horizontal (independent of g). The vertical motion (free fall) and the horizontal translational motion (with a = 0) are represented as vertical and horizontal components. The projectile is generally fired at some angle to the horizontal, and the motion is parabolic (Fig. 7-48).

Vertical component (free fall—note that here $g = -32$ ft/sec^2):

Initial vertical component of velocity: $\quad\quad\quad\quad\quad v_{0y} = v_0 \sin \theta$

Vertical displacement from the origin at time t: $\quad y = v_{0y}t + \dfrac{1}{2}gt^2$

Vertical component of velocity at time t: $\quad\quad v_y = v_{0y} + gt$

Horizontal components (straight-line motion with constant veocity v_{0x}):

Constant horizontal component of velocity: $\quad\quad v_{0x} = v_0 \cos \theta$

Horizontal displacement from the origin at time t: $\quad x = v_{0x}t$

Relationship of lengths of vectors (|v| denotes the length of the vector v):

$$|v_0|^2 = |v_{0y}|^2 + |v_{0x}|^2 \quad (Pythagorean\ Theorem)$$

$$\tan (\theta) = \frac{|v_{0y}|}{|v_{0x}|}$$

Relationships to note:

1. The horizontal component of velocity remains constant ($=v_0 \cos \theta$)
2. At the highest point of the trajectory, y_{max}, the vertical component of velocity must be zero. Hence the time (t), taken to reach the highest point is given by

$$0 = v_{0y} + gt \Rightarrow v_{0y} = -gt \Rightarrow t_{max} = \frac{|v_{0y}|}{|g|}$$

3. At O and F the vertical components of velocity are equal in magnitude and opposite in direction while the horizontal components are equal in both magnitude and direction.
4. The maximum range is attained when $\theta = 45°$

APPLIED CONCEPTS

1. Analyze the construction, design, and working of a ballistocardiography unit. The displacement, velocity, and acceleration of a platform are used to measure several cardiac parameters to diagnose abnormalities in the cardiovascular system. Find information from an encyclopedia on how science problems are constructed from such a device.
2. Measure velocities and acceleration of a walker, a jogger, and a runner. Try to plot motion trajectories and analyze the concept of positive and negative acceleration.
3. Read articles on biomechanics of running and other athletic activities, e.g., trampoline jumps, tennis, discus throw, and javelin throw.

TRANSLATIONAL MOTION: REVIEW QUESTIONS

1. Which of the following does not depend on direction?
   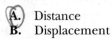
   A. Distance
   B. Displacement

C. Acceleration
D. All of the above

2. Which of the following is a vector?

   A. Distance
   B. Speed
   C. Velocity
   D. All of the above

3. The variable with the dimension of length/time^2 is:

   A. displacement.
   B. velocity.
   C. acceleration.
   D. force.

4. A constant acceleration is caused by a:

   A. constant force.
   B. changing force.
   C. constant displacement.
   D. combination of constant and changing force.

5. A force was applied for 10 seconds to an object moving at 10 m/sec. The final velocity was 60 m/sec. What was the acceleration?

   A. 3 m/sec^2
   B. 5 m/sec^2
   C. 7 m/sec^2
   D. None of the above

6. An object initially moving at 15 m/sec is accelerated at the rate of 5 m/sec^2 for 5 seconds. What is the final velocity of the object?

   A. 15 m/sec
   B. 25 m/sec
   C. 40 m/sec
   D. 100 m/sec

7. An object starts 5 m from a reference point with an initial velocity of 10 m/sec and an acceleration of 5 m/sec^2. How far is the object from the reference point after 5 seconds?

   A. 75 m
   B. 80 m
   C. 117.5 m
   D. 180.5 m

$$d = d_0 + V_0 t + \tfrac{1}{2} a t^2$$
$$5 + (10)5 + \tfrac{1}{2}(5)(5)^2$$
$$5 + 50 + 125/2$$
$$5 + 62.5$$

$$\begin{array}{r} 62.5 \\ 55 \\ \hline 117.5 \end{array}$$

Questions 8–12
Use the following velocity-time graph to answer this group of questions. The motion is in a straight line.

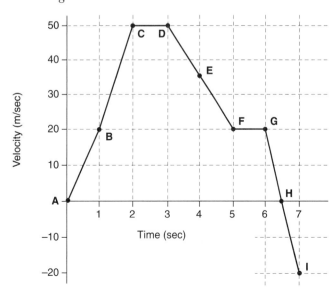

8. The slope of the graph at any point represents:

   A. acceleration.
   B. displacement.
   C. force.
   D. kinetic energy.

9. What is the instantaneous velocity at point B?

   A. 20 m/sec
   B. 25 m/sec
   C. 10 m/sec
   D. 35 m/sec

10. What is the instantaneous acceleration at point E?

    A. 15 m/sec^2
    B. -15 m/sec^2
    C. 30 m/sec^2
    D. -30 m/sec^2

11. The total displacement of the particle between t = 0 to t = 7 seconds is approximately:

    A. -145 m.
    B. 125 m.
    C. 185 m.
    D. 350 m.

12. The average speed from 0 to 2 seconds is:

    A. 12.5 m/sec.
    B. 20 m/sec.
    C. 22.5 m/sec.
    D. 25 m/sec.

13. Which of the following steps greatly simplifies the analysis of projectile motion?

    I. Using the formula for describing the motion as a parabola
    II. Realizing that the time of ascent is one-half the time of descent
    III. Neglecting the effect of gravity if the object is considered a point mass
    IV. Separating the motion into vertical (free fall) and horizontal (uniform accelerated motion) components

    A. I and II
    B. II, III, and IV
    C. I and III
    D. I, II, and IV

14. The maximum horizontal distance an object can attain is when the object is thrown at an angle to the horizontal. What is the value of that angle?

    A. 15°
    B. 30°
    C. 45°
    D. 60°

15. An unbalanced force acting on an object causes:

    A. a change in mass.
    B. acceleration of the object.
    C. it to maintain a constant velocity.
    D. none of the above.

16. An object is thrown vertically at an initial velocity of 49 m/sec. To what height will it rise?

    A. 122.5 m
    B. 245 m
    C. 490 m
    D. Cannot determine without knowing time

17. An object is dropped from the edge of a cliff. How far will it fall in 10 seconds?

A. Cannot be determined without knowing mass of object
B. 98 m
C. 980 m
D. 490 m

Questions 18 and 19
An object is thrown with an initial speed of 19.6 m/sec at an angle of 30° with the horizontal.

18. The maximum height the object reaches is:

A. 2.45 m.
B. 4.9 m.
C. 9.8 m.
D. 98 m.

19. The range (horizontal distance) of the object is:

A. 19.6 m.
B. $19.6\sqrt{3}$ m.
C. 9.8 m.
D. $9.8\sqrt{3}$ m.

ANSWERS AND EXPLANATIONS

1–4. 1-A, 2-C, 3-C, 4-A. See text for explanation.

5. **B** Use the formula for acceleration (a):

$$a = \frac{\Delta v}{\Delta t} = \frac{(v_f - v_i)}{(t_f - t_i)} = \frac{(60 - 10)}{(10 - 0)} = \frac{50}{10} = \frac{5 \text{ m}}{\text{sec}^2}$$

6. **C** The final velocity (v_f) is:

$$v_f = \text{initial velocity} + \text{velocity change due to acceleration}$$

$$= \frac{15 \text{ m}}{\text{sec}} + at = 15 + \left(\frac{5 \text{ m}}{\text{sec}^2}\right)(5 \text{ sec})$$

$$= 15 + 25 = \frac{40 \text{ m}}{\text{sec}}$$

7. **C** Use the formula for distance:

$$d = d_o + v_o t + \tfrac{1}{2} at^2 = 5 + (10)(5) + \tfrac{1}{2}(5)(5)^2$$

$$= 5 + 50 + (\tfrac{1}{2})(5)(25) = 55 + \tfrac{1}{2}(125)$$

$$= 55 + 62.5 = 117.5$$

8. **A** The slope of the curve of any graph is the ratio of the change in the y-axis (Δy) to the corresponding change in the x-axis (Δx). In this case:
Δy = change in speed = Δv
Δx = change in time = Δt
then:
Slope = $\Delta y / \Delta x = \Delta v / \Delta t$ = acceleration

9. **A** Instantaneous velocity is the velocity at a given point in time.

10. **B** Because E is on line DF, the instantaneous acceleration (i.e., the slope at a given point) at E is the same as the slope of line DF:

$$\text{Acceleration at E} = \frac{(20 - 50)}{(5 - 3)} = \frac{-30}{2} = -\frac{15 \text{ m}}{\text{sec}^2}$$

11. **C** The area of the graph for each time interval is the displacement. Review equations for area of a triangle and a trapezoid to calculate values.

Triangle AB 0–1 sec $20 \times \tfrac{1}{2} = 10$ m

Trapezoid BC 1–2 sec $(20 + 50) \times \tfrac{1}{2} = 35$ m

Rectangle CD 2–3 sec $50 \times 1 = 50$ m

Trapezoid DE 3–4 sec $35 + \frac{1}{2}(15) = 42.5$ m

Trapezoid EF 4–5 sec $20 + \frac{1}{2}(15) = 27.5$ m

Rectangle FG 5–6 sec $20 \times 1 = 20$ m

Triangle G-H-I 6−7 sec $20 \times (\frac{1}{2}) − 20 \times (\frac{1}{2}) = 0$ m (area H-I is negative)

Total of all displacements from $t = 0$ to $t = 7$: $10 + 35 + 50 + 42.5 + 27.5 + 20 = 185$ m

12. **C** The average speed = total distance/total time. The total distance is the area under the graph from A to C.

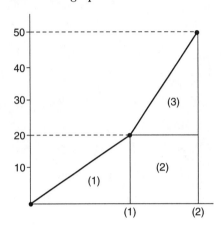

Total area = distance = Area 1 + Area 2 + Area 3

$$= (\tfrac{1}{2})(20)(1) + (20)(1) + (\tfrac{1}{2})(30)(1)$$

$$= 10 + 20 + 15 = 45 \text{ m}$$

Average speed $= 45 \text{ m}/2 \text{ sec} = 22.5$ m/sec. The formula $v = \dfrac{v_f + v_i}{2}$ cannot be used because the acceleration is not constant over this interval.

13–15. **13-D, 14-C, 15-B.** See text for explanation.

16. **A** The velocity at the top $= v_y = 0$

$$v_y = v_{oy} − gt = 0$$

therefore, $v_{oy} = gt$

$$t = \frac{v_{oy}}{g} = \frac{\dfrac{49 \text{ m}}{\text{sec}}}{\dfrac{9.8 \text{ m}}{\text{sec}^2}} = 5 \text{ sec}$$

Then, using the formula for uniform accelerated motion:

$$y = y_o + v_{oy} + \tfrac{1}{2} gt^2 = 0 + 49(5) + \tfrac{1}{2}(−9.8)(5)^2 = 245 − 122.5$$

$$d = 122.5 \text{ m}$$

17. **D** In this example of free fall motion, use the equations for accelerated motion and the fact that gravity is the acceleration (taking the downward direction as positive):

$$y = y_o + v_{oy}t + \tfrac{1}{2} gt^2$$

$$= 0 + (0)(10) + (\tfrac{1}{2})(9.8)(10)^2 = (4.9)(100) = 490 \text{ m}$$

18. **B** The maximum height would correspond to the height reached if the object was thrown upward with the vertical component of the initial velocity (v_o):

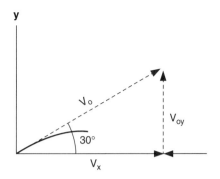

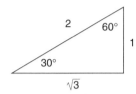

Note: For future reference, memorization of these lengths for the triangle is suggested.

$$v_{oy} = v_o \sin 30° = (19.6)(½) = \frac{9.8 \text{ m}}{\text{sec}}$$

$$v_{ox} = v_o \cos 30° = (19.6)\left(\frac{\sqrt{3}}{2}\right) = 9.8 \frac{\sqrt{3}\text{m}}{\text{sec}}$$

Remember: sin θ = opposite/hypotenuse; cos θ = adjacent/hypotenuse. The height can be calculated using the formula for accelerated motion:

$$y = y_0 + v_{oy}t + ½ gt^2$$

where g = -32 ft/sec^2

Time is found by reasoning that the object continues to rise until its upward motion is offset by the downward acceleration of gravity g (note that here g = -9.8 m/sec^2). At the highest point, v_y = 0 so that $v_y = v_{oy} + gt = 0$ implies

$$t = \frac{v_{oy}}{g} = -\frac{9.8 \text{ m/sec}}{(-9.8 \text{ m/sec}^2)} = 1 \text{ sec}$$

to reach the top of the trajectory.

Note that 1 second is the time required for half the trajectory. Using the formula for accelerated motion:

$$y = y_0 + v_{oy}t + ½ gt^2$$

$$y = 0 + (9.8)(1) + ½(-9.8)(1)^2 = 9.8 - 4.9 = 4.9 \text{ m}$$

19. B If the time for half the trajectory is 1 sec (see question 18), the total time is 2 seconds. To find the range, use the horizontal component of the initial velocity (v_x) as calculated in question 18. There is no force in the horizontal direction so the acceleration is zero in this direction. Using the equation for accelerated motion applied in the horizontal direction:

$$d = d_x + v_xt + ½ a_xt^2$$

$$d = 0 + (9.8\sqrt{3})(2) + (½)(0)(2)^2$$

$$d = 19.6 \sqrt{3} \text{ m}$$

Force and Motion, Gravitation

Self-Managed Learning Questions

1. Conceptualize force in real-life situations. Construct diagrams to understand the direction and magnitude of several forces, e.g., on a swimmer, on an airplane, on

a seatbelt in a car, on objects during an earthquake, that cause chemical reactions, etc.

2. Draw free-body diagrams for complex situations:
   - Forces on the hook when you catch a fish
   - Forces on your body when you run uphill
   - Forces on a bird flying from point A to point B
   - Forces on an ant's body dragging a piece of bread on the wall
   - Forces on a beetle swimming in a cup of water
   - Forces on the space shuttle astronauts at takeoff, 15 seconds after takeoff, 1 minute after takeoff, and 10 minutes after takeoff
3. List several types of forces acting on a red blood cell as it enters the heart and as it leaves the heart.
4. How will you estimate the forces acting on plasma in a blood centrifuge? Draw a rough sectional view of a blood centrifuge. Read the specifications on the machine and the actual working mechanisms of such a machine.

Note: The terms "body" and "object" are used interchangeably in physics. A body generally refers to a rigid body. A body consists of a large number of particles.

MASS, CENTER OF MASS, AND WEIGHT

The center of mass (COM) of a body is the point at which motion can be described like a particle (e.g., as linear, circular, parabolic), even if the motion of the object cannot be so described. In collisions, the COM velocity (of the system) is not changed. The **center of gravity** (COG) is the COM, but it is conceptualized as the point at which the sum of gravitational forces acting on an object can be represented by a summation force (acting at the COM). An object suspended from the COG is in rotational equilibrium (see subsequent discussion of equilibrium and momentum). The COG can be determined experimentally by suspending an object by a string at different points and noting that the direction of the string passes through the COG. The intersections of the projected lines in the different suspensions is the COG. The COG of a regular geometric object is the geometric center. The COG of an irregular object may be inside or outside the object.

An object is in **stable equilibrium** if the COG is as low as possible, and any change in orientation would lead to an elevation of the COG. In **unstable equilibrium**, the COG is high (relative to a surface supporting it), and any change in orientation would lead to a lowering of the COG. **Neutral equilibrium** is an intermediate location of the COG and a change in orientation would not change the level of the COG.

A force acting through the COG causes translational motion. A force acting off the COG causes rotational and translational motion. **Mass** (a scalar) is a dimension that cannot be broken down into simpler units. This fact is in contrast to **weight**, which is a force, hence, a vector. Units of mass are slugs (weight in pounds divided by $g = 32$ ft/$\sec^2$), kilograms, grams, etc. Units of weight are pounds, dynes ($g \cdot cm/\sec^2$), and newtons ($kg \cdot m/\sec^2$).

NEWTON'S SECOND LAW

Newton's second law relates an unbalanced force acting on an object, producing an acceleration in the direction of the force that is directly proportional to the force and inversely proportional to the mass of the body:

$$a = \frac{F}{m}$$

$$\text{or, } F = ma$$

Or, Force = mass $\times$ acceleration. Notice that for uniformly accelerated motion, Newton's second law can be written in the form:

$$F = ma = m \frac{v_f - v_i}{t_f - t_i}$$

Applications and uses of this important law include driving a nail into the wall, putting your foot on the accelerator of the car while driving, freely falling objects, inclined plane motion with friction, running compared to jogging, and the movement of blood and drugs in arteries and veins. Draw a "free-body" diagram to solve problems that involve the second and third laws of motion.

Momentum (a vector) is defined by the equation:

$$\text{Momentum} = \text{mass} \times \text{velocity}$$

The **impulse–momentum principle** relates the effect a force exerted on a mass (m) has on the velocity of the mass and is defined, in the case of a fixed force and fixed mass, by the equation:

$$F\Delta t = m\Delta v$$

or

$$F(t_f - t_i) = m(v_f - v_i)$$

which is just another way to write Newton's second law for uniformly accelerated motion. Note that if either F or v vary with time, these equations no longer hold, and the analysis would require calculus.

NEWTON'S THIRD LAW

This law states that for every action, there is an equal and opposite reaction. If one object exerts a force, F, on a second object, the second object exerts a force, $-F$, on the first. These forces cannot neutralize each other because they act on different objects. Every force relates to three basic forces: gravitational (see subsequent discussion), electromagnetic (see section concerning electrostatics and electromagnetism), and nuclear (see section concerning nuclear and atomic structure).

LAW OF GRAVITATION

Newton's law of gravitation:

$$F = G\left(\frac{m_1 m_2}{r^2}\right)$$

G = Gravitational constant (do not confuse with Gibbs' free energy, ΔG)

states that a gravitational force exists between any two bodies of masses m_1 and m_2. The magnitude of force is proportional to the product of the masses:

$$F \propto m_1 m_2$$

and inversely proportional to the square of the distance between them:

$$F \propto \frac{1}{r^2}$$

The forces act along the line joining the centers of the masses. (G is the universal constant of gravitation. Its value depends on the units being used.)

UNIFORM CIRCULAR MOTION AND CENTRIPETAL FORCE

In **uniform circular motion** (UCM), an object rotates around a fixed point at a constant speed. The velocity is constant in magnitude, but is not constant in direction, and its acceleration is directed toward the center of the circle (also known as centripetal acceleration). UCM also can be described by specifying the period rather than the speed. Period is equal to the amount of time required for the object to travel once around the circle. Consider the formula:

$$v = \frac{2\pi r}{T} = \frac{\text{circumference}}{\text{time period}}$$

in which the velocity vector is tangential to the circle.

Angular velocity, ω, is measured in radians per second, and it can be connected to the rpm (revolutions per minute) of a moving rotor or a centrifuge (Fig. 7-49).

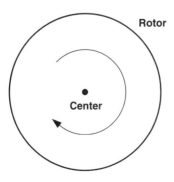

Fig. 7-49.   1 revolution = 360° = 2π radius

If N = RPM of rotor = revolutions/minute, then

$$\omega = 2\pi(\text{radians}) \times \frac{\text{N revolutions/minute}}{60 \text{ seconds/minute}} = 2\pi\frac{\text{N}}{60} \text{ (radians/second)}.$$

The velocity of an object with angular velocity ω is given by

$$v = \omega r$$

where r is the radius of the circle.

For a rotating object, m is constant, r is usually constant, and ω and v can vary with time. Hence, force is proportional to the radial distance from the center.

Centripetal force is the force exerted on the rotating object and is directed toward the center of the circle. Centripetal force must be present to achieve UCM. The magnitude of the force is given by the equation:

$$F = \frac{mv^2}{r} = \frac{m}{r}(\omega r)^2 = m\omega^2 r$$

FRICTION

Frictional forces are illustrated in Figure 7-50. $F = \mu N$, which is the maximal frictional force; μ = coefficient of friction; and N = normal (perpendicular) force to the surface on which the object rests.

Friction is the resistance offered to the motion between two bodies. Friction depends on the texture (roughness) of the contact surface of two bodies.

Frictional forces are nonconservative (mechanical energy is not conserved) and are caused by molecular adhesions between tangential surfaces, but they are independent of the area of contact of the surfaces. Frictional forces always oppose motion. Static friction exists when the object is not moving, and it must be overcome for motion to begin. The **coefficient of static friction**, μ_s, is expressed as:

$$\mu_s = \tan \theta$$

in which θ is the angle at which the object first begins to move. On an inclined plane, as the angle is increased from 0° to θ, the object slips initially and then slides down the plane (Fig. 7-51).

A **coefficient of kinetic friction**, μ_k, exists when surfaces are in motion. Note that the static coefficient is always greater than the kinetic coefficient ($\mu_s > \mu_k$).

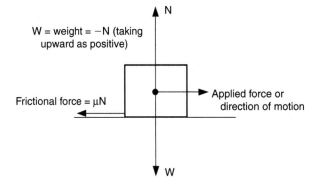

Fig. 7-50. Frictional forces related to normal forces.

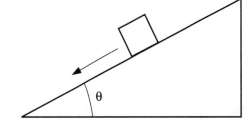

Fig. 7-51. Inclined plane.

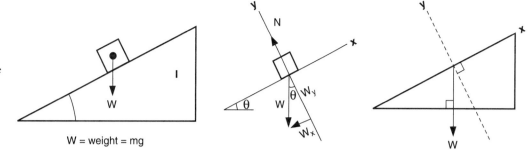

Fig. 7-52. Motion on an incline I (neglecting friction).

W = weight = mg

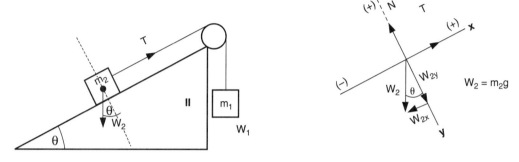

Fig. 7-53. Motion on an incline II.

$W_2 = m_2g$

INCLINED PLANES

The analysis of **motion on an incline** is shown in Figure 7-52. The components of forces are as follows:

N = normal (perpendicular) force to the surface on which the object rests

$W_y = W\cos\theta$, $W_x = W\sin\theta$

The weight (W), related to gravity (g), may be sufficient to cause motion if friction is overcome. The reference axes are usually chosen as shown such that one (axis) is along the surface of the incline. In Figure 7-53, additional forces, such as tension (T), on the object are added. In this illustration, $m_2 > m_1$ and the free-body diagram is for mass m_2. Note that N is the reactive force to W_{2y}, and the axes are assigned (+) and (−) as one desires.

In Figure 7-53, let F denote the net force on m_2 and let its components be F_x, F_y with the coordinate axes as shown. Note that $T = w_1 = m_1g$, and this is directed in the + x-direction. The x-component of the force due to m_2 is w_{2x} and is directed in the negative x-direction. Hence

$$F_x = T - w_{2x} = m_1g - w_{2x} = m_1g - w_2 \sin \theta$$

Because m_2 is not moving in the y-direction (recall Newton's second law $F_y = ma_y$), the forces in the y-direction must sum to zero. The upward force is N and the downward force is $-w_{2y}$ so that

$$0 = F_y = N - w_{2y} = N - w_2 \cos \theta$$

The resultant of the forces on m_2 has magnitude

$$F = \sqrt{(F_x)^2 + (F_y)^2}$$

PULLEY SYSTEMS

Pulleys are used in several traction devices. The basic components in two traction mechanisms are illustrated in Figures 7-54 and 7-55.

APPLIED CONCEPTS

1. Understand the design working and sources of error for the goniometer and accelerometer and other biomechanical instruments, such as the electromyography apparatus.

2. Construct free-body diagrams for forces acting on a golf ball, basketball, football, and tennis ball during motion.

3. Draw and analyze the major bones of the human skeleton—understand the bone shape, size, basic structure, and its use for biomedical functions.

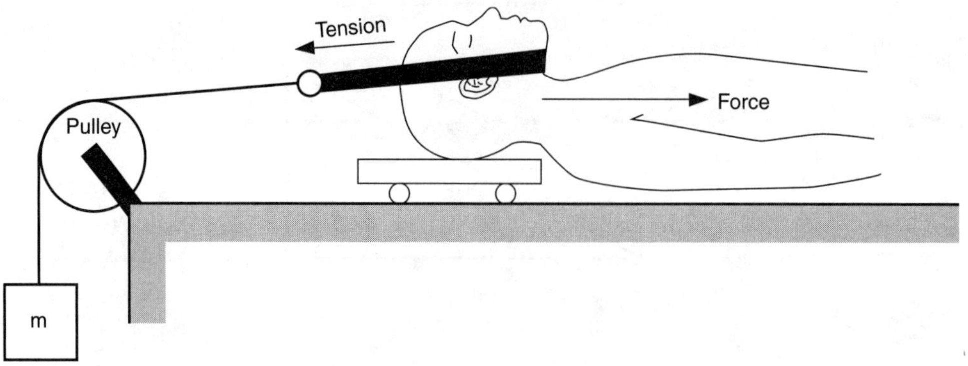

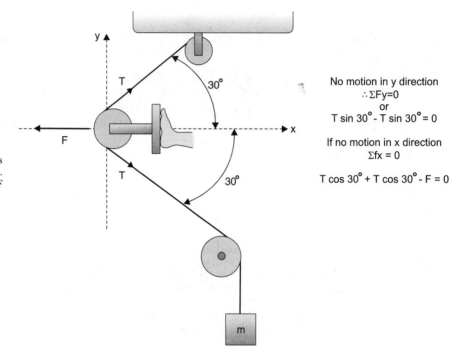

Fig. 7-54. Neck injury requires traction to keep cervical vertebrae under tension.

Tension

Force

Pulley

m

y

T

30°

x

F

T

30°

m

No motion in y direction
∴ ΣFy=0
or
T sin 30° - T sin 30° = 0

If no motion in x direction
Σfx = 0

T cos 30° + T cos 30° - F = 0

Fig. 7-55. Foot injury requires traction device with three pulleys. The force at the foot plate is F along the x-axis.

FORCE AND MOTION, GRAVITATION: REVIEW QUESTIONS

1. One of Newton's laws of motion states that:

   A. an unbalanced force acting on an object produces an acceleration of that object.
   B. objects moving in circles at constant tangential velocity have no force acting on them.
   C. the square of the period of revolution is proportional to the cube of the radius of revolution.
   D. objects falling to earth describe a hyperbolic trajectory.

2. For any object to undergo an acceleration, it must:

   A. lose energy.
   B. gain energy.
   C. be acted on by balanced (net zero) forces.
   D. be acted on by unbalanced forces.

3. Newton's second law is mathematically represented by which of the following expressions?

   A. $E = \frac{1}{2}mv^2$
   B. $F = -kx$
   C. $U = mgh$
   D. $F = ma$

4. Frictional forces exist between an object and the surface it is on, and they:

   A. are proportional to the normal force to the surface.

B. are dependent on the area of contact between the surfaces.

C. always augment the motion of the object.

D. are conservative forces.

5. Which of the following expressions best represents the relationship between μ_s (coefficient of static friction) and μ_k (coefficient of kinetic friction)?

A. $\mu_s > \mu_k$

B. $\mu_s = \mu_k$

C. $\mu_s < \mu_k$

D. $\mu_s \cdot \mu_k = 1$

6. The motion of the center of mass is like:

A. the motion of a particle.

B. the motion of an extended object.

C. the motion of a rigid body.

D. none of the above.

7. The force of gravitation between two objects is:

A. inversely proportional to the products of the masses.

B. inversely proportional to the distance between the objects.

C. directly proportional to the square of the radius.

D. inversely proportional to the square of the distance between the objects.

8. A force of 15 newtons (N) acting on a 5-kg object will produce an acceleration equal to:

A. $\frac{1}{3}$ m/sec².

B. $\frac{1}{75}$ m/sec².

C. 3 m/sec².

D. 75 m/sec².

9. An object has an acceleration of 2 m/sec² and a mass of a 5 kg. What is the force (in newtons) necessary to impart this acceleration?

A. 0.4

B. 2.5

C. 5

D. 10

10. An object first begins to slip down an inclined plane when the angle with the horizontal is 45°. What is the coefficient of static friction (μ_s) of the object–surface?

A. 0.5

B. 1.0

C. $\frac{\sqrt{2}}{2}$

D. Insufficient information provided

Questions 11–15

The following speed–time graph is for a 2-kg object moving along a straight line to the right.

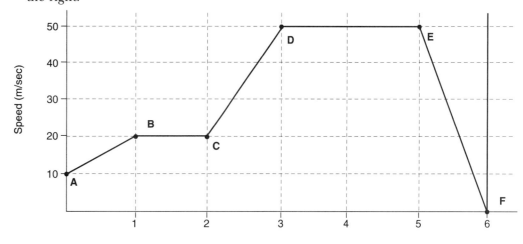

11. The area under the graph represents:

    A. distance.
    B. acceleration.
    C. force.
    D. velocity.

12. The greatest force is acting at:

    A. AB.
    B. BC.
    C. CD.
    D. EF.

13. No net force is acting along:

    A. AB.
    B. BC.
    C. CD.
    D. EF.

14. What is the distance (in meters) traveled from A to B?

    A. 5
    B. 10
    C. 15
    D. 20

15. At point F, the object is:

    A. motionless.
    B. moving backward.
    C. moving forward.
    D. at the origin.

16. What value of weight (W_1) is required such that the object (A) in the following diagram does not move down the incline (assume no friction)?

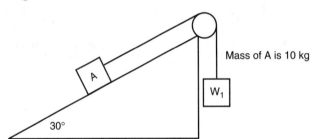

Mass of A is 10 kg

30°

    A. 5 newtons
    B. 10 newtons
    C. 49 newtons
    D. None of the above

17. The wheel of a car has a radius of 12 inches and is being rotated at 750 rpm on an automotive tire-balancing machine. Determine the angular velocity and the tangential velocity at which the wheel periphery is moving.

    A. 750 sec^{-1}, 88 fps
    B. 78 · 5 sec^{-1}, 78 · 5 fps
    C. 750 fps, 88 sec^{-1}
    D. 12 · 5 sec^{-1}, 78 · 5 fps

ANSWERS AND EXPLANATIONS

1–7. **1-A, 2-D, 3-D, 4-A, 5-A, 6-A, 7-D.** See text for explanation.

8. **C** $F = ma$

$$a = \frac{F}{m} = \frac{15 \text{ newtons}}{5 \text{ kg}} = 3(\text{nts/kg})$$

$$= 3 \left[\frac{\frac{kg \cdot m}{sec^2}}{kg} \right] = \frac{3 \text{ m}}{sec^2}$$

9. D $F = ma = (5\ kg)(2\ m/sec^2) = 10\ kg \cdot m/sec^2 = 10$ newtons

10. B   Use the following to find μ_s:

$$\mu_s = \tan \theta$$

$$\mu_s = \tan 45°$$

$$\mu_s = \frac{1}{1} = 1$$

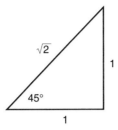

tan θ = opposite/adjacent.

11. A   The area under any curve is proportional to the product of the quantities represented by the axes:

y-axis is speed (v)

x-axis is time (t)

Product = (v)(t) = distance

12. D   The greatest force acts where the greatest acceleration (positive or negative) acts, because:

$$F = ma \text{ and } F \propto a$$

The greatest acceleration is where the slope $\Delta v / \Delta t$ is the greatest in absolute value (neglecting signs). For each of these line segments, the slope and acceleration is:

$$a = \frac{\Delta v}{\Delta t} = \frac{(v_f - v_i)}{(t_f - t_i)}$$

$$AB: a = \frac{(20 - 10)}{(1 - 0)} = \frac{10}{1} = 10$$

$$BC: a = \frac{(20 - 20)}{(2 - 1)} = \frac{0}{1} = 0$$

$$CD: a = \frac{(50 - 20)}{(3 - 2)} = \frac{30}{1} = 30$$

$$EF: a = \frac{(0 - 50)}{(6 - 5)} = \frac{-50}{1} = -50$$

Hence, EF has the greatest acceleration and the greatest force.

13. B   Because $F = ma$ and $F \propto a$, a zero acceleration gives a zero force. A zero acceleration occurs where the slope is zero (see discussion in question 12 for the slopes of the segments). BC and DE are the only segments with a zero slope and, therefore, a zero acceleration and a zero force.

14. C   (I) By geometry:

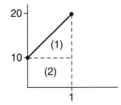

$$\text{Area (1)} = (\tfrac{1}{2})(10)(1) = 5 \text{ m}$$

$$\text{Area (2)} = (10)(1) = 10 \text{ m}$$

$$\text{Total} = 5 + 10 = 15 \text{ m}$$

(II) By formulas:

$$d = d_o + v_o t + \tfrac{1}{2} at^2$$

$$d_o = 0 \qquad v_o = \frac{10 \text{ m}}{\text{sec}}$$

$$a = \frac{\Delta v}{\Delta t} = \frac{(20 - 10)}{(1 - 0)} = \frac{10}{1} = \frac{10 \text{ m}}{\text{sec}^2}$$

$$t = 1 \text{ sec}$$

$$d = 0 + (10)(1) + (\tfrac{1}{2})(10)(1)^2 = 10 + 5 = 15 \text{ m}$$

15. A The speed is zero at point F, so the object must not be moving. Also, note that at no point is the speed negative, so the object could not have returned to the origin.

16. C The forces are shown as follows:

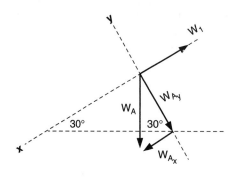

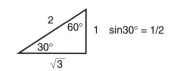

$$W_A = mg = (10)(9.8) = 98 \text{ N}$$

$$W_{A_x} = W_A \sin 30° = (98)(1/2) = 49 \text{ N}$$

$$\sin 30° = 1/2$$

W_1 should balance W_{Ax}. W_{Ay} has no effect on motion along x (the incline). Therefore, W_1 of 49 newtons is required. The mass would be: $m = W_1/g = 49/9.8 = 5$ kg.

17. B $r = 12$ inches $= 1$ foot

$$N = 750 \text{ RPM} = \frac{750}{60} = 12.5 \text{ RPS}$$

$$T = \frac{\text{seconds}}{\text{revolution}} = \frac{1}{12.5} \text{ sec} = 0.08 \text{ sec}$$

$$v_T = \text{tangential velocity} = \frac{2\pi r}{T} = \frac{2\pi(1)}{0.08} = 78.5 \text{ fps}$$

$$\omega = v_T r = 78 \cdot 5(1) = \frac{78 \cdot 5 \text{ radians}}{\text{sec}} = 78.5/\text{sec}$$

Equilibrium and Momentum

Self-Managed Learning Questions

1. Draw free-body diagrams for several situations to analyze problems using equilibrium or momentum principles; for example, a diver jumping off a diving board, an airplane taking off and landing, or a car coming to a screeching stop in a sudden traffic jam. List all the variables involved in solving such problems using impulse-momentum or energy principles.

2. Observe the concept of collision by obtaining several colored balls from a toy store and using rigid and elastic collisions. Use a steel ball hitting a tennis ball at several speeds or use a pool table to understand the concept of elastic and inelastic collisions.

3. Understand the concepts of resistance, viscosity, and friction as they apply to exter-

nal surface forces (e.g., soles of shoes used by walkers and runners) and internal forces (e.g., blood viscosity), and how a simple model (experimental) can be proposed to measure and analyze blood viscosity. Relate the blood viscosity concept to momentum of blood in arteries (linear or angular) and friction measurements.

EQUILIBRIUM

Translational Equilibrium

When a force (see previous section concerning force and motion, gravitation) acts on an object, the object undergoes translational or rotational motion. Translational motion is the motion of the object through space when the force is acting along an axis and/or the center of mass (that point for which motion can be described like a particle). For translational equilibrium:

$$\sum Fx = \text{sum of all forces in } x\text{-direction} = 0$$

$$\sum Fy = \text{sum of all forces in } y\text{-direction} = 0$$

Rotational Equilibrium, Torques, and Lever Arms

Rotational motion is the rotation of an object about an axis caused by a force not directed along that axis. The effective force causing rotation about an axis is the torque (L) (Fig. 7-56). To determine the direction of rotation caused by the torque, imagine the direction in which the object would rotate if the force is pushing against its moment arm (at right angles). The net forces acting on an object is best determined by resolving them into the x and y components. The net torques acting on an object is obtained by summing the counterclockwise ($+$) and clockwise ($-$) torques. An object is at equilibrium when the net forces and torques acting on it are zero. There is no acceleration, but that does not mean there is no velocity. Rather, either the object is motionless or it is moving with a constant velocity.

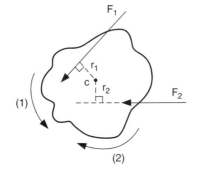

Fig. 7-56. Torque (rotational moment).

L = (force) x (moment arm);
   moment arm is the perpendicular
   distance from the force to the axis
F = force
r = moment arm
c = center of mass or an axis
$L_1 = (F_1)(r_1)$ = counterclockwise (1) = positive
$L_2 = (F_2)(r_2)$ = clockwise (2) = negative

For rotational equilibrium:

$$\sum L = 0 \text{ (in a given geometric plane, must hold for three}$$
mutually perpendicular planes)

If the torques sum to zero about one point in an object, they will sum to zero about any point in the object. If the point chosen as reference includes the line of action of one of the forces, that force need not be included in calculating the torques.

The offset between two parallel forces is the **lever arm** (Fig. 7-57). When the lever arm increases, the rotation of the object occurs more readily. Torque depends on the size of the force and on the lever arm. Note that a small force and a large lever arm can cause the same rotation as a large force and a small lever arm.

Newton's First Law

Newton's first law states that objects at rest or in motion tend to remain as such unless acted on by an outside force; that is, objects have inertia (resistance to a **change** in

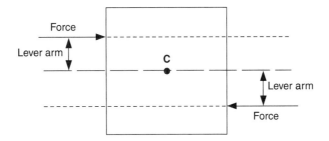

Fig. 7-57. Lever arm.

motion). For translational motion, the mass (m) is a measure of inertia. For rotational motion, a quantity derived from mass called the moment of inertia (I) is the measure of inertia. Thus, in general, $I = \sum mr^2$, but its exact formulation depends on the structure of the object (see previous discussion of solid and fluid properties for compressive and tensile forces).

MOMENTUM

Momentum (P) is a vector quantity. It is defined by:

$$P = mv$$

in which m = mass and v = velocity. Be sure to understand impulse and momentum concepts as they relate to a human situation.

The **impulse** (I) generated by a force F acting over a time Δt is defined to be $I = F\Delta t$. The impulse–momentum principle states that

$$I = F\Delta t = m\Delta v = mv_f - mv_i$$

$$= \text{final momentum} - \text{initial momentum}$$

Conservation of Linear Momentum

Linear momentum is a measure of the tendency of an object to maintain motion in a straight line. Notice that P is directly proportional to the mass of the object and its velocity (not acceleration). The larger the P, the greater the tendency of the object to remain moving along a straight line (in the same direction). Momentum is also a measure of the force needed to stop or change direction of the object. Just like energy, **momentum is also conserved**. The total linear momentum of a system is constant when the resultant external force acting on the system is zero.

Remember the three conservation laws for all states of matter:

1. Law of conservation of mass
2. Law of conservation of momentum
3. Law of conservation of energy

Elastic and Inelastic Collisions

Collisions are a form of interaction of matter during which momentum (which is a vector) is conserved. During an elastic collision (objects do not stick), there is conservation of momentum and conservation of kinetic energy. During an inelastic collision (objects stick together), there is conservation of momentum but not of kinetic energy (the remainder of the energy is lost as heat or sound, so total energy is conserved).

It is important to mention two special collisions. In the explosion of an object at rest, the total momentum of all the fragments must sum to zero (original momentum was zero). If one object collides elastically with a second identical object that is at rest, the first object comes to rest and the second moves off with the momentum of the first. (Newton's second and third laws of motion are discussed in the preceding section concerning force and motion, gravitation.)

APPLIED CONCEPTS

1. Understand the working and design of a centrifugal sample analyzer as an application of rotational equilibrium and angular momentum. Usually the centrifugal rotor spins at 300 rpm. Mixing takes place by bubbles or by alternate acceleration and deceleration. Samples are measured at approximately 200 msec.
2. Understand the concept of angular momentum as it applies to the knee joint, which is the center of rotation for body movements, as well as the elbow angle variations for different movements. Draw a basic diagram illustrating the joint movements at the wrist of a tennis player, a softball pitcher, and a golf player. Consider how to relate momentum and equilibrium principles to the movements of these sports players.

EQUILIBRIUM AND MOMENTUM: REVIEW QUESTIONS

1. Rotational motion represents:

   A. movement of an object along a curved line.
   B. movement of an object through space.
   C. motion of an object about a fixed point.
   D. motion of an object about an axis.

2. Newton's first law states, "An object at rest tends to remain at rest while objects in motion tend to remain in motion . . . " It reflects the property of:

   A. velocity.
   B. weight.

C. potential energy.
   D. inertia.

3. If a force is acting on an object, but off an axis, what type of motion results? Assume the axis is fixed in space.

   A. Rotational
   B. Translational
   C. Frictional
   D. Projectile

4. The product of force times the perpendicular moment arm is the:

   A. energy.
   B. work.
   C. torque.
   D. force.

5. The net force in newtons (N) on the following object is:

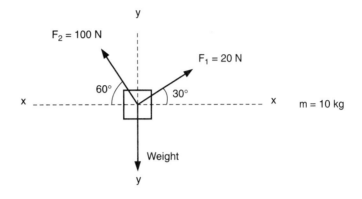

   A. zero
   B. 32.7
   C. 99.5
   D. 127.9

6. What is the net force on the following object?

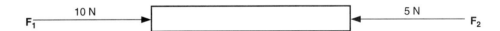

   A. 15 N
   B. 5 N to the right
   C. 5 N compressive force
   D. None of the above

7. What is the net torque acting about the axis through the center A (perpendicular to the page) of the square with sides equal to 4 m?

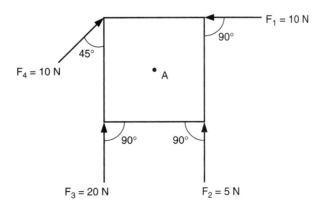

A. 38.2 N·m — counterclockwise
B. 76.4 N·m — clockwise
C. 38.2 N·m — clockwise
D. None of the above

8. The following object is in static and rotational equilibrium. What are the components of the force, F_1?

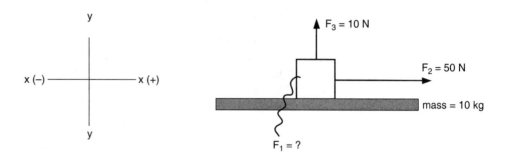

A. $F_x = -50$ N; $F_y = -10$ N
B. $F_x = -50$ N; $F_y = +88$ N
C. $F_x = +50$ N; $F_y = -108$ N
D. None of the above

9. The following object is in rotational equilibrium. What force, F_1 (along the dashed line), is required for this equilibrium (neglect the weight)?

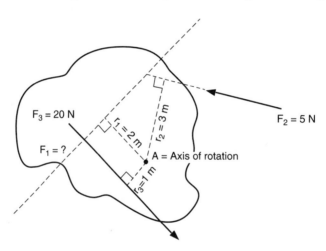

A. Counterclockwise, 17.5 N
B. Clockwise, 5 N
C. Clockwise, 35 N
D. None of the above

ANSWERS AND EXPLANATIONS

1–4. 1-D, 2-D, 3-A, 4-C. See text for explanation.
5. B The forces may be rediagrammed as:

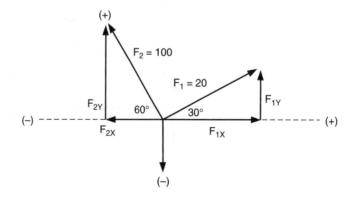

$W_y = 10(-9.8) = -98N$
(Weight has no x-component in this case.)

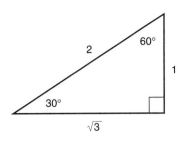

Let F_x, F_y be the resultant forces in the x and y directions. Then:

$$F_x = F_{1x} + F_{2x}$$

and

$$F_y = W_y + F_{1y} + F_{2y}$$

Since:

$$\frac{1}{2} = \sin 30° = \frac{F_{1y}}{20} \Rightarrow F_{1y} = 10 \text{ N},$$

$$\frac{\sqrt{3}}{2} = \cos 30° = \frac{F_{1x}}{20} \Rightarrow F_{1x} = \frac{\sqrt{3}}{2}(20) = 10\sqrt{3} \text{ N}$$

$$\frac{\sqrt{3}}{2} = \sin 60° = \frac{F_{2y}}{100} \Rightarrow F_{2y} = 50\sqrt{3} \text{ N},$$

$$\frac{1}{2} = \cos 60° = \frac{-F_{2x}}{100} \Rightarrow F_{2x} = -50 \text{ N}.$$

Thus with $\sqrt{3} \approx 1.73$:

$$F_x = 10\sqrt{3} \text{ N} - 50 \text{ N} \approx 17.3 \text{ N} - 50 \text{ N} = -32.7 \text{ N}$$

and

$$F_y = -98 \text{ N} + 10 \text{ N} + 50\sqrt{3} \text{ N} \approx -1.5 \text{ N}.$$

Hence the magnitude of the resultant is:

$$\sqrt{F_x^2 + F_y^2} = \sqrt{(-32.7)^2 + (-1.5)^2} = 32.7 \text{ N}.$$

6. **B** Opposing forces are acting along the same line of action. The net force is the algebraic sum (assume positive is to the right):
Net force $= +10 \text{ N} - 5 \text{ N} = +5 \text{ N}$

7. **C** The forces, their moment arms (r), and directions of rotation (R) are:

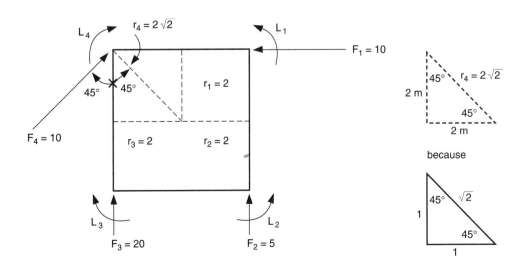

The torques are:
Counterclockwise ($+$)

$$L_1 = F_1 \times r_1 = (10)(2) = + 20 \text{ N} \cdot \text{m}$$
$$L_2 = F_2 \times r_2 = (5)(2) = + 10 \text{ N} \cdot \text{m}$$

Clockwise ($-$)

$$L_3 = F_3 \times r_3 = -(20)(2) = -40 \text{ N} \cdot \text{m}$$
$$L_4 = F_4 \times r_4 = -(10)(2\sqrt{2}) = -20\sqrt{2} = -28.2 \text{ N} \cdot \text{m}$$

The net torque (L) is:

$$L = L_1 + L_2 + L_3 + L_4 = +20 + 10 - 40 - 28.2 = +30 - 68.2$$
$$L = -38.2 \text{ N} \cdot \text{m} \text{ (which is clockwise)}$$

8. B The force diagram is:

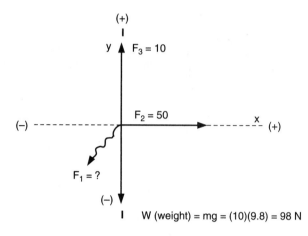

Components of forces:

$$F_1: F_{1x} = ?, F_{1y} = ?$$
$$F_2: F_{2x} = +50 \quad F_{2y} = 0$$
$$F_3: F_{3x} = 0, F_{3y} = +10$$
$$W: W_x = 0, W_y = -98$$
$$\text{Net force (F): } \sum F_x = 0 =$$
$$F_{1x} + F_{2x} + F_{3x} + W_x = F_{1x} + 50 + 0 + 0 = F_{1x} + 50$$

Then: $F_{1x} + 50 = 0$

$$F_{1x} = -50 \text{ N}$$
$$\sum F_y = 0 = F_{1y} + F_{2y} + F_{3y} + W_y = F_{1y} + 0 + 10 - 98 = F_{1y} - 88$$

Then: $F_{1y} - 88 = 0$

$$F_{1y} = 88 \text{ N}$$

Practice using the quick graphic method shown in the section concerning translational motion.

9. D The directions of rotations are:

F_2 causes counterclockwise ($+$) motion

F_3 causes counterclockwise ($+$) motion

The individual torques are:

$$L_1 = F_1 \times r_1 = (F_1)(2) = 2F_1 \text{ (sign unknown)}$$
$$L_2 = + F_2 \times r_2 = + (5)(3) = + 15 \text{ N} \cdot \text{m}$$

$$L_3 = + F_3 \times r_3 = + (20)(1) = + 20 \text{ N} \cdot \text{m}$$

Because rotational equilibrium exists, the torques sum to zero:

$$\sum L = L_1 + L_2 + L_3 = 0$$

$$2F_1 + 15 + 20 = 0$$

$$2F_1 + 35 = 0$$

$$2F_1 = -35$$

$$F_1 = -17.5 \text{ N pointing lower left to upper right and motion is clockwise}$$

Work and Energy

Self-Managed Learning Questions

1. Understand concepts related to different types of potential energy, e.g., chemical energy, biochemical energy, electrostatic energy stored as charge, thermal energy. Work on the actual types as they relate to the human body and what formulas or equations are applicable to humans and other mammals.
2. Relate the concepts of potential and kinetic energy to athletics, e.g., for the high jump or long jump, wherein kinetic energy is transformed into the potential energy as height of the jump.
3. Understand potential and kinetic energy concepts for astronomical bodies and the subatomic particles and how these work under conservative gravitational or nuclear forces.
4. Calculate your mechanical power by going up 10 or 15 stairs and timing yourself. Calculate the power using your weight, height, and time taken to travel the steps. Relate that to the number of calories lost or burned.

Energy is a scalar and is generally conceptualized as the ability to do work. If displacement results when objects exert forces on other objects, work is performed that is not contained within the object. Energy, by contrast, is contained by the object (or system); if work is performed, this energy either increases or decreases (for negative or positive work, respectively).

WORK

$$\text{Work} = \text{Force times distance} = F \times d$$

Work (W) is a scalar. Work results when a force (F) causes displacement (d) (Fig. 7-58). Note that $F \cos \theta$ is the component of F along the displacement (d). When $\theta = 0°$, then $\cos 0° = 1$, and $W = Fd$, which is the result for forces in the same direction as the displacement. When $\theta = 90°$, then $\cos 90° = 0$ and $W = 0$; that is, forces perpendicular to the displacement do no work. Remember, walking a dog illustrates the concept of work.

Work can also be defined in terms of the change in mechanical energy of an object. The potential energy between two points (or positions) is the amount of work that would be required to move an object between those two points. The change in kinetic energy of an object is the work performed by the object, assuming all the energy goes into work. To summarize:

$$W = E_f - E_i = \Delta E$$

$$E = K + U = \text{mechanical energy} = \text{kinetic energy} + \text{potential energy}$$

$$f = \text{final}; i = \text{initial}; \Delta = \text{change}$$

Note that work and energy have the same units:

$$W = (\text{force})(\text{distance}) = \text{newtons} \cdot \text{meters} = \text{joules} = \text{dynes} \cdot \text{cms} = \text{ergs}$$

Joules and ergs are units of work or energy. Pressure (P) times volume (V) also yields work (W): $W = PV$. This concept is used to study heat engines.

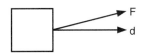

Fig. 7-58.

KINETIC ENERGY AND POTENTIAL ENERGY

Mechanical energy is divided into kinetic energy (K) and potential energy (U). **Kinetic energy** is the energy associated with the motion of objects. **Potential energy** is the energy that results by position or configuration (of a system); no motion is involved. When motion begins, potential energy is converted into kinetic energy.

The formulation of potential energy depends on the system.

U = mgh = gravitational potential energy
k = (½)mv^2 = kinetic energy
m = mass
h = height above earth's surface
v = speed of object

Additional features of potential energy are: (1) potential energy cannot be defined for frictional forces; (2) the potential energy of a system is independent of the path to reach that system; (3) potential energy can be of many types, such as gravitational, magnetic, electric, and chemical; (4) potential energy is a **field** that exists around molecules.

CONSERVATION OF ENERGY

The total mechanical energy of a system is defined by

Total Mech Energy (TE) = Kinetic Energy (K) + Potential Energy (U)
+ energy related to dissipative forces (e.g., friction).

In the absence of dissipative forces the equation takes the form:

TE = K + U.

The **law of conservation of mechanical energy** states that the total mechanical energy of a system is conserved (remains constant). Thus, if a system goes from state 1, with total mechanical energy $K_1 + U_1$, to state 2, with total mechanical energy $K_2 + U_2$, then:

$$K_1 + U_1 = K_2 + U_2.$$

As an example, given a particle of mass m moving along a path from point 1 to point 2 (Fig. 7-59), with velocities and heights indicated by subscripts, conservation of mechanical energy yields the equation:

$$\frac{1}{2}mv_1^2 + mgh_1 = \frac{1}{2}mv_2^2 + mgh_2$$

so that

$$\frac{v_1^2}{2} + gh_1 = \frac{v_2^2}{2} + gh_2.$$

Potential and kinetic energy are scalar quantities.

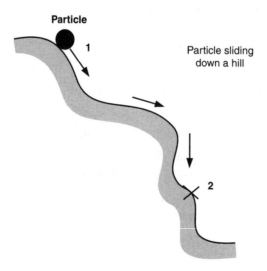

Particle

1

Particle sliding
down a hill

2

Fig. 7-59.

CONSERVATIVE FORCES

A **conservative force** is one for which the work done (or ΔE) when moving from one state to another depends only on the endpoints, and not on the intermediate process. Gravity, for example, is a conservative force because the change in gravitational potential energy of a body moving from one point to another depends only on the endpoints, and not on the path taken. Common examples are the elastic force of a spring, and the electrical force between electrically charged particles. Conservative forces are related to the elasticity of your muscles. Exercise and athletic activity help you flex your muscles and store potential energy. Calcium ions (Ca^{++}) and several other ions are related to muscle physiology as elastic potential energy, which is stored in the muscles.

POWER

Power (P) is a scalar and is the rate at which work is done:

$$P = \frac{work(W)}{time(t)} = \frac{W}{t}$$

The units of power are $P = work/time = joules/sec \equiv watts$. Horsepower is used for measuring power generated by electric motors and internal combustion engines. The efficiency of an engine is output/input.

APPLIED CONCEPTS

1. Understand the concept of metabolic rate, which measures the rate at which energy is consumed.

$$Metabolic\ rate = M_R = \frac{power}{efficiency} = \frac{P}{e}$$

Several methods are used to determine metabolic rate. Examine the oxygen consumption method and try to perform an experiment to measure it.

2. The oxygen consumed during metabolism reacts with bioorganic molecules, e.g., proteins, carbohydrates, and fats, releasing approximately 20,000 joules of energy per liter of oxygen consumed. Review metabolic rate tables from an exercise physiology book.

3. Look at several applications of work-energy principle in every day life with a focus on conservative and nonconservative forces. Examples include a man riding an escalator, a woman with a baby riding an elevator, sky diving, basketball in a court (smooth floor) versus football in a stadium (rough turf), movement of a train on a track or rail versus movement of a car on a highway. Analyze sources of potential and kinetic energy, application of work-energy principle, and how to deal with friction.

WORK AND ENERGY: REVIEW QUESTIONS

1. When a system does work or work is done on a system, what aspect of the system changes?

   A. Force
   B. Momentum
   C. Torque
   D. Energy

2. All of the following statements concerning potential energy (PE) are correct EXCEPT:

   A. PE depends on the configuration rather than the motion of a system.
   B. PE may be converted to kinetic energy.
   C. PE cannot be defined for frictional forces.
   D. PE depends on the path taken to reach a certain state.

3. The law of conservation of mechanical energy takes into account all of the following EXCEPT:

   A. conversion of mass into energy
   B. potential energy
   C. kinetic energy
   D. energy loss due to dissipative forces

4. If W = work and t = time, what is power (P)?

   A. $P = W/t$
   B. $P = t/W$
   C. $P = Wt$
   D. $P = 1/Wt$

5. At what angle to the direction of the displacement would a force perform no work?

    A. 0°
    B. 45°
    C. 90°
    D. 180°

6. All of the following are expressions of work EXCEPT:

    A. changes in mechanical energy
    B. momentum times mass
    C. force times distance
    D. pressure times volume

7. A 5-kg object is moving in a straight line at a velocity of 4 m/sec. What is the kinetic energy (K)?

    A. 40 joules $K = \frac{1}{2}mv^2$
    B. 20 joules
    C. 10 joules
    D. 80 joules

8. An object weighing 10 kg is at a distance of 10 m above the earth's surface. What is the potential energy (U) of this object?

    A. 980 joules $U = mgh$
    B. 100 joules
    C. 9.8 joules
    D. 1000 joules

9. If a 5-kg object is 20 m above the earth's surface and it falls to 10 m above the surface, what is the change in potential energy (U)?

    A. Gains 490 joules $U_2 - U_1$
    B. Loses 490 joules
    C. Loses 50 joules
    D. No change. Only the kinetic energy changes.

10. The shaded area under the following graph represents:

    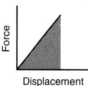

    A. momentum.
    B. force field.
    C. work.
    D. pressure.

11. A person does 20 joules of work in 10 seconds. The power (P) generated is:

    A. 2000 watts
    B. 200 watts
    C. 2 watts
    D. 0.5 watts

12. A force of 20 newtons is used to move an object 20 m in 10 seconds. How much power (P) is used?

    A. 40,000 watts
    B. 4,000 watts
    C. 400 watts
    D. 40 watts

13. A force of 10 newtons pushes a 5-kg object 20 meters. The work performed is:

    A. 200 joules.
    B. 40 joules.

C. 10 joules.
D. 2.5 joules.

14. How much work is performed in the following diagram?

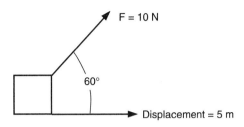

A. 50 joules
B. 50 cos 30° joules
C. 25 joules
D. 50 sin 60° joules

15. A 5-kg object moving at 4 m/sec strikes a second object. After the collision, the first object is moving at 2 m/sec. Assuming all the energy (E) was used to perform work (W) on the second object, the work performed is:

A. 30 joules. $\frac{1}{2}mv_f^2 - \frac{1}{2}mv_i^2$
B. 60 joules.
C. 90 joules.
D. 120 joules.

16. If F = force, ΔU = potential energy change, and Δx = displacement over which ΔU occurs, then:

A. $F = \Delta U \Delta x$.
B. $F = 1/\Delta U \Delta x$.
C. $F = -\Delta x/\Delta U$.
D. $F = -\Delta U/\Delta x$.

ANSWERS AND EXPLANATIONS

1–6. 1-D, 2-D 3-A, 4-A, 5-C, 6-B. See text for explanation.

7. **A** $K = \frac{1}{2}mv^2 = (\frac{1}{2})(5)(4)^2 = (\frac{5}{2})(16) = 40$ joules

8. **A** $U = mgh = (10 \text{ kg})(9.8 \text{ m/sec}^2)(10 \text{ m}) = 980$ joules

9. **B** $U = U_2 - U_1 = mgh_2 - mgh_1 = mg(h_2 - h_1)$

   $= (5)(9.8)(10 - 20) = (5)(9.8)(-10) = -490$ joules

   The minus sign means U is lost.

10. **C** The shaded area represents the product of the quantities on the axes: (force)(displacement), which is work (or energy).

11. **C** $P = \text{work/time} = 20 \text{ joules}/10 \text{ sec} = 2 \text{ joules/sec} = 2$ watts

12. **D** $P = \text{work/time} = 400 \text{ joules}/10 \text{ sec} = 40 \text{ joules/sec} = 40$ watts
    Work = (force)(distance) = (20)(20) = 400 joules

13. **A** $W = Fd \cos \theta$

    For: $\theta = 0°, \cos \theta = 1$

        $W = Fd = (10)(20) = 200$ joules

14. **C** According to the 30°–60°–90° triangle rules, the side lengths are shown:

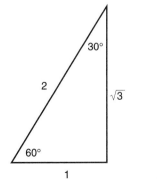

cos60° = 1/2

Then: $W = Fd \cos \theta = (10)(5) \cos 60° = 50(\frac{1}{2}) = 25$ joules

15. **A** $\Delta E = W = E_f - E_i$
$E = \frac{1}{2} mv^2$
$W = \frac{1}{2} mv_f^2 - \frac{1}{2} mv_i^2 = \frac{1}{2} m(v_f^2 - v_i^2)$
$W = \frac{1}{2}(5)(4^2 - 2^2) = (\frac{5}{2})(16 - 4) = (\frac{5}{2})(12) = 30$ joules

16. **D** If you do not know the relationship, it may be determined (in this case) by knowing unit interrelations (i.e., by doing dimensional analysis):

- Energy = work = Fd (see subsequent section concerning work and energy
- Force = energy/displacement, which is the **form** of answer (D)
- Force = newtons and energy = joules = **newtons · meters** and d = meters

The only way to combine the units of energy and displacement to yield the units of force follows:

$$\text{Newtons (force)} \propto \frac{\text{newtons · meters (energy)}}{\text{meters (displacement)}} = \text{newtons}$$

or

$$\text{Force} \propto F(\text{energy, displacement})$$

Force is proportional to energy/displacement.

Wave Characteristics and Periodic Motion

Self-Managed Learning Questions

1. Examine how animals use waves as valid information sources to communicate. How does the anatomy of the bee permit this insect to detect both the frequency and polarization of light? Check animal physiology articles and books on waves and animals.

2. Construct a simple pendulum. Determine the frequency and check against the theoretic equation: $T = \frac{1}{f} = 2\pi\sqrt{\frac{L}{g}}$. Does the shape or size of the suspended object affect the results? Trace the path of the harmonic motion as a sine wave corresponding to the to and fro motion of the pendulum and plot a graph between theoretic versus observed frequency. How do you account for the differences?

3. Visit a cardiologist's office and obtain some information on spectral Doppler echocardiography. Learn the basic functions to measure amount and speed of blood passing through the cardiac valves and chambers. Leaky valves and mitral stenosis can be detected.

WAVE CHARACTERISTICS

Transverse and Longitudinal Motion

A wave is a disturbance in a medium such that each particle in the medium vibrates about an equilibrium point in a simple harmonic motion (see subsequent discussion). If the direction of vibration is perpendicular to the direction of propagation of the wave, the wave is called a **transverse wave** (e.g., light) (Fig. 7-60A). If the direction of vibration is in the same direction as propagation of the wave, the wave is called a **longitudinal wave** (e.g., sound). Longitudinal waves are characterized by condensations (regions of crowding of particles) and rarefactions (regions in which particles are far apart) along the wave in the medium (Fig. 7-60B).

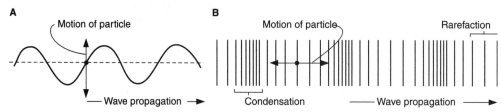

Fig. 7-60. (A) Transverse wave; (B) longitudinal wave.

Wavelength, Frequency, Velocity, Amplitude, and Intensity

The **wavelength** (λ) is the distance from crest to crest (or valley to valley) of a transverse wave. It may also be defined as the distance between two particles with the same displacement and direction of displacement. In a longitudinal wave, the wavelength can be taken as the distance from one rarefaction (or condensation) to another. The **amplitude** (A) is the maximum displacement of a particle from its equilibrium point. **Frequency** (f) is the number of wavelengths (cycles) that pass a point per unit time. **Period** (T) is the time required for one wavelength to pass a point. **Speed** (v) of a wave refers to its propagation through the medium. Generally, speed increases as the inertia of the medium decreases (e.g., as density decreases). **Intensity** is defined as the average rate at which a wave transmits its energy per unit area in the direction of propagation.

Superposition of Waves, Phase, Interference, and Addition

Phase (ϕ) is the difference in displacement and direction of a particle because of two different waves. Two waves are in phase if each particle has the same displacement and direction of motion ($\phi = 0$) [Fig. 7-61]. (That is, if crests and valleys coincide.)

The **superposition principle** states that the effects of two or more waves on the displacement of a particle are independent. This implies that the resultant displacement of a particle in a medium by simultaneous waves is obtained by algebraically adding the displacements from the separate waves.

Interference is the summation of the displacements of different waves in a medium. **Constructive interference**, when the waves add to a larger resultant wave than either original, occurs maximally when the phase difference (ϕ) is a whole wavelength (λ)—that is, when the peaks and valleys of the two waves coincide (see Fig. 7-62). If the wavelength is 2π, then maximal constructive interference occurs when $\phi = 0, 2\pi, 4\pi$, etc. **Destructive interference** occurs when the waves add to a smaller resultant wave than either original wave, and occurs maximally when the waves are out of phase by odd multiples of $\lambda/2$ (see Fig. 7-63).

Compare Figures 7-62 and 7-63. In Figure 7-62, waves 1 and 2 have the same λ but different A. The summation wave is maximal, because $\Delta L = \lambda$. In Figure 7-63, $\Delta L = \lambda/2$. Waves 1 and 2 begin as shown and have the same λ and the same A. The summation wave is the horizontal line (or the minimum) because $\Delta L = \lambda/2$.

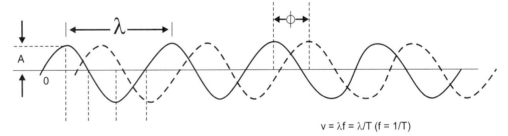

Fig. 7-61. Characteristics of waves.

$$v = \lambda f = \lambda/T \ (f = 1/T)$$

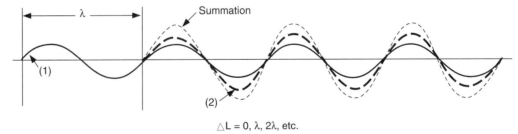

Fig. 7-62. Maximal constructive interference.

$$\triangle L = 0, \lambda, 2\lambda, \text{etc.}$$

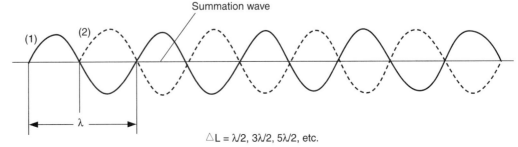

Fig. 7-63. Maximal destructive interference.

$$\triangle L = \lambda/2, 3\lambda/2, 5\lambda/2, \text{etc.}$$

Resonance

Forced vibrations occur when a series of waves impinge on an object and cause it to vibrate. Natural frequencies are the intrinsic frequencies of vibration of a system. If the forced vibration causes the object to vibrate at one of its **natural frequencies**, the body will vibrate at maximal amplitude. This situation is called **resonance**. Note also that **energy** and **power** are proportional to the amplitude squared, so energy and power are also at a maximum.

Standing Waves and Nodes

Standing waves result when waves are reflected off a stationary object back into the oncoming waves of the medium, resulting in superimposition (Fig. 7-64). **Nodes** are points at which there is no particle displacement; they are similar to points of maximal destructive interference. Nodes occur at fixed end points (points that cannot vibrate). **Antinodes** are points that undergo maximal displacements and are similar to points of maximal constructive interference. Open or free endpoints must be antinodes.

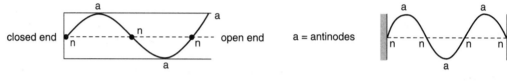

Fig. 7-64. Standing waves.

String fixed at one end   a = antinodes   String fixed at both ends

Stringed musical instruments are an obvious application of these concepts because they produce standing waves by their very nature. Two important properties of stringed instruments are implied by the relation (f_0 = fundamental frequency)

$$f_0 = \frac{1}{2L} \sqrt{\frac{T}{\mu}}.$$

This indicates that natural frequency increases with increasing tension (tuning a guitar) and also that natural frequency decreases as the "thickness" (mass/unit length) of a string increases.

The speed at which a wave travels down a string is given by the relation:

$$v = \sqrt{\frac{T}{\mu}}.$$

Beats

When sounds of different frequencies are heard together, they interfere. Constructive interference results in beats. The number of beats per second is the absolute value of the difference of the frequencies ($|f_1 - f_2|$). Hence, the new frequencies heard include the original frequencies and the arithmetic average, as $(f_1 + f_2)/2$ is the average frequency heard.

PERIODIC MOTION

Hooke's Law, Simple Harmonic Motion, and Pendulum Motion

The particles undergoing displacement when a wave passes through a medium undergo **simple harmonic motion** (SHM) (Fig. 7-65) and are acted on by a force described by **Hooke's law**. Simple harmonic motion is caused by an inconstant force (a restoring force) and as a result has an inconstant acceleration. The force is proportional to the displacement (distance from the equilibrium point) but opposite in direction:

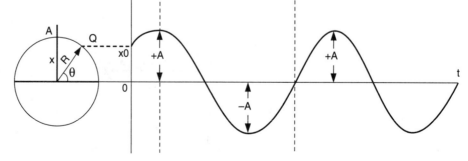

Fig. 7-65. Simple harmonic motion.

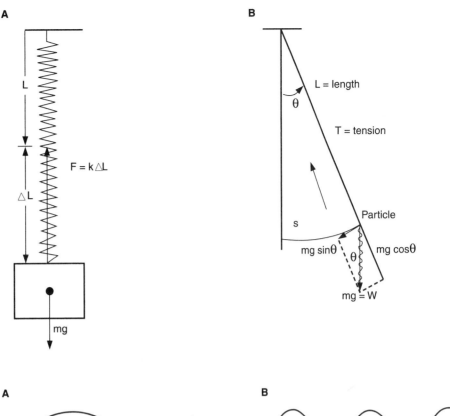

Fig. 7-66. (A) Simple harmonic motion (oscillator); (B) simple harmonic motion (pendulum).

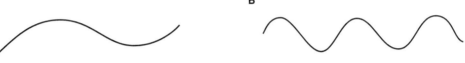

Fig. 7-67. (A) Long waves; (B) short waves.

Hooke's law: $F = -kx$

in which k = constant and x = displacement from equilibrium.

Pendulum motion is an example of simple harmonic motion. If an object is swinging back and forth by a string, and if the angle made by the string with the vertical is not too great, then the motion of the object is simple harmonic (Fig. 7-66).

Features of SHM and Hooke's law are as follows:

1. Force and acceleration are always in the same direction.
2. Force and acceleration are always in the opposite direction of the displacement.
3. Force and acceleration have their maximal values at $+A$ and $-A$; they are zero at the equilibrium point.
4. Velocity direction has no constant relation to displacement or acceleration.
5. Velocity is maximum at equilibrium and zero at A and $-A$.

The **electromagnetic spectrum** has the sequence from long wavelength (λ) and low frequency (f) to short wavelength and high frequency (Figure 7-67). Many regions overlap.

Long λ Short λ
radiowaves/microwaves/infrared/visible/ultraviolet/X-rays/gamma rays
Low f   High f

Planck developed the relation between energy (E) and the frequency (f) of electromagnetic radiation:

$E = hf$

h = Planck's constant

Because $f \propto 1/\lambda$, then, $E \propto 1/\lambda$. That is, high frequencies but short wavelengths correspond to high energy and vice versa.

APPLIED CONCEPTS

1. Obtain an EKG from a doctor's office. Analyze the complex wave pattern as a series of superimposed waves. Determine the period, frequency, amplitude, energy, and power for each simple sine or cosine component.

Problem Solving in the Physical Sciences   333

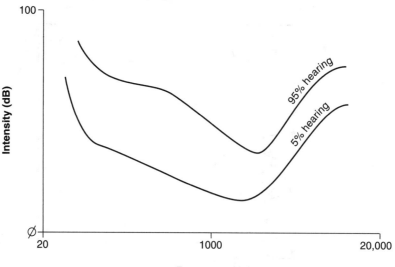

Fig. 7-68.

2. Visit a clinic where a ballistocardiograph is installed to plot displacement, velocity, or acceleration of the platform. Compare the normal ECG of the subject with the ballistocardiogram and see if any abnormalities are detected. The ballistocardiograph is a useful diagnostic tool to detect heart disease in some individuals. Look at the displacement, velocity, and acceleration plots to see if they are in phase and how the positive and negative peaks show an abrupt or gradual change relative to the P, QQ, R, S, and T on the ECG.

3. Perform a graphic analysis of the following intensity versus frequency plots for several levels of hearing (Fig. 7-68). Dissect the slope, shape of each frequency segment, and the sharp change in higher frequencies.

WAVE CHARACTERISTICS AND PERIODIC MOTION: REVIEW QUESTIONS

1. If the direction of vibration of particles of a medium is in the direction of propagation of a wave, the wave is called:

   A. longitudinal.
   B. transverse.
   C. both.
   D. neither.

2. Condensations and rarefactions would be found in:

   A. light waves.
   B. water waves.
   C. transverse waves.
   D. longitudinal waves.

3. "The effects of two or more waves on the displacement of a particle are independent" is a statement of:

   A. interference principle.
   B. Huygens' principle.
   C. correspondence principle.
   D. superposition principle.

4. At the node of a wave:

   A. the displacement is maximal.
   B. there is no displacement.
   C. there may be an open or a free point.
   D. both A and C are true.

5. Select the incorrect relationship between the energy (E) of a wave and the parameters given (f = frequency, l = wavelength, A = amplitude):

   A. $E \propto f$
   B. $E \propto A^2$

C. $E \propto 1/\lambda$

D. All are correct

6. The restoring force that causes an object to undergo simple harmonic motion is:

   A. a constant force.
   B. inversely proportional to the displacement (from equilibrium) and in the same direction.
   C. directly proportional to the displacement but opposite in direction.
   D. both A and B.

7. All of the following statements are true about simple harmonic motion except:

   A. force and acceleration have their maximum values at the equilibrium point.
   B. force and acceleration are always in the same direction.
   C. velocity direction has no constant relation to displacement or acceleration direction.
   D. velocity is maximal at the equilibrium point.

8. Which of the following colors of visible light has the shortest wavelength?

   A. Green
   B. Blue
   C. Yellow
   D. Red

9. Which of the following colors of visible light has the longest wavelength?

   A. Yellow
   B. Orange
   C. Blue
   D. Green

10. If f = frequency and λ = wavelength of light, then the speed of light (c) is:

    A. $c = 1/f$.
    B. $c = \lambda/f$.
    C. $c = f/\lambda$.
    D. $c = f\lambda$.

11. The relation $E = hf$ was put forth by:

    A. Planck.
    B. Einstein.
    C. Newton.
    D. Maxwell.

12. Given 2 waves of the same wavelength (λ), constructive interference occurs when:

    A. phase differences are $\frac{\lambda}{2}$, $3\frac{\lambda}{2}$, $5\frac{\lambda}{2}$, etc.
    B. phase differences are 0, λ, 2λ, 3λ, etc.
    C. neither A nor B are correct.
    D. both A and B are correct.

13. If the frequency of a wave is 10,000 hertz and it is traveling at 5000 m/sec, what is its wavelength?

    $\frac{c}{f} = \lambda$

    A. 5 m
    B. 2 m
    C. 0.5 m
    D. 0.2 m

14. The speed of light (c) is 3.0×10^{10} cm/sec. If the wavelength of (λ) of blue-light is approximately 400 nm (nm $= 10^{-9}$ m), what is the frequency (f) of blue-light?

    A. 7.5×10^{12}/sec
    B. 7.5×10^{14}/sec
    C. 1.2×10^{4}/sec
    D. 1.2×10^{6}/sec

     $\frac{c}{\lambda} = f$

15. Electromagnetic radiation (e.g., light) with frequency (f) of 50,000 hertz (hertz = 1 cycle/sec) would have a wavelength (λ) of:

   A. 1/50,000 cm.
   B. 6.0×10^{-5} cm.
   C. 6.0×10^5 cm.
   D. Cannot be determined

16. In a vibrating column of air:

   A. open ends can only have nodes.
   B. nodes can occur at open or closed ends.
   C. open ends can only have antinodes.
   D. antinodes may only occur at closed ends.

Questions 17–22
The particle of mass = 2 kg in this illustration is oscillating about the fixed point O. Given are some values of the force on the particle at different values of displacement (x) from O. The maximal displacement from O in any one direction is O ± A and A = 5 m.

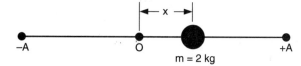

m = 2 kg

x (meters)	+3	+1	-2	-4
F (newtons)	-0.6	-0.2	+0.4	+0.8

17. This type of motion is called:

   A. rigid body translation.
   B. simple harmonic motion.
   C. projectile motion.
   D. free fall motion.

18. The force is described by:

   A. Faraday's law.
   B. Newton's first law.
   C. Hooke's law.
   D. none of the above.

19. If the motion and force in this example follow Hooke's law, what is the value of k (neglect the units)?

   A. 0.1
   B. 0.2
   C. 0.5
   D. 1.0

   $F = -kx$

20. What is the value (in nts) of F at A = −5 m?

   A. 0.2
   B. 0.5
   C. 1.0
   D. 5

21. The force has a value of zero at x = ?

   A. 0 m
   B. +5 m
   C. −5 m
   D. O ± 2 m

22. At x = −2 m, what is the acceleration (a) (in m/sec²)?

   A. 4.0
   B. 2.0

C. 1.0
D. 0.2

23. A standing wave is established in a string fixed at both ends between two points 1 m apart. Which of the following is NOT a possible wavelength for this system?

   A. 4 m
   B. 2 m
   C. 1.0 m
   D. 0.5 m

24. A standing wave is established in a pipe that is open at one end and is 2 m long. All of the following are possible wavelengths for this system EXCEPT:

   A. 8 m.
   B. 6 m.
   C. $2\frac{2}{3}$ m.
   D. All are possible.

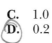

25. The wavelength of ultraviolet waves is 10^3 angstroms. Find the energy of the ultraviolet waves, given Planck's constant $= 6.626 \times 10^{-34}$ joule-sec (1 angstrom = 1Å $= 10^{-10}$ m):

   A. 6.626×10^{-31} J
   B. 6.626×10^{-41} J
   C. 2×10^{18} J
   D. 2×10^{-18} J

ANSWERS AND EXPLANATIONS

1–11. 1-A, 2-D, 3-D, 4-B, 5-D, 6-C, 7-A, 8-B, 9-B, 10-D, 11-A. See text for explanation.

12. **B**   See text on page 331 and Figure 7-62.

13. **C** $v = \lambda f$
   $\lambda = v/f = 5,000/10,000 = 0.5$ m

14. **B** $c = f\lambda$

   $f = \dfrac{c}{\lambda} = \dfrac{(3.00 \times 10^{10} \text{ cm/sec})}{4 \times 10^{-5} \text{ cm}} = 0.75 \times 10^{15} \text{ sec}^{-1} = 7.5 \times 10^{14} \text{ sec}^{-1}$

   ($\lambda = 400 \times 10^{-9}$ m $= 4.0 \times 10^{-7}$ m $= 4 \times 10^{-5}$ cm)

15. **C** $c = f\lambda = 3.00 \times \dfrac{10^{10} \text{ cm}}{\text{sec}}$

   $f = 50,000/\text{sec} = 5.0 \times \dfrac{10^4}{\text{sec}}$

   $\lambda = \dfrac{c}{f} = \dfrac{3.00 \times 10^{10}}{5.0 \times 10^4} = .60 \times 10^6$ cm

   $\lambda = 6.0 \times 10^5$ cm

16. **C**   See text for explanation.

17. **B**   The particle oscillating about a fixed point (O) is simple harmonic motion.

18. **C**   The force is a restoring force and the motion is simple harmonic. Hooke's law, as $F = -kx$, determines the restoring force.

19. **B**   The motion follows Hooke's law: $F = -kx$. To find the k, any set of F and x may be substituted in the equation:

   $$k = -\left(\frac{F}{x}\right) = -\left(\frac{-0.6 \text{ nts}}{+3 \text{ m}}\right) = \frac{+0.2 \text{ nt}}{\text{m}}$$

   $$k = -\left(\frac{F}{x}\right) = -\left(\frac{-0.2 \text{ nts}}{+1 \text{ m}}\right) = \frac{+0.2 \text{ nt}}{\text{m}}$$

20. **C**   Using the data from question 19:

   $$F = -kx$$

   $$F = -(0.2)(-5) = +1.0 \text{ nts}$$

   Note at $\pm A$, F has its maximal value

21. A $F = -kx = 0$

$-kx = 0$

$x = 0$ because k is not equal to zero

22. D $F = +0.4$ nts from chart at $x = -2$, $a = F/m = 0.4/2 = 0.2$ m/sec^2

or

$F = -kx$ from Hooke's law

$F = ma$ from Newton's second law (see section concerning

force and motion, gravitation)

$ma = -kx$

$$a = -\frac{kx}{m} = -\frac{(0.2)(-2)}{2} = +\frac{0.2 \text{ m}}{\text{sec}^2}$$

23. A   Given that the string is fixed on both ends, both ends must be nodes. The smallest number of nodes that can occur is two—one at each end point, which yields the wave shown in the figure below. For this wave $\lambda = 2$m. Any wave with longer wavelength cannot have a node at both endpoints. Therefore, the correct response is A. It is clear that any number of equidistantly spaced points will yield a wavelength that will work.

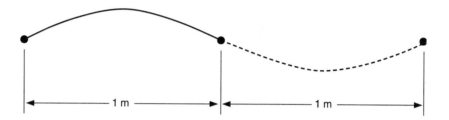

Looking at the question more generally, let the distance between the two end-points be L. Because any wave with fixed endpoints must have an integer multiple of half the wavelength (otherwise the endpoints would not be fixed), any n for which $n(\lambda/2) = L$ will do. Hence:

$$\lambda = \frac{2}{n}L, \qquad n = 1, 2, 3, \cdots.$$

are the permissible wavelengths. (Please note that any set of equidistantly placed points that include the endpoints will give a waveform that will work.)

If the wave has a propagation velocity v then, because $v = f\lambda$ where f is the frequency,

$$f = \frac{v}{\lambda} = \frac{v}{\frac{2}{n}L} = \frac{nv}{2L}.$$

24. B   A node must be at the closed end of the pipe and an antinode must be at the open end. The shortest fraction of a wave that has a node and antinode in sequence is $\frac{1}{4}\lambda$, which must equal the 2 m:

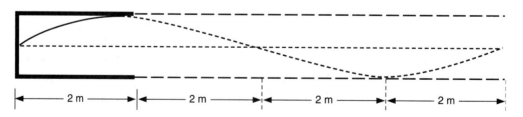

If $\frac{1}{4}\lambda = 2$ m, $\lambda = 8$ m as the longest wavelength possible.

Because an antinode can be present at the open end only if an odd number of quarter cycles are present,

$$2 = n\left(\frac{\lambda}{4}\right) \Rightarrow \lambda = \frac{8}{n}, \qquad n = 1, 3, 5, \cdots .$$

and hence, λ cannot be 6. Reasoning as in the previous problem, if the open pipe is of length L, then the possible wavelengths must satisfy:

$$L = n\left(\frac{\lambda}{4}\right) \Rightarrow \lambda = \frac{4L}{n}, \qquad n = 1, 3, 5, \cdots .$$

25. D $E = hf$, $v = f\lambda$

$v = 2.998 \times 10^8$ m/sec = speed of light

1 J = 1 Newton-meter

$\lambda = 10^3 \, \text{Å} = 10^3 \, 10^{-10} = 10^{-7}$ m

$$f = \frac{v}{\lambda} = \frac{2.998 \times 10^8}{10^{-7}} = 2.998 \times 10^{15} \text{ Hz}$$

$$E = \text{Planck's constant} \times f = hf$$

$$= 6.626 \times 10^{-34} \times 2.998 \times 10^{15}$$

$$= 1.99 \times 10^{-18} \text{ joules}$$

Sound

Self-Managed Learning Questions

1. Read the following passage: "A 300-lb ultrasound machine could view damaged organs to locate internal bleeding using low-intensity sound waves. High intensity ultrasound could generate enough heat to coagulate blood and cause coagulation." What are the underlying assumptions in this passage? What is the frequency of low-intensity sound waves? What sentence in the passage weakens the entire research hypothesis?
2. Find out the speed of sound in several solids, liquids, and gases and explain why the speeds are higher in solids than gases. Draw a diagram that explains physical properties that alter the speed of sound in several mediums.
3. Identify equipment and procedures used to detect ultrasonic ($>20,000$ Hz) and infrasonics (<20 Hz).
4. Using all appropriate laboratory precautions, breathe a lungful of helium gas. Remember that speed of sound in helium is 2.9 times the speed in air. In a normal man, the first three formants to make the sound "ah" are approximately 730, 1090, and 2440 Hz. When helium is involved, the answers can be multiplied by 2.9. Recite "ah" and "oo" sounds. How can these data be compiled and plotted?
5. Test several musical string instruments using several frequency ranges of tuning forks. Understand nodes, antinodes, and standing waves with low-frequency tuning forks.

PRODUCTION

Sound is a longitudinal (see previous section concerning wave characteristics and periodic motion) mechanical wave that travels through an elastic medium. Sound is thus produced by vibrating matter. No sound occurs in a vacuum (because there is no matter). Compressions (condensations) are regions in which particles (of matter) are close together and are high pressure regions. Rarefactions are regions in which particles are sparse and are low pressure regions of sound waves.

RELATIVE SPEED IN SOLIDS, LIQUIDS, AND GASES

The **speed** (v) of sound in a medium is proportional to the square root of the elastic restoring force and inversely proportional to the square root of the inertia of the particles (e.g., density, ρ, is a measure of inertia):

$$v \propto \sqrt{F}$$

$$v \propto \frac{1}{\sqrt{\text{inertia}}}$$

The speed in various substances is calculated as follows.

For solid wire or rod: $\sqrt{\dfrac{Y}{\rho}}$, Y = Young's modulus

For fluid or liquid: $\sqrt{\dfrac{B}{\rho}}$, B = bulk modulus

For gas: $\sqrt{\dfrac{\gamma p}{\rho}}$, $\gamma = \dfrac{c_p}{c_v}$ and p = undisturbed pressure = 1.4

The speed of sound in solids and liquids is considerably higher than the speed in air. The speed of sound in air at 0°C is 331.5 m/sec, and it increases with temperature at approximately 0.6 m/sec per degree celsius. The speed of sound in water at 0°C is 1402 m/sec and is 6000 m/sec in granite.

INTENSITY AND PITCH

Hearing is subjective, but its characteristics are closely tied to the physical characteristics of sound. These relations are sensory, including loudness, pitch, and quality, as well as physical, including intensity (I), frequency (f), and waveforms.

The **quality** depends on the number and the relative intensity of the overtones of the waveforms. Frequency, and, therefore, **pitch**, are perceived by the ear from 20 to 20,000 Hz (Hertz = cycles/second). Frequencies below 20 Hz are called infrasonic. Frequencies above 20,000 Hz are called ultrasonic. Sound **intensity** (I) is the rate of energy (power) propagation through space:

$$I = \frac{\text{Power}}{\text{area}} \propto f^2 A^2$$

in which f = frequency and A = amplitude.

DOPPLER EFFECT

The Doppler effect is the effect on the observed frequency caused by the relative motion of the observer (o) and the source (s). If the distance is decreasing between them, a shift occurs to higher frequencies and shorter wavelengths (to higher pitch for sound and toward blue-violet for light). If the distance is increasing between them, a shift occurs to longer wavelengths and lower frequencies (to lower pitch for sound and toward red for light). A summary equation in terms of frequency f is:

$$f_o = f_s \frac{(V \pm v_o)}{(V \mp v_s)}$$

in which the upper signs are used if observer and source are moving toward each other and the lower signs are used otherwise.

Choose the (+) or (−) such that the frequency varies as you would predict. If the o or s is moving toward the other, the f should increase and vice versa. Predict the results and select the sign for the s and o independently of the motion of the other.

RESONANCE IN PIPES AND STRINGS, HARMONICS

Resonance

Organ pipes (closed and open tubes) produce tones by establishing standing waves in cylindric and longitudinal cavities (Fig. 7-69). To understand **resonance**, remember a standing wave in a tube necessitates that the air vibrate with a frequency near one of the characteristic frequencies of the pipe or tube. Consider the following equations for open and closed pipes.

Consider the frequencies of various organ pipes. Let L = length of the pipe and let c = 345 m/sec = speed of sound in air.

Pipes open at both ends:

Wavelengths: $\lambda_n = \dfrac{2L}{n}$

Natural frequencies: $f_n = n \dfrac{c}{2L}$

where $n = 1, 2, 3, \cdots$.

Pipes closed at one end:

$$\lambda_n = \frac{4L}{n},$$

$$f_n = n \frac{c}{4L}$$

where $n = 1, 3, 5, 7, \cdots$.

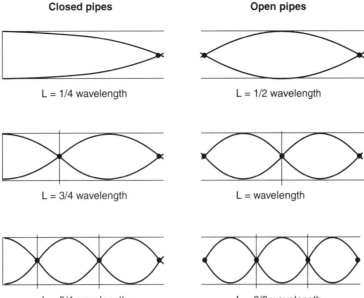

Closed pipes	Open pipes
L = 1/4 wavelength	L = 1/2 wavelength
L = 3/4 wavelength	L = wavelength
L = 5/4 wavelength	L = 3/2 wavelength

Fig. 7-69. Production of tones in organ pipes (open and closed) by standing waves in cylindric and longitudinal cavities.

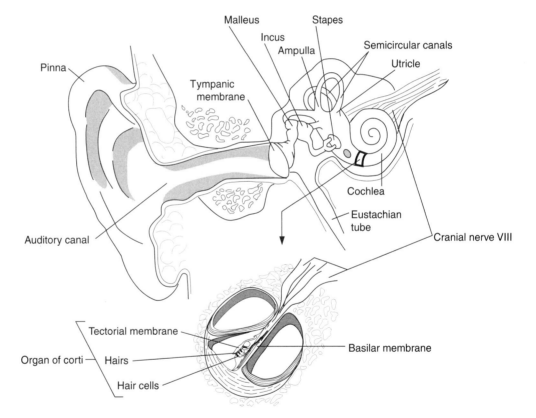

Fig. 7-70. The human ear.

Harmonics

If a string is fixed at both ends, it has not only one but also a series of natural frequencies. These frequencies are integral multiples of the lowest frequency at which the string can vibrate, called the **fundamental frequency**. Organ pipes and other musical instruments produce tones by establishing standing waves in pipes. Human voice also emits tones when the vocal cords vibrate at several frequencies. Typically f_i is the fundamental frequency and $f_n = nf_i$ are the possible harmonics.

HEARING

The divisions of the human ear (Fig. 7-70) are the **external ear** (pinna and auditory canal), the **middle ear** (the tympanic membrane and three bones—malleus or hammer, incus or anvil, and stapes or stirrup), and the **internal ear** (the cochlea, the semicircular canals, and the origin of the vestibulocochlear nerve). The **tympanic membrane** (eardrum) is attached to the **malleus**, which attaches to the **incus**, which attaches to the **stapes**, which attaches to the **oval window** of the cochlea. The function of the outer and middle ear is to match the impedance of the air outside and the fluid of the cochlea inside. This mechanism results in more efficient transmission of sound.

Sound waves are transmitted from the stapes via the oval window to the fluid in the **cochlea**. This fluid sets up vibrations in the **basilar membrane** that cause special hair cells to send impulses to the auditory part of the vestibulocochlear (VIII) nerve, which in turn transmits them to the auditory cortex in the temporal lobe of the cerebrum. The basilar membrane, tectoral membrane, and hair cells run the full length of the cochlea and together constitute the **organ of Corti**. The distance between the oval window and the point of maximum vibration of the basilar membrane determines the **frequency (pitch)** of the sound—highest frequencies are closest to the oval window. The **round window**, at the other end of the cochlea, serves as a release of pressure imparted to the cochlear fluid by the stapes.

The **vestibular system** is continuous anatomically but not functionally with the cochlea. The system is filled with fluid (endolymph) and contains the sacculus, the utricle, and three perpendicular **semicircular canals**. Each semicircular canal has an **ampulla,** which contains hair cells sensitive to changes in angular acceleration. The **utricle** and **sacculus** contain a special sensory region called the **macula,** which has crystals of calcium carbonate on it. These regions are sensitive to changes in gravity (position) and linear acceleration. Impulses travel from these special regions via the vestibular portions of the vestibulocochlear nerve (cranial nerve VIII) to the central nervous system. The vestibular system helps maintain posture, balance, spatial orientation, and stabilization of eye movements.

Loudness varies with amplitude. The ears are most sensitive (hear sounds of lowest intensity) at approximately 2,000 to 4,000 Hz. I_o, taken to be 10^{-12} watts/m^2, is barely audible and is assigned a value of 0 (zero) dB (decibels). Then, the intensity level (I) of a sound wave in dB is:

$$dB = 10 \log\left(\frac{I}{I_o}\right)$$

in which I = intensity at a given level and I_o = threshold intensity.

Examples of some dB values are: whisper (20), normal conversation (60), subway car (100), pain threshold (120), and jet engine (160). Continual exposure to sounds greater than 90 dB can lead to hearing impairment (Fig. 7-71).

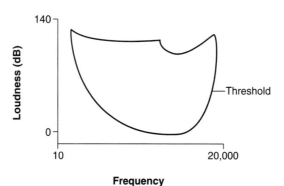

Fig. 7-71. Audible sound intensities.

APPLIED CONCEPTS

1. In a biology laboratory, compare ears of humans, cats, dogs, and birds. Use plastic model ears to closely examine the anatomy and how each organism hears. Can animals hear frequencies humans cannot hear? How?
2. Observe ultrasonic generators (design and working) and ultrasonic devices used in hospitals to break kidney stones, create blood clots, and other clinical applications.
3. Examine hearing devices of various types and how they work. Understand the workings of a microphone, speakers, and digital devices.

SOUND: REVIEW QUESTIONS

1. Sound waves are:

    A. transverse waves.
    B. produced by vibrating matter.
    C. transmitted in a vacuum.
    D. all of the above.

2. The speed of sound is:

    A. proportional to the square root of the elastic restoring force of the medium.
    B. inversely proportional to the square root of the inertia of the particles of the media.
    C. neither A nor B.
    D. both A and B.

3. The speed of sound is _____ by an increase of temperature and _____ in density of the medium.

    A. decreased, decrease
    B. increased, increase
    C. decreased, increase
    D. increased, decrease

4. What is the effect when an object is forced to vibrate at one of its natural frequencies?

    A. Resonance
    B. Minimum energy
    C. Minimum work
    D. Minimum amplitude of vibration

5. Which sensory (as interpreted by the brain) aspect of sound is incorrectly paired with its physical correlate of sound?

    A. Loudness — intensity
    B. Pitch — frequency
    C. Quality — waveforms
    D. All are correctly paired

6. A human with normal hearing probably could not hear sound at:

    A. 100,000 Hz
    B. 20,000 Hz
    C. 5,000 Hz
    D. 20 Hz

7. The intensity (power per unit area) of a sound is:

    A. inversely proportional to the square of the frequency.
    B. directly proportional to the square of the frequency.
    C. inversely proportional to the frequency.
    D. directly proportional to the frequency.

8. Decibels are used in describing:

    A. light.
    B. sound.
    C. electricity.
    D. magnetism.

9. The effect on the frequency of sound observed when the source of the sound is moving relative to the observer is explained by the:

    A. Doppler effect.
    B. Compton effect.
    C. theory of relativity.
    D. Compton and Doppler effects.

10. If the density of a gas is quadrupled ($\times 4$), the speed (v) of sound through it is:

    A. decreased by one half of its initial value.
    B. multiplied by a factor of 2.
    C. multiplied by a factor of 4.
    D. decreased to one quarter of its initial value.

11. If the elasticity (restoring force) of medium 1 is four times the elasticity of medium 2, then the sound will travel:

    A. twice as fast in 1 as in 2.
    B. twice as fast in 2 as in 1.

C. four times as fast in 1 as in 2.
D. four times as fast in 2 as in 1.

12. If the tension (F) in a string is increased by a factor of 4, the speed (v) of a wave in that string will be:

A. quadrupled ($\times 4$).
B. doubled.
C. reduced by one half.
D. reduced to one quarter of the original.

13. Three notes of 128, 256, and 512 are sounded; the frequencies heard are:

A. 128, 256, 384, 512, 640, 768.
B. 512, 640, 768.
C. 128, 256, 384, 512.
D. 128, 256, 512.

14. A sound has an intensity 100 times that of the standard intensity. How many decibels is it?

A. 10 $dB = 10 \log \left[\frac{I}{I_0} \right]$
B. 20
C. 50
D. 100

15. If a source that is emitting sound is moving toward an observer, the frequency of sound heard by the observer is _____ the frequency emitted by the source, caused by _____ _____.

A. the same as, Doppler effect
B. less than, mutual interference
C. greater than, Doppler effect

16. If a source that is emitting light is moving away from an observer, the wavelength of light seen by the observer is _____ the wavelength emitted by the source, due to _____ _____.

A. the same as, Planck's constant
B. shorter than, increased frequency
C. longer than, decreased frequency

17. An observer is moving toward a source at 170 m/sec. The source is moving toward the observer at 130 m/sec and is emitting sound at a frequency of 10,000 hertz (Hz). The frequency of sound heard by the observer (assume speed of sound is 330 m/sec) is:

A. 15,000 Hz. $f_o = 10,000 hz \frac{(330 + 170)}{(330 - 130)}$
B. 7,500 Hz.
C. 25,000 Hz.
D. 5,000 Hz.

18. The threshold of human hearing lies between:

A. 20 Hz and 20,000 Hz.
B. 10 Hz and 10,000 Hz.
C. 18 Hz and 8,000 Hz.
D. 12 Hz and 1,200 Hz.

19. Assume $I_o = 10^{-12}$ watts/m^2. Find the intensity in watts/m^2 of sound, given the intensity in dB = 100.

A. 100 W/m^2 $100 = 10 \log \left[\frac{I}{10^{12}} \right]$
B. 1000 W/m^2
C. 10^{-10} W/m^2
D. 10^{-2} W/m^2

20. Determine loudness in decibels at the threshold of human hearing:

A. 0
B. 20
C. 200
D. 2,000

21. The intensity of sound of a subway car (I_1) is 100 dB and the intensity of sound of a whisper (I_2) is 20 dB. Compare their intensities in watts/cm$_2$.
   A. $I_1 = 10^8 I_2$
   B. $I_1 = \frac{1}{5} I_2$
   C. $I_1 = 5 I_2$
   D. $I_2 = 5 I_1$

22. An ambulance traveling 24 m/sec is moving toward an approaching car that is traveling at a speed of 14 m/sec. If the siren emits a frequency of 1000 Hz, what is the frequency heard by the driver of the car? Speed of sound = 350 m/sec.
   A. 1000 Hz
   B. 1116 Hz
   C. 1350 Hz
   D. 1038 Hz

23. Frequency (pitch) of sound is determined in the ear by the:
   A. oval window.
   B. basilar membrane.
   C. tympanic membrane.
   D. medial geniculate body.

24. Which of the following structures is NOT found in the middle ear of humans?
   A. Cochlea
   B. Tympanic membrane
   C. Anvil
   D. Incus

25. Hearing is localized in which lobe of the cerebral cortex?
   A. Frontal
   B. Parietal
   C. Temporal
   D. Occipital

ANSWERS AND EXPLANATIONS

1–9. 1-B, 2-D, 3-B, 4-A, 5-D, 6-A, 7-B, 8-B, 9-A. See text for explanation.

10. A $v \propto \dfrac{1}{\sqrt{\rho}}$ $\quad \rho$ = density, $\rho_2 = 4\rho_1$

$$\frac{v_2}{v_1} = \frac{\dfrac{1}{\sqrt{\rho_2}}}{\dfrac{1}{\sqrt{\rho_1}}} = \frac{1}{\sqrt{\rho_2}} \cdot \frac{\sqrt{\rho_1}}{1} = \frac{\sqrt{\rho_1}}{\sqrt{\rho_2}} = \sqrt{\frac{\rho_1}{\rho_2}} = \sqrt{\frac{\rho_1}{4\rho_1}} = \sqrt{\tfrac{1}{4}} = \tfrac{1}{2}$$

$$\frac{v_2}{v_1} = \tfrac{1}{2}$$

$$v_2 = \tfrac{1}{2} v_1$$

11. A Speed of sound (v) $\propto \sqrt{\text{restoring force}}$ = F, $F_1 = 4F_2$

$$\frac{v_2}{v_1} = \frac{\dfrac{1}{\sqrt{F_2}}}{\dfrac{1}{\sqrt{F_1}}} = \sqrt{\frac{F_2}{F_1}} = \sqrt{\frac{F_2}{4F_2}} = \sqrt{\tfrac{1}{4}} = \tfrac{1}{2}$$

$$\frac{v_2}{v_1} = \tfrac{1}{2}$$

$$2v_2 = v_1$$

12. B $v \propto \sqrt{F}$

$$F_2 = 4F_1$$

$$\frac{v_2}{v_1} = \frac{\sqrt{F_2}}{\sqrt{F_1}} = \sqrt{\frac{F_2}{F_1}} = \sqrt{\frac{4F_1}{F_1}} = \sqrt{4} = 2$$

$$v_2 = 2v_1$$

13. C The frequencies heard are the original frequencies plus all new frequencies resulting from the differences of the original frequencies:

$$512 - 128 = 384 \text{ (the only new frequency)}$$

14. B $\text{dB} = 10 \log\left(\dfrac{I}{I_o}\right) = 10 \log\left(\dfrac{100}{1}\right)$

$$= 10 \log 100 = 10(2) = 20 \ (\log 100 = 2)$$

15. C As the observer and source move together, the observed frequency increases.

16. C If the distance between observer and source is increasing, the wavelength observed increases as the frequency decreases.

17. C Use Doppler's relation as shown in the text:

$$f_o = f_s \frac{V \pm v_o}{V \mp v_s} f_s$$

For this problem:

$$f_o = \frac{f_s(V + v_o)}{(V - v_s)}$$

$$f_o = \frac{(10{,}000)(330 + 170)}{(330 - 130)} = (10{,}000)\left(\frac{500}{200}\right) =$$

$$f_o = (10{,}000)\left(\frac{5}{2}\right) = 25{,}000 \text{ hertz}$$

18. A Review the loudness–frequency graph (Fig. 7-71).

19. D $\text{dB} = 10 \log \dfrac{I}{I_o}$

$$100 = 10 \log \frac{I}{10^{-12}}$$

$$10 = \log I + \log 10^{12} = \log I + 12$$

$$-2 = \log I, \ I = \frac{10^{-2} \text{ watts}}{\text{m}^2}$$

20. A $I = I_o$ for threshold hearing

$$\text{dB} = 10 \log \frac{I}{I_o}$$

$$= 10 \log \frac{I_o}{I_o} = 0$$

21. A For subway car: $100 = 10 \log \dfrac{I_1}{I_o}$

For the whisper: $20 = 10 \log \dfrac{I_2}{I_o}$

$$10 = \log \frac{I_1}{I_o} \text{ and } 2 = \log \frac{I_2}{I_o}$$

$$10 = \log I_1 - \log I_o \text{ and } 2 = \log I_2 - \log I_o$$

$$10 - \log I_1 = -\log I_o \text{ and } 2 - \log I_2 = -\log I_o$$

$$10 - \log I_1 = 2 - \log I_2$$

$$8 = 10 - 2 = \log I_1 - \log I_2 = \log \frac{I_1}{I_2}$$

$$10^8 = \frac{I_1}{I_2}$$

The subway car is 100 million times louder than the whisper or the sound level of the subway car is 100 million times that of the whisper.

22. B If v = sound speed:

$$f_o = f_s \left(\frac{v + v_o}{v - v} \right)$$

$$= 1000 \, \frac{(350 + 14)}{(350 - 24)}$$

$$= 1000 \, \frac{(364)}{(326)} = 1{,}116 \text{ Hz}$$

23–25. 23-B, 24-A, 25-C. See text for explanation.

Light and Geometric Optics

Self-Managed Learning Questions

1. Define light. Explain the particle and wave theories of light.
2. Why does light travel in straight lines?
3. Using everyday observations, prove that light travels in straight lines (law of rectilinear propagation of light).
4. How can the concept of light be used in chemistry (general and organic)?
5. How can the concept of light be used in biology?
6. What is photosynthesis?
7. What is a shadow?
8. What is an eclipse?
9. Prove that white light is made up of seven colors (e.g., Newton's disk).
10. What are the differences between colors in the ''white light spectrum'' and ''paints and pigments?''

VISUAL SPECTRUM AND COLOR

Remember the colors in the visible light spectrum by the mnemonic, ROY G. BIV: red, orange, yellow, green, blue, indigo, violet (Figs. 7-72 and 7-73).

POLARIZATION

Unpolarized light waves have electric fields that, although confined to the planes perpendicular to the direction of light, are directed randomly throughout those planes. **Polarized light** displays asymmetry in its electric field distribution in the plane perpendicular to

Fig. 7-72. Visible spectrum.

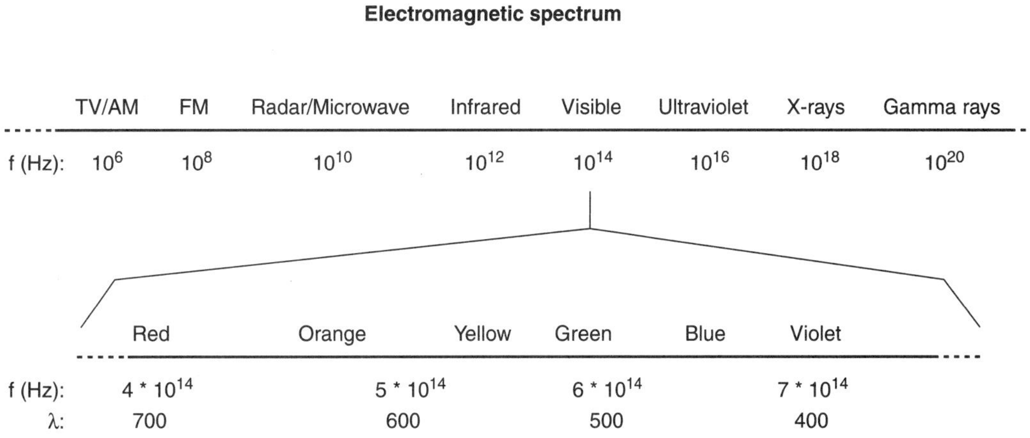

White light → Prism → Red, Orange, Yellow, Green

Electromagnetic spectrum

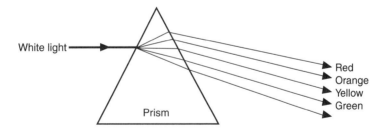

	TV/AM	FM	Radar/Microwave	Infrared	Visible	Ultraviolet	X-rays	Gamma rays
f (Hz):	10^6	10^8	10^{10}	10^{12}	10^{14}	10^{16}	10^{18}	10^{20}

Fig. 7-73. Electromagnetic spectrum.

	Red	Orange	Yellow	Green	Blue	Violet	
f (Hz):	$4 * 10^{14}$	$5 * 10^{14}$		$6 * 10^{14}$		$7 * 10^{14}$	
λ:	700	600		500		400	

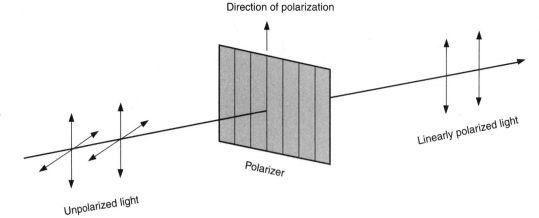

Fig. 7-74. Polarization of light.

Direction of polarization

Linearly polarized light

Polarizer

Unpolarized light

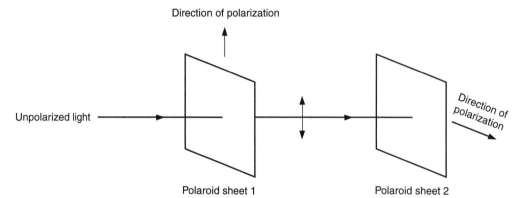

Fig. 7-75. How a polaroid sheet works.

Direction of polarization

Unpolarized light

Direction of polarization

Polaroid sheet 1

Polaroid sheet 2

the propagation direction (Fig. 7-74). The types of polarization include **plane polarized** light (or linearly polarized light), in which the oscillation of the electric field is along a line; **circularly polarized** light, which has waves that move along the path in a circular motion; and **elliptically polarized** light, which has waves that move in a elliptical motion along the path.

Four phenomena produce polarized light from unpolarized light. **Absorption** occurs when light strikes a material which does not allow transmission equally in all directions. A so-called "Polaroid"—a crystal or substance that allows light to pass along only one axis—is the usual example of this. In Figure 7-75, a beam of light is passed through two polaroids in succession. The first allows transmission of the light ray only along a certain axis. If the second polaroid is now oriented so that it does not allow transmission along the same axis, then no light is transmitted. **Reflection** of light from a plane surface, such as glass, usually causes partial polarization. The degree of polarization depends on the angle of incidence. Brewster's law states that when reflected and refracted light rays are 90° apart, or perpendicular to each other, the reflected light is completely polarized. **Scattering** is a combination of absorption and reradiation. Scattering centers are closely spaced (compare with the wavelength). For example, because of random changes in air density, clusters of air molecules scatter the short wavelengths of visible light more than the long wavelengths, making the sky blue. **Double refraction** (or **birefringence**) occurs in materials that are **anisotropic**, or have different optical characteristics along different directions. The indices of refraction are different for the different directions.

REFLECTION

Reflection is the process by which light rays (imaginary lines drawn perpendicular to advancing wave fronts) bounce back into a medium from the surface of another medium (versus being refracted or absorbed). The **laws of reflection** are: (1) The angle of incidence (I) equals the angle of reflection (R) at the normal (N, perpendicular to surface), and (2) The I, R, and N all lie on the same plane (Fig. 7-76).

Mirrors may have a plane surface or a curved surface. This discussion focuses on spherical curved mirrors. For a plane mirror, all parallel incident light is reflected off in parallel, and all images seen are virtual, erect, left-right reversed, and appear to be just as far (perpendicular distance) behind the mirror as the object is in front of the mirror.

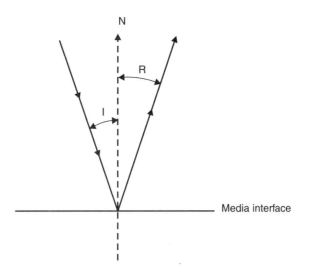

Fig. 7-76.

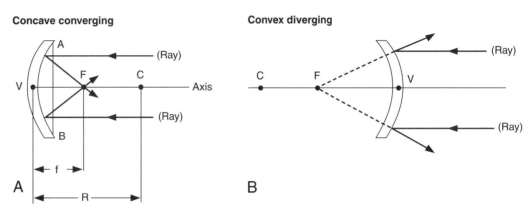

Concave converging

Convex diverging

A

B

Fig. 7-77.

A **virtual image** has no light rays passing through it and cannot be projected on a screen. A **real image** has light rays passing through it and can be projected on a screen.

Spherical mirrors may have a reflecting surface that is either convex (diverges light) or concave (converges light) [Fig. 7-77]. Note that the images formed by a converging mirror (concave) are similar to those formed by a converging lens (convex), and that diverging mirrors (convex) and diverging lens (concave) also form similar images. Terminology for spherical mirrors is as follows:

R = radius of curvature = radius of sphere of which mirror is a part
C = center of curvature = center of sphere of which mirror is a part
F = focal point
V = center of the mirror (mirror is assumed to have zero thickness)
Axis = line drawn through F and V
f = focal length = distance between F and V
i = image distance = distance of image from V measured along the axis
o = object distance = distance of object from V measured along the axis
AB = **Linear Aperture** = length of chord joining ends of mirror
s, s′ = symbols used for object/image distance from mirror.

Note that i, s, and s′ are signed quantities and can be negative (with a convex mirror). The positive direction along the axis is taken to be from V to F.

With **concave (spherical) mirrors,** the incident light is converged toward the axis (Fig. 7-78). The path of light rays is (1) incident rays parallel to the axis reflect through F, (2) incident rays along a radius (of curvature) reflect back on themselves (rays through C), and (3) incident rays through F reflect parallel to the axis.

The image formed by an object depends on the position of the image relative to the F and C (or f and R). Study the general rules for image formation:

1. If s < f, then image is virtual, erect, and enlarged (note that o in this case is negative). (See Fig [7-78(1)])
2. If s = f then the rays are reflected parallel to the axis and no image is formed (mathematically, the image is at infinity) [Fig 7-78(2)].

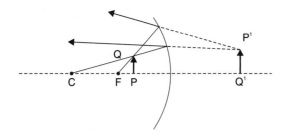

1) o < f → image virtual, upright

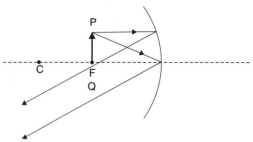

2) o = f → image = ±∞, reflected rays parallel

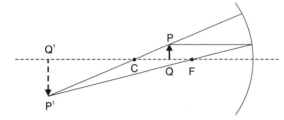

3) C < o < f → image real, inverted, magnified

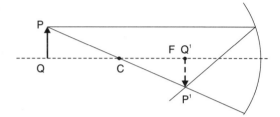

4) o > C → image real, inverted, diminished

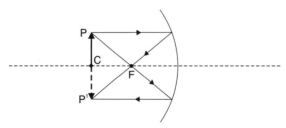

5) o = C → image real, inverted, same size

Fig. 7-78. Reflection from concave spherical mirror for which $F = \frac{c}{2}$.

3. If $f < s < R$ the image is real, inverted, and enlarged [Fig 7-78(3)].
4. If $s > R$ the image is real, inverted, and reduced in size [Fig 7-78(4)].
5. If $s = R$ the image is real, inverted, and the same size [Fig 7-78(5)].

These relations are similar to those for a converging lens (convex).

With **convex (spherical) mirrors**, the incident light is diverged from the axis after reflection. It is the backward extension (dotted lines above) that may pass through the F. The path of light rays are (1) incident rays parallel to the axis have backward extension of their reflections through F (see Fig. 7-78), (2) incident rays along a radius (that would pass through C if extended) reflect back along themselves, and (3) incident rays that pass through F (if extended) reflect parallel to the axis. The image formed for a convex mirror is always virtual, erect, and smaller than the object.

The **mirror equation** and derivations from it allow you to calculate the relations between object and image. The following equation is valid for convex and concave mirrors:

$$\frac{1}{i} + \frac{1}{o} = \frac{1}{f}$$

in which $f = R/2$ and M = magnification = $-i/o$. If i is negative, then the image is on the same side of the lens as the object.

Consider the following questions:

1. What are the assumptions and limitations behind the mirror equation?
2. Do you know the inverse relationship, viz. if focal length increases, $1/f$ decreases?

3. $\dfrac{1}{i} + \dfrac{1}{o} = \dfrac{1}{f}$

$\dfrac{o + i}{io} = \dfrac{1}{f}$

$f = \dfrac{io}{i + o}$

What does this formula tell you? Draw a graph between i and o.
Remember the following conventions in regard to the mirror equation:

For i positive values mean real, negative values mean virtual.

For f, a positive value means converging (concave), a negative value means diverging (convex).

For M, positive means erect, negative is inverted

REFRACTION

Refraction is the bending of light as it passes from one transparent medium to another, and is caused by the different speeds of light in the two media. The **index of refraction** of a medium is defined as the ratio of the speed of light in a vacuum to the speed of light in the medium (note this will always be greater than 1).

If θ_1 is taken as the angle (to the normal) of the incident light, θ_2 is the angle (to the normal) of the refracted light, and subscripts 1 and 2 represent the two media, then the following relations hold **(Snell's Law)** [Fig 7-79]:

$$\frac{\sin \theta_1}{\sin \theta_2} = \frac{v_1}{v_2} = \frac{n_2}{n_1} = \frac{\lambda_1}{\lambda_2}$$

where

v_i = velocity of light in medium$_i$

λ_i = wavelength of light in medium$_i$

n_i = index of refraction of medium$_i$ = $\dfrac{c}{v_i}$

and $c = 3 \times 10^{10}$ cm/sec = 186,000 m/sec. Another way of writing Snell's law, which may be easier to remember, is the more symmetric form:

$n_1 \sin \theta_1 = n_2 \sin \theta_2.$

Examples of indices of refraction for some common substances include:

n = 1.0 for air

n = 1.33 for H_2O

n = 1.5 for glass at λ = 589 m

as well as those shown in Table 7-8.

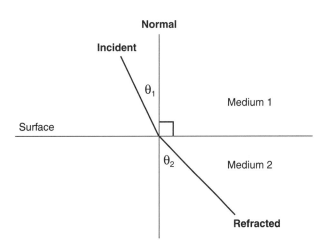

Fig. 7-79. Refraction.

TABLE 7-8. Typical Refraction Indices of Transparent Materials

Gases	
Air	1.0003
Carbon dioxide	1.0005

Liquids	
Carbon disulfide	1.64
Carbon tetrachloride	1.46
Ethyl alcohol	1.35
Water	1.33

Solids	
Diamond	2.42
Glass	1.50–1.66
Quartz	1.46

Note that the θ is smaller (closer to the normal) in the more optically dense (higher n) medium. From Snell's law:

$$\frac{\sin \theta_1}{\sin \theta_2} = \frac{n_2}{n_1} \Rightarrow \sin \theta_2 = \frac{n_1}{n_2} \sin \theta_1$$

Hence in the more optically dense media ($n_1/n_2 < 1$), the refracted ray is closer to the normal (θ_2 is smaller than θ_1). Note also from Snell's law that

$$\sin \theta_2 = \frac{\lambda_2}{\lambda_1} \sin \theta_1.$$

This equation indicates that light rays of different wavelengths are differently refracted. Because white light consists of light of different wavelengths (colors), it follows that a ray of white light can be separated into its component colors by refraction. A prism does just this, separating white light into its components. The **laws of refraction** are (1) The incident ray, the refracted ray, and the normal ray all lie in the same plane, and (2) The path of the ray (incident and refracted parts) is reversible (Fig. 7-80).

When light passes from a more optically dense (higher n) medium into a less optically dense medium, an angle of incidence exists such that the angle of refraction θ_2 is $90°$. This special angle of incidence is called the critical angle θ_c, because when the angle of incidence is less than θ_c, refraction occurs. As θ_1 approaches θ_c, reflection begins and refraction is reduced. As θ_1 moves to θ_c, reflection becomes predominate until it is total at θ_c. If $\theta_1 \geq \theta_c$, then **internal reflection** (ray is reflected back into the more dense medium) occurs. The θ_c is found from Snell's law.

$$n_1 \sin \theta_c = n_2 \sin \theta_2 \text{ (Snell's law)}$$

$$n_1 \sin \theta_c = n_2(1) \text{ (because } \theta_2 = 90° \text{ and } \sin 90° = 1)$$

$$\sin \theta_c = \frac{n_2}{n_1} \Rightarrow \theta_c = \arcsin\left(\frac{n_2}{n_1}\right).$$

$$\text{e.g., } \theta_c = 42° \text{ for glass and air}$$

When looking at an object under water from above the surface, the object appears closer than it actually is because of refraction. In general:

$$\frac{\text{Apparent depth}}{\text{actual depth}} = \frac{n_1}{n_2}$$

where

$$n_1 = \text{refractive index of observer's medium}$$

$$n_2 = \text{refractive index of object's medium.}$$

DISPERSION

Dispersion is the wave speed in a medium that depends on the wavelength and frequency of the light. When a beam of white light strikes a glass surface, such as a prism, at an angle, the angle of refraction of the shorter wavelengths (the violet end of the spectrum) is smaller than the angle of refraction of the longer wavelengths (the red end of the spectrum). The result is the dispersion of white light into the different wavelengths, each a different color. Another example of the dispersion of white light is the refraction of white light in water droplets during a rain storm, which causes a rainbow.

LENSES

A lens is a transparent material that refracts light. Converging lenses refract light toward the axis and diverging lenses refract light away from the axis. A converging lens is wider at the middle than at the ends, and a diverging lens is thinner at the middle than at the ends (Fig. 7-80).

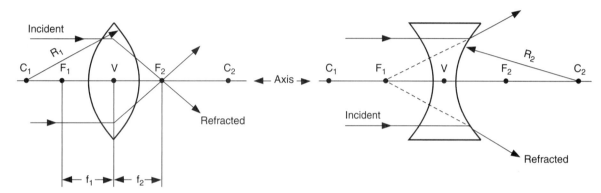

Fig. 7-80. If the surface of the lens is convex, then R (radius of curvature) is positive (e.g., R_1). If the surface is concave, then R is negative (e.g., R_2). Subscript 1 refers to the incident side, subscript 2 refers to the refracted side. C = center of curvature, F = focal point, f = focal length is distance between V and F, V = optical center of the lens, i = image distance (from V to image), axis = line through C and V, o = object distance (from V to object).

The path of rays through a lens is (1) incident rays parallel to the axis refract through F_2 of a converging lens, and appear to come from F_1 of a diverging lens (backward extensions of the refracted ray; see the dotted line in Fig. 7-80); (2) an incident ray through F_1 of a converging lens is refracted parallel to the axis; and (3) incident rays through V are not deviated (refracted).

Converging Lens

For a converging lens (e.g., biconvex), the image formed depends on the object distance relative to the focal length (f). Compare the following relations to those of the converging mirror (Fig. 7-81):

1. If o < f, the image is virtual, erect, and enlarged
   If f < o < 2f, the image is real, inverted, and enlarged
2. If o = f, no image is formed
3. If o > 2f, image is real, inverted, and reduced in size
   If o = 2f, image is the same size

Diverging Lens

For a diverging lens (e.g., biconcave), the image is always virtual, erect, and reduced in size as for a diverging mirror. The preceding relations can be calculated by using the **lens equation** (similar to the mirror equation) and derivations from it. First, $1/o + 1/i = 1/f$ (lens equation, same as mirror equation). Second, **diopters** (D) = $1/f$, in which f is in meters, represents a measurement that is indicative of the refractive power of the lens; the larger the diopters (D), the stronger the lens. It has a $+D$ for converging lens and a $-D$ for diverging lens. To determine the refractive power (D) of lenses in series, add the diopters, which can then be converted into focal length: $D_T = D_1 + D_2 = 1/f_T$. Third, note that you cannot add focal lengths except as reciprocals: $1/f_T = 1/f_1 + 1/f_2$; and fourth M = magnification = $-i/o$, M = M_1M_2 for lenses in series.

Remember the following conventions:

1. For i, positive values are real, negative values are virtual

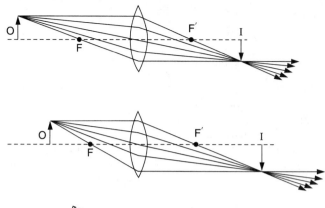

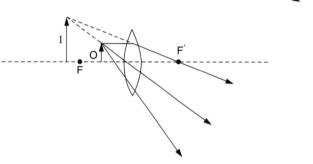

Fig. 7-81. Refraction through a convex lens.

2. For f, positive means converging, negative is diverging
3. For M, positive means erect, negative is inverted

The lens equation holds only for thin lenses—the thickness is small relative to other dimensions.

Lens Combinations and Aberrations

For a combination of lenses not in contact with each other, the image is found for the first lens (nearer the object) and then this image is used as the object of the second lens to find the image formed by it.

An **aberration** occurs when all the rays from a point object are not focused at a single point, causing a blurry image. Spherical lenses refract light somewhat differently from the outer edges of the lens compared to the center of the lens. Consequently, the image of a point on the object is slightly blurred This inherent limitation of a spherical lens is called **spherical abberation.** A **coma** is when rays from a point off the axis fail to form a point image after the rays are refracted by a lens. Coma is named because an off-axis image of a point is shaped like a comet. An **astigmatism** is the imaging of a point source off the axis into two perpendicular lines at different locations. **Chromatic aberrations** occur because of a variation in the index of refraction of a lens material with wavelength, causing the rays of different colors from an object to form images at different points. This problem can be corrected by using a combination of lenses made from materials with different dispersion characteristics.

PREMEDICAL CONCEPTS IN OPTICS

Emmetropia means that light is focused on the retina (by the cornea–lens system) when objects are near or far. **Myopia**, or nearsightedness, means that light is focused on the retina when objects are near but is focused in front of the retina when objects are far away (Fig. 7-82). One cause of myopia is that an eyeball is too long, and an ophthalmologist may prescribe diverging (concave) glasses (i.e., lens). **Hypermetropia**, or farsightedness, means that light is focused on the retina when objects are far away and behind the retina when they are near (see Fig. 7-82). In this situation, an eyeball is too short, and an ophthalmologist may prescribe converging (convex) glasses for correction.

OPTICAL INSTRUMENTS

It is important to understand the anatomy (structure) and physiology (working and functions) of the following instruments:

• Microscope (several types)
• Telescope
• Binoculars
• Polarimeter
• LASER and MASER guns

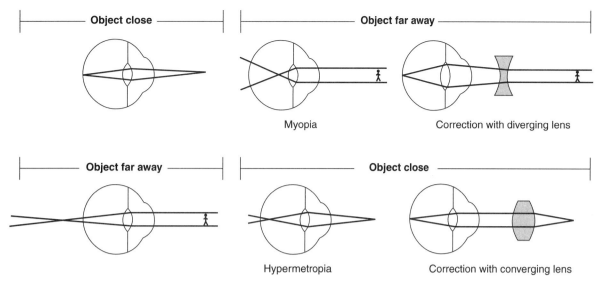

Fig. 7-82. Myopia and hypermetropia.

Be sure to note the major physical differences and similarities among these instruments.

APPLIED CONCEPTS

1. Contact lenses
2. Radial keratotomy surgery. In people with myopia, images come into focus before they reach the retina. Radial keratotomy (RK) reshapes the curvature of the cornea, which allows images to be focused farther back on the retina. Doctors make tiny, spokelike incisions in the cornea. Because every cornea is different, successful RK depends on precise predictive formulas to determine the optimum number, length, and depth of incisions. This operation usually involves only one eye; a second procedure may be required. Also on the horizon is widespread use of ultraviolet laser surgery. Instead of making a tiny incision, the laser removes tiny amounts of tissue from the surface of the cornea to correct myopia.
3. Making blind people "see" by stimulating rods and cones with electric impulses.

The following information is presented in passage format to test your reading comprehension.

Anatomically, the eye is separated by the lens into an anterior region filled by the **aqueous humor** and a posterior region filled by the **vitreous humor** (Fig. 7-83). The eye has three layers. The **sclera** (dense connective tissue) is the outermost. It is covered anteriorly by the conjunctiva (whites of the eyes). It is continuous with the clear portion called the **cornea**, which is important in focusing light. Inside the sclera is the **choroid**, which contains blood vessels and black pigment to prevent light scattering. Continuous with the choroid in front are the **iris**, which gives the eye its color and opens and shuts

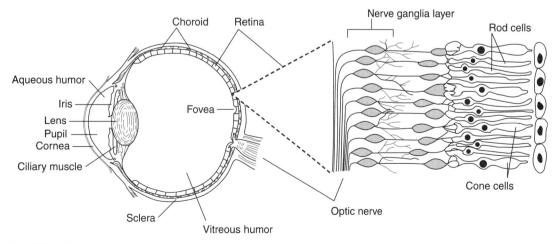

Fig. 7-83. The human eye.

to let light in through the pupil, and the **ciliary muscle**, which controls the shape of the lens and helps to focus the eye for distance. The innermost layer is the **retina**, which is light sensitive and contains a mixture of rods and cones. **Rods** are concentrated more peripherally in the eye, are concerned with vision in dim light and peripheral vision, and contain **rhodopsin** (retinal from vitamin A and a protein called opsin). Light converts retinal from a **cis** to a **trans** form, which causes rhodopsin to fall apart, and sets up an impulse that is transmitted to the optic nerve (cranial nerve II). Cones are concentrated more centrally, are more sensitive to bright light, are responsible for color vision, contain **iodopsin** (light-sensitive substance), and are maximally concentrated at the **fovea** (or macula area), which has the highest visual acuity (i.e., the ability to see clearly points that are close together).

   Light passes through the cornea, where it is refracted (bent). Next, it passes through the aqueous humor and then through the pupil. Pupil size is regulated by the iris, which is regulated by the parasympathetic system (which causes the pupil to get smaller) and the sympathetic system (which causes the pupil to get larger). The light then passes through the lens, where it is refracted further and focused on the retina after it passes through the vitreous humor. The lens is flat for far away objects (the ciliary muscle is relaxed) and is rounded for nearby objects (the ciliary muscle is contracted—parasympathetic). Light then stimulates the cones and rods of the retina. From there, nerve impulses are transmitted via the ocular nerve (II) to the visual center in the occipital cortex of the cerebrum. (This section may also be used for solving biologic sciences problems.)

LIGHT AND GEOMETRIC OPTICS: REVIEW QUESTIONS

1. Using the following diagram, select the INCORRECT statement of the laws of reflection of light from surfaces:

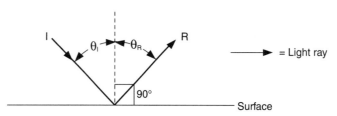

   A. $\theta_I = \theta_R$
   B. $\theta_I + \theta_R = 90°$
   C. I, N, and R all lie in the same plane
   D. Both A and C

2. All of the following statements about images seen in plane (flat) mirrors are true EXCEPT:

   A. they are always virtual.
   B. they appear at a distance behind the mirror equal to the distance (perpendicular) of the object in front of the mirror.
   C. they are right-left reversed.
   D. they are inverted.

3. The reflected light rays from a smooth concave mirror:

   A. converge.
   B. diverge.
   C. are parallel.
   D. are diffused.

4. In terms of reflected light and images, a convex mirror is most like a:

   A. convex lens.
   B. concave lens.
   C. triangular prism.
   D. square prism.

5. For the following spherical convex mirror:

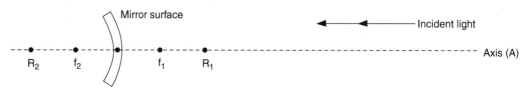

   ($f_1 = f_2$; $R_1 = R_2$; f = focal length; R = radius of curvature)

A. incident rays parallel to A reflect through f_1.
B. incident rays passing through R_1 reflect through R_2.
C. the forward extensions of incident rays that reflect through f_2 pass through f_1.
D. the backward extensions of reflected rays that result from incident rays parallel to A pass through f_2.

6. For a convex mirror with f = focal length, R = radius of curvature, and o = object distance (along the axis) from the mirror:

   A. the image is always virtual, erect, and reduced in size.
   B. if o > f, the image is virtual and inverted.
   C. if o = R, the image and object are the same size.
   D. if o > R, the image is larger than the object.

7. The mirror equation is (f = focal length, o = object distance, I = image distance):

   A. f = o + I.
   B. f = 1/o + 1/I.
   C. 1/f = o + I.
   D. 1/f = 1/o + 1/I.

8. The phenomenon of refraction ("bending" of light rays) is attributable to:

   A. the particle character of light.
   B. the varying speeds of light in different media.
   C. the longitudinal wave character of light.
   D. none of the above.

9. Given the following diagram for refraction of light, the correct relationship between the angles (θ) shown and the indices of refraction (n) in the media is:

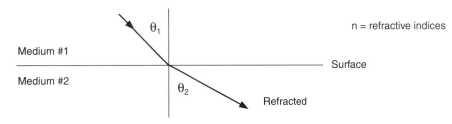

   A. $n_2 \sin\theta_1 = n_1 \sin\theta_2$.
   B. $n_1\theta_1 = n_2\theta_2$.
   C. $\sin\theta_1/\sin\theta_2 = n_2/n_1$.
   D. $\theta_1/\theta_2 = n_1/n_2$.

10. The index of refraction of a medium is:

    A. the speed of light in free space divided by the speed of light in that medium.
    B. the density of the medium divided by the density of air.
    C. the absorption of light in the medium divided by the absorption of light in water.
    D. none of the above.

11. Dispersion of white light into its component colors (as through a prism) occurs by the process of:

    A. diffraction.
    B. polarization.
    C. refraction.
    D. reflection.

12. A critical angle of incidence (θ_c):

    A. is reached when light passes from a lower optically dense medium into a higher optically dense medium.
    B. means that the angle of refraction is 90°.
    C. means that at all angles of incidence less than θ_c, light is reflected.
    D. is all of the above.

13. For the following lens, in which V = vertex, F = focal point, and C = center of curvature, which of the following statements is correct?

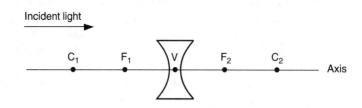

Incident light

A. If the incident rays are parallel to the axis, the backward extensions of the refracted rays pass through C_1.
B. If the forward extension of an incident ray would pass through F_2, then the backward extension of the refracted ray would pass through F_1.
C. Incident rays through V are not refracted.
D. All of these statements are correct.

14. Concerning the image formed by a converging lens, select the incorrect statement (f = focal length, o = object distance):

A. If o < f, the image is virtual and erect.
B. If o = f, no image is formed.
C. If o > f, the image is real and inverted.
D. If o < 2f, the object is reduced in size.

15. Diopters are defined as:

A. the number of degrees of visual acuity.
B. a type of lens that corrects astigmatism.
C. the refractive power of a lens.
D. the reflective power of a mirror.

16. A concave mirror with a focal length (f) = 4 cm forms an image (I) of an object (O) placed 10 cm from it. What is the magnification (M) of this image?

A. ⅓ of the object
B. ⅔ of the object
C. ⅚ times the object
D. 3 times the object

$\frac{1}{f} + \frac{1}{O} + \frac{1}{i}$

$M = -\frac{i}{O}$

17. An object (O) is placed 10 cm from a concave mirror with focal length (f) = 2 cm. The image is:

A. real, inverted, reduced, and 2.50 cm from the mirror.
B. virtual, erect, enlarged, and 8 cm from the mirror.
C. virtual, erect, enlarged, and 20 cm from the mirror.
D. real, erect, enlarged, and 2.50 cm from the mirror.

18. Optically dense media have high indices of refraction. Referring to the following diagram, select the correct statement:

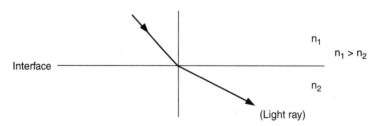

A. $\theta_1 < \theta_2$
B. $\theta_1 = \theta_2$
C. $\theta_1 > \theta_2$
D. Insufficient data provided

19. If violet light and red light both have the same angle of incidence, which of the following statements is correct concerning the angles of refraction?

A. The angles of refraction are equal.
B. The angle of refraction of the violet light is larger than that of the red light.

C. The angle of refraction of the red light is larger than that of the violet light.

D. The velocities in the media are needed to evaluate the angles of refraction.

20. A fish is 8 m from the surface in a tank of water. Looking from the air surface, the fish would appear to be how deep? (n of air = 1.00, n of water = 1.33)

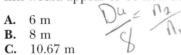

   A. 6 m
   B. 8 m
   C. 10.67 m
   D. Angles of incidence and refraction needed to determine

21. An object is 15 cm from a converging lens with a focal length of 5 cm. The image formed is:

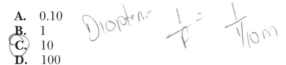

   A. virtual, erect, enlarged.
   B. virtual, erect, reduced.
   C. real, erect, enlarged.
   D. real, inverted, reduced.

22. A lens with a focal length of 10 cm is how many diopters?

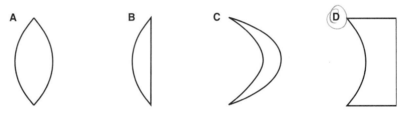

   A. 0.10
   B. 1
   C. 10
   D. 100

23. Which of the following diagrams does not represent a converging lens?

24. Which structure is anterior to the lens in the human eye?

   A. Aqueous humor
   B. Vitreous humor
   C. Retina
   D. Choroid

25. Select the incorrect association of structure and function in the eye:

   A. Cornea—scatters light
   B. Choroid—prevents light scattering
   C. Iris—regulates amount of light that enters eye
   D. Ciliary muscle—controls shape of the lens

26. Which of the following statements concerning rods and cones of the eye is incorrect?

   A. Rods are for vision in dim light.
   B. Rods are located peripherally in the eye.
   C. Cones are for color vision.
   D. Cones contain rhodopsin.

27. Select the correct path of light through the eye (anterior to posterior):

   A. Cornea, aqueous humor. lens, vitreous humor, retina
   B. Lens, aqueous humor, cornea, vitreous humor, retina
   C. Cornea, vitreous humor, lens, aqueous humor, retina
   D. Retina, cornea, aqueous humor, lens, vitreous humor

28. Which of the following statements is incorrect?

   A. Converging lenses are corrective for myopic eyes.
   B. Light focuses in front of the retina when objects are distant in myopic eyes.
   C. Light is focused behind the retina.
   D. A convex lens will correct hypermetropic eyes.

1–15. **1-B, 2-D, 3-A, 4-B, 5-D, 6-A, 7-D, 8-B, 9-C, 10-A, 11-C, 12-B, 13-C, 14-D, 15-C.** See text for explanation.

16. B Use the mirror equation:

$$\frac{1}{f} = \frac{1}{o} + \frac{1}{i}$$

$f = +4$ cm because of converging mirror

$$\frac{1}{4} = \frac{1}{10} + \frac{1}{i}$$

$$20i\left(\frac{1}{4}\right) = 20i\left(\frac{1}{10}\right) + 20i\left(\frac{1}{i}\right)$$

(note 20i is the least common denominator)

$$5i = 2i + 20$$

$$3i = 20$$

$$i = \frac{20}{3} \text{ cm from the mirror and is real}$$

$$m = -\frac{i}{o} = \frac{\left(\frac{-20}{3}\right)}{10} = \left(-\frac{20}{3}\right)\left(\frac{1}{10}\right) = -\frac{2}{3} \text{ of the object}$$

The image is inverted (because it is negative).

17. A Use the mirror equation:

$$\frac{1}{f} = \frac{1}{o} + \frac{1}{i}$$

$f = +2$ m because of converging mirror

$$\frac{1}{2} = \frac{1}{10} + \frac{1}{i}$$

$$10i\left(\frac{1}{2}\right) = 10i\left(\frac{1}{10}\right) + 10i\left(\frac{1}{i}\right)$$

$$5i = i + 10$$

$$4i = 10$$

$$i = \frac{10}{4} = +\frac{5}{2} = 2.50 \text{ cm from the mirror}$$

Because o (10 cm) > f (2 cm), the image is real and inverted.
Because o (10 cm) > R (4 cm), the image is reduced.

$$R = 2f = 2 \cdot 2 = 4$$

18. A The angle to the normal is smaller in the more optically dense medium for refraction of light.

19. C For light, the smaller the wavelength, the closer the refracted ray to the normal. Because violet light has a shorter wavelength than red, red light will be refracted through a larger angle.

20. A Apparent depth (D_a)/actual depth = n_2/n_1

$$n_2 = \text{of observer} = 1.00$$

$$n_1 = \text{of object} = 1.33$$

$$\frac{D_a}{8} = \frac{1.00}{1.33} = \frac{1}{\left(\frac{4}{3}\right)} = \frac{3}{4}$$

$$D_a = \left(\frac{3}{4}\right)(8) = 6 \text{ m}$$

21. D Because the object distance is greater than the focal length, the image is real and inverted. Because the object distance is more than twice the focal length, the image is reduced in size.

Electrostatics and Electromagnetism

Self-Managed Learning Questions

1. What is an electroscope? Why do the leaves of an electroscope separate as a positively charged rod is brought closer? Propose a hypothesis that can be verified experimentally.
2. What is electroplating? How is the concept used in painting large objects, such as an automobile?
3. What is bioelectricity and what is biomagnetism? Is it true that a cell membrane behaves as a capacitor? Propose a hypothesis with experimental evidence.
4. What is the right-hand rule for an electromagnetic field? Draw a diagram to illustrate the principle.
5. Is it possible to make a small motor to produce power using lemon juice? Explain.
6. Understand the working of an electron microscope and a mass spectrograph. What errors can be made by using these instruments incorrectly?

ELECTROSTATICS

The elementary charges are positive (+) or negative (−). Each has a charge of 1.6×10^{-19} coulombs but differ in sign. The electron is the negative charge carrier, and the proton is the positive charge carrier. Substances with an excess of electrons have a net negative charge. Substances with a deficiency of electrons have a net positive charge. One way of charging substances is by rubbing them (i.e., by contact). For example, glass rubbed on fur becomes positive and rubber rubbed on fur becomes negative. Objects can also be charged by **induction**, which occurs when one charged object brought near another causes a charge redistribution in the latter to give net charge regions. **Conductors** transmit charge readily. **Insulators** resist the flow of charge.

Coulomb's Law

Charges exert forces on each other. Like charges repel each other and unlike charges attract. For two charges, the force is given by Coulomb's law (Fig. 7-84).

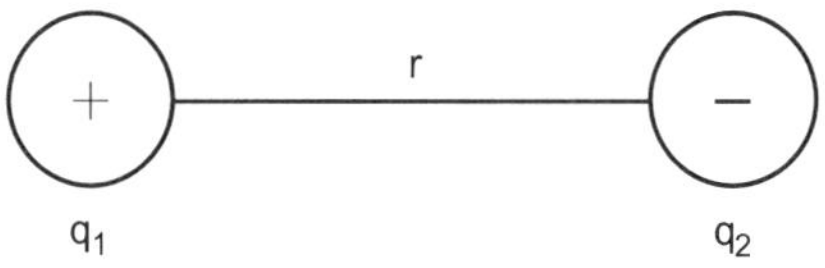

Fig. 7-84. Coulomb's law. q_1, q_2 = charges; k = constant = 9.0×10^9 nt · m²/coul²; ε_0 = permitivity of air to the forces = 8.85×10^{-12} coul²/(nt · m²); r = distance between the charges.

$$F = k \frac{q_1 q_2}{r^2} = k q_1 q_2 / r^2 = \frac{1}{4\pi\varepsilon_0} \frac{q_1 q_2}{r^2} = q_1 q_2 / (4\pi\varepsilon_0 r^2)$$

Electric Field

A charge generates an electric field (E) in the space around it. Fields (force fields) are vectors (have direction and magnitude). The electric field generated by a charge (Q) is characterized by the force it produces on a test charge brought into the field. The electric field is defined as the force per unit charge exerted on the test charge (q),

$$E = \frac{F}{q} = \frac{k \dfrac{qQ}{r^2}}{q} = k \frac{Q}{r^2}$$

where the second equality follows from Coulomb's law. Note that the **field intensity** is directly proportional to Q and inversely proportional to r^2, implying that the field extends in all directions to infinity (E, F, Q are vectors). Also note that E and F are in the same direction; the direction of an electric field is the direction in which a positive charge would move if placed in the field.

Charges exert forces on each other through fields. The direction of a field is the direction a positive charge would move if placed in it. **Electric field** lines are imaginary

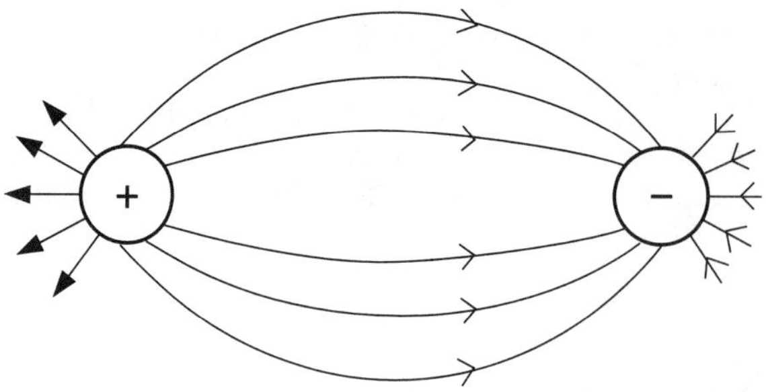

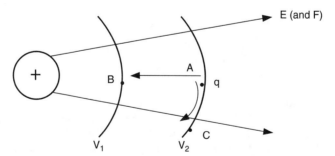

Fig. 7-85. Electric field lines.

lines that are in the same direction as E at that point (Fig. 7-85). The direction is away from positive charges and toward negative charges.

The **electrical potential energy** (PE) of a charge q in an electric field generated by a charge Q is defined as the work done on charge q in bringing it from infinity to its position in the electric field, and can be shown to be

$$PE = k\frac{qQ}{r}$$

where r is the distance between Q and q. Note that the potential energy so defined can be positive or negative, depending on whether the charges are the same or opposite in value. For example, if Q and q are both positive or both negative, then work must be done on q because of the repulsive forces between two like charges. If one is positive and one is negative, however, work is done by the charges because of the attractive force.

Potential Difference, Absolute Potential, and Equipotential Lines

Given a charge (Q), the **electric potential** (V) at a point in the electric field generated by Q at a distance (r) from Q is given by:

$$V = volts = k\frac{Q}{r} = \frac{joules}{coulombs}.$$

V is a scalar and represents the work done in bringing a unit positive charge (a positive charge with a magnitude of 1) from infinity to any point r units in distance from Q. The value of V is independent of the path taken by the unit positive charge. Note that if Q is a positive charge, V will be positive, and vice versa. Note also that the **electric potential** (V) at a point is the **potential energy** (PE) per unit charge at that point

$$V = \frac{PE}{q}.$$

Note also that given a charge Q, the potential at any point of the surface of a sphere with Q at its center is the same. Such surfaces are called equipotential surfaces.

Fig. 7-86. Electric potential.

As an example, consider Fig 7-86. Suppose that V_1 and V_2 are two equipotential surfaces, and that the difference in potential between them can be measured. If a charge q is moved from point A to point B, the work done (the change in electrical potential energy of q) is given by:

$$W = q(V_1 - V_2).$$

Note that the work in moving q from point A to point C is zero because the electrical potential of these two points is the same.

The **potential difference** (PD) between point A and B is the difference in V between the points, and is the work done by moving a unit positive charge from point A to B. This relationship is demonstrated by the following equation:

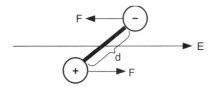
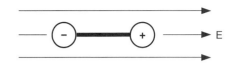

Fig. 7-87. Dipoles.

Dipole with equal and opposite charges
E = electric field
F = forces exerted by E on the dipole
d = distance

Alignment of dipole with E

$$PD = V_B - V_A = volts = \frac{work}{charge} = \frac{joules}{coulomb}$$

$$Work = q(V_B - V_A) = q \cdot PD.$$

Electric Dipole

An **electric dipole** (Fig. 7-87) consists of two charges separated by some finite distance (d). Usually, the charges are equal and opposite. The laws of forces, fields, etc., as described previously, apply to dipoles. A dipole is characterized by its **dipole moment (D.M.)**, which is the product of the charge (q) and d. Dipoles tend to line up with the electric field. Motion of dipoles against an electric field requires energy, as discussed previously.

ELECTROMAGNETISM

This discussion links magnetism and its numerous applications to electronic structure and the periodic properties of elements; interaction of mechanical, electric, and magnetic fields; and electromagnetic wave spectrum related to accelerating electric charges. Concepts related to electromagnetism are divided into the following categories:

1. Definition and applications
2. Types of magnetic materials
3. Dimensions of common electromagnetic properties
4. Fundamental rules and laws
5. Electromagnetic wave spectrum

Definition and Applications

A magnet has two poles, similar to an electric dipole. Unlike an isolated resting electron that can exist as a monopole, the simplest magnetic structure that can exist is the magnetic dipole. Magnetism is caused by the arrangement of individual atoms in a substance. The applications of magnetism range from stick-on refrigerator magnets to the design of highly sophisticated particle accelerators. Other applications include mechanisms inside galvanometers, voltmeters, ammeters, running of supermagnetic levitation trains, brain wave analysis related to hearing, storing data on floppy computer diskettes, walkman radio/tape recorders, credit card strips, and cabinet door locks. As Blackmore discovered, bacteria are guided by the north-end of the magnetic compass, which allows the bacteria to orient themselves in chaotic waters. These **magnetotactic bacteria** have led to advanced research in microbiology.

Types of Magnetic Materials

Common household magnets are made of Fe_3O_4 molecules (composed of 2 FeO and Fe_2O_3 molecules). These molecules appear as reddish brown rust when iron objects are exposed to both air and water for long time periods. Magnetic materials are of three types.

Diamagnetic substances are the weakest magnetic materials. The atoms of these materials do not have inherent magnetic dipoles. Magnetic polarities or moments can be induced in them by external fields (e.g. bismuth, copper).

Paramagnetic substances are relatively stronger than diamagnetic materials. Paramagnetism is the tendency of individual atoms (each with a magnetic dipole) to align along the magnetic field. Atoms of these materials have inherent magnetic dipoles. The stronger the magnetic field, the higher the magnetic tendency toward atomic alignment within the substance.

Ferromagnetic substances are highly magnetic, even without an external magnetic field. These substances have strong inherent magnetic dipoles. Each surrounding or neighboring atom has a strong interaction with the strong dipoles. The arrangement is more permanent in ferromagnetic materials (e.g., lodestone).

Dimensions of Common Electromagnetic Properties

Electromagnetic properties are represented by a combination of electric and magnetic variables and constants.

$$\textbf{Magnetic field (B) units} = \frac{1N}{1C \cdot 1m/s} = \frac{1 \text{ Newton}}{1 \text{ Coulomb} \cdot 1m/\text{second}}$$

Since $1 \text{ ampere} = \dfrac{1C}{s}$,

$$\therefore \text{ units} = \frac{1N}{m \cdot A} = \frac{1 \text{ Newton}}{\text{meter} \cdot \text{ampere}}$$

$$\text{Unit of measure} = \text{Tesla} = 1T = \frac{1N}{m \cdot A} = 10^4 \text{ gauss}$$

Permeability constant $[\mu_o]$ $\mu_o = 4\pi \times 10^{-7} \dfrac{T \cdot m}{A}$

Magnetic flux (Wb)

$1 \text{ Wb} = 1 \text{ Weber} = 1 \text{ Tesla} \cdot m^2$

Bohr Magneton $[\mu_B]$ $1\mu_B = \dfrac{he}{4\pi m}$

in which m = mass of electron; h = Planck constant = $6.63 \times 10^{-34} J \cdot s$; and e = unit charge on one electron $(-)$.

Fundamental Rules and Laws

1. Opposite magnetic poles attract each other and like magnetic poles repel each other.

2. A moving electric charge or a current in a conductor produces a magnetic field that is perpendicular to the direction of motion of the charge. The strength of the magnetic field is related to the charge and its velocity; this property is used in the design of motors and other electrical devices. Changing electric fields also give rise to magnetic fields.

   In addition, a magnetic field exerts a force on a moving charge, the force being perpendicular to the direction of the magnetic field. As a result, a magnetic field can alter the direction of motion of a moving electron (proton), but cannot change its velocity; this characteristic is utilized in the design of televisions, cathode ray tubes, and computer terminals.

   Given a moving charge q with velocity vector v that makes an angle ϕ with a magnetic field B, the force tending to deflect the charge is given by

   $$F_B = qvB \sin \phi.$$

   Hence the maximal deflecting force occurs when the charge is moving at right angles to the magnetic field and the force is then

   $$F_B = qvB$$

3. Given a magnetic field B perpendicular to an electric field E, if a charge q moves with velocity v perpendicular to both of these fields without being deflected, the force exerted by the electric field is given by qE and the force exerted by the magnetic field is given by qvB. Since the charge is not deflected,

   $$qE = qvB \Rightarrow v = \frac{E}{B}.$$

   If a charge of mass m moves with velocity v in a circular path of radius r and the path is perpendicular to a magnetic field B, then centripetal force = the force of the magnetic field,

   $$F = ma = \frac{mv^2}{r} = qvB$$

   and hence the radius of the path must be

   $$r = \frac{mv}{qB}.$$

The angular velocity in this case is

$$\overline{\omega} = \frac{v}{r} = \frac{qB}{m}$$

and so the angular velocity of the charge is independent of particle velocity—that is, as velocity increases, radius increases equally.

4. **Biot and Savart law** states that in a long straight wire conducting current I, the magnetic field is proportional to the current and inversely proportional to the perpendicular distance r from the center of the wire. $B = \frac{\mu_o I}{2\pi r}$ gives the magnitude of the magnetic field for the simple case of a straight wire. Given a length of wire of length L carrying a current I in a magnetic field of strength B, the force developed on the wire by the magnetic field is given by:

$$F = ILB.$$

If the magnetic field B is generated by a current in another wire, the force F will be attractant if the current in both wires flows in the same direction, repellant otherwise.

5. **Right-hand rule** helps you determine the direction of the magnetic field set up by an electric current in a wire. Grasp the wire in your right hand with your thumb laid out in the direction of the current. Your four fingers will curl around, indicating the direction of the lines of the magnetic field.

6. **Faraday's law of electromagnetic induction** states that the induced electromotive force in an electric circuit is equal in magnitude to the time rate of change of magnetic flux. Faraday's law was followed by Lenz's law to determine the direction of an induced current. Refer to a physics reference book to understand Lenz's law.

7. **Gauss' law for magnetism** states that isolated magnetic poles (monopoles) do not exist.

Electromagnetic Spectrum and X-Rays

The electromagnetic spectrum is discussed in the section reviewing wave characteristics and periodic motion. It is important to realize that electric fields and magnetic fields are further interrelated. If a magnetic field changes, an electric field is produced. From the principle of symmetry, the reverse is true. An electric field produced by a changing magnetic field is expressed by Faraday's law, and a magnetic field produced by a changing electric field (or by a current or both) is expressed by the Ampere-Maxwell law. Gauss' law, Faraday's law, and the Ampere-Maxwell law can be combined, yielding the so-called "Maxwell's equations." With S = distance, m = magnetic dipole, and I = current, electromagnetic waves can be generated with widely varying wavelengths. Notice that x-rays are at the lower end of the electromagnetic spectrum, visible light toward the middle, and radio bands toward the upper end of the spectrum.

APPLIED CONCEPTS

1. Read research articles to understand how birds and turtles orient themselves with the Earth's magnetic field. Understand the working of Helmholtz cells.
2. Read more on the magnetic field produced around the heart and in the human brain.
3. Review the working of a voltmeter, ammeter, and a galvanometer. How can these instruments be calibrated in the laboratory?
4. Explain the working and structural features of an electromagnetic rail gun to shoot projectiles.

ELECTROSTATICS AND ELECTROMAGNETISM: REVIEW QUESTIONS

1. Which of the following statements concerning fields is incorrect?
   A. They exist in space and are generated by objects (e.g., mass).
   B. Gravitational and electric fields are examples.
   C. They are scalars.
   D. They exist independently of other objects.

2. Coulomb's law of electric forces (q = charge, r = distance between charges, k = constant, F = force) is expressed as:
   A. $F = k(q_1 q_2 / r_2)$.
   B. $F = k(q / r_2)$.
   C. $F = k(q_1 q_2 / r)$.
   D. $F = k(q_2 / r)$.

3. If F = force = kq_1q_o/r^2 and q_o = an electric charge, what is F/q_o?

   A. The electric field generated by q_1.
   B. The force acting on q_o.
   C. The electric potential set up by q_o.
   D. The work done by the force on q_1.

4. All of the following formulations, in which q = charge, r = distance, E = electric field, F = force, and ϵ_0 = permitivity, express electric potential (V) EXCEPT:

   A. $V = (\frac{1}{4}\epsilon_0)(q/r)$.
   B. V = potential energy/charge.
   C. V = Er/q.
   D. V = Fq.

5. Which of the following phrases best describes electric work?

   A. Depends on the path taken by a charge between equipotential surfaces
   B. Zero when a charge is moved along an equipotential (electric potential) line
   C. Zero when a charge moves between surfaces of different electric potential
   D. Both A and C

6. The potential difference as used in electrostatics is:

   A. the difference in potential energy between two points.
   B. the difference in electric potential between two points.
   C. the difference in work between two points.
   D. both A and C.

7. Which of the following is a correct formulation of electric work (W) done on moving a charge (q) in an electric field (E) (V = electric potential, PD = potential difference, F = electric force, r = distance between charges)?

   A. W = q(PD)
   B. W = Fq
   C. W = Vr
   D. W = Eq

8. All of the following statements about electric dipoles are true EXCEPT:

   A. they consist of two charges separated by a finite distance.
   B. the dipole moment is a product of the charge and the distance between them.
   C. the motion of dipoles against an electric field requires no energy.
   D. the positive end of the dipole points in the direction of the electric field.

9. If the distance between two electric charges is doubled, the force between them is:

   A. decreased by one quarter.
   B. decreased by one half.
   C. doubled.
   D. quadrupled.

10. If the charge (q) on each of two objects is doubled and they are moved twice as far apart (r), what is the force between them?

    A. Multiplied by a factor of 8
    B. Quadrupled
    C. Doubled
    D. Unchanged

11. As two electric charges move further apart, the force between them:

    A. increases proportionally to the inverse square of the distance between them.
    B. increases proportionally to the distance between them.
    C. decreases proportionally to the inverse square of the distance between them.
    D. decreases proportionally to the distance between them.

12. If charge 1 (q_1) is doubled, charge 2 (q_2) is tripled, and the distance (r) between them is not changed, the force (F) between them:

    A. divides by a factor of 36.
    B. multiplies by a factor of 36.

C. multiplies by a factor of 6.

D. does not change.

13. What is the force between charge 1 (q_1) and charge 2 (q_2) in the following diagram?

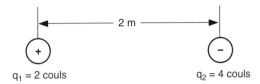

q_1 = 2 couls q_2 = 4 couls

    A. Repulsive, 2 N

    B. Attractive, 2 N

    C. Repulsive, 2 kN

    D. Attractive, 2 kN

14. The net force on charge C (q_c) is:

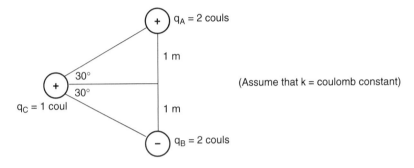

(Assume that k = coulomb constant)

    A. zero.

    B. horizontal and to the right, 0.5 kN

    C. horizontal and to the left, 0.5 kN

    D. vertical and down, 0.5 kN

15. The electric field (E) generated by a charge:

    A. is constant at all distances from the charge.

    B. decreases directly as distance from the charge increases.

    C. decreases proportional to the inverse square of the distance from the charge.

    D. decreases proportional to the inverse distance from the charge.

16. All of the following formulas for the potential energy (PE) of a charged object (q) in an electric field (F = force on charge, V = electric potential, E = electric field, r = distance of charge from object setting up the electric field) are correct EXCEPT:

    A. PE = Vq.

    B. PE = Fr.

    C. PE = Eq.

    D. PE = qEr.

17. A positive charge is moved against (in the opposite direction of) an electric field. The potential energy of this positive charge:

    A. remains the same.

    B. decreases.

    C. increases.

    D. cannot be evaluated from the information given.

18. A negative charge is moved against (in the opposite direction of) an electric field. The potential energy of this negative charge:

    A. stays the same.

    B. increases.

    C. decreases.

    D. cannot be evaluated from the information given.

19. What is the electric potential (V) at point A?

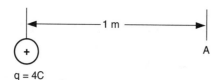

A. +4 volts
B. −4 volts
C. +4k volts
D. −4k volts

20. What is the work done in moving a charge q_1 from A to B?

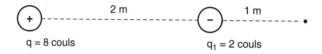

(A) ⟶ (B)

A. −10π joules
B. +10π joules
C. +(8k/3) joules
D. −(8k/3) joules

21. Using Gauss' law of magnetism, which of the following statements is NOT true?

A. The simplest magnetic structure is a dipole.
B. Magnetic flux varies with the charge.
C. Magnetic flux is not related to change in surface area of the magnetic field.
D. Magnetic flux varies with the velocity of the charge.

22. Some of the shortest electromagnetic waves are:

A. microwaves.
B. x-rays.
C. AM-radio waves.
D. FM-radio waves.

ANSWERS AND EXPLANATIONS

1–8. 1-C, 2-A, 3-A, 4-D, 5-B, 6-B, 7-A, 8-C. See text for explanation.

9. A From Coulomb's law, in which f = final and o = original:

$$\frac{F_f}{F_o} = \frac{k\dfrac{q_1 q_2}{r_f^2}\cdot\dfrac{1}{r_f^2}}{k\dfrac{q_1 q_2}{r_o^2}\cdot\dfrac{1}{r_o^2}} = \frac{1}{r_f^2}\cdot\frac{r_o^2}{1} = \frac{r_o^2}{r_f^2} = \frac{r_o^2}{(2r_o)^2} = \frac{r_o^2}{4r_o^2} = \frac{1}{4}$$

$$(r_f = 2r_o)$$

$$\frac{F_f}{F_o} = \frac{1}{4}$$

$$F_f = \frac{1}{4}F_o$$

Or reason from Coulomb's law that force is proportional to the inverse square of distance $(1/r^2)$, which is $(\frac{1}{2})^2 = \frac{1}{4}$ for this case. Hence the force difference:

$$F_o - F_f = F_o - \frac{1}{4}F_o = \frac{3}{4}F_o$$

10. D From Coulomb's law, in which f = final and o = original:

$$q_{1f} = 2q_{1o}; \qquad q_{2f} = 2q_{2o}; \qquad r_f = 2r_o;$$

$$\frac{F_f}{F_o} = \frac{k\dfrac{q_{1f}q_{2f}}{r_f^2}}{k\dfrac{q_{1o}q_{2o}}{r_o^2}} = \frac{q_{1f}q_{2f}}{r_f^2} \cdot \frac{r_o^2}{q_{1o}q_{2o}} = \frac{(2q_{1o})(2q_{2o})}{(2r_o)_2} \cdot \frac{r_o^2}{q_{1o}q_{2o}}$$

$$= \frac{2 \cdot 2 \cdot q_{1o} \cdot q_{2o} \cdot r_o^2}{4 \cdot r_o^2 \cdot q_{1o} \cdot q_{2o}} = 1$$

Reasoning from Coulomb's law shows that force is directly proportional to the product of the charges; the doubling of each charge would increase the force by a factor of $(2)(2) = 4$. Because force is proportional to the inverse square of the separation, the increase in separation decreases the force by $(\frac{1}{2})^2 = \frac{1}{4}$. Multiplying these factors together to get the net change as $(4)(\frac{1}{4}) = 1$ or no change.

11. C From Coulomb's law: $F \propto 1/r^2$. Hence, the force decreases proportionally to the square of the distance.

12. C From Coulomb's law, in which f = final and o = original:

$$q_{1f} = 2q_{1o} \qquad q_{2f} = 3q_{2o}$$

$$\frac{F_f}{F_o} = \frac{k\dfrac{q_{1f}q_{2f}}{r^2}}{k\dfrac{q_{1o}q_{2o}}{r^2}} = \frac{q_{1f}q_{2f}}{q_{1o}q_{2o}} = \frac{(2q_{1o})(3q_{2o})}{(q_{1o})(q_{2o})} = \frac{2 \cdot 3}{1} = 6$$

$$F_f = 6F_o$$

Reasoning from Coulomb's law shows force is directly proportional to the product of the charges. This product is increased $(2)(3) = 6$ times, so the force must also be multiplied with 6.

13. D From Coulomb's law:
$$F = k\left(\frac{q_1 q_2}{r^2}\right) = \frac{k(+2)(-4)}{(2)2} = -2 \, k \, N.$$ Because the sign is negative, the force is attractive.

14. D Solve this problem by using the symmetry of the system, Coulomb's law, and geometry. The forces (vectors) and their components exerted by $q_A(F_A)$ and $q_B(F_B)$ on q_c are:

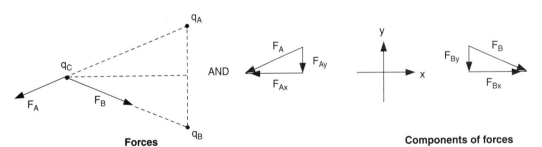

Forces AND **Components of forces**

The x-components (F_{Ax} and F_{Bx}) cancel (because they are equal and opposite by the symmetry of the system) and the y-components sum to a vertically downward force. So, by elimination, the answer is D. Alternatively, apply Coulomb's law:

$$F_A = k\left(\frac{q_A q_c}{r^2}\right) = k\left[\frac{(+2)(+1)}{(2)^2}\right] = \frac{k}{2}$$

$$F_B = k\left(\frac{q_B q_c}{r^2}\right) = k\left[\frac{(-2)(+1)}{(2)^2}\right] = -\frac{k}{2}$$

r = 2 m (meters) is derived by:

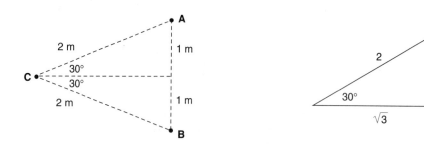

The side opposite the 30° angle is one half the hypotenuse (which must then be 2 m). The x-components still cancel and the y-components are:

$$F_{Ay} = +(\tfrac{1}{2})F_A = -\tfrac{1}{2}\left(\frac{k}{2}\right) = -\frac{k}{4}$$

$$F_{By} = (\tfrac{1}{2})F_B = \tfrac{1}{2}\left(-\frac{k}{2}\right) = -\frac{k}{4}$$

$$F_y = F_{Ay} + F_{By} = -\frac{k}{4} - \frac{k}{4} = -\frac{k}{2}N$$

(minus sign means F_y is directed down the y-axis)

15. C The formula for the electric field (E) is:

$$E = \frac{F}{q_o} = \frac{kq}{r^2}; \text{ hence, } E \propto \frac{1}{r^2}$$

16. C Eq = force generated by E on q.

17. C The direction of the lines of an electric field is the direction a positive charge would move if placed in it. To move a positive charge in the opposite direction requires energy. This energy is stored as the potential energy, which increases. The potential energy of the system may be used to move any charge along the direction of the field lines.

18. C The direction of the field lines of an electric field is the direction a positive charge would move if placed in it. So, a negative charge would normally move in the opposite direction or against the field. When a charge moves in the expected direction in an electric field, the potential energy of the charge system decreases. As an example, the potential energy of a rock decreases as it falls toward earth, because this expected direction makes it move in the gravitational field.

19. C The formula for V is:

$$V = \frac{kq}{r} = k\left(+\frac{4}{1}\right) = +4k \text{ volts}$$

20. C The work done can be calculated by using the following formulations:

$$W = q_1(V_B - V_A) = q_1(PD)$$

$$V_B = k\left(\frac{q}{r_B}\right) = k(+\tfrac{8}{3}) = (+\tfrac{8}{3}) k \text{ volts}$$

$$V_A = k\left(\frac{q}{r_A}\right) = k(+\tfrac{8}{2}) = +4 k \text{ volts}$$

(q is generating the potential for both points A and B)

PD (Potential difference) =

$$V_B - V_A = \left(\frac{8}{3}\right)k - 4k = \frac{(8-12)k}{3} = -\frac{4k}{3} \text{ volts}$$

$$W = q_1(PD) = (-2)\left(-\frac{4k}{3}\right) = \left(+\frac{8}{3}\right)k \text{ joules}$$

The positive sign means that work must be put into (done to) the system.

21–22. **21-C, 22-B.** See text for explanation.

Electric Circuits

Self-Managed Learning Questions

1. What is the difference between + and − charged objects? What makes them different?
2. What is the difference between charge and current in a conductor?
3. Why does charge not accumulate on an insulator and why does current not flow through an insulator?
4. How can a conductor become a capacitor?
5. What is electric induction? How can a charged conductor attract substances without touching them?
6. Is this a valid statement: "All substances are either conductors or dielectrics (insulators)." What makes this claim correct or incorrect? Why?
7. Explain the working of a bimetallic strip flasher (Fig. 7-88). (Hint: Heat is generated when electric charge flows through a resistor.)

The main elements in an electric (DC = direct current) circuit are the electromotive force (emf) source (V) and the resistors (R). The current (I) results from their interaction. These three quantities are interrelated in **Ohm's law** as: V = IR. Capacitors may also be used in electronic circuits.

CURRENT

Current (I) is the amount of charge (Q) that flows past a point in a given amount of time (t):

$$I = \frac{Q}{t} = amperes = \frac{coulombs}{sec}$$

Current is the movement of electrons. The velocity of electrons is slowed by impurities in the conductor and by the thermal motion of atoms. According to Ohm's law, if specific conducting impurities are added to a semiconductor, the resistance of the semiconductor drops. This change results in increased flow of current. A transient current is set up when a capacitor discharges. A continuous current is set up when a source of emf is present to replace the energy lost by moving electrons. The direction of current is taken as the direction in which a positive charge moves, by convention. It is represented on a circuit diagram by arrows. Ammeters are used to measure the flow of current and are symbolized as shown in Figure 7-89.

BATTERIES, ELECTROMOTIVE FORCE, VOLTAGE, TERMINAL POTENTIAL, AND INTERNAL RESISTANCE

Electromotive force (V) maintains a constant potential difference and thereby maintains a continuous current. The emf source replaces energy lost by the moving electrons. Sources of emf are batteries (conversions of chemical energy to electric energy) and generators (conversion of mechanical energy to electric energy). A source of emf is symbolized in a circuit as in Figure 7-90.

The source of emf works on each charge to raise it from a lower potential to a higher potential. Then, as the charge flows around the circuit (naturally from higher to lower

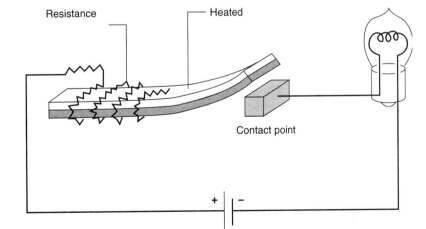

Fig. 7-88. Bimetallic strip flasher.

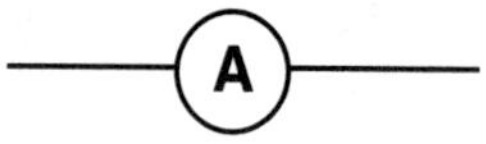

Fig. 7-89.

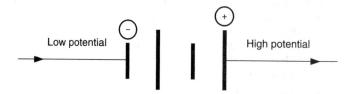

Fig. 7-90. Electromotive force.

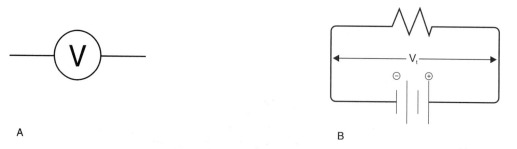

Low potential

High potential

(Arrows show normal current direction)

potential), it loses energy, which is replaced by the emf source again, etc. Therefore, work (energy) must be supplied at the rate energy is lost by the current flowing through the circuit:

Energy supplied = energy lost

Energy is lost whenever a charge (as current) passes through a resistor. A voltmeter is used to measure voltages (potential differences) in circuits and is symbolized as shown in Figure 7-91(A).

The **units of emf** (E) are volts (see previous section concerning electrostatics and electromagnetism). In Fig. 7-91(B), the actual voltage delivered to the external circuit is less than the total voltage, V_T (called the emf of the source), developed by the source because of the internal resistance of the source, which leads to a voltage drop (energy loss). If the internal resistance of the source is r and the current flowing in the circuit is I, then by Ohm's law:

$$V_t = V_T - Ir.$$

Another way of stating this is the equation

$$V_T = I(r + R)$$

where R is the resistance of the external circuit. The emf source also has resistance and accounts for a (usually small) voltage drop.

Normally, a charge gains energy as it flows through a source of emf. But when two sources of emf are connected in opposition (positive pole to positive pole), the charge flows from the higher emf source to the lower emf source. In this instance, it loses energy when passing through the smaller emf because it passes in the opposite direction to normal. With more than one source of emf in a circuit, the total emf is the sum of these by taking into account the differences in polarity (i.e., reversed emf's are negative):

$$V_t \text{ (total)} = \sum V_{ti}, i = 1, 2, \ldots.$$

Fig. 7-91.   A

B

V_t

RESISTANCE, OHM'S LAW, SERIES AND PARALLEL CIRCUITS, AND RESISTIVITY

The **resistivity** (ρ) of a material is a property that inherently reflects the opposition to the flow of electrons in the material. In a wire, resistance varies directly with resistivity and length, and varies inversely with cross-sectional area (diameter). The resistance of a material increases with increasing temperature because the increasing thermal motions of atoms impedes the flow of electrons. The unit of resistance of a material, symbolized by Ω, is the ohm. The following are important relations:

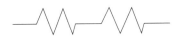

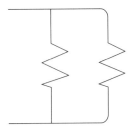

Fig. 7-92.   Series   Parallel

Ω increases as the length of a conductor increases
Ω increases as temperature increases
Ω decreases as cross-sectional area increases

Power (P) is defined as the rate at which work is done. If q coulombs pass through a conductor which has across it a potential difference V, then the work done in moving these charges is Vq. If this occurs over time t, then the work per unit of time is

$$P = \frac{Vq}{t} = VI$$

because $I = q/t$.
Since $V = IR$ this also yields:

$$P = (IR)I = I^2R$$

and

$$P = V\left(\frac{V}{R}\right) = \frac{V^2}{R}.$$

A variable resistance (as with a rheostat) is symbolized as shown in Figure 7-93.

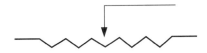

Fig. 7-93.

Total resistance (R) in a series circuit is the sum of the resistances:

$$R = R_1 + R_2 + R_3 + \ldots$$

Total resistance in a parallel circuit is:

$$\frac{1}{R} = \frac{1}{R_1} + \frac{1}{R_2} + \frac{1}{R_3} + \ldots$$

Circuit elements may be in series, in parallel, or in combinations of both. Two components are in series when they have only one point in common; that is, the current traveling from one of them back to the emf source must pass through the other. In a complete series circuit, or for individual series loops of a larger mixed circuit, the current (I) is the same over each component and the total voltage (V_T is the sum of all the emf sources) is the sum of voltages across each resistor (including the internal resistances of emf sources). Two components are in parallel when they are connected to two common points in the circuit; that is, the current traveling from one such element back to the source of emf (assume current started at source of emf) need not pass through the second component because there is an alternate path. In a parallel circuit, the total current is the sum of currents for each path (i.e., each path has a different current), and the voltage is equal for all paths and thus equals V_T. Circuits can be simplified into subunits that are either series or parallel, and the rules just described are applied to each subunit.

CAPACITOR AND DIELECTRICS

Capacitance (C) is an inherent property of two adjacent conductors and is formulated as:

$$C = \frac{\text{charge}}{\text{electric potential}} = \frac{Q}{V} = \text{farad} = \frac{\text{coulomb}}{\text{volt}}$$

Capacitance is a measure of the ratio of the charge on a capacitor to the voltage difference between the conductors. One conductor has charge $+Q$ and the other has $-Q$. The amount of charge that can be stored is determined by the size, shape, and surroundings of the conductor. A smaller conductor usually has a smaller capacitance. Capacitance depends directly on the area of the conductors and inversely as the separation distance. The higher the dielectric strength of the medium between the conductors, the greater the capacitance.

A **capacitor** is two or more conductors with opposite but equal charges placed near each other. A common example is the parallel plate capacitor. The formulas of importance for capacitors are as follows:

1. $C = Q/V$
   V = potential difference between the plates
2. $V = Ed$
   E = electric field strength
   d = distance between the plates
3. C is directly proportional to the area of the plates
   C is inversely proportional to the distance between the plates
   i.e., $C_o = \epsilon_o A/d$ for air and vacuum (as the medium) between the plates

The **energy associated with each charged capacitor** is:

$$V_{avg} = \tfrac{1}{2} V$$

$$\text{Potential Energy (PE)} = W = (\tfrac{1}{2}V)(Q) = \tfrac{1}{2} QV = \tfrac{1}{2}(CV)(V)$$

$$= \tfrac{1}{2}CV^2 = \tfrac{1}{2}Q\left(\frac{Q}{C}\right) = \frac{\tfrac{1}{2}Q^2}{C}$$

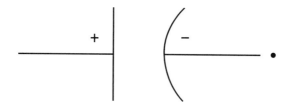

Fig. 7-94.

The symbol for a capacitor is shown in Figure 7-94.

When a voltage V is applied to a capacitor with capacitance C, the charge on the two plates builds up over a finite period of time determined by the characteristics of the capacitor. The maximal charge is $Q_{max} = VC$, and the time it takes to reach this charge is related to a the **capacitive time constant** (τ = seconds) of the capacitor. The time rate of change of the charge buildup satisfies:

1. The capacitor takes approximately 5τ to reach full charge or discharge fully
2. In one τ the capacitor is about 63% charged
3. The capacitor will discharge down to 37% of Q_{max} in τ seconds.

If an alternating voltage is applied to a capacitor, the plates are alternately charged either positive or negative, depending on the nature of the alternating applied voltage. In this situation a current flows even though no transfer of charge occurs between the plates of the capacitor.

In a series circuit consisting of a resistor R and a capacitor C, because

$$C = \frac{Q}{V_c} \Rightarrow V_c = \frac{Q}{C},$$

the total voltage drop will be

$$V_t = \text{drop across resistor} + \text{drop across capacitor} = IR + \frac{Q}{C}.$$

Concept of Capacitance

The net charge on the capacitor as a whole is zero and "the charge on a capacitor" is understood to mean the charge on either conductor, without regard to sign. From the definition, note that capacitance is expressed in coulombs per volt. Because 1 volt is equivalent to 1 joule per coulomb, 1 coulomb per volt is equivalent to 1 coul²/joule. A capacitance of 1 coulomb per volt is called 1 farad (for Faraday). The capacitance of a capacitor is 1 farad if 1 coulomb is transferred from one conductor to the other, per volt of potential difference between the conductors.

Capacitors find many applications in electric circuits. A capacitor is used to eliminate sparking when a circuit containing inductance is suddenly opened. The ignition system of the automobile engine contains a capacitor for this purpose. Capacitors are used in radio circuits for tuning, and for "smoothing" the rectified current delivered by the power supply. The efficiency of alternating current power transmissions can often be increased by the use of large capacitors.

Dielectric Coefficient

For most capacitors, a solid, nonconducting material or dielectric is used between their plates. A common type is the paper and foil capacitor, in which strips of metal foil form the plates and a sheet of paper impregnated with wax is dielectric. By rolling up such a capacitor, a capacitance of several microfarads can be obtained in a relatively small volume. The "Leyden jar," constructed by cementing metal foil over a portion of the inside and outside surfaces of a glass jar, is essentially a parallel-plate capacitor, with the glass forming the dielectric.

Electrolytic capacitors have as their dielectric an extremely thin layer of nonconducting oxide between a metal plate and a conducting solution. Because of the small thickness of the dielectric, electrolytic capacitors of relatively small dimensions may have a capacitance on the order of 50 μF. Placing a dielectric material between the plates of a capacitor can alter the capacitance significantly. The **dielectric constant** (K) of a material is defined as the ratio

$$K = \frac{C}{C_0}$$

where C is the capacitance with the material between the plates and C_0 is the capacitance with air between the plates. With similar interpretation of the subscript the dielectric constant can also be expressed as:

$$K = \frac{V}{V_0} = \frac{E}{E_0}.$$

The **dielectric substances** set up an opposing electric field to that of the capacitor, which decreases the net electric field and allows the capacitance of the capacitor to increase (C = Q/Ed). The molecules of the dielectric are dipoles that line up in the electric field (Figs. 7-95 and 7-96).

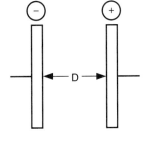

Fig. 7-95. Capacitor without dielectric. E = electric field, D = dielectric, C = capacitor, N = net, C = total capacitance.

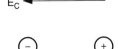

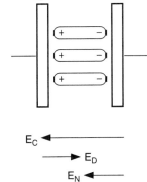

Fig. 7-96. Capacitor with dielectric. E = electric field, D = dielectric, C = capacitor, N = net, C = total capacitance.

ELECTRIC POWER

Power is work per unit time. When a current (I) is in a circuit, resulting from voltage (V), the formula for the electric power delivered to the circuit is P = IV. Power transmission is affected only by the vector component of the voltage in the direction of the flow of the current.

ALTERNATING ELECTRIC CURRENTS

Alternating current (AC) electricity constitutes 99% of that used in the United States. It is made by converting mechanical energy to electric energy. An armature, which is a loop of wire, is rotated in a magnetic field using mechanical energy. A current is induced (see discussion of inductance) in the wire of the armature. This current changes direction because the direction of the velocity of the loop and the magnetic field changes. Slip rings are fused to each end of the wire loop and rotate with it. Because the direction of the current alternates, the slip rings alternate in conducting the current away from the loop (hence AC). Graphite brushes on the slip rings brush against conducting materials, which carry away from the generator AC that looks like a sine wave (Fig. 7-97).

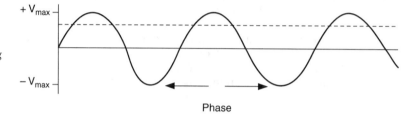

Fig. 7-97. EMF or alternating voltage curve.

Note that the maximum voltages (V) are not the same as V_{eff} (effective voltage, or root-mean square voltage). Similarly, the maximum current is not the effective (root-mean square) current delivered (I_{eff}):

$$V_{eff} = 0.707 \, V_{max}$$

$$I_{eff} = 0.707 \, I_{max}$$

One effective volt of AC will develop one effective ampere of current through a resistance of one ohm. The frequency of alternation of the cycle is also important in determining the V and I values. A typical frequency is 60 cycles/second. Note: $\omega = 2\pi f$ = angular frequency. In a capacitive circuit, the capacitive reactance is defined as $X_c = 1/(\omega C)$; in an inductive circuit, the inductive reactance is defined as $X_L = \omega L$.

The combined effect of a resistance and an inductive reactance is apparent resistance, or **impedance** (usually represented by the letter Z). Thus, in an AC circuit, we can write Ohm's law as:

$$I \text{ (amperes)} = \frac{V \text{(volts)}}{Z \text{(Ohms)}}$$

Impedance can be represented vectorially as the hypotenuse of the right triangle, the

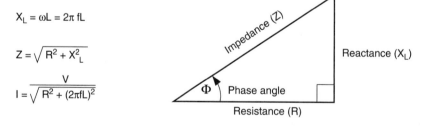

Fig. 7-98. Vector triangle relating resistance, reactance, and impedance.

$$X_L = \omega L = 2\pi \, fL$$

$$Z = \sqrt{R^2 + X_L^2}$$

$$I = \frac{V}{\sqrt{R^2 + (2\pi fL)^2}}$$

two sides of which are the ohmic resistance and the reactance (Fig. 7-98). The angle ϕ between R and Z is called the phase angle and is equal to the lag of the current behind the voltage, in degrees.

APPLIED CONCEPTS

1. Evaluate the working of an x-ray tube and determine what, if any, errors should be avoided in acquiring a radiograph of a patient.
2. Compare and contrast a cathode ray tube (CRT) from a television tube. (Hint: electric versus magnetic.)
3. Compare the structure and the working of an electrolytic cell, Galvanic cell, and concentration cell used in the human physiology laboratory. List the advantages

and disadvantages of each cell to determine fluid and electrolyte concentrations in the human body.

4. Give applications and major limitations of Ohm's law and Kirchhoff's laws as they apply to cell membranes.

5. Understand the application of resistors in parallel or series to blood vessels in the human body (arteries and veins in series and in parallel). Viscosity and fluid resistance follow similar laws as current flow in a conductor. Apply Nernst equation to concentration cells and explain the limitations of the equation. Read more on how the Nernst equation is applicable to an electric eel.

ELECTRIC CIRCUITS: REVIEW QUESTIONS

1. The following graph represents which type of current(s)?

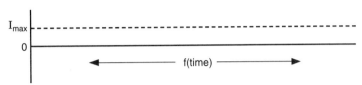

 A. AC only
 B. DC only
 C. AC or DC
 D. Neither AC nor DC

2. Ohm's law is represented by which of the following formulas (V = potential difference, I = current, R = resistance, C = capacitance, Q = charge, L = inductance, t = time)?

 A. $C = Q/V$
 B. $L = -\Delta V/\Delta I/\Delta t)$
 C. $V = IR$
 D. $V = QLt$

3. Which of the following describes the actual voltage output of an electromotive source relative to the expected voltage of the source?

 A. May be equal to, less than, or greater than
 B. Always equal to
 C. Always greater than
 D. Always less than

4. All of the following statements concerning electromotive force (emf) are correct EXCEPT:

 A. units are microfarads.
 B. maintains constant potential differences in a circuit.
 C. replaces energy lost by the moving electrons in a circuit.
 D. sources include both batteries and generators.

5. Normally, a charge gains energy as it moves through a source of emf, but it can lose energy if the emf source:

 A. has an internal resistance.
 B. has a reversed polarity.
 C. is a generator.
 D. is of low voltage.

6. Resistance, as used in electricity, is:

 A. the opposition to flow of electrons in a substance.
 B. the opposition to the generation of emf.
 C. the location of storage of energy of electrons.
 D. in the units of farads.

7. Resistance (electric) has a fixed value for a given material and depends on all of the following factors EXCEPT:

 A. size of a conductor.
 B. current in a conductor.
 C. shape of a conductor.
 D. temperature.

8. To set up a continuous, as opposed to a transient, current in a circuit, it is possible to use a:

A. source of emf.
B. capacitor.
C. capacitor and resistor.
D. capacitor and inductor.

9. An increase in all of the following factors is associated with increased capacitance of a conductor EXCEPT:

A. inducibility.
B. size.
C. separation.
D. dielectric strength of the medium.

10. A capacitor will charge up to a certain point and then will cause the current to stop in which of the following circuits?

A. DC
B. AC
C. Both DC and AC
D. Neither DC nor AC

11. In an AC circuit, a capacitor is placed in series with a resistor. The voltage of the AC generator (neglecting internal resistance) is:

A. (capacitor voltage)(resistor voltage).
B. voltage across the capacitor minus voltage across the resistor.
C. voltage across the resistor minus voltage across the capacitor.
D. voltage across the resistor plus voltage across the capacitor.

12. If total resistance is 9 ohms and total voltage is 3 volts, what is the current?

A. $\frac{1}{27}$ ampere
B. $\frac{1}{3}$ ampere
C. 3 amperes
D. 27 amperes

13. A battery has a voltage of 6V marked on it and an internal resistance of 0.5 ohm. If it is placed in the following circuit, what is the actual voltage it is producing in that circuit?

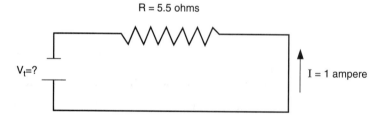

R = 5.5 ohms

V_t=?

I = 1 ampere

A. 10 volts
B. 8.5 volts
C. 5.5 volts
D. 5 volts

14. Calculate the internal resistance of the 20-volt battery in the following circuit:

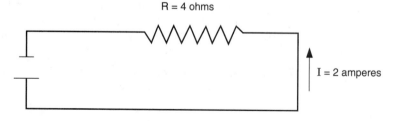

R = 4 ohms

I = 2 amperes

A. 16 ohms
B. 10 ohms

C. 6 ohms

D. 2 ohms

15. All of the following are formulations of power (P) in a circuit with an emf (V) source and a resistor (R) with a current (I), EXCEPT:

    A. $P = VI$.

    B. $P = IR/V$.

    C. $P = I^2R$.

    D. $P = V^2/R$.

16. A DC circuit has a current of 2 amperes and a resistance of 4 ohms. What is the DC power delivered to the resistance?

    A. 16 watts $P = I^2R$

    B. 8 watts

    C. 2 watts

    D. ½ watt

17. If the cross-sectional area of a conductor is quadrupled ($\times 4$), the resistance:

    A. increases 16 times.

    B. increases 4 times.

    C. decreases to ¼.

    D. decreases to ¹⁄₁₆.

18. In a DC circuit with a voltage of 10 volts, a resistance of 10 ohms, and a current passing for 10 seconds, what is the maximum number of joules of heat that could be produced?

    A. 100 $P = V^2/R$

    B. 1000 $\frac{100}{10} = 10$

    C. 1   (power)(time) = joules

    D. 10

19. What is the voltage (V) of the following battery (neglect internal resistance of battery)?

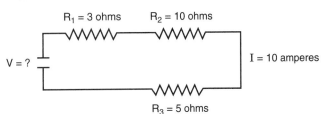

    A. 180

    B. 18

    C. 1.8

    D. 0.55

20. A current of 8 amperes will deliver what charge in 4 seconds?

    A. 2 statcoulombs $I = \dfrac{q}{t}$

    B. 2 coulombs

    C. 32 statcoulombs

    D. 32 coulombs

21. A conductor attains maximal charge when 40 coulombs is placed on it at a voltage of 10 volts. What is its capacitance?

    A. 4000 farads $C = \dfrac{q}{v} = \dfrac{40}{10} = 4$

    B. 400 farads

    C. 0.25 farads

    D. 4 farads

22. The capacitance of a parallel plate capacitor in air is 20 farads. What is the capacitance when this capacitor is placed in a medium with a dielectric constant equal to 5?

    A. 20 farads   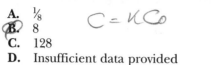 $C = K C_0$
    B. 4 farads
    C. 400 farads
    D. 100 farads

23. In air, a parallel plate capacitor has a capacitance of 4 farads. In medium A, the capacitance is 32 farads. What is the dielectric constant of medium A?

    A. ⅛ $C = KC_0$ $\dfrac{32}{4}$
    B. 8
    C. 128
    D. Insufficient data provided

ANSWERS AND EXPLANATIONS

1–11. 1-B, 2-C, 3-D, 4-A, 5-B, 6-A, 7-B, 8-A, 9-A, 10-A, 11-D. See text for explanation.

12. B From Ohm's law:

$$V = IR$$

$$I = \frac{V}{R} = \frac{3 \text{ volts}}{9 \text{ ohms}} = \frac{1}{3} \text{ amp}$$

13. C The terminal voltage (V_t) of an emf source is determined by taking into account the internal resistance:

$$r = 0.5 \text{ ohms } V_t = V_T - Ir = IR$$

$$R = 5.5 \text{ ohms } V_T = I(R + r)$$

$$V_T = 6 \text{ volts } 6 = I(5.5 + 0.5)$$

$$I = 1 \text{ amp}$$

Hence, $V_t = V_T - Ir = 6 - 1(0.5) = 5.5$ volts

14. C See text for an explanation of the formula:

$$V_T = 20 \text{ volts, } r = ?, V_T = I(R + r)$$

$$R = 4 \text{ ohms, } 20 = 2(4 + r)$$

$$I = 2 \text{ amps, } 20 - 2r = 8$$

$$r = 6 \text{ ohms}$$

15. B Try to remember how to convert it to the others using Ohm's law.

16. A The appropriate formula is:

$$P = I^2 R = (2)^2(4) = 16 \text{ watts}$$

The units are determined as follows:

$$P = (\text{amperes})^2(\text{ohms}) = (\text{amps})^2\left(\frac{\text{volts}}{\text{amps}}\right) = (\text{amps})(\text{volts})$$

$$= \left(\frac{\text{coulomb}}{\text{sec}}\right)\text{volts} = \text{volt} \cdot \frac{\text{coulomb}}{\text{sec}} = \frac{\text{joules}}{\text{sec}} = \text{watts}$$

Remember: joule = volt · coulomb.

17. C Resistance (R) $\propto$ 1/Area(A). If A increases by a factor of 4, the R decreases to one quarter of the original value, or:

$$\frac{R_2}{R_1} = \frac{\left(\frac{\rho L}{A_2}\right)}{\left(\frac{\rho L}{A_1}\right)} = \frac{A_1}{A_2} = \frac{A_1}{4A_1} = \frac{1}{4} \Rightarrow R_2 = \frac{1}{4} R_1$$

18. A $P = \dfrac{V^2}{R}$ (see text)

$$P = \dfrac{(10)^2}{10} = 10 \text{ watts}$$

(Power)(time) = joules = (10)(10) = 100 joules

19. A This battery represents a series circuit because the current (I) must pass through each resistor (R) before returning to the voltage source (V). The total resistance (RT):

$$R_T = R_1 + R_2 + R_3 = 3 + 10 + 5 = 18 \text{ ohms}$$

Calculate V using Ohm's law: V = IR = (10 amps)(18 ohms) = 180 volts

20. D $I = \dfrac{q}{t}$

$$q = (I)(t) = (8 \text{ amps})(4 \text{ seconds}) = 32 \text{ coulombs}$$

21. D C = q/V = 40 coulombs/10 volts = 4 farads

22. D $C = K C_o$, C_o = capacitance of air

$$C = (5)(20) = 100 \text{ farads}$$

23. B C = K Co

$$K = \dfrac{C}{Co} = \dfrac{32}{4} = 8$$

Nuclear and Atomic Structure

An atom is made of a **nucleus** containing protons (mass = 1 a.m.u., charge +1) and neutrons (mass = 1 a.m.u., charge = 0). The **atomic number** (Z) is the number of protons in the nucleus of an atom. An **element** is a group of atoms with the same Z. The **mass number** (A) is the sum of protons and neutrons in a given atom (not element!). Note that it is the number of protons that distinguishes one element from another, and it is the electron configuration (see section concerning the electronic structure of the atom) of a given element that determines its chemical reactivity.

Coulomb repulsive forces (between protons) in the nuclei are overcome by **nuclear forces**. The nuclear force is a nonelectric type of force that binds nuclei together and is equal for protons and neutrons. The **nuclear binding energy** (E_b) is a result of the Coulomb and nuclear binding forces. Einstein derived the relation between energy and mass changes associated with nuclear reactions:

$$\Delta E = \Delta mc^2 = \text{ergs, if } m = \text{grams and } c = \dfrac{cm}{sec}$$

ΔE = energy released or absorbed

Δm = mass lost (**mass deficit**) or gained, respectively

c = speed of light = 3.0×10^{10} cm/sec

Conversions:

$$1 \text{ gram} = 9 \times 10^{20} \text{ ergs}$$

$$1 \text{ amu (atomic mass unit)} = 931.4 \text{ MeV}$$

$$1 \text{ amu} = \tfrac{1}{12} \text{ the mass of } C_6^{12}$$

The preceding is a statement of the **law of conservation of mass and energy**. The value of E_b depends on the mass number (A) as shown in Figure 7-99. Note that the peak

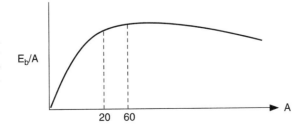

Fig. 7-99. Binding energy diagram. E_b/A = binding energy per nucleon, which is the energy released by the formation of a given nucleus.

E_b/A is at $A = 60$. Also, the E_b/A is relatively constant after $A = 20$. **Fission** is when a nucleus splits into smaller nuclei. **Fusion** is when small nuclei combine to form a larger nucleus. Energy is released from a nuclear reaction (see Fig. 7-99) when nuclei with mass number $>> 60$ undergo fission or nuclei $<< 60$ undergo fusion.

NEUTRONS, PROTONS, AND ISOTOPES

Not all combinations of protons and neutrons are equally likely or stable. The **most stable nuclei** are those with an even number of protons and an even number of neutrons. The **least stable nuclei** are those with an odd number of protons and an odd number of neutrons. Also, as the atomic number (Z) increases, more neutrons (N) are needed for the nuclei to be stable (Fig. 7-100). Up to $Z = 20$ (calcium), the protons equal the neutrons. After this point, the number of neutrons exceeds that of protons. If an atom is in region 1 (see Fig. 7-100), it has too many protons or too few neutrons and must decrease its protons or increase its neutrons to become stable. The reverse is true for region 2 (see Fig. 7-100). Also, all nuclei after $Z = 84$ (polonium) are unstable.

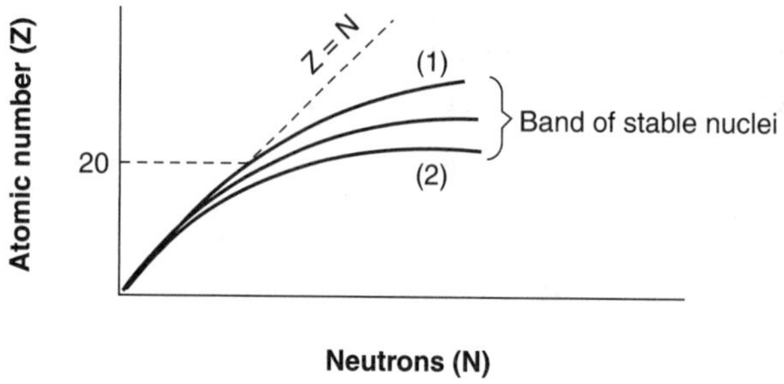

Fig. 7-100. Stability of atoms.

Isotopes are atoms of the same element with different A, i.e., they have the same number of protons but different numbers of neutrons. The **atomic weight** is the weighted average of all naturally occurring isotopes of an element.

RADIOACTIVE DECAY AND HALF-LIFE

Unstable nuclei can become stable nuclei by fission (splitting) to smaller nuclei or by absorbing or emitting small particles. Spontaneous fission is rare. **Spontaneous radioactivity** (emitting particles) is common. Common particles are (1) **alpha (α) particle**: $_2He^4$ (helium nucleus); (2) **beta (β) particle**: 1e (an electron); (3) a **positron** $+1e$; (4) gamma (γ) ray—no mass, just energy; and (5) **orbital electron capture**—nucleus takes electrons from K shell and converts a proton to a neutron. In the event of a flux of particles, such as neutrons ($_0^1n$), the nucleus can absorb these also.

Nuclear reactions involve changes in nuclear composition. An example of a nuclear reaction and the terminology follows:

$$_{92}^{238}U + _1^2H \rightarrow _{93}^{238}Np + 2_0^1n$$

Note: $238 \leftarrow$ mass number $\rightarrow ^{238}U$

$92 \leftarrow$ atomic number $\rightarrow _{92}U$

the sum of the lower (higher) numbers on one side of the equation equals the sum of the lower (higher) numbers on the other side. Writing this reaction another way:

$$_{92}^{238}U \,(_1^2H, 2_0^1n)\, _{93}^{238}Np$$

Each type of radioactive atom (radioisotope) is characterized by its own specific fractional decay rate. Activity (A) is directly proportional to the number of atoms available for decay (N). The rate of decay, $\Delta N/\Delta t$, can be expressed as:

$$A = \frac{\Delta N}{\Delta t} = -\lambda N$$

in which A is the activity in nuclear disintegrations per unit time and λ is a proportional factor called the decay constant (a specific constant for each radioisotope). The minus ($-$) sign is used to indicate that the total number of radioactive atoms is decreasing with time. Integrating the preceding equation yields:

$$A = N_0 e^{-\lambda t}$$

in which N_0 is the number of atoms present at $t = 0$, and e is the base of the natural logarithm.

To compare relative strengths of radioactivity, the basic unit of activity, the curie (Ci), is used. The curie equals 3.7×10^{10} disintegrating atoms per second (dps). A millicurie (mCi) is therefore 3.7×10^7 dps, a microcurie (μCi) is 3.7×10^4 dps. Because each radioisotope has a specific decay constant, a useful way of comparing relative isotope activity is the **half-life**, which represents the time required for the radioactivity to decrease to one-half of its initial value or, $T\frac{1}{2} = 0.693/\lambda$. Note: time can be expressed in any unit (seconds, minutes, hours, days, years).

The amount left after n half-lives is:

$$\text{Amount left} = (\tfrac{1}{2})^n A$$

$$A = \text{beginning activity}$$

$$n = \text{number of half lives} = \frac{\text{elapsed time}}{T\frac{1}{2}}$$

Or, the amount that has disappeared can be calculated using λ from the preceding equation:

$$\text{Amount decayed} = \Delta A = (\lambda)(\Delta t)(A)$$

$$\lambda = \text{decay constant}$$

$$\Delta t = \text{elapsed time}$$

$$A = \text{beginning activity}$$

ENERGY LEVELS FOR ELECTRONS

The energy that an atom contains is not continuous over the whole range of possible energies. Rather, electrons in an atom may contain only discrete energies and occupy certain orbits. Electrons of each atom are restricted to these discrete energy levels. These levels have an energy below zero, which means energy is released when an electron moves from infinity into these energy levels. Figure 7-101 illustrates a representative set of energy levels of an electron in an atom. If there is one electron in this atom, its **ground state** will be in the n = 1, or lowest energy level available. Any other energy level, such as n = 2 or n = 3, is considered an **excited state** for that electron. The difference in energies (E) between the levels gives the energy and, hence, frequency (f) of light necessary to cause the excitation (see Fig. 7-101, absorption, electron A):

$$E_3 - E_1 = hf$$

in which E_1 = energy level one, E_3 = energy level three, h = Planck's constant, and f = frequency of light absorbed.

If light is passed through a substance (e.g., gas), certain wavelengths (because $\lambda = c/f$, c = speed of light, λ = wavelength) will be absorbed, corresponding to the energy

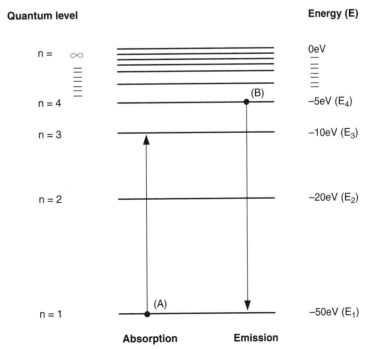

Fig. 7-101. Absorption and emission spectra.

needed for the electron transitions. An **absorption spectrum** will result that has dark lines against a light background. Multiple lines result because of possible transitions from all quantum levels occupied by electrons to any unoccupied levels (e.g., n = 1 to n = 2, n = 3, etc., n = 2 to n = 3, n = 4, etc.).

An **emission spectrum** results when an electron is excited to a higher level by another particle or by an electric discharge, for example. Then, as the electron falls from the excited state to lower states, light is emitted that has wavelength (frequency) corresponding to the energy differences between the levels. As an example (see Fig. 7-101, emission, electron B):

$$E_1 - E_4 = hf$$

The resulting spectrum will have light lines against a dark background.

The absorption and emission spectra should have the same number of lines but often they do not. In the absorption spectrum, there is rapid radiation of the absorbed light in all directions, and transitions are generally from the ground state initially. These factors result in fewer lines in the absorption than in the emission spectrum.

FLUORESCENCE

Fluorescence is an emission process that occurs after light absorption excites electrons to higher electronic and vibrational levels. The electrons spontaneously lose excited vibrational energy to the electronic level and then emit light as they fall to the ground vibrational and electronic states. Certain molecular types possess this property, e.g., some amino acids (tryptophan). The fluorescence process is depicted in Figure 7-102.

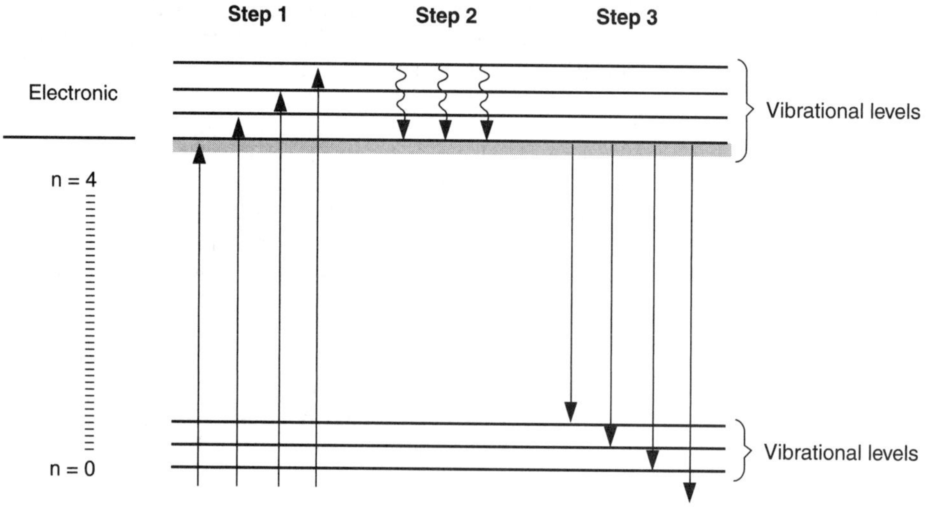

Fig. 7-102. Fluorescence emission. Step 1: absorption of light; step 2: spontaneous deactivation of vibrational levels to zero vibrational level for electronic state; step 3: fluorescence with light emission (longer wavelength than absorption).

APPLIED CONCEPTS

1. Explore the design, maintenance, and working of a clinic located inside a nuclear reactor plant. Explain risks of opening a clinic in such surroundings.
2. Review the working of a Geiger counter and what sources of error are possible. Do Geiger counters detect photons?
3. Why is NaI used in a scintillation counter? How does a scintillation counter differ from a Geiger counter?
4. What is "rad" in nuclear medicine? Is dosimetry a risky branch of science? Why or why not?
5. What genetic defects are caused by long-term exposure to low-level radiation?
6. What are the main components of an Anger Gamma-Scintillation camera? What are the sources of error in such a camera?

NUCLEAR AND ATOMIC STRUCTURE: REVIEW QUESTIONS

1. A proton is _____ charged and has a mass of _____ amu(s).

    A. positively, 1
    B. negatively, $\frac{1}{1845}$
    C. neutral, 1
    D. None of the above

2. The sum of protons and neutrons in a nucleus is called the:

    A. electron number.
    B. atomic number.

C. atomic weight.

D. mass number.

3. Isotopes have the _____ atomic numbers and _____ mass numbers.

   A. same, same

   B. same, different

   C. different, same

   D. different, different

4. The particles that distinguish one element from another are the:

   A. neutrons.

   B. protons.

   C. electrons.

   D. mesons.

5. The subnuclear particle that has mass and is neutral is called the:

   A. neutron.

   B. proton.

   C. neutrino.

   D. meson.

6. Which particle has no mass?

   A. Neutron

   B. Meson

   C. Neutrino

   D. Electron

7. The nuclear binding energy of nuclei depends on:

   A. coulomb forces.

   B. nuclear forces.

   C. both forces.

   D. neither force.

8. If ΔE = the energy change, Δm = mass change, and c = the speed of light, the correct relation for describing the conversion of mass and energy is:

   A. $\Delta E = \Delta m/c$.

   B. $\Delta E = c^2/\Delta m$.

   C. $\Delta E = \Delta mc$.

   D. $\Delta E = \Delta mc^2$.

9. Which of the following statements is correct concerning binding energy (E_b)?

   A. Binding energy depends on protons only.

   B. Binding is relatively constant at all mass numbers.

   C. The peak in binding energy per nucleon is at mass number = 60.

   D. None of the above.

10. Which of the following particles is emitted by nuclei in spontaneous radioactivity?

    A. α-particle

    B. β-particle

    C. γ-ray

    D. All of the above

11. The particle composed of two protons and two neutrons is the:

    A. γ-ray.

    B. α-particle.

    C. neutrino.

    D. positron.

12. Which of the following statements describes the rate of radioactive decay relative to the amount of radioactive atoms present?

    A. It is independent of the radioactive atoms.

    B. It is inversely proportional.

    C. It varies unpredictably, depending on the amount of atoms.

    D. It is directly proportional.

13. The radioactive decay constant is:

    A. the fraction of radioactive atoms that decay in a given amount of time.
    B. the number of radioactive atoms that decay in one half-life.
    C. not related to the half-life.
    D. none of the above.

14. The atomic number is the number of _____ contained in the nucleus.

    A. neutrons
    B. electrons
    C. protons
    D. positrons

15. The atomic weight of an element is:

    A. the weighted average of naturally occurring isotopes.
    B. the sum of protons and neutrons.
    C. twice the number of protons.
    D. none of the above.

16. Carbon has an atomic number (Z) of 6. One of its isotopes has a mass number (A) of 13. The number of neutrons in this isotope is:

    A. 6.
    B. 7.
    C. 13.
    D. 19.

17. An isotope of boron has 5 protons and 6 neutrons. What is the atomic number (Z) of boron?

    A. 11
    B. 10
    C. 6
    D. 5

18. Suppose the natural abundance of the isotopes of beryllium (atomic number = 4) is 90% of mass number = 8; 10% of mass number = 9. The atomic weight (AW) is:

    A. 9.00.
    B. 8.50.
    C. 8.10.
    D. 8.00.

19. An atom has an atomic number (Z) = 18 and a mass number (A) = 38. Letting P = number of protons and N = number neutrons, which of the following atoms is an isotope of this atom?

    A. P = 18, N = 20
    B. P = 20, N = 19
    C. P = 19, N = 18
    D. None of the above

20. A nuclear reaction proceeds with a mass deficit (mass loss) of 5×10^{-5} g. What is the amount of energy released?

    A. 1.5×10^{6} erg $E = mc^2$
    B. 4.5×10^{16} erg
    C. 9.0×10^{20} erg
    D. None of the above

21. A radioactive substance has a half-life ($T\frac{1}{2}$) of 10 seconds. What is the decay constant (λ)?

    A. 1.4 sec^{-1} $\lambda = .693/T\frac{1}{2}$
    B. 0.069 sec^{-1}
    C. 6.9 sec^{-1}
    D. None of the above

22. How much of a substance with a half-life of 5 days is left after 20 days if 10 mCi was present initially?

A. 2.50 mCi
B. 2 mCi
C. ⅝ mCi
D. None of the above

23. How much of 5 mCi of radioactive substance with a half-life of 10 seconds has decayed in 2 seconds?

    A. 1.38 mCi
    B. 1.0 mCi
    C. 0.69 mCi
    D. None of the above

24. What is the missing particle in the following reaction?

$$^{59}_{27}\text{Co} + ? \rightarrow ^{60}_{27}\text{Co}$$

    A. Proton
    B. Electron
    C. Neutron
    D. None of the above

25. What is the missing particle in the following reaction?

$$^{238}_{92}\text{U} + ? \rightarrow ^{239}_{94}\text{Pu} + 3\text{ n}$$

    A. β-particle
    B. Proton
    C. γ-ray
    D. None of the above

26. Determine the amount of phosphorus left after 4 weeks if initially given 100 mCi of $^{32}_{15}\text{P}$ (half-life = 14 days).

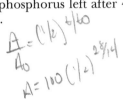

    A. 50 mCi
    B. 37.5 mCi
    C. 25 mCi
    D. 12.5 mCi

27. The half-life of a substance called JUNKIUM is 11.5 hours. How much time (in hours) will it take to lose 25% of its original starting mass?

    A. 2.88
    B. 46
    C. 5.75
    D. 4.77

ANSWERS AND EXPLANATIONS

1–15. 1-A, 2-D, 3-B, 4-B, 5-A, 6-C, 7-C, 8-D, 9-C, 10-D, 11-B, 12-D, 13-A, 14-C, 15-A. See text for explanation.

16. **B**   A = protons (P) + neutrons (N)

    13 = 6 + N (Z = P)

    7 = N

17. **D**   Z is the number of protons in an atom.

18. **C**   To determine the atomic weight, which is the weighted average of the naturally occurring isotopes, multiply the percent abundance (as a decimal) of each isotope by the mass number of that isotope and add:

    AW = (0.90)(8) + (0.10)(9) = 7.2 + 0.9 = 8.1

19. **A**   Z = the number of protons, and this number must be the same because isotopes are of the same element.

20. **B** $\Delta E = \Delta mc^2 = (5 \times 10^{-5}\text{ g}) \, 3 \times 10^{10}\text{ cm/sec}$

    $= (5 \times 10^{-5})(9 \times 10^{20}) = 45 \times 10^{15} = 4.5 \times 10^{16}\text{ ergs}$

21. **B** $\lambda = 0.693/T_{1/2} = 0.693/10\text{ sec} = 0.0693\text{ sec}^{-1}$

22. C Amount decayed $= (\frac{1}{2})^n A = \left(\frac{1}{2}\right)^{20/5}(10) = (\frac{1}{2})^4(10)$

$$= \left(\frac{1}{16}\right)(10) = \frac{10}{16}$$

$$= \frac{5}{8} \text{ mCi}$$

23. C Use $T\frac{1}{2}$ or λ to find the amount left. In this problem, it is easier to use λ:

$$\lambda = \frac{0.693}{T\frac{1}{2}} = \frac{0.693}{10} \text{ sec} = 0.069 \text{ sec}^{-1}$$

Amount left $= (\lambda)(\Delta t)(A)$

$$= (0.069)(2)(5) = (0.069)(10) = 0.69 \text{ mCi}$$

24. C Adding the top numbers (the sum of protons and neutrons):

$$59 + x = 60$$

$$x = 1$$

Adding the bottom numbers (the number of protons):

$$27 + y = 27$$

$$y = 0$$

The particle is then: $^1_0?$, which fits the neutron: $^1_0 n$.

25. D See explanation for question 24 for steps:

Top numbers:

$$238 + x = 239 + 3(1) = 242$$

$$x = 242 - 238 = 4$$

Bottom numbers:

$$92 + y = 94 + 3(0) = 94$$

$$y = 94 - 92 = 2$$

The particle is: $^4_2?$, which fits the α-particle (or helium nucleus): $^4_2 He$.

26. C $\frac{A}{A_0} = (\frac{1}{2})^{t/t_0}$

$A_0 = 100 \text{ mCi}$

$t_0 = 14 \text{ days} = \text{half-life}$

$t = 4 \text{ weeks} = 28 \text{ days}$

$A = \text{activity left} = A_0(\frac{1}{2})^{t/t_0}$

$$= 100(\frac{1}{2})^{28/14}$$

$$= 100(\frac{1}{2})^2 = 25 \text{ mCi}$$

27. D $\qquad t_0 = 11.5 \text{ hours}$

$$A_0 = \text{starting activity}$$

Activity lost $= 0.25 A_0$

Activity left $= A = A_0 - 0.25 A_0 = 0.75 A_0$

$$\frac{A}{A_0} = (\frac{1}{2})^{t/t_0}$$

$$\frac{0.75 A_0}{A_0} = (\frac{1}{2})^{t/11.5}$$

$$0.75 = (\frac{1}{2})^{t/11.5}$$

$$\log 0.75 = \left(\frac{t}{11.5}\right)\log(\tfrac{1}{2})$$

$$\log 3 - \log 4 = \left(\frac{t}{11.5}\right)(\log 1 - \log 2)$$

$$0.4771 - 0.6021 = \left(\frac{t}{11.5}\right)(0 - 0.3010)$$

$$-0.1249 = \left(\frac{t}{11.5}\right)(-.3010)$$

$$t = 4.77 \text{ hours}$$

Bibliography

Tippens PE: Applied Physics, 3rd ed. New York, McGraw-Hill, 1985.

Masterson WL, Slowinski EJ: Chemical Principles, with Qualitative Analysis, 6th ed. Philadelphia, WB Saunders College Publishing, 1986.

Kotz JC, Purcell KF: Chemistry and Chemical Reactivity, 2nd ed. Philadelphia, WB Saunders College Publishing, 1991.

Halliday D, Resnick R: Fundamentals of Physics, 4th ed. New York, John Wiley & Sons, 1993.

Petrucci RH, Wismer RK : General Chemistry with Qualitative Analysis, 2nd ed. Edited by Peter Gordon. New York: Macmillan, 1987.

Harris NC, Hammerling EM: Introductory Applied Physics, 4th ed. New York, McGraw-Hill, 1980.

Tipler PA: Physics, 2nd ed., vols. 1 and 2. New York, Worth, 1982.

Stanford, Jr., AL, Tanner, JM: Physics for Students of Science & Engineering. Philadelphia, WB Saunders College Publishers, 1985.

Mahan B: University Chemistry, 4th ed. Redwood City, CA, Benjamin-Cummings, 1987.

8

Problem Solving in the Biological Sciences

Review Chapter 2 before beginning to work in this chapter. According to the *MCAT Student Manual*, problem solving in the biological sciences focuses on application and understanding of basic premedical concepts. This chapter should be reviewed to develop a conceptual understanding of scientific facts and their application to medical- or health-related situations.

Introduction

MEDICAL KNOWLEDGE AND TECHNOLOGY REFLECTED ON THE MCAT

The MCAT is based on premedical concepts and problem-solving strategies according to AAMC guidelines. Review the following statements to get a clearer picture of the nature of the MCAT.

1. The knowledge base and technologies of medicine are rapidly changing and expanding.
2. The basic concepts and principles of medicine are applied to the solution of scientific and clinical problems.
3. Applicants are encouraged to broaden their undergraduate education.
4. Students are encouraged to investigate a wide variety of course offerings outside the natural sciences.
5. If you need to retake the MCAT, it may be that course work was inadequate for the materials included in the test.
6. While passages may discuss advanced-level topics, the questions accompanying the passages will not require knowledge of these topics.
7. The content outline focuses primarily on areas necessary for the study of medicine.
8. Some of the topics included in the outline may not have been emphasized in your school's introductory undergraduate courses.
9. The materials assume the appropriate background knowledge, but they also contain new information or new uses of information.
10. Research studies are incorporated in passages, documenting all or part of the rationales, methods, and results of research projects. The questions test your understanding of the projects and are designed to convince the reader that particular perspectives, methodologies, pieces of evidence, or products are correct.
11. The content outline may differ in several important ways from the content of your introductory biological sciences courses.
12. Topics may focus on some aspect of the structure or function of a given body system, on the interaction of two or more body systems, or on the effects of an external factor (for example, a disease or an environmental influence) on the total physiology of an organism.
13. These concepts include basic principles of molecular biology, cellular structure and function, and genetics and evolution.
14. The passages call upon your knowledge of organic compounds and reactions

and ask you to explain results, arguments, and experimental procedures in terms of reactions or principles of organic compounds.

15. The passages require you to solve basic chemistry problems and evaluate research in general chemistry.

16. The questions may deal with situations or problems you have not previously encountered.

17. You should be prepared to apply your knowledge of these concepts to experimental situations.

18. Check course descriptions in catalogues and syllabi; review class notes and laboratory exercises.

19. If you find that the basic science courses at your school do not address the required skills and content, then you may need additional course work or outside reading. Supplemental activities might include reading selected parts of basic science texts, reading science journals, or working in laboratories where you can be involved in research planning or analysis.

PROBLEM SOLVING IN THE BIOLOGICAL SCIENCES USING THIS BOOK

In this chapter, each section begins with self-managed learning questions to get you "warmed up" to the topic. At the end of each section is a discussion entitled Applied Concepts in which modern and sophisticated instruments, medical terms, and related medical disorders are briefly discussed. Biological sciences and medical research are changing rapidly and this discussion provides an overview of these changes.

The biological sciences include problems both in applied biology and applied organic chemistry. It is fairly easy to relate topics in biology and organic chemistry, e.g., molecular structure and spectroscopy of ACTH or PTH (organic chemistry of a biological compound) or biological structure and function of lipids or proteins (biology of an organic compound). As a premedical student, you should relate various biologically important compounds—molecular structure and biological function. This permits you to understand scientific articles related to medicine, to review laboratory experiments, and to become a better problem solver who is well equipped to read long passages and make appropriate connections.

The arrangement of subtopics within a major topic in this book is based on interdisciplinary and sequential learning. Biology is presented in four levels: molecular, cellular, tissues, and systems. Organic chemistry is presented first at a molecular level followed by discussion of complex biological molecules. This arrangement of subject matter covers the entire AAMC *MCAT Student Manual* outline, but not in the same order. To help make your learning process easier, complete pedagogical flow charts are included (Figures 8-1 through 8-3).

Molecular Structure of Organic Compounds

Self-Managed Learning Questions
Focus on the following experimental issues:

1. Are there any clinical tests or applications of the molecular structure of organic compounds related to specimen collection, specimen classification and type, collection time for specimens, specimen handling, or experimental errors?

2. Are there any graphs, diagrams, reaction mechanisms, or sketches that require quantitative analysis? Which mathematical concepts will help in interpreting graphical data?

3. The physical and chemical properties (including chemical reactions) of organic and biological compounds are connected to the molecular structure, the types of bonds, and the strengths of chemical bonds. This section presents classification and nomenclature (how to name an organic molecule) techniques for organic compounds. These nomenclature techniques include a brief discussion of hybrid orbitals, resonance in bonds, and chemical rigidity. Students should learn six to eight basic rules in naming organic compounds. Learn these rules with at least three to five applications of each rule. Molecular structure is also determined using (1) laboratory instruments such as various types of polarimeters (working and design of polarimeters is required for the MCAT), and (2) special laboratory procedures such as preparing racemic mixtures.

Building Blocks for Studying MCAT Biology

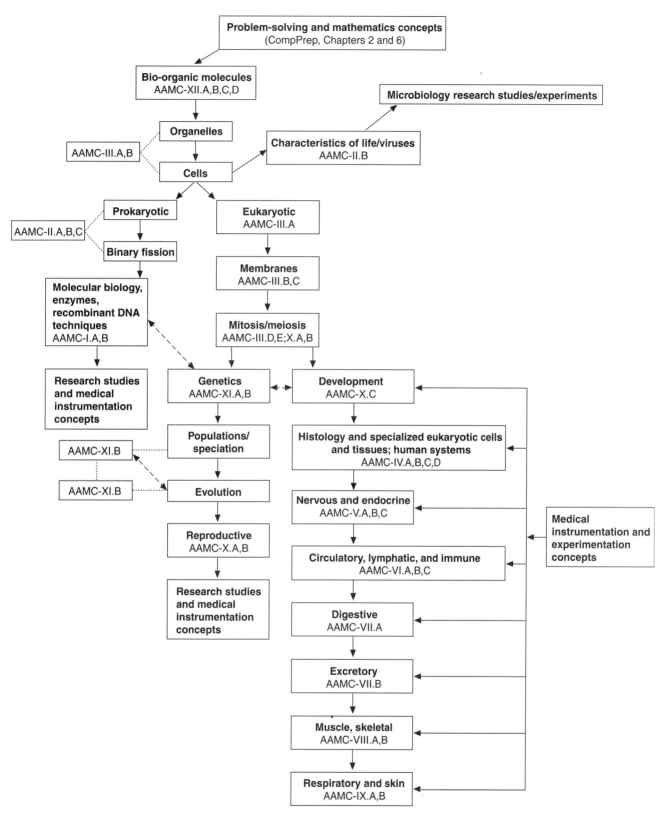

Fig. 8-1. Building blocks for studying biology. The flowchart presents a logical method for reviewing biology, beginning with bio-organic molecules and eukaryotic and prokaryotic cells, then molecular biology, and finally, tissues and systems in the human body. The chart will facilitate your review and make it more methodical. You will find that the AAMC manual and *A Complete Preparation for the MCAT* do not present topics in the same order as this chart. For your review, start with molecules, cells, and tissue, and then work with physiologic systems and other medical sciences.

Building Blocks for Studying Organic Chemistry

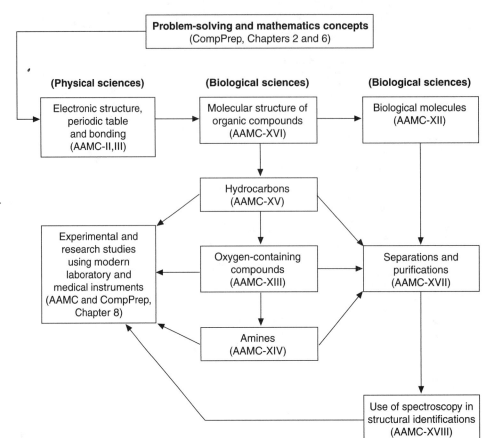

Fig. 8-2. Building blocks for studying organic chemistry.

Building Blocks for Studying Biological Sciences

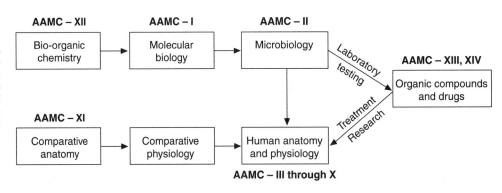

Fig. 8-3. Building blocks for studying biological sciences. Shown are major topics according to the *AAMC Student Manual* that form the learning structure for biological sciences. When visiting the library, find books in the subject areas shown and try to interrelate various topics within each subject. Do not take advanced courses in these subjects.

SIGMA AND PI BONDS

Refer to Chemical Bonding in Chapter 7.

STEREOCHEMISTRY OF COVALENTLY BONDED MOLECULES

Isomers

Isomers are compounds that have the same molecular formula but different structural formulas. The structural formulas may differ in the arrangement of atoms and bonds (structural isomers) or the arrangement of the atoms in space (stereoisomers). For example, ethanol and dimethyl ether are structural isomers, but *cis*-2-butene and *trans*-2-butene are stereoisomers. In the pair of structural isomers, the carbon and oxygen atoms are arranged differently: C—C—O and C—O—C; in the pair of stereoisomers, the carbon atoms are arranged identically: C—C=C—C (Figure 8-4).

Stereoisomers are divided into two categories: **enantiomers** and **diastereomers.** Stereoisomers that are nonsuperimposable mirror images of each other are called **enantiomers.** If any object is not superimposable on its mirror image, for example, a hand or shoe, the object is chiral or it displays chirality. A pair of gloves is a pair of chiral objects; the chirality of each glove is designated by "left" or "right." Enantiomers are chiral molecules whose chirality is designated by different notations. An object or molecule is not chiral if it has a plane of symmetry (it is achiral).

A left ear has no plane of symmetry; it is chiral and it has an enantiomer—a right ear. A nose has a plane of symmetry bisecting it vertically; it is achiral and has no enantiomer. A tetrahedron has several planes of symmetry; it is achiral. A tetrahedron whose corners are painted four different colors, however, does not have a plane of symmetry. There are two permutations for the corners of a tetrahedron with four different colors; these painted tetrahedrons are enantiomers. Because carbon atoms with single bonds have tetrahedral geometry, a molecule in which a carbon atom is attached to four different groups is a chiral molecule, and there are two stereoisomers (enantiomers) of the molecule (Figure 8-5). (Note: In the drawings in this book, a heavy line means that the bond is coming toward you; a broken line means the bond is going away from you.)

The chirality of a compound may be specified in one of two ways: absolute configuration, which requires a set of rules that are applied to the substituents on the chiral carbon, and relative configuration, in which the configuration is compared with a standard reference compound. Stereoisomers that are not enantiomers are **diastereomers**. That means that geometric (*cis-trans*) isomers are diastereomers, whether in alkenes or in cyclic compounds, but other diastereomers are the result of more than one chiral atom in a molecule. An example is 3-chloro-2-butanol, which has two chiral carbons and four stereoisomers, whose Fischer projections are shown (Figure 8-6). The absolute configuration is determined for each chiral center as described, giving the stereoisomers shown as *A, B, C,* and *D* on Figure 8-6.

If compounds have more than one chiral center, then enantiomers have opposite configurations at every chiral center; diastereomers have at least one chiral center with the same configuration. Figure 8-6 shows the relationships among the stereoisomers.

Epimers are diastereomers that have several chiral carbons, but have opposite configurations at only one chiral center. Epimers are commonly found in carbohydrates, but may be found in any kind of compound. **Meso compounds** are compounds that have more than one identically substituted chiral carbons, which are symmetrically arranged

Structural isomers

$CH_3 - CH_2 - OH$ $CH_3 - O - CH_3$

Fig. 8-4. Isomer comparisons.

Stereoisomers

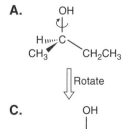

Mirror

Fig. 8-5. Enantiomers.

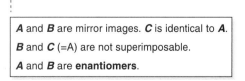

A and B are mirror images. C is identical to A.

B and C (=A) are not superimposable.

A and B are **enantiomers**.

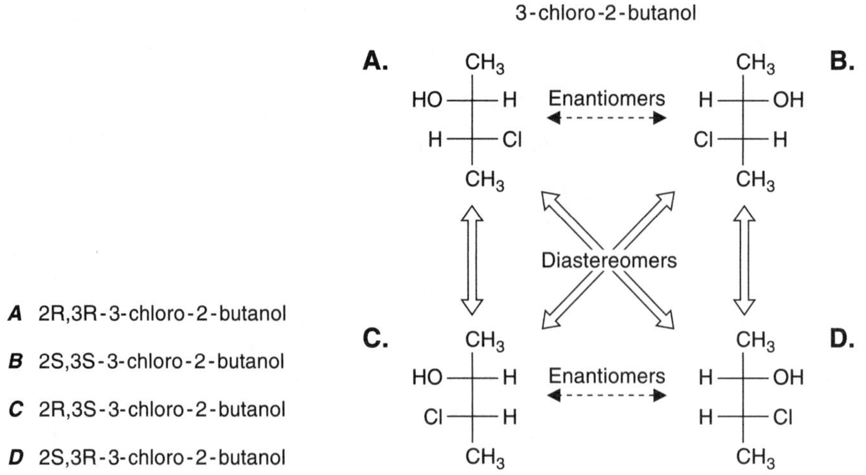

3-chloro-2-butanol

A.

CH₃
HO—|—H
H—|—Cl
CH₃

Enantiomers ←------→

B.

CH₃
H—|—OH
Cl—|—H
CH₃

Diastereomers

C.

CH₃
HO—|—H
Cl—|—H
CH₃

Enantiomers ←------→

D.

CH₃
H—|—OH
H—|—Cl
CH₃

Fig. 8-6. Diastereomer-enantiomer interrelationship.

A 2R,3R-3-chloro-2-butanol

B 2S,3S-3-chloro-2-butanol

C 2R,3S-3-chloro-2-butanol

D 2S,3R-3-chloro-2-butanol

(plane of symmetry in molecule) so that the molecule is achiral. Meso compounds do not have enantiomers (they are superimposable on their mirror images) and are not optically active. Meso compounds do have diastereomers, which may be optically active. Examples of stereoisomers that include enantiomers, diastereomers, and a meso compound are shown for 2,3-butanediol (Figure 8-7).

The following are the Fischer projection rules for diastereomers:

1. Rotation of 180° retains configuration.
2. Interchanging any two groups on one chiral carbon converts to another diastereomer.
3. Interchanging two groups on every chiral carbon converts to the enantiomer.

Separation of Stereoisomers

Because diastereomers have different physical properties, they may be separated by physical means used to separate any compound (e.g., fractional distillation, chromatography, crystallization). Special techniques must be used to separate enantiomers because their physical properties are identical. The separation of a racemic mixture into pure enantiomers is called **resolution**.

Reactions of Chiral Stereoisomers

MCAT Tip: Chiral centers may be formed or destroyed in chemical reactions. A molecule that has no chiral carbon may be converted to a racemic mixture (pair of enantiomers), or an enantiomer may be converted into a pair of diastereomers in a reaction (Figure 8-8).

A pure enantiomer with a single chiral carbon may undergo a reaction in which the configuration is unchanged (retention) or inverted or racemized. If the chiral carbon is not at the reaction center, the configuration is retained. In an S_N2 reaction (bimolecular nucleophilic substitution), the configuration is inverted. In a reaction in which a trivalent carbon species (carbocation, free radical, carbanion) is an intermediate, the product is racemic (Figure 8-9).

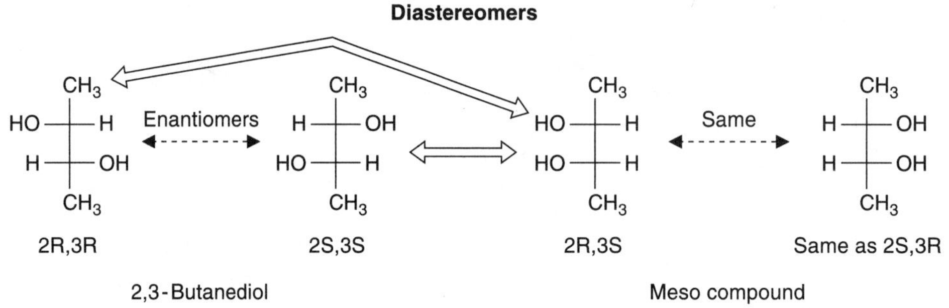

Diastereomers

CH₃
HO—|—H
H—|—OH
CH₃
2R,3R

Enantiomers ←------→

CH₃
H—|—OH
HO—|—H
CH₃
2S,3S

CH₃
HO—|—H
HO—|—H
CH₃
2R,3S

Same ←------→

CH₃
H—|—OH
H—|—OH
CH₃
Same as 2S,3R

Fig. 8-7. Meso compounds.

2,3-Butanediol

Meso compound

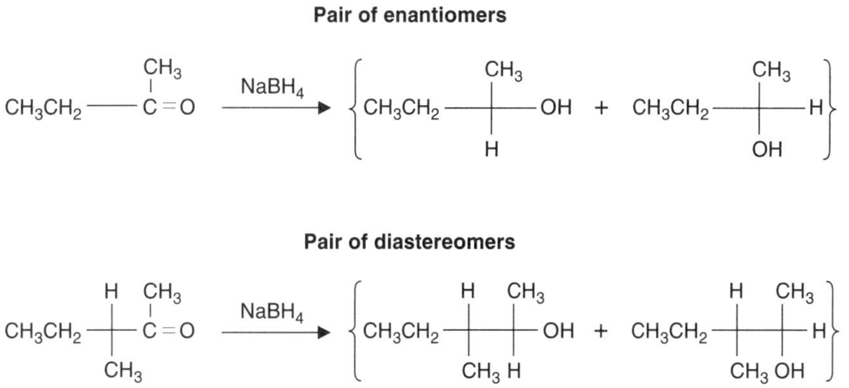

Pair of enantiomers

Pair of diastereomers

Retention

Inversion

Racemic mixture reactions

Planar carbocation

Pair of diastereomers

Fig. 8-8. Chiral stereoisomer reactions I.

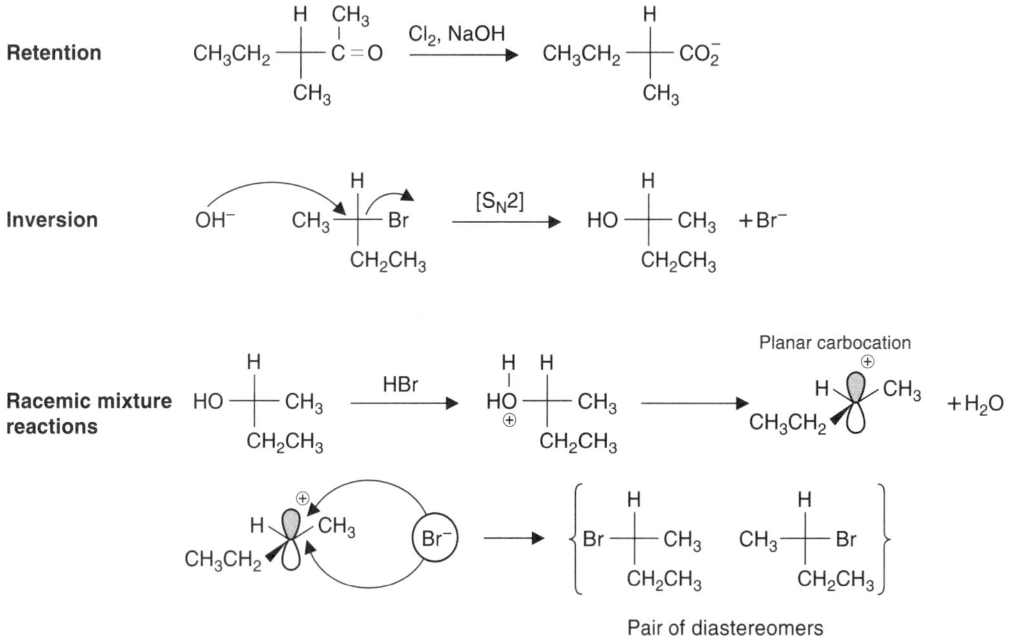

Fig. 8-9. Chiral stereoisomer reactions II.

Polarization of Light, Specific Rotation

Optical Activity as Related to Enantiomers

Structural isomers usually have different physical properties, such as melting points, boiling points, and solubilities. Enantiomers have the same physical properties with one important exception: they rotate the plane of polarized light to an equal and opposite extent. Because of this property, which is an optical effect, enantiomers are called **optical isomers,** and the ability to rotate the plane of polarized light is called **optical activity**. The instrument used to measure the rotation of polarized light by an optical isomer is a polarimeter. Rotation is measured in degrees as either positive [clockwise (+), dextrorotatory (D)] or negative [counterclockwise (−), levorotatory (L)]. There is no correlation between direction of rotation of polarized light and absolute configuration. That is, a molecule with R configuration may have either + or − observed rotation. There is no correlation between the relative configuration (D or L) and the observed rotation (+ or −), except in glyceraldehyde in which the D enantiomer has the + rotation.

To find the observed rotation, use the equation a = [a] (l × C), where a = observed rotation (degrees), [a] = specific rotation (degrees), l = path length (decimeters), and C = concentration (g/mL of solution).

Absolute and Relative Configuration

Absolute Configuration

To determine the absolute configuration, it is necessary to assign priorities to the four groups attached to the chiral carbon according to the sequence rules. In general, the higher atomic number has priority over the lower. When two atoms have the same atomic number, continue down the chain until there is a difference. For example:

$$Br > Cl > O > N > C > H, CH_2CH_3 > CH_3, and CCl_3 > CH_2Cl$$

Fig. 8-10

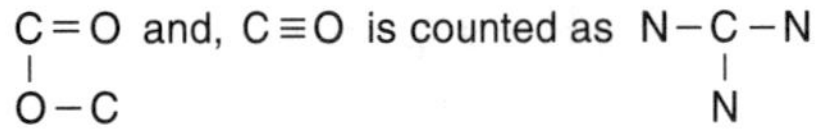

$C=O$ and, $C\equiv O$ is counted as

$$C=O \text{ (with } O-C\text{)} \qquad C\equiv O \to N-C-N \text{ (with } N\text{)}$$

Double bonds are treated as two substituents, and triple bonds as three substituents (Figure 8-10).

Consider $CH=O > CH_2OCH_3 > CH_2OH$. After priorities 1 through 4 have been assigned to the groups, the molecule must be oriented so that the group of lowest priority (4) is pointed away from you. When the molecule has been oriented in this way, groups 1, 2, and 3 will be toward you and the direction that turns 1 into 2 and 2 into 3 is determined. If that direction is clockwise, the chiralty designation is rectus (R); if it is counterclockwise, the chirality designation is sinister (S). One enantiomer always has the R configuration and the other has the S configuration.

Fischer Projections

The stereochemistry around a chiral carbon may be represented in a useful shorthand way developed by Emil Fischer. The groups are written at the ends of a cross or plus sign with groups on the vertical axis going away from you and groups on the horizontal axis coming toward you. There is no rule for representing a molecule like 2-butanol as a specific Fischer projection; that is, there are several projections for the R enantiomer and several for the S enantiomer. The following are useful rules for Fischer projections with one chiral carbon:

1. Turning the drawing 180° retains the configuration (R stays R).
2. Turning the drawing 90° inverts the configuration (R becomes S). Interchanging any two groups inverts the configuration.

The following are rules to determine absolute configuration (R or S) from Fischer projections:

1. Determine order of priority as before.
2. Determine direction (clockwise or counterclockwise) of $1 \to 2 \to 3$.
3. Determine whether group 4 is on a horizontal or vertical axis.
4. Use the following chart:

	Axis of group 4	
$1 \to 2 \to 3$	*Vertical*	*Horizontal*
Clockwise	R	S
Counterclockwise	S	R

(Figure 8-11) shows several Fischer projections of 2-butanol and their absolute configurations.

Determination of absolute configuration from Fischer projection

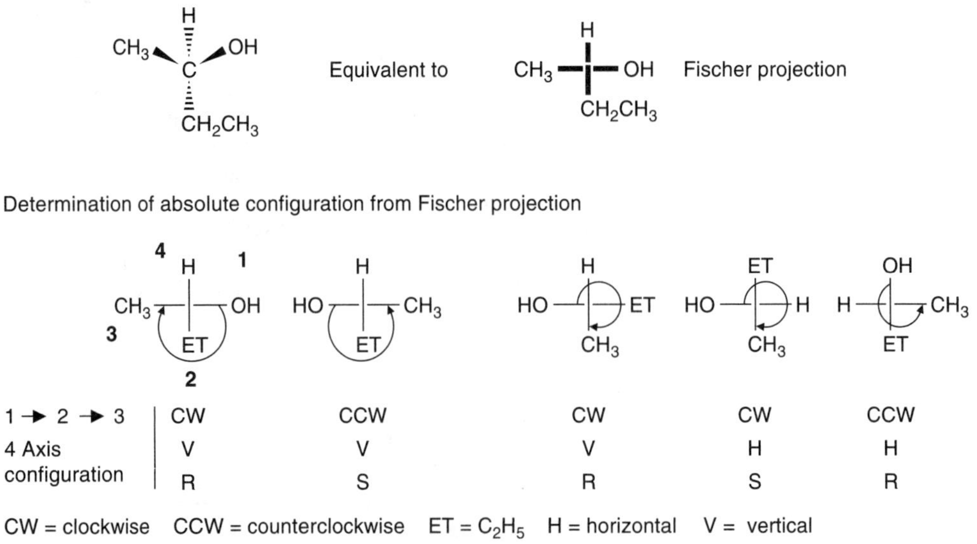

Fig. 8-11. Fischer projections and their absolute configurations.

$1 \to 2 \to 3$	CW	CCW	CW	CW	CCW
4 Axis configuration	V	V	V	H	H
	R	S	R	S	R

CW = clockwise   CCW = counterclockwise   ET = C_2H_5 H = horizontal   V = vertical

Relative Configuration

Before rules for absolute configuration were adopted, chemists used standard compounds and related other configurations to the standards. At the time, the actual configurations of the standards were not known, but they are known now. The relative configuration system is still used extensively in carbohydrate and amino acid chemistry. The symbols used to denote configuration in the relative system are dextrorotatory (D) and levorotatory (L). The reference compounds are the enantiomers of glyceraldehyde (Figure 8-12).

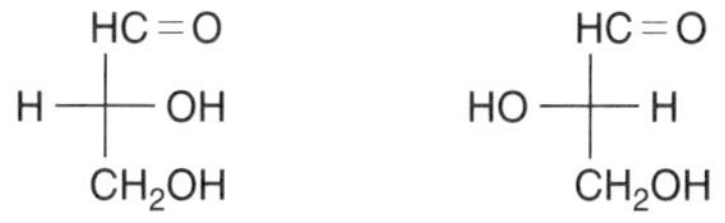

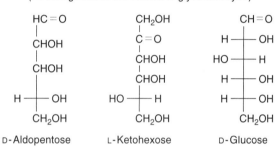

(All configurations are related to glyceraldehyde)

Fig. 8-12. Relative configurations and carbohydrates.

It is easy to determine the configuration with a model of the molecule, but it takes more effort to determine R or S from a drawing. In the compounds shown for 2-butanol (Figure 8-13), the priorities are OH=1 > CH₂CH₃=2 > CH₃=3 > H=4. The molecules are oriented with the H pointing away from you, as shown in the figure, and the direction of rotation of the groups is noted. From this it is determined that enantiomer *A* has the R configuration and enantiomer *B* has the S configuration. *A* is R-2-butanol; *B* is S-2-butanol. Any other drawing of 2-butanol that indicates stereochemistry must be treated as shown for *A* or *B* and its configuration will be R or S. For example, structure *D* is rotated as shown in (Figure 8-14) to determine its configuration. *D* must be oriented so that group 4 is away from you, which can be done by rotating around the bond between the chiral carbon and the ethyl group. The correct orientation leads to the R configuration, which means that *D* (see Figure 8-14) and *A* (see Figure 8-13) are different drawings of the same compound.

Racemic Mixtures

Because enantiomers have opposite and equal rotations, an equimolar mixture of the two enantiomers does not show rotation: this is a racemic mixture or racemate. Racemiza-

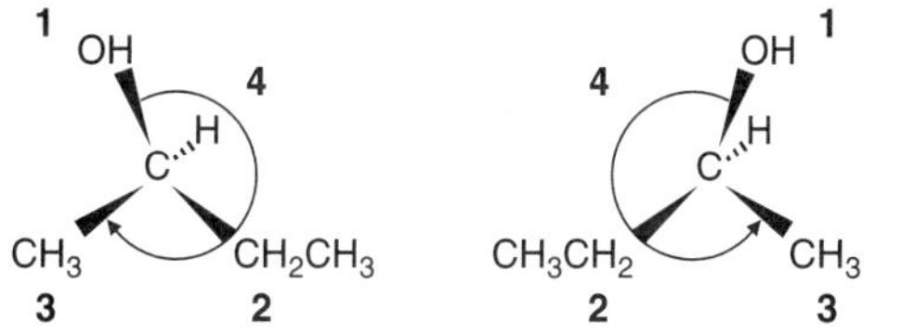

Fig. 8-13

A.

B.

Fig. 8-14

D.

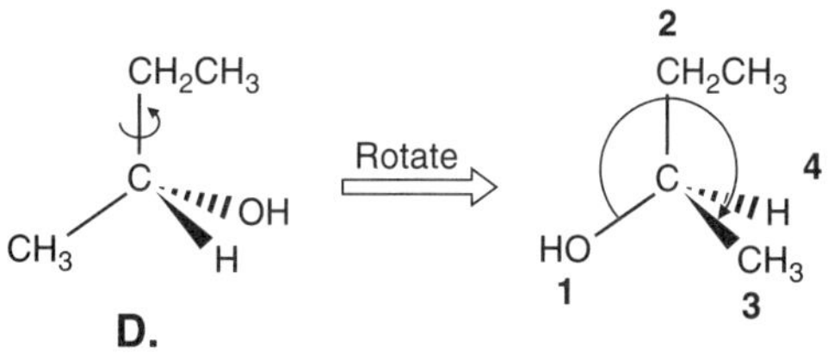

Rotate

tion is the process in which an optically active compound loses optical activity because of a chemical reaction.

APPLIED CONCEPTS

- Relate chirality of molecules to the formation of enzyme-substrate complexes and to hormonal action and feedback inhibition.
- Examine laboratory methods and research techniques in developing racemic mixtures for biological hormones, steroids, and complex molecules.
- Understand properties of organic and biological compounds as related to varying percentages of components in a racemic mixture.
- Review stereoselective reactions.
- Review the historical work done by Louis Pasteur on using a polarimeter to study the structure of tartaric acid. Appraise the experimental evidence and decide whether the research was valid (use various reasoning patterns discussed in Chapter 4).
- Learn the naming conventions of rectus (R) and sinister (S) forms of enantiomers. Check your understanding of conventions by applying them to biologically important enantiomers.

MOLECULAR STRUCTURE OF ORGANIC COMPOUNDS: REVIEW QUESTIONS

1. *Cis*-2-pentene and *trans*-2-pentene are:

   A. structural isomers.
   B. optical isomers.
   C. enantiomers.
   D. diastereomers.

2. Which compound may be optically active?

   A. 2-Methyl-2-pentanol
   B. 2-Methyl-3-pentanol
   C. 2-Methyl-3-pentanone
   D. 3-Methyl-3-pentanol

3. Which is the enantiomer of compound A?

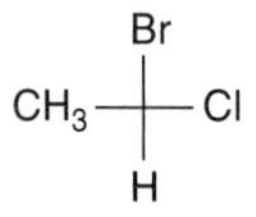

$$CH_3 \overset{Br}{\underset{H}{|}} Cl$$

Compound A

A. 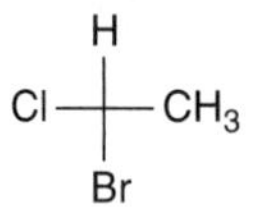 $Cl \overset{H}{\underset{Br}{|}} CH_3$

B. 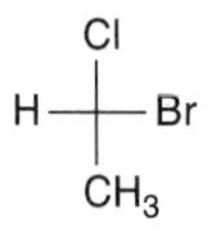 $H \overset{Cl}{\underset{CH_3}{|}} Br$

C. 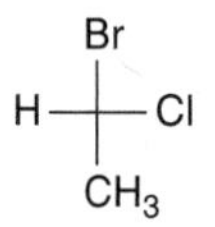 $H \overset{Br}{\underset{CH_3}{|}} Cl$

D. 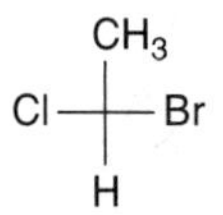 $Cl \overset{CH_3}{\underset{H}{|}} Br$

4. Which structure represents 2R, 3R-3-bromo-2-pentanol?

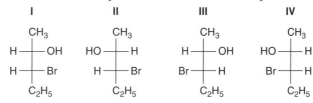

    A. I and II only
    B. I and III only
    C. II and IV only
    D. II and III only

5. Compounds I and III in question 4 are:

    A. enantiomers.
    B. diastereomers.
    C. structural isomers.
    D. racemic.

6. Compounds B and C in question 4 are:

    A. enantiomers.
    B. diastereomers.
    C. structural isomers.
    D. meso compounds.

7. The specific rotation of compound W is $-37°$.

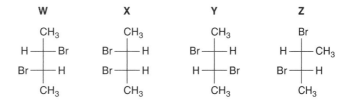

    What is the specific rotation of compound X?

    A. $+37°$
    B. $-37°$
    C. $0°$
    D. Cannot be determined

8. In question 7, what is the specific rotation of compound Y?

    A. $+37°$
    B. $-37°$
    C. $0°$
    D. Cannot be determined

9. In question 7, what is the specific rotation of compound Z?

    A. $+37°$
    B. $-37°$
    C. $0°$
    D. Cannot be determined

10. 2-Methylcyclohexanol has _____ stereoisomers, and _____ of these are optically active.

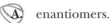

    A. 2; 0
    B. 2; 2
    C. 4; 2
    D. 4; 4

11. 4-Methylcyclohexanol has _____ stereoisomers, and _____ of these are optically active.

    A. 2; 0
    B. 2; 2

C. 4; 2

D. 4; 4

12. If a single, pure stereoisomer of 2-methylcyclohexanone is reduced to 2-methylcyclohexanol, the product will be:

A. a single enantiomer.

B. a racemic mixture.

C. a pair of diastereomers.

D. a mixture of four stereoisomers.

13. Two grams of an amino acid is dissolved in 10 mL water. The solution is placed in a 5-cm long polarimeter tube and shows an observed rotation of $-12°$. What is the specific rotation of the amino acid?

A. $-1.2°$

B. $-12°$

C. $-120°$

D. Some other value

$$\frac{-12}{(.2)(.5)}$$

14. D-Lyxose is an aldopentose. We know that in the Fischer projection of D-lyxose:

A. the OH on carbon 2 is on the right.

B. the OH on carbon 3 is on the right.

C. the OH on carbon 4 is on the right.

D. all the OH groups are on the right.

15. A reaction produces a mixture of amino acids D-alanine and L-alanine. One could obtain the pure D-alanine by:

A. fractional crystallization.

B. electrophoresis.

C. biological separation.

D. ultracentrifugation.

1. D *Cis/trans* isomers are a type of diastereomer.

2. B Only B has a chiral carbon (carbon-3).

3. C From the rules concerning configuration of Fischer projections, compound A has the R configuration [Br > Cl > CH_3 > H], as do all the others except C.

4. B Assign configurations to each chiral carbon. For carbon-2, the order is OH > carbon-3 > CH_3 > H, and for carbon-3 the order is Br > carbon-2 > CH_3 > H. From the rules, I is 2R, 3R; II is 2S, 3R; III is 2R, 3R; IV is 2S, 3R.

5. B Options I and II have the same configuration at carbon-2, and opposite configurations at carbon-3; therefore, they are diastereomers.

6. A They have opposite configurations at each chiral carbon atom.

7. C Compound X is a meso compound (plane of symmetry) and shows no optical activity.

8. A Compound Y is the enantiomer of W and must have opposite specific rotation.

9. D Compound Z is the diastereomer of W because two groups on the top chiral carbon have been interchanged. In this case, the diastereomer of W is Z (not a meso compound), so the rotation cannot be determined. If the diastereomer was also a meso compound, the rotation will be 0°.

NOTE FOR QUESTIONS 10–12: Two possible configurations at each chiral carbon R and S produce 2^n possible stereoisomers and 2^{n-1} enantiomers for n chiral carbon atoms if all chiral carbons have different substituents. If some carbons have identical substituents, meso compounds will exist (i.e., $< 2^n$ stereoisomers).

10. D There are two non-identical chiral carbons, so there are $2^2 = 4$ stereoisomers; all of them are chiral.

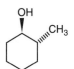

cis Enantiomers   *trans* Enantiomers

11. A There is a plane of symmetry through the molecule, and there are no chiral carbons. There is a *cis* and a *trans* form, neither optically active.

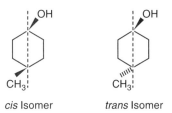

cis Isomer   trans Isomer

12. C The products will have the same configuration at the carbon bearing the methyl and opposite configurations at the alcohol; they are diastereomers.

13. C Observed rotation = specific rotation $\times$ (concentration of solid or density of liquid) $\times$ length of polarimeter tube (1 dm = 10 cm), $\alpha = [\alpha]Cl$. From formula: observed rotation = $-12°$; C = 2g/10 ml = 0.2; L = 5 cm = 0.5 dm spec rot = $(-12°)/(0.2)(0.5) = -120°$.

14. C From convention about relative configuration of carbohydrates.

15. C Organisms will metabolize the L isomer and ignore the D isomer.

Bioorganic Molecules

AMINO ACIDS

Biologically important macromolecules (proteins, nucleic acids, and polysaccharides) are composed of repeating monomeric subunits, often referred to as "building blocks," that polymerize to form these compounds. Amino acids are the building blocks of proteins. There are 20 different amino acids, each found at least once in most proteins. Those rare amino acids found in proteins in excess of 20 are formed by modification of one or more of the standard 20 after the protein has been formed, a change usually referred to as a post-translational modification.

All of the amino acids found in proteins are α-amino substituted carboxylic acids (in this system of nomenclature, the Greek alphabet is used to designate the position of a substituent . . . the α-carbon is the first substitutable carbon adjacent to the functional group for which the compound is named; i.e., an acid. The β-carbon is next, etc.). In all but one of the 20 amino acids commonly found in proteins, the α-carbon is chiral. Glycine is the exception, because it contains two hydrogens on the α-carbon. Only the L-isomers are found in proteins. These compounds are therefore optically active (will rotate plane polarized light). With only one exception (proline), the amino acids all conform to the structure shown in Figure 8-15 in a perspective formula, differing only in the R group. When written in the projection formula, the chiral carbon, by convention, is considered in the plane of the page. The vertical bonds project behind the page and the horizontal bonds project in front of the page. If the structure is rotated 90°, the bonds must be changed if the absolute configuration of the chiral center is to be represented.

$$H_2N - \overset{COOH}{\underset{R}{C}} - OH \quad = \quad R - \overset{H}{\underset{NH_2}{C}} - COOH$$

Fig. 8-15

The types and sequences of amino acids in proteins determine their structural properties and acid-base behavior. The amino acids shown in Figure 8-16 have R groups that are hydrocarbon in nature, are hydrophobic, and are found in the interiors of proteins.

Ionic amino acids, polar amino acids, or both are hydrophilic and tend to be found on the exterior of proteins (Figure 8-17).

Certain amino acids can be found on the exterior or interior of proteins (these are polar also) as shown in Figure 8-18.

Cysteine forms sulfur-sulfur covalent bonds with itself to stabilize the tertiary structure of proteins (Figure 8-19).

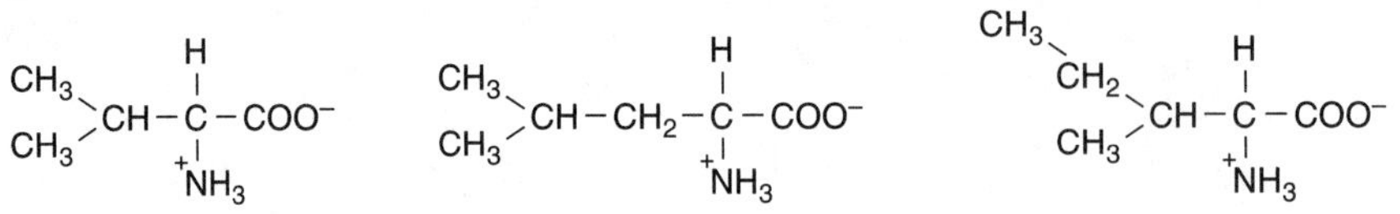

Fig. 8-16

Valine   Leucine   Isoleucine

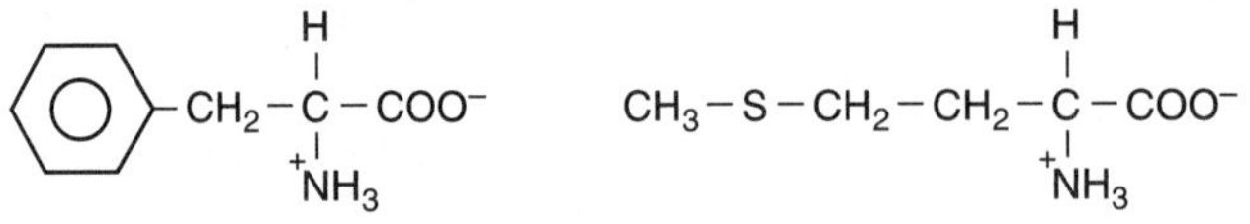

Phenylalanine   Methionine

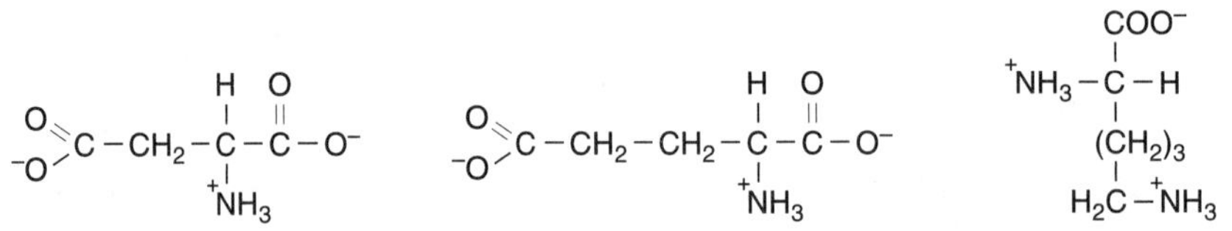

Aspartic acid and its amide   Glutamic acid and its amide   Lysine

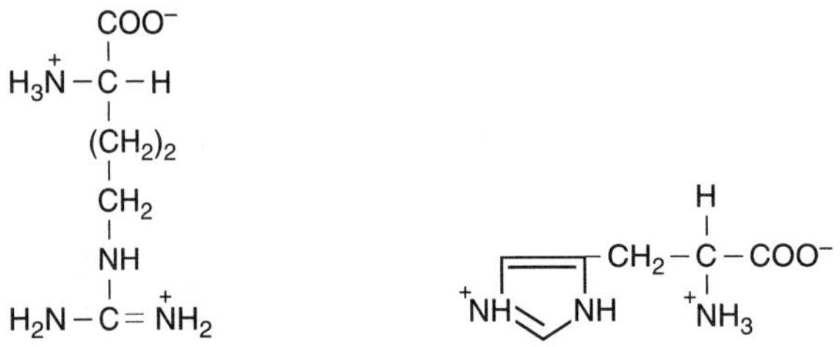

Fig. 8-17

Arginine   Histidine

Fig. 8-18

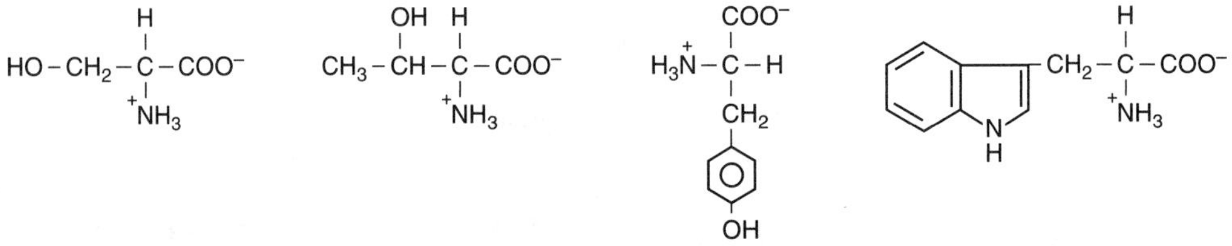

Serine   Threonine   Tyrosine   Tryptophan

Fig. 8-19

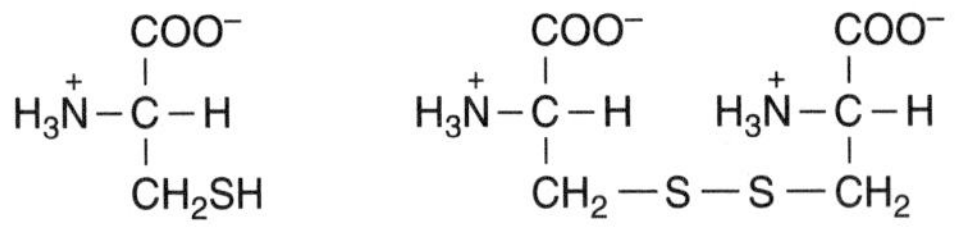

Cysteine   Cystine

Glycine, the smallest amino acid and the only one that is not optically active, is often found at the "corners" of proteins (Figure 8-20).

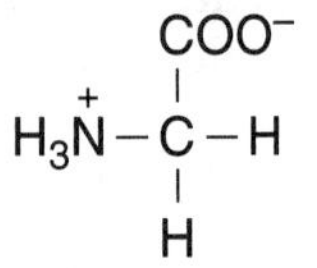

Fig. 8-20   Glycine

Proline breaks the α-helix structure of proteins as shown in Figure 8-21.

Alanine, being small, is usually found on the surface of proteins even though it is hydrophobic (Figure 8-22).

The basic amino acids are lysine and arginine, which have extra amino ($-NH_2$) groups. The acidic amino acids are aspartic acid and glutamic acid, which have extra carboxyl ($-CO_2H$) groups. Histidine can act as a base or an acid depending on the pH,

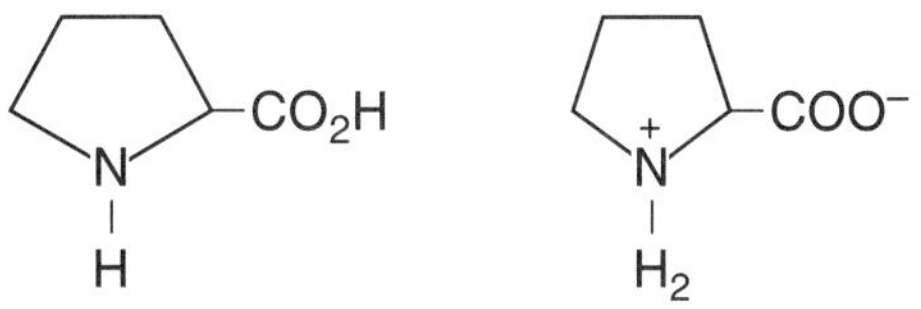

Fig. 8-21   Proline

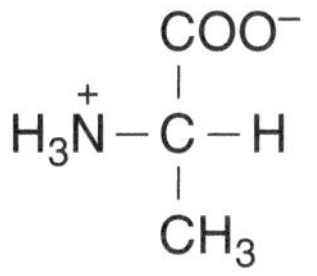

Fig. 8-22   Alanine

and it is the best physiologic buffer of the amino acids. All of the others are considered neutral amino acids.

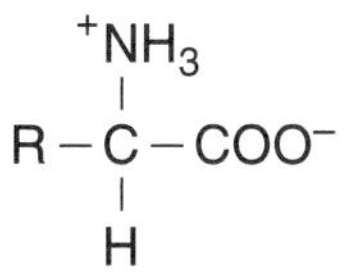

Fig. 8-23   Dipolar ion

Amino acids exist as dipolar ions (Figure 8-23) because they have both a basic part (the $-NH_2$) and an acidic part (the $-CO_2H$).

The charge on the amino acid varies with the pH and the isoelectric point. The isoelectric point (pI) of an amino acid is the pH at which the amino acid has no net charge (Figure 8-24).

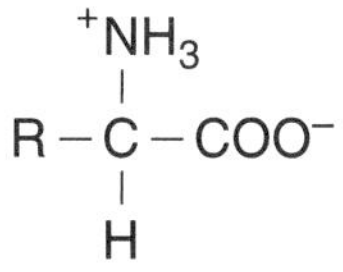

Fig. 8-24   No *net* charge at isoelectric points

If the pH is above the isoelectric point, amino acids have a net negative charge (anions) [Figure 8-25].

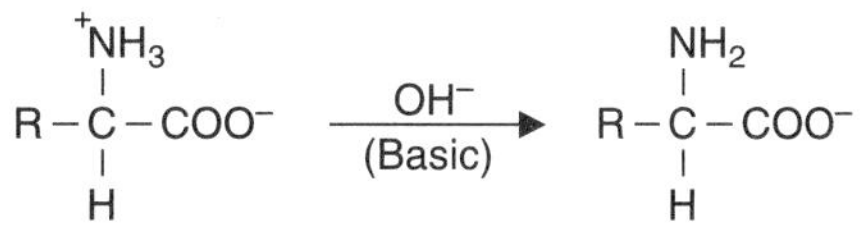

Fig. 8-25   Uncharged form   Anionic form

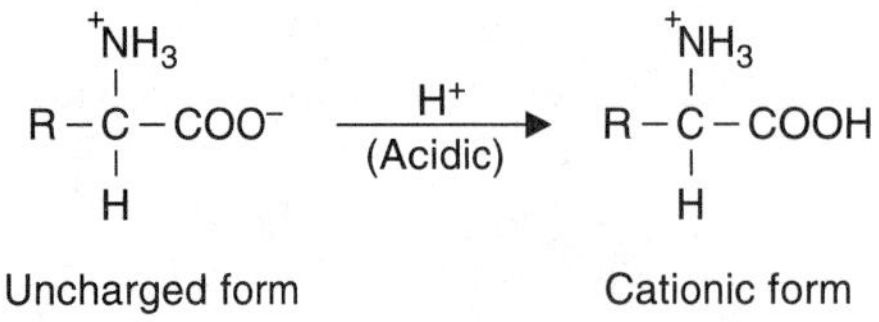

Fig. 8-26

Uncharged form   Cationic form

If the pH is below the isoelectric point or very acidic, amino acids have a net positive charge (cations) [Figure 8-26].

At neutral pH, the free amino acid is polar because these molecules exist as zwitterions (there is a full negative charge on the carboxyl, which is completely dissociated, and a full positive charge on the amino group, which is protonated). Once protonated, the amino group becomes a proton donor (in the reverse direction); hence, it is the conjugate acid of the base. (Amino acids follow the same rules of dissociation as weak acids; review Acids and Bases in Chapter 7 for their behavior at differing pH levels.) These charges are not present when the amino acids are polymerized into a polypeptide chain; hence, the R groups largely determine the properties of the protein.

Classification

Amino acids are both acids and bases because they possess both carboxyl and amino groups. These two groups are ionized at the pH values commonly found in cells; the carboxyl group has lost a proton and the amino group has gained a proton.

Amino acids can be classified as hydrophobic or hydrophilic depending on whether their side chains are electrically charged, polar but uncharged, or hydrophobic. The two groups of amino acids with electrically charged side chains are those with positive charges and those with negative charges. The four amino acids with polar but uncharged chains readily form hydrogen bonds with water and with other molecules; they are hydrophilic. Eight other amino acids have side chains that are either hydrocarbon or are modified from hydrocarbons; they are hydrophobic.

Reactions

Two cysteine side chains have the ability to lose hydrogen atoms so that their sulfur atoms are joined in a disulfide bridge by a covalent bond (a disulfide bridge helps to determine how a protein chain folds). When cysteine is not part of a disulfide bridge, its side chain is hydrophobic (Figure 8-27).

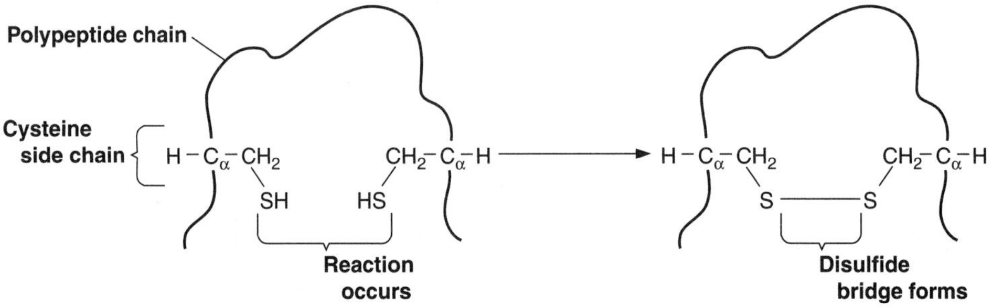

Fig. 8-27. Formation of a disulfide bridge.

In proteins or fragments of proteins (oligopeptides), the α-amino acids are linked through peptide bonds into a linear sequence. These bonds are formed by a condensation reaction in which water is removed from the α-carboxyl of one acid and the α-amino group of another, which makes them chemically similar to a substituted amide. These peptide bonds have special properties because resonance structures exist across the peptide bond, giving partial double-bond character to the C—N bond, as shown in Figure 8-28.

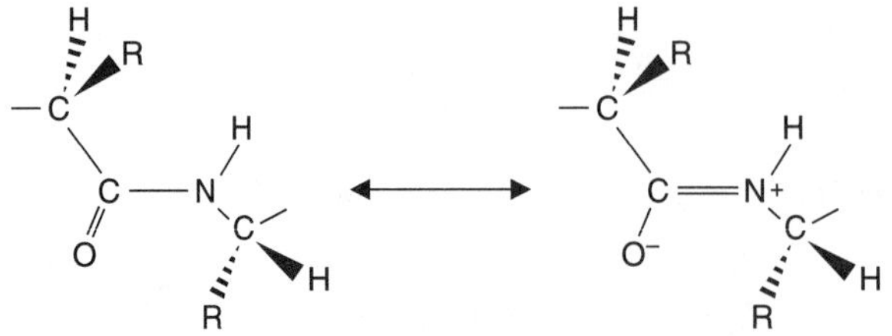

Fig. 8-28. Peptide bond characteristics.

Due to the partial positive charge on the amino nitrogen in a peptide bond, these amino nitrogens do not bind protons. These amino nitrogens are not completely charged even in the presence of high proton concentrations. This partial double-bond character of the peptide bond also makes it rigid and planar. It is unable to rotate as a typical single bond, because the bond has the characteristics of an sp^2 hybrid orbital. Figure 8-28 shows the planar nature of the peptide bond. The six atoms in the shaded area all lie within the same plane.

In a peptide chain, only the free amino group and the free carboxyl can contribute to the charge of the peptide except in the R groups. These side chains, or R groups, therefore determine the charge on a polypeptide chain. If there is a high concentration of nonpolar amino acids (based strictly on the polarity of the side chain), the protein will be insoluble. If the protein contains a high concentration of polar amino acids, it will usually be soluble in water. Basic proteins have more basic amino acids than acidic amino acids; acidic proteins have a preponderance of aspartic and glutamic acids.

By convention, peptide notation is written with the free amino group to the left and the free carboxyl group to the right (they are also numbered and named left to right). The tetrapeptide shown in Figure 8-29 demonstrates this principle.

Fig. 8-29. Peptide illustration.

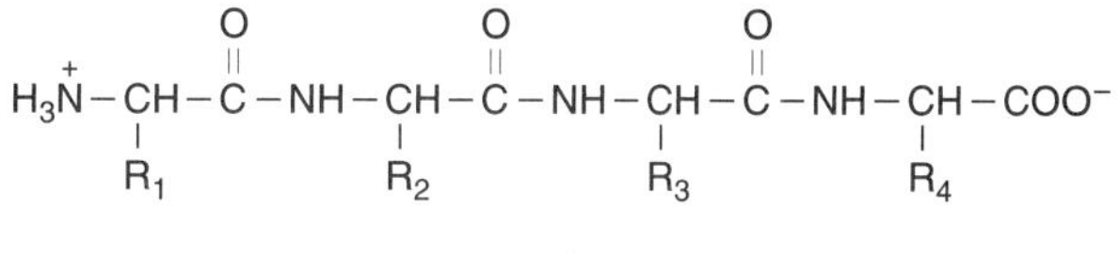

$$H_3\overset{+}{N}-\underset{\underset{R_1}{|}}{CH}-\overset{\overset{O}{||}}{C}-NH-\underset{\underset{R_2}{|}}{CH}-\overset{\overset{O}{||}}{C}-NH-\underset{\underset{R_3}{|}}{CH}-\overset{\overset{O}{||}}{C}-NH-\underset{\underset{R_4}{|}}{CH}-COO^-$$

To determine the total charge for an oligopeptide, write the amino acid, including the amino-terminal and the carboxyl-terminal groups, at a given pH; then determine the net charge by taking the algebraic sum of the charged groups. The changes that occur when amino acids are polymerized are seen when the amino-terminal group of a protein has a pK_a near 8.0 and the carboxyl-terminal is near 3.0.

Proteins are destroyed by hydrolysis (water is added) of the peptide bond. There are many enzymes that hydrolyze the peptide bond, including trypsin, chymotrypsin, pepsin, carboxypeptidase, and aminopeptidase, which are found in the gastrointestinal tract of higher-order animals. Their normal function is to hydrolyze ingested proteins to their constituent amino acids so that they may be absorbed across the intestinal wall and into the bloodstream. These enzymes and certain chemicals such as cyanogen bromide are used by protein chemists to experimentally hydrolyze proteins to determine their amino acid sequence (Figure 8-30).

Fig. 8-30. Hydrolysis of a peptide bond.

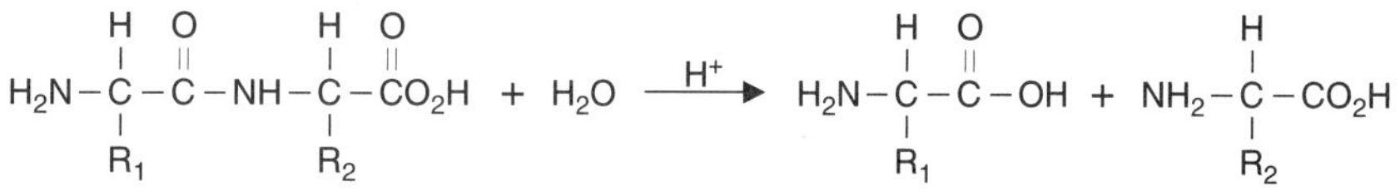

$$H_2N-\underset{\underset{R_1}{|}}{\overset{\overset{H}{|}}{C}}-\overset{\overset{O}{||}}{C}-NH-\underset{\underset{R_2}{|}}{\overset{\overset{H}{|}}{C}}-CO_2H \ + \ H_2O \ \xrightarrow{H^+} \ H_2N-\underset{\underset{R_1}{|}}{\overset{\overset{H}{|}}{C}}-\overset{\overset{O}{||}}{C}-OH \ + \ NH_2-\underset{\underset{R_2}{|}}{\overset{\overset{H}{|}}{C}}-CO_2H$$

General Principles

Proteins are classified according to biological function, shape, chemical composition, or the number of constituent peptide chains. Proteins function as transport proteins, contractile proteins, structural proteins, storage proteins, regulatory proteins, protective proteins, or enzymes. Proteins may be globular (usually soluble and biologically active) or fibrous (highly asymmetric and often insoluble). Some proteins are simple (contain only amino acids); others are conjugated (contain other non-amino acid components such as metals, phosphates, heme, flavin, or sugars). Some proteins are monomeric (contain only one polypeptide chain) or are oligomeric (contain 2 or more peptide chains, e.g., dimers, trimers, tetramers).

Protein structures may be described at several different levels of organization as follows:

1. Primary (1°) structure—describes the sequence of amino acids within a chain.
2. Secondary (2°) structure—describes the regular, repeating pattern of folding that is stabilized primarily by hydrogen bonds between groups close together in the sequence (e.g., α-helix, β-pleated sheet).
3. Tertiary (3°) structure—describes the folding of the chains in three dimensions, stabilized by interactions between segments far apart in sequence. Hydrophobic side chains on the inner sides of the helices ensure that the helices correctly fold against each other as the molecule is formed.
4. Quaternary (4°) structure—describes interactions between different polypeptide chains in an oligomeric protein, stabilized solely by noncovalent bonds.

Biologically active proteins spontaneously assume a unique structure that is referred to as the native conformation. Renaturation experiments have demonstrated that the information necessary to correctly fold into the proper 2° and 3° structure that will yield a biologically active molecule resides in the sequence of amino acids in the chain. A number of different forces stabilize globular proteins, including (1) hydrogen bonds, (2) electrostatic interactions, (3) hydrophobic interactions, (4) van der Waals forces, and (5) disulfide bonds. Individually, many of these forces are relatively weak, but because they act cooperatively, the structure of proteins is relatively stable.

Most proteins with intense biological activity are globular and active in aqueous solution. The folding of the polypeptide chain that results in 2° and 3° structure brings certain functional groups (side chains) into close proximity even though they may be separated by long distances in the sequence of amino acids. Interaction of these side chains may create the active site of enzymes, antibodies, or toxins in a cleft or pocket on the protein. The active site occupies only a small part of the total volume of the molecule. Globular proteins exclude water from the internal structure, and the nonpolar side chains tend to aggregate in this nonpolar environment, whereas the polar amino acid side chains tend to be found on the surface of the protein in contact with water.

Stability of the 2°, 3°, 4° structure can be disrupted by heat, extremes of pH, detergents, urea, acetone, and ethanol. Such agents are termed "denaturing agents." Denaturation results in changes in conformation, which causes the native proteins to unfold, and results in loss of the shell of water surrounding the molecule. Denatured proteins often precipitate from solution. For example, when an enzyme unfolds, the active site is thus distorted so that biological activity is lost.

The isoelectric point of an amino acid is the pH at which the acid molecule exists only as a bipolar ion with zero net charge.

$$pI = \frac{pK_{a1} + pK_{a2}}{2}$$

If pH > pI, the anion migrates to the anode. If pH = pI, the amino acid exists as a zwitterion with no migration. If pH < pI, the cation migrates to the cathode. The following is a list of pI values for some amino acids:

Alanine, 6.00
Glutamine, 5.65
Glycine, 5.97
Isoleucine, 6.02
Leucine, 5.98
Threonine, 5.60
Tryptophan, 5.89
Serine, 5.68
Valine, 5.96

CARBOHYDRATES

Carbohydrates is the name given to the family of organic molecules that is composed of sugars (saccharides). The basic units are **monosaccharides,** given general names ending in *-ose* according to the number of carbons (e.g., pentose, hexose), the nature of the carbonyl group (aldose or ketose), or a combination of both. For example, ribose is an aldopentose (five-carbon aldehyde), and fructose is a ketohexose (six-carbon ketone). Chemically, they are polyhydroxyaldehydes or ketones of the formula $(CH_2O)n$, with a hydroxy group on each carbon other than the carbonyl.

Monosaccharides are frequently drawn to emphasize stereochemical relationships, with the aldehyde (C-1) at the top. Examples of hexoses are shown in Figure 8-31.

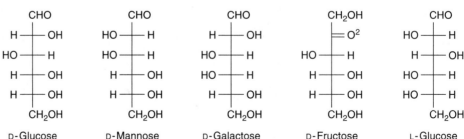

Fig. 8-31   D-Glucose   D-Mannose   D-Galactose   D-Fructose   L-Glucose

Stereoisomerism

Aldohexoses contain four asymmetric centers (carbons 2–5), so there are $2^4 = 16$ stereoisomers, or eight pairs of enantiomers. Each of the eight has a distinct common name. The sugars found in nature are pure enantiomers, optically active. Stereochemical descriptors common in carbohydrates include D and L, and epimers.

D and L symbols refer to the absolute configuration of the highest numbered asymmetric center, that is, the bottom asymmetric carbon in the Fischer projection (C-5 in glucose). When the OH lies on the right, the sugar is D; if the OH is on the left, the sugar belongs to the L series. Most common sugars of nature have the D configuration. L-glucose, the enantiomer of D-glucose, must have the opposite configuration at every asymmetric center.

The simplest chiral carbohydrate is the aldotriose glyceraldehyde, and the higher-order sugars can be considered as homologs of either D- or L-glyceraldehyde (Figure 8-32).

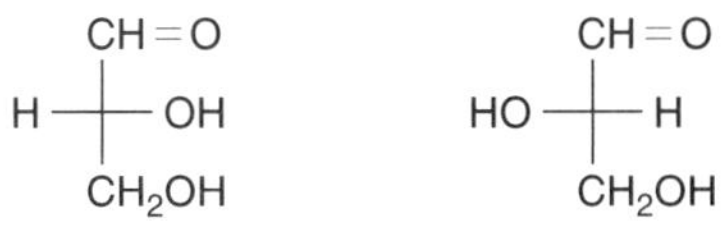

Fig. 8-32   D-Glyceraldehyde   L-Glyceraldehyde

Cyclic Structures

Hydroxyl groups suitably situated can add intramolecularly to the carbonyl group, forming cyclic hemiacetals or hemiketals. These cyclic structures predominate at equilibrium, and monosaccharides exist almost totally in ring forms. Two relatively unstrained ring sizes are possible, five-membered (named **furanose**) and six-membered (named **pyranose**). Figure 8-33 shows the pyranose form of glucose illustrated in several ways.

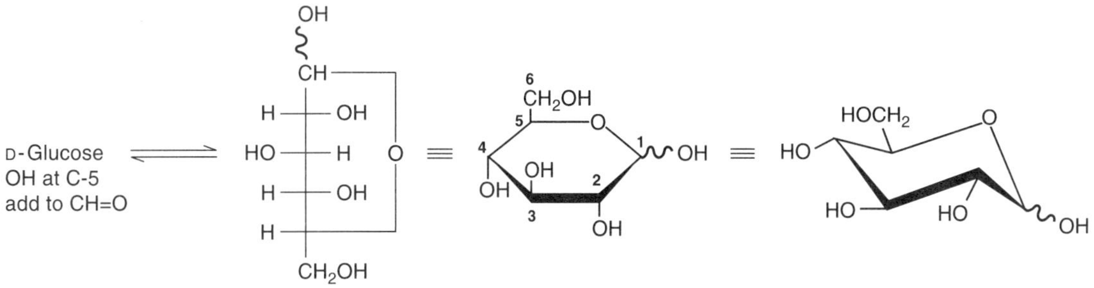

Fig. 8-33

Fischer   Haworth   Conformation

Fischer projections clearly show the relationship to the aldose structure but are awkward in representing the configuration at C-1. Haworth formulas depict the ring as a planar hexagon, with substituents oriented either on the top or bottom of the ring. The most geometrically accurate representation is a conformational drawing, showing the six-membered ring in the familiar chair conformation with substituents either equatorial or axial. Aldopentoses (e.g., arabinose) are usually drawn as Haworth formulas (Figure 8-34).

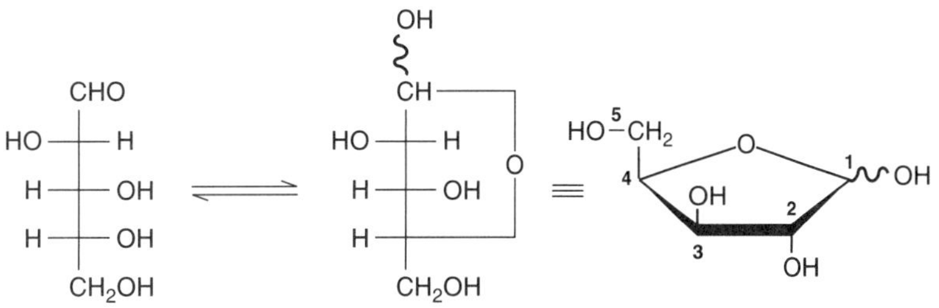

Fig. 8-34   D-Arabinose   Furanose structure   Haworth

Epimers are a kind of diastereomer with two sugars that differ in configuration at only one of several asymmetric centers. Glucose and mannose are epimers at C-2; glucose and galactose are C-4 epimers.

Cyclic Hemiacetal Equilibria

The cyclic hemiacetals possess a new asymmetric center at C-1, in addition to the four already present in the aldohexoses, so two diastereomers (called **α-** and **β-anomers**) are possible. In the conventional Haworth or conformational drawings, the C-1 OH is down in the α-anomer and up in the β-anomer. A wavy bond indicates that the OH may be either α or β. The cyclic structure of β-D-glucose is the one in which all substituents are equatorial in the chair conformation (Figure 8-35).

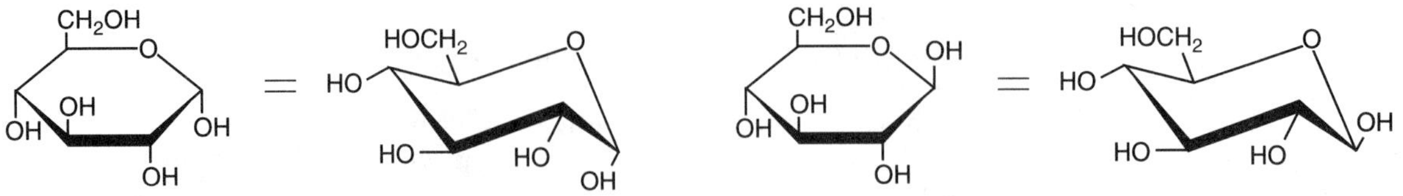

α-D-Glucose   β-D-Glucose

Fig. 8-35

Although the cyclic structures predominate and can be crystallized as pure solids, in aqueous solution they are in equilibrium with the open-chain carbonyl forms. The structural formulas of cyclic hemiacetals do not show an aldehyde group, but they exhibit all the characteristic aldehyde reactions, such as is seen with the Fehlings test (Figure 8-36). Experimental evidence for this equilibrium comes from the phenomenon of mutarotation; the optical rotation of a freshly prepared solution or pure α- or β-D-glucose changes with time until an equilibrium value is reached starting from either anomer.

$$\text{α-D-Glucose} \rightleftharpoons \text{Equilibrium mixture} \rightleftharpoons \text{β-D-Glucose}$$
$$[a]_D + 112° \qquad\qquad [a]_D + 52.7° \qquad\qquad [a]_D + 19°$$

Fig. 8-36

At equilibrium in aqueous solution, D-glucose exists as approximately 39% of the α-pyranose anomer, 61% as the β-pyranose anomer, and approximately 0.15% each of the α- and β-furanose rings, with no detectable aldehyde.

Oxidation of Monosaccharides

Periodate Cleavage
HIO_4 (periodic acid) cleaves the carbon-carbon bond between vicinal hydroxyl groups to leave carbonyl groups. It also cleaves α-hydroxy aldehydes and ketones (imagine the carbonyl group as its hydrate). The examples in Figure 8-37 show how this oxidation can be used to determine the ring size in methyl glucoside: periodate cleavage of the pyranoside gives one equivalent of formic acid, whereas cleavage of the furanoside gives one equivalent of formaldehyde.

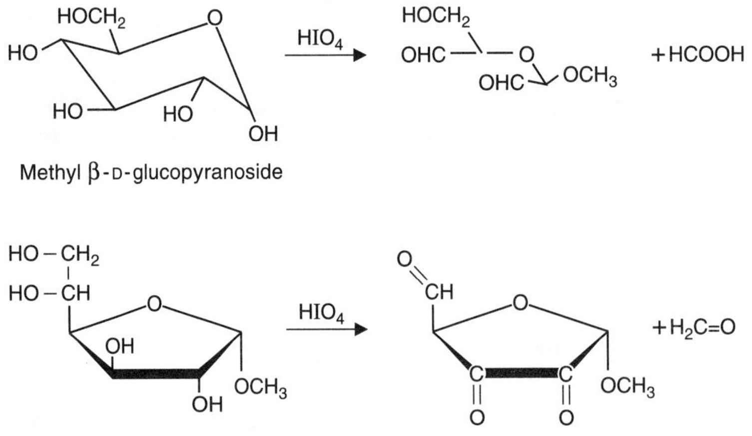

Methyl β-D-glucopyranoside

Fig. 8-37   Methyl α-D-glucofuranoside

Natural Monosaccharides
L-Ascorbic acid (vitamin C) is a natural monosaccharide found in citrus fruits and many vegetables, important for the prevention of scurvy. It is a lactone in which C-1 of a hexose has been oxidized to the carboxylic acid level, and with a double bond between carbons 2 and 3. This enediol moiety is easily oxidized, and vitamin C is believed to serve a

protecting role by reducing some biological oxidants, such as free radicals and hydro-peroxides.

Ribose is the aldopentose unit in ribonucleic acid (RNA), and 2-deoxyribose is the sugar unit in deoxyribonucleic acid (DNA). The related ketopentose ribulose plays a crucial role in photosynthesis as the acceptor of carbon dioxide (Figure 8-38).

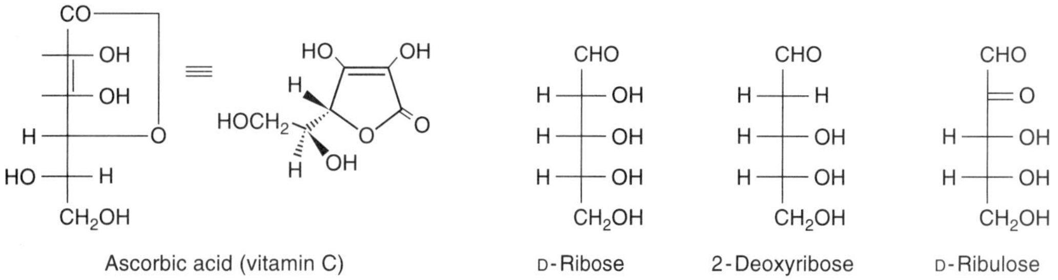

Ascorbic acid (vitamin C)   D-Ribose   2-Deoxyribose   D-Ribulose

Fig. 8-38

Disaccharides are molecules composed of two monosaccharides connected by an acetal bond; one of the five OH groups of one hexose, for example, is used to bond to the carbonyl carbon (usually C-1) of a second hexose in its cyclic form. Examples of three common disaccharides are shown in Figure 8-39.

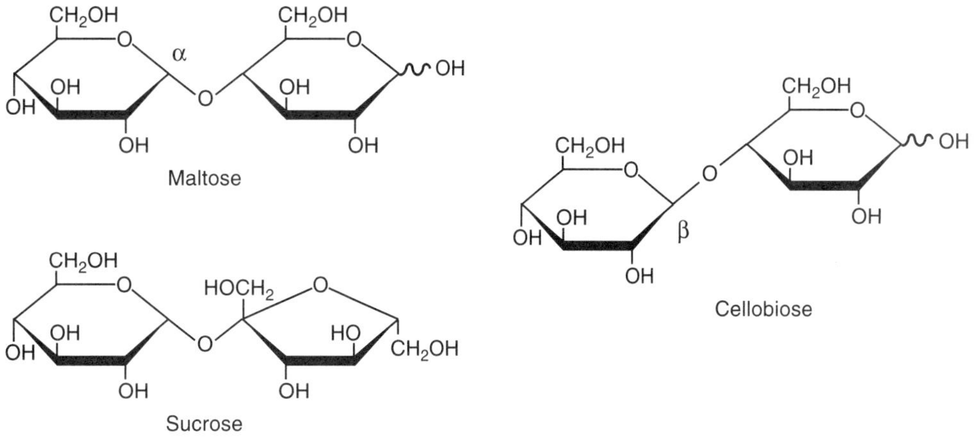

Maltose

Cellobiose

Sucrose

Fig. 8-39

Maltose, the repeating unit of starch, and cellobiose, the repeating unit of cellulose, are both composed of two D-glucose units, the second attached by the hydroxyl at C-4. The sole difference is the configuration at the anomeric carbon C-1, maltose being α (α-1,4 bond) and cellobiose β (β-1,4 bond). Although the oxygen that links the rings is part of an acetal group, the right-hand ring in each is still a cyclic hemiacetal, in equilibrium with an aldehyde, so that maltose and cellobiose are reducing sugars. Sucrose, on the other hand, is a non-reducing sugar; the bridging oxygen atom connects an acetal carbon (C-1) in a d-glucose unit with a ketal carbon (C-2) in a fructose unit. The right-hand ring is an example of a ketose in its cyclic furanose structure. Lactose (milk sugar) is made of galactose and glucose (β-1,4 bond).

Hydrolysis of the Glycoside Linkage

Polysaccharides are large polymeric molecules, containing as many as hundreds or thousands of repeating monosaccharides linked together by acetal (glycoside) bonds. The most important are starch, glycogen, and cellulose. Cellulose, the most abundant organic compound and the main structural component of vegetable matter, is a 1,4-β-polymer of glucose (or cellobiose). Starch and glycogen, also 1,4-polymers of glucose but with α-links, store glucose to meet energy needs; both are relatively insoluble but can be hydrolyzed on demand by enzymes (α-glycosidases) to release soluble glucose units. When more glucose is available than is needed, animals store it in the liver as glycogen. Starch, the polysaccharide found in plants, is a mixture of amylose, an unbranched polymer, and amylopectin, which has branching chains formed by acetal formation with the C-6 hydroxyl.

LIPIDS

The term **lipids** denotes several types of organic compounds of biological origin. Almost all lipids are soluble in organic solvents and insoluble in water. They are unlike carbohydrates and proteins that have specific chemical structures. Important classes of lipids are fats and oils, steroids, prostaglandins, terpenes, glycolipids, and phospholipids. Simple lipids do not undergo hydrolysis reactions (e.g., steroids and terpenes), whereas complex lipids may be hydrolyzed (e.g., fats and oils, phospholipids). Lipids are obtained from plant or animal tissue by extraction with organic solvents.

Fatty acids (carboxylic acids) do not usually occur in the free state. They are bound as esters of glycerol (triacylglycerols). The common fatty acids are straight-chain (non-branched) carboxylic acids that contain an even number of carbons between 12 and 20. The acids may be saturated (no double bonds) or unsaturated (contain double bonds). The saturated fatty acids have higher melting points than the unsaturated acids that have *cis* double bonds. This is due to irregularity in the geometry of the unsaturated molecule, leading to difficulty in stacking in the crystal. Compare stearic acid with oleic acid as follows:

$$CH_3(CH_2)_{16}COOH \qquad (cis)\ CH_3(CH_2)_7CH = CH(CH_2)_7COOH$$

Stearic acid mp 70°   Oleic acid mp 4°

(Saturated)   (Unsaturated)

The biosynthesis of fatty acids involves a series of reactions in which the chain is built from acetate, that is, two carbons at a time. Acetate is derived from pyruvate in carbohydrate metabolism or from metabolism of fats. Some fatty acids are called **essential fatty acids** because mammals cannot synthesize them from acetate and must obtain them from plants. An important essential fatty acid is linoleic acid (9, 12-octadecadienoic acid), which is converted by mammals to arachidonic acid (5, 8, 11, 14-icosatetraenoic acid). Arachidonic acid, obtained from human fat, is the starting compound in the biosynthesis of prostaglandins, which have important physiologic functions.

Soaps are sodium or potassium salts of fatty acids obtained from basic hydrolysis of triacylglycerols. Soaps solubilize dirt and grease particles because the hydrocarbon chain of the molecule (hydrophobic) interacts with the organic grease while the carboxylate anion end of the molecule (hydrophilic) interacts with the water solvent. The soap thereby emulsifies the grease and brings it into the water (Figure 8-40).

[Grease] ------ /\/\/\/\/\/\/\/\ CO_2^- ------ [H_2O]

Fig. 8-40   Soap micelles

Hard water contains metal ions (Fe^{3+}, Ca^{2+}), which form insoluble salts with fatty acid soaps. Synthetic detergents substitute the sulfonic acid anion $R—SO_3^{-2}$ for the carboxylate anion RCO_2^-. Detergents are soluble in hard water.

Triacylglycerols (triglycerides, glycerides, glyceryl trialkoanoates) are triesters of fatty acids. Fats are solid triacylglycerols that contain mostly saturated fatty acids, and oils are liquid triacylglycerols that contain mostly unsaturated fatty acids. Two commercial reactions of triacylglycerols are hydrogenation and saponification. In hydrogenation, unsaturated fatty acid groups in oils are converted to saturated groups, thereby raising the melting point and producing fats used in shortening (Figure 8-41).

$$R-CH=CH-R'-CO_2-CH_2$$
$$R-CH=CH-R'-CO_2-CH \xrightarrow{\text{Excess } H_2, \text{catalyst}} R-CH_2-CH_2-R'-CO_2-CH$$
$$R-CH=CH-R'-CO_2-CH_2$$

Fig. 8-41

(resulting in)

$$R-CH_2-CH_2-R'-CO_2-CH_2$$
$$R-CH_2-CH_2-R'-CO_2-CH$$
$$R-CH_2-CH_2-R'-CO_2-CH_2$$

In saponification, a triacylglycerol (triester) is hydrolyzed with base to give the sodium salts of the fatty acids and glycerol. The salts are soaps (Figure 8-42).

$$RCO_2-CH_2$$
$$RCO_2-CH \xrightarrow{3\text{ NaOH}} 3\ RCO_2Na\ +\ HOCH_2-CH(OH)-CH_2OH$$
$$RCO_2-CH_2$$

Fig. 8-42   Soap   Glycerol

Triacylglycerols (fats) are used to store chemical energy. Twice as much energy per gram is released when fats are oxidized to CO_2 and water than when carbohydrates are oxidized. The major cause is the hydrocarbon nature of the fats (many C—H bonds).

Steroids are complex tetracyclic molecules of physiologic significance. The general steroid structure consists of four rings designated A, B, C, and D. The most significant biological steroid is cholesterol, which is most abundant in humans. It is the starting compound for other steroids. Other steroids include bile acids, which assist in the digestion of fats, corticosteroids, such as cortisone, and sex hormones, which are secreted by endocrine glands. Ergosterol is a steroid derived from yeast, which may be converted to vitamin D by irradiation. Synthetic steroids are used as oral contraceptives and for other medicinal purposes. The structure of cholesterol is shown in Figure 8-43, with the numbering system used for steroids.

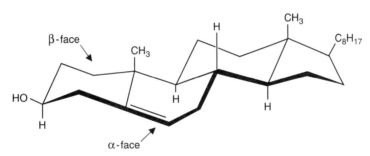

Fig. 8-43   Steroid structure   Cholesterol

Stereochemistry of steroids is complex. Cholesterol has eight chiral carbon atoms, which means that 256 possible stereoisomeric forms are possible. Cholesterol has unique stereochemistry. Studies on conformation of steroids show that cyclohexane rings have the chair conformation, with substituent groups on axial or equatorial positions. Cholesterol is almost a planar molecule, and the face on the same side as the methyl substituent (19 in the formula) is the β face; the side opposite the methyl group is the α face. The OH group on carbon 3 is *cis* to the reference methyl group: it is referred to as 3-β-hydroxy. The conformational structure of cholesterol is shown in Figure 8-44.

Fig. 8-44   Cholesterol conformation

PHOSPHORUS COMPOUNDS

Some bioorganic compounds are derivatives of phosphoric acid. Organic esters of phosphoric acids are compounds in which one or more of the acid hydrogens are replaced by an organic group.

HO	RO	RO	RO
HO—P=O	HO—P=O	RO—P=O	RO—P=O
HO	HO	HO	RO
Phosphoric acid	Alkyl phosphate	Dialkyl phosphate	Trialkyl phosphate

Phosphoric Acid— Chemistry and Structure of Anhydrides and Esters

Organic phosphate esters are hydrolyzed to phosphoric acid and the corresponding alcohol in acid solution. Only trialkyl phosphates are hydrolyzed in basic solution, and only one alkyl group is removed. The acidic hydrogens are removed by base and the resulting anions are not susceptible to basic hydrolysis:

$$(RO)_3PO + H_3O^+ \rightarrow 3\ ROH + (HO)_3PO$$

$$(RO)_3PO + OH^- \rightarrow ROH + (RO)_2PO_2^-$$

Phosphorous esters are important in the biosynthesis of triacylglycerols. Two fatty acid residues are joined to L-glycerol-3-phosphate as shown in Figure 8-45.

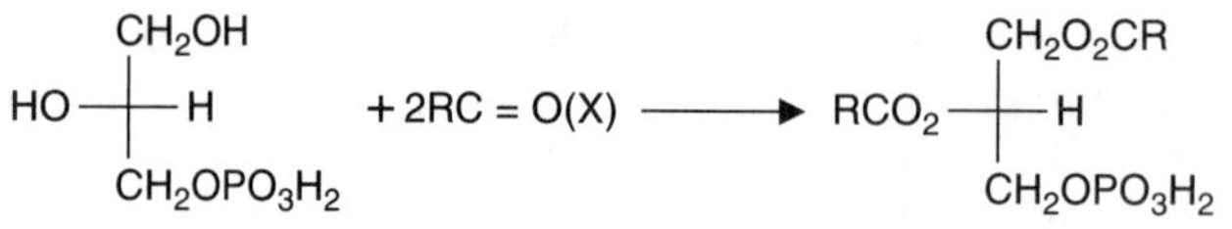

Fig. 8-45

Phosphatidic acid

The product is called **phosphatidic acid**. Phosphatidic acid is hydrolyzed to give a diacylglycerol, which is then acylated to give the triacylglycerol as shown in Figure 8-46.

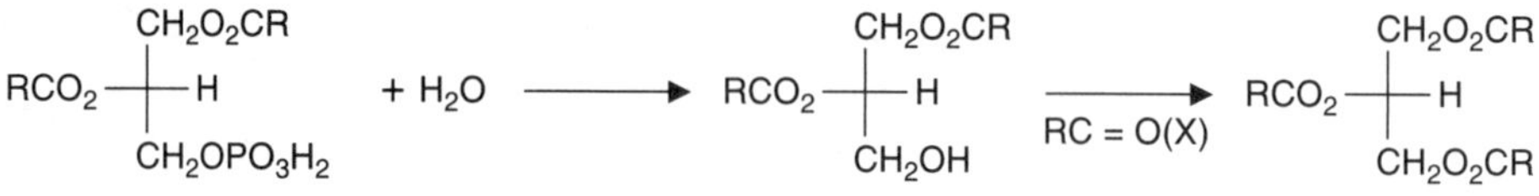

Fig. 8-46

Diacylglycerol   Triacylglycerol

Phosphatidic acids are also precursors to another class of compounds called **phosphatides**. These compounds are dialkyl phosphates in which one alkyl group is diacylglycerol and the other contains an amino group as an ammonium ion. These compounds are present in cell membranes, nerve, and brain tissue. In addition to esters of phosphoric acids, organic groups may be bonded to phosphoric acid anhydrides, as in the compounds adenosine diphosphate (ADP) and adenosine triphosphate (ATP), which are involved in energy transfer in metabolism. The structures are shown in Figure 8-47. At physiologic pH, phosphorus esters and anhydrides are converted to their corresponding anions and are inert to hydrolysis; however, enzymes catalyze the hydrolysis in living cells.

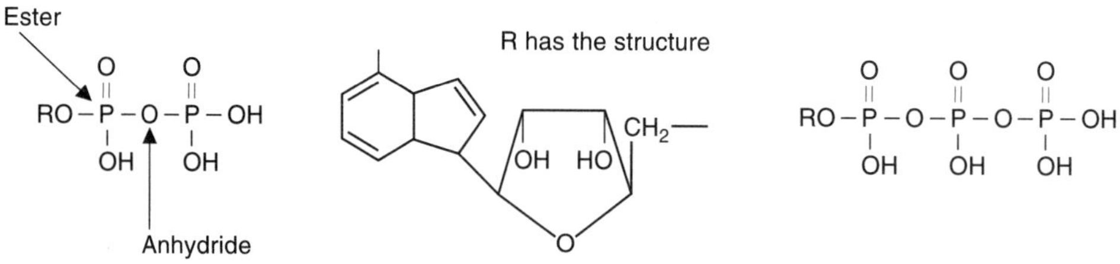

Fig. 8-47   **ADP**   **R**   **ATP**

APPLIED CONCEPTS

Read research papers and journals to familiarize yourself with new bioorganic molecules, their current physiologic applications, and recent experimental procedures to study structure and chemical reactions. Types of compounds in the following list are amino acids (A), carbohydrates (C), and lipids (L).

- Study electrophoresis showing difference between anionic and dicationic ions; racemic resolutions of amino acids; role of globular proteins as antibodies; ninhydrin reaction to produce colors with special understanding of reliability and error analysis of ninhydrin test (compound type A).
- Understand complete theory, design, functions, and reactions of amino acids in the automatic amino acid analyzer, two-dimensional gel scanner, DNA sequencer and synthesizer, and protein sequencer; chromatography of amino acids (only paper chromatography) [compound type A].
- Study theory, design, and functions of thin-layer chromatography applied to polypeptides (e.g., hemoglobin and insulin).
- Measure mutarotation of D-glucose using a polarimeter and determine equilibrium constant and relation between α-D-glucose and β-D-glucose; understand thin-layer chromatography of saccharides, working with Benedict's test accuracy and Barfoed's test accuracy, both linked to special anomers and epimers (compound type C).
- Compare and contrast Ruff degradation (makes chain shorter) and Fischer synthesis (makes chain longer) [compound type C].
- Understand the role of cellulose, cellobiose, glycogen, lactose, and starch in cellular metabolism using stereochemistry of each to illustrate metabolic biochemical reactions (compound type C).

- Study biological functions and stereochemistry of lipids (e.g., cholesterol, reproductive hormones, phospholipids and sphingolipids) [compound type L].

BIOORGANIC MOLECULES: REVIEW QUESTIONS

1. What characteristics of amino acids determine the primary structure of proteins?

   A. Acid-base properties
   B. Side chain composition
   C. Hydrogen-bonding properties
   D. Sequence in proteins

2. Which of the following is an α-amino acid?

   A.

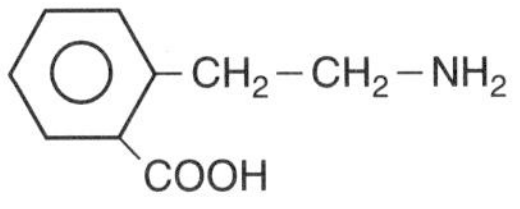

   B.

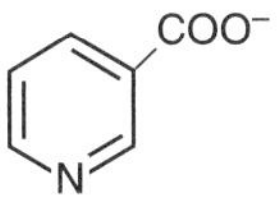

   C.

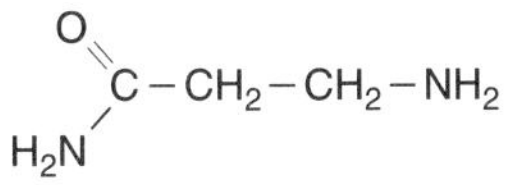

   D.

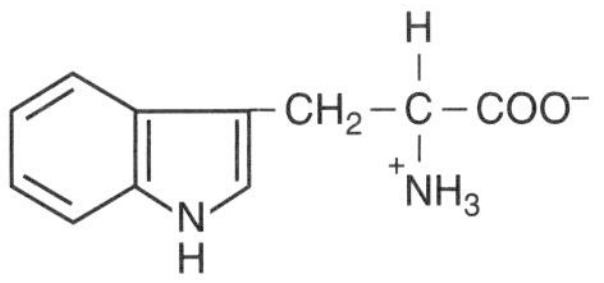

3. The peptide bond would be described chemically as which type of bond?

   A. Ester
   B. Amide
   C. Ether
   D. Anhydride

4. When a peptide bond is hydrolyzed (split):

   A. water is released from the peptide bond.
   B. water is added to the peptide bond.
   C. oxidation of the peptide bond occurs.
   D. reduction of the peptide bond occurs.

5. Primary structure of amino acids is:

   A. the sequence of amino acids.
   B. not found in quaternary proteins.
   C. coded for by DNA.
   D. all of the above.

6. Secondary structure of proteins is associated with:

   A. sequence of amino acids.
   B. not in globular proteins.
   C. coded for by DNA.
   D. α-helix.

7. Select the type(s) of bonding important in maintenance of tertiary structure of proteins.

   A. Hydrophobic
   B. van der Waals
   C. Covalent
   D. All are important

Problem Solving in the Biological Sciences   415

8. The highest level of protein structure found in monomeric globular proteins is:
   A. primary.
   B. secondary.
   C. tertiary.
   D. quaternary.

9. Which of the following would be considered a hydrophilic amino acid?

   A.

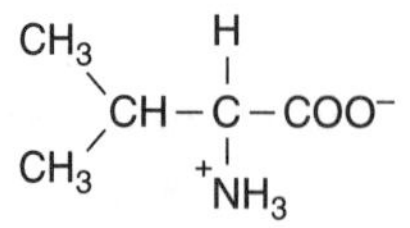

   B.

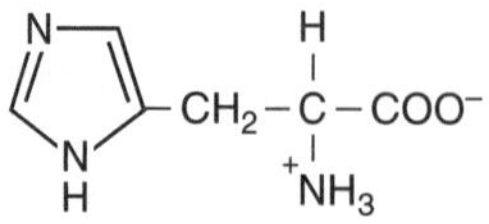

   C.

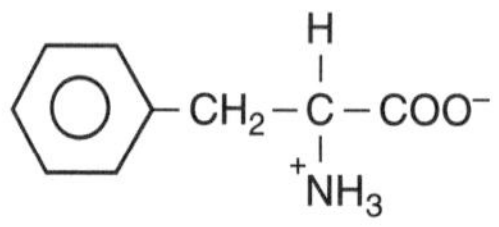

   D. None of the above

10. Select the basic amino acid.

    A. 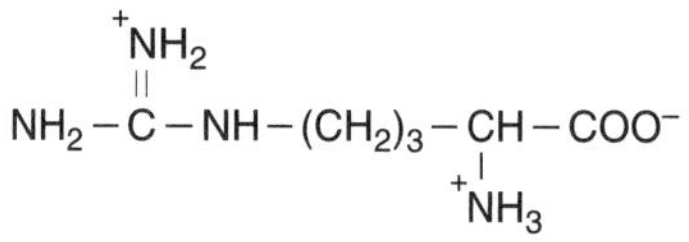 $NH_2 - \overset{\overset{+}{N}H_2}{\overset{\|}{C}} - NH - (CH_2)_3 - \underset{\overset{|}{\overset{+}{N}H_3}}{CH} - COO^-$

    B. $^-OOC - CH_2 - \underset{\overset{|}{\overset{+}{N}H_3}}{CH} - COO^-$

    C. $CH_3 - S - CH_2 - CH_2 - \underset{\overset{|}{\overset{+}{N}H_3}}{CH} - COO^-$

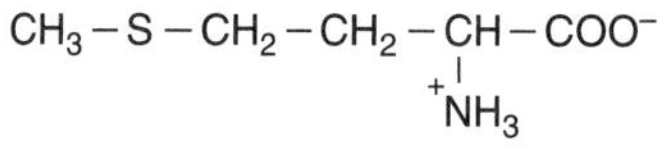

    D. None of the above

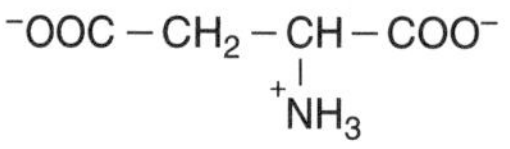

11. Select the acidic amino acid.

    A. 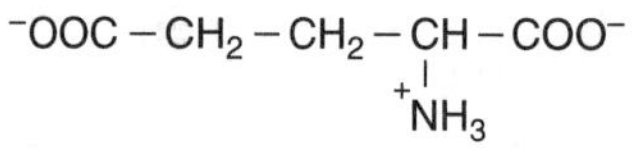 $^-OOC - CH_2 - CH_2 - \underset{\overset{|}{\overset{+}{N}H_3}}{CH} - COO^-$

    B. 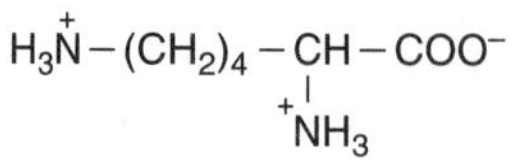 $H_3\overset{+}{N} - (CH_2)_4 - \underset{\overset{|}{\overset{+}{N}H_3}}{CH} - COO^-$

    C.

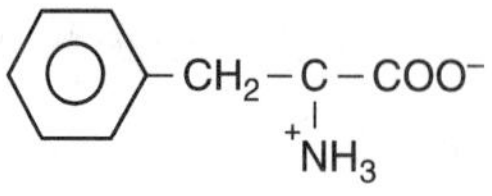

    D. None of the above

12. Which amino acid in question 11 will most likely be found on the interior of globular proteins?

A. A
B. B
C. C
D. D

13. Which of the following peptides has the highest pI?

A. 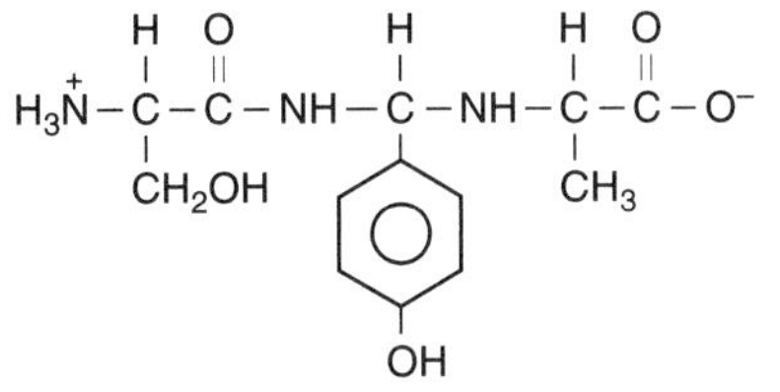 $H_3\overset{+}{N}-\underset{\underset{CH_2OH}{|}}{\overset{\overset{H}{|}}{C}}-\overset{\overset{O}{||}}{C}-NH-\underset{\underset{\bigcirc-OH}{|}}{\overset{\overset{H}{|}}{C}}-NH-\underset{\underset{CH_3}{|}}{\overset{\overset{H}{|}}{C}}-\overset{\overset{O}{||}}{C}-O^-$

B. $H_3\overset{+}{N}-\underset{\underset{CH_2COO^-}{|}}{\overset{\overset{H}{|}}{C}}-\overset{\overset{O}{||}}{C}-NH-\underset{\underset{\underset{COO^-}{|}}{\underset{CH_2}{|}}}{\overset{\overset{H}{|}}{C}}-\overset{\overset{O}{||}}{C}-NH-\underset{\underset{CH_2-imidazole}{|}}{\overset{\overset{H}{|}}{C}}-\overset{\overset{O}{||}}{C}-O^-$

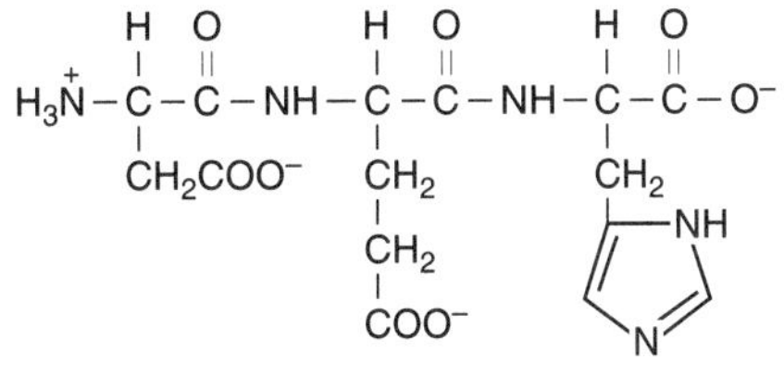

C. $H_3\overset{+}{N}-\underset{\underset{CH(CH_3)_2}{|}}{\overset{\overset{H}{|}}{C}}-\overset{\overset{O}{||}}{C}-NH-\underset{\underset{HO-CH-CH_3}{|}}{\overset{\overset{H}{|}}{C}}-\overset{\overset{O}{||}}{C}-NH-\underset{\underset{CH_2OH}{|}}{\overset{\overset{H}{|}}{C}}-\overset{\overset{O}{||}}{C}-O^-$

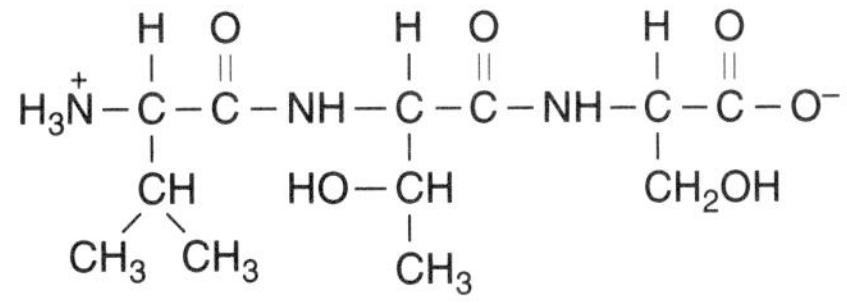

D. 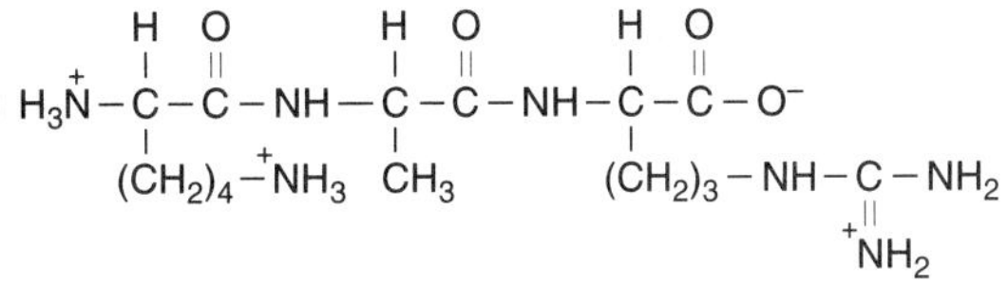 $H_3\overset{+}{N}-\underset{\underset{(CH_2)_4-\overset{+}{N}H_3}{|}}{\overset{\overset{H}{|}}{C}}-\overset{\overset{O}{||}}{C}-NH-\underset{\underset{CH_3}{|}}{\overset{\overset{H}{|}}{C}}-\overset{\overset{O}{||}}{C}-NH-\underset{\underset{(CH_2)_3-NH-C(=\overset{+}{N}H_2)-NH_2}{|}}{\overset{\overset{H}{|}}{C}}-\overset{\overset{O}{||}}{C}-O^-$

14. Which of the peptides in question 13 will migrate to the cathode at pH = 7.0?

A. A
B. B
C. C
D. D

15. Which of the peptides in question 13 will migrate to the anode at pH = 7.0?

A. A
B. B
C. C
D. D

16. Which disaccharide has the incorrect monosaccharide components listed beside it?

A. Maltose: mannose and glucose
B. Lactose: galactose and glucose
C. Sucrose: fructose and glucose
D. Cellobiose: two glucoses

17. Which compound is the reference for the relative configuration of sugars and amino acids?

A. D-glucose
B. D-glyceraldehyde
C. L-glycine
D. D-alanine

18. Both glycogen and cellulose are polymers of glucose. The main factor that makes them different is:

    A. cellulose has more glucose units.
    B. glycogen has more branch points.
    C. glycogen has α-1,4 bonds and cellulose has β-1,4 bonds between glucose units.
    D. cellulose has more glucose units and more branch points.

19. For monosaccharides, the ring forms (pyranose or furanose) are:

    A. acetals.
    B. hemiacetals.
    C. carbonyls.
    D. esters.

20. A triacylglycerol (TG-1) is hydrolyzed and the only fatty acid obtained has molecular formula $C_{16}H_{33}CO_2H$. The molecular formula of TG-1 is:

    A. $C_{53}H_{100}O_6$.
    B. $C_{51}H_{100}O_6$.
    C. $C_{56}H_{102}O_6$.
    D. $C_{54}H_{104}O_6$.

21. The most likely structural formula of the fatty acid from TG-1 is:

    A. $CH_3(CH_2)_{15}CO_2H$.
    B. $CH_3(CH_2)_6CH = CH(CH_2)_7CO_2H$.
    C. $CH_3(CH_2)_6CH(CH_3)(CH_2)_7CO_2H$.
    D. not determinable from the above information.

22. A second triacylglycerol (TG-2) is hydrolyzed and yields only one fatty acid whose molecular formula is $C_{16}H_{27}CO_2H$. In comparing the melting points of the acids from TG-1 and TG-2, melting point of TG-1 would be:

    A. higher.
    B. lower.
    C. about the same as the acid from TG-2.
    D. unpredictable; any result is possible.

23. The infrared spectrum of TG-1 would show absorption at which frequencies (cm^{-1})?

    A. 3500 and 1700
    B. 3500 and 2900
    C. 2900 and 1700
    D. 3500, 2900, and 1700

24. TG-1 is allowed to undergo partial hydrolysis to give a mixture of monoacyl and diacylglycerols (R is $C_{16}H_{33}$) as follows: I = $RCO_2 CH_2 CH(OH) CH_2OH$; II = $HOCH_2CH(O_2CR)CH_2OH$; III = $RCO_2 CH_2 CH(O_2CR) CH_2OH$; IV = $RCO_2CH_2 CH(OH)CH_2O_2CR$. Which of the glycerides can exist in enantiomeric forms?

    A. I and II
    B. III and IV
    C. I and III
    D. II and IV

25. The principal constituent of beeswax is $CH_3(CH_2)_{14}CO_2(CH_2)_{29}CH_3$. This compound is a lipid because it:

    A. has the ester functional group.
    B. is obtained from an animal.
    C. has a high molecular weight.
    D. can be extracted by organic solvents.

26. The hydroxyl group on carbon-3 of cholesterol is on an equatorial bond. If cholesterol is oxidized to a ketone and the ketone is reduced to an alcohol with an axial hydroxyl on carbon-3, what is the relationship between the isomeric alcohols?

    A. Enantiomers
    B. Diastereomers

    C. Anomers

    D. Meso compounds

27. The structures of the male hormone testosterone and the female hormone estradiol are shown. Which statement is true about the chemistry of these hormones?

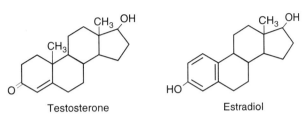

Testosterone   Estradiol

    A. Testosterone is the stronger acid; it has more stereoisomers than estradiol.

    B. Testosterone is the weaker acid; it has more stereoisomers than estradiol.

    C. Testosterone is the stronger acid; it has fewer stereoisomers than estradiol.

    D. Testosterone is the weaker acid; it has fewer stereoisomers than estradiol.

28. Which conditions are most favorable for the hydrolysis of an alkyl phosphate?

    A. Strongly acidic

    B. Strongly basic

    C. Neutral pH

    D. Strongly acidic or strongly basic

29. In a phosphorylation reaction, ATP reacts with an alcohol: ATP + ROH → ADP + ROP(OH)$_2$. In this reaction phosphorus is transferred from:

    A. an anhydride to an anhydride.

    B. an anhydride to an ester.

    C. an ester to an anhydride.

    D. an ester to an ester.

ANSWERS AND EXPLANATIONS

1–8. **1-D, 2-D, 3-B, 4-B, 5-C, 6-D, 7-D, 8-C.** See text for explanation.

9–11. **9-B, 10-A, 11-A.** Look at the R groups to determine the neutrality, basicity, acidity or hydrophilicity. See text for explanation.

12. C Hydrophobic amino acids are found on the interior. The amino acid in option C with the phenyl group is hydrophobic.

13. D A and C have only polar or hydrophobic amino acids, so their pI is around 7. B has two acidic amino acids and one amino acid that may be basic or acidic; therefore, its pI is less than 7. D has two basic amino acids and, therefore, has a pI greater than 7.

14. D The cathode attracts the positive ion. Therefore, the peptide must be positively charged at pH = 7.0. This means that the pI must be greater than 7 and must contain basic amino acids.

15. B The anode attracts the negative ion. Therefore, the peptide must be negatively charged at pH = 7.0. This means that the pI must be less than 7 and there must be an excess of acidic amino acids.

16–19. **16-A, 17-B, 18-C, 19-B.** See text for explanation.

20. D The triacylglycerol contains three C$_{16}$H$_{33}$CO$_2$ units and one CH$_2$CHCH$_2$.

21. A The common fatty acids are unbranched chains.

22. A The acid from TG-2 has three double bonds. Saturated acids have higher melting points.

23. C The infrared spectrum will show absorption for C—H (2900) and C=O (1700).

24. C The second carbon atoms are chiral in I and III only.

25. D Definition of a lipid.

26. B Only one chiral center is changed; others are unchanged.

27. B The phenol in estradiol is more acidic than the alcohol in testosterone; testosterone has more chiral carbon atoms.

28. A Base or neutral conditions change the esters to anions, which cannot be hydrolyzed.

29. B ATP is an anhydride (also ADP); the alcohol is converted to an ester of phosphoric acid.

Molecular Biology—DNA and RNA, Protein Synthesis

Self-Managed Learning Questions

1. How is information passed from deoxyribonucleic acid (DNA) to ribonucleic acid (RNA)?
2. How is information passed from RNA to proteins?
3. How is experimental research done to determine evidence for hydrogen bonds in DNA?
4. Analyze the denaturation and melting curves to determine the structure of DNA. Review experimental procedures and equipment related to:
   a. denaturation of DNA in alkali.
   b. denaturation of DNA by helix-destabilizing proteins.
   c. preparing filter-binding assays for renaturation.
   d. purification of complementary strands of DNA.
5. Understand concepts related to fragments in the replication fork. How are fragments detected?
6. Review several articles reflecting persuasive arguments in *Scientific American* magazine about molecular machines that control genes, genetic basis of cancer, and genetics of colon cancer. Review claims, evidence, and conclusions of each article and implied assumptions in each argument.

STRUCTURE AND COMPOSITION

DNA has the information that is the key of life. DNA remains constant and unchanged during mitosis and is responsible for transmitting genetic and hereditary information. DNA molecules contain biologically coded information that instructs cells to perform polypeptide synthesis. This information codes for the sequence of amino acids in proteins and is the sequence of nucleotides in DNA. DNA has a **helical structure** with sugar-phosphates as the backbone and with the nitrogen bases sticking off at more-or-less right angles (Figure 8-48). It is composed of two strands of nucleic acids running in antiparallel fashion (i.e., one strand goes 5′ → 3′ and the other 3′ → 5′). The nitrogen bases pair by hydrogen bonding, which holds the strands together. The nitrogen bases are paired by the matching up of hydrogen bonding sites and by space limitations in the double helix (proposed by James Watson and Francis Crick), which require a purine (two rings) and pyrimidine (one ring) to bond to each other. The more hydrogen bonds, the more stable is the nucleic acid. Hydrophobic bonds between the stacked nitrogen bases also stabilize the double helix. Most naturally occurring DNA molecules are right-handed helixes; that is, each strand follows a clockwise path.

Base-Pair Specificity

The bases of DNA are adenine (A), thymine (T), guanine (G), and cytosine (C), from which [A + G] = [T + C], or [purines] = [pyrimidines]. Adenine and thymine pair, forming two hydrogen bonds. Guanine and cytosine pair, forming three hydrogen bonds. The bases of one strand of DNA are hydrogen-bonded to the bases of the other DNA strand. Uracil replaces thymine in RNA, which may occasionally have pairing of strands. **Base pairing** is one of the most important features of DNA structure, because the base sequences of the two strands are complementary. If one strand has the base sequence AATGCT, the other has TTACGA, reading in the same direction. This is important for the replication of DNA because the replica of each strand is given the base sequences of its complementary strand. The base-pairing rule states that adenine always pairs with thymine (A:T or T:A) and cytosine always pairs with guanine (G:C or C:G).

DNA—THE GENETIC CODE

The **genetic code** is universal (all living organisms have the same code). The genetic code (triplet code) is 64 sets of sequences of three nucleotides each. Sixty-one of these

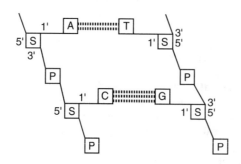

Fig. 8-48. Base pairing.

.... = Hydrogen bond

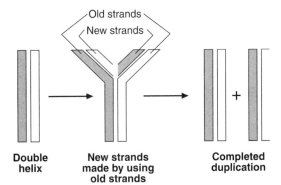

Fig. 8-49. Semiconservative replication.

Old strands
New strands

Double
helix

New strands
made by using
old strands

Completed
duplication

code for amino acids and three are punctuation marks (terminate protein chains). Some amino acids have only one triplet (methionine, tryptophan), whereas others have six (leucine). A gene or cistron is the sequence of triplets that codes for a single polypeptide chain. DNA is duplicated semiconservatively (using each strand as a template for the new DNA strand) by DNA polymerase from the 5′ to the 3′ end. Information on DNA is passed to mRNA (messenger RNA) by the process called **transcription**. Only one of the DNA chains is used, the enzyme is called **RNA polymerase**, and the direction of synthesis is from 5′ to 3′.

DNA is **duplicated** in a semiconservative fashion. That is, each strand serves as the template on which a new complementary strand is made (Figure 8-49). The actual process is very complicated and may occur at multiple sites along the DNA strand simultaneously.

RNA is involved in the manufacture of proteins. RNA molecules are much shorter than DNA molecules, but there are structural similarities between DNA and RNA. The important differences between DNA and RNA structures are as follow:

1. RNA usually has only one strand of nucleotides. The strand does not bond to a complementary strand as in a DNA molecule and hence does not form a helix.
2. The four bases in RNA are uracil, guanine, cytosine, and adenine. The base thymine is not found in RNA. Instead, uracil forms a complementary pair with adenine.
3. RNA nucleotides contain ribose sugars instead of deoxyribose sugars. The ribose sugars contain an extra oxygen atom.

The three types of RNA are mRNA (messenger RNA), tRNA (transfer RNA), and rRNA (ribosomal RNA). RNA is synthesized as a complementary copy of a DNA sequence.

Protein Synthesis

Protein synthesis (also called **biosynthesis)** is made of two subprocesses: transcription and translation. Link biological molecules (structure and chemistry) to the mechanics of transcription and translation. Each process of transcription and translation consists of three major steps: initiation, elongation, and termination or release of the biochain. The emphasis is to comprehend Crick's law of molecular biology. The law states that DNA information is passed onto the RNA, which, in turn, transfers it to the proteins.

Scientists have found that at least 20 different amino acids are used to make proteins. The following reasoning was used to justify that each codon is made up of three bases. If a codon was only one base long, mRNA could code for only four amino acids (both DNA and RNA have four bases). If a codon was two bases long, only $4^2 = 16$ amino acids could be coded. However, if a codon is three bases, $4^3 = 64$ arrangements are possible. Review in this book the math section on permutations, combinations, and probability to understand the fundamental principles of arranging four letters, three at a time. Scientific experiments also support the concept of a three-base codon. Table 8-1 lists amino acids and DNA codons, and Figure 8-50 shows the genetic code dictionary.

Transcription is the enzymatic process that uses genetic information in one DNA strand to specify a complementary sequence of bases in an RNA molecule. The three stages are initiation, elongation, and termination.

Initiation begins when a specific location is defined by short nucleotide sequences called **promotes**. Then, the protein subunit of RNA polymerase binds to the promoter, and strands of the DNA double helix start to separate and form mRNA. Elongation takes place when the RNA polymerase continues to catalyze the formation and elongation of mRNA. Termination occurs when nucleotide sequences serve to stop the reaction for RNA polymerase. A DNA molecule carries a series of regulatory commands throughout

TABLE 8-1. Amino Acids and DNA Codons

Terminaton Codons	ATT, ATC, ACT
Valine	CAA, CAG, CAT, CAC
Tyrosine	ATA, ATG
Tryptophan	ACC
Threonine	TGA, TGG, TGT, TGC
Serine	AGA, AGG, AGT, AGC, TCA, TCG
Proline	GGA, GGG, GGT, GGC
Phenylalanine	AAA, AAG
Methionine	TAC
Lysine	TTT, TTC
Leucine	AAT, AAC, GAA, GAG, GAT, GAC
Isoleucine	TAA, TAG, TAT
Histidine	GTA, GTG
Glycine	CCA, CCG, CCT, CCC
Glutamine	GTT, GTC
Glutamic Acid	CTT, CTC
Cysteine	ACA, ACG
Aspartic Acid	CTA, CTG
Asparagine	TTA, TTG
Arginine	TCT, TCC, GCA, GCG, GCT, GCC
Alanine	CGA, CGG, CGT, CGC

Fig. 8-50. The genetic code dictionary. *Ala* = alanine; *Arg* = arginine; *Asn* = asparagine; *Asp* = aspartic acid; *Cys* = cysteine; *Gln* = glutamine; *Glu* = glutamic acid; *Gly* = glycine; *His* = histidine; *Ile* = isoleucine; *Leu* = leucine; *Lys* = lysine; *Met* = methionine; *Phe* = phenylalanine; *Pro* = proline; *Ser* = serine; *STOP* = nonsense codons (UAA, UAG, UGA); *Thr* = threonine; *Trp* = tryptophan; *Tyr* = tyrosine; *Val* = valine.

	U	C	A	G	
5' end	Uracil	Cytosine	Adenine	Guanine	3' end
First position	Second position	Second position	Second position	Second position	Third position
U Uracil	UUU Phe UUC Phe UUA Leu UUG Leu	UCU Ser UCC Ser UCA Ser UCG Ser	UAU Tyr UAC Tyr UAA STOP UAG STOP	UGU Cys UGC Cys UGA STOP UGG Trp	U C A G
C Cytosine	CUU Leu CUC Leu CUA Leu CUG Leu	CCU Pro CCC Pro CCA Pro CCG Pro	CAU His CAC His CAA Gln CAG Gln	CGU Arg CGC Arg CGA Arg CGG Arg	U C A G
A Adenine	AUU Ile AUC Ile AUA Ile AUG Met	ACU Thr ACC Thr ACA Thr ACG Thr	AAU Asn AAC Asn AAA Lys AAG Lys	AGU Ser AGC Ser AGA Arg AGG Arg	U C A G
G Guanine	GUU Val GUC Val GUA Val GUG Val	GCU Ala GCC Ala GCA Ala GCG Ala	GAU Asp GAC Asp GAA Glu GAG Glu	GGU Gly GGC Gly GGA Gly GGG Gly	U C A G

First — Second — Third

all its stages. The final products of transcription are mRNA, tRNA, and rRNA (Figure 8-51).

Translation is the decoding of information that is contained in the mRNA transcript. The DNA code information in the nucleotide sequence of mRNA consists of sets of three nucleotides, or triplets, called **codons.** One end of individual tRNA molecules contains complementary triplet nucleotide sequences, called **anticodons,** that attach to specific codons during protein synthesis. The mRNA directs the sequence that links specific amino acids together to form proteins and related molecules. The three types of RNA have specific roles in the translation process. mRNA transfers the DNA code from the eukaryotic nucleus to the ribosomes, rRNA makes up a part of the ribosomes, and tRNA carries amino acids to the mRNA at the ribosomes. Ribosomes are complex, bead-like structures composed of three subunits of RNA and protein. One subunit has a binding site for mRNA and is the site of synthesis in the cytoplasm of polypeptides encoded by the mRNA. The other two subunits have tRNA binding sites. Translation follows a sequence including amino acid activation, initiation, elongation, and termination (Figure 8-52).

The **amino acid activation** process takes place in two steps (Figure 8-53). First, an amino acid reacts with ATP to create an enzyme-linked intermediate form, aminoacyl adenylic acid. In the second step, this acid is transferred to the amino acid accepting site of a specific tRNA molecule, and the activated amino acid is ready to participate in the

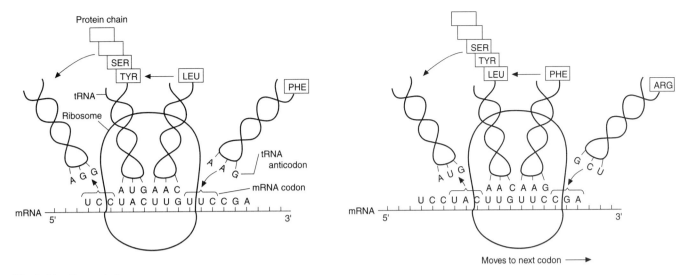

Fig. 8-51. Transcription.

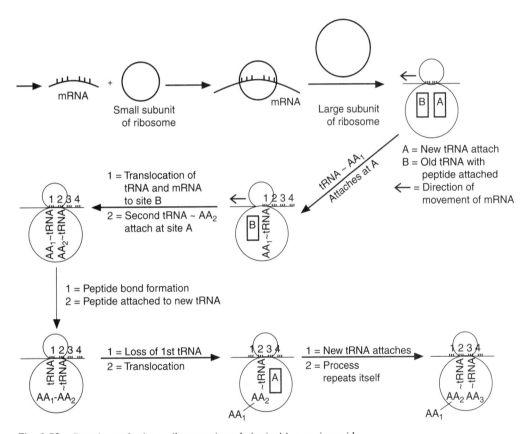

Fig. 8-52. Protein synthesis on ribosome (translation). *AA* = amino acid.

translation process. To begin the initiation step, an initiation complex must be formed. This involves binding a methionine carrying tRNA to the small ribosomal subunit. Proteins called **initiation factors** position the tRNA to ensure that the groups of three nucleotides (or reading frames) will be translated into protein. This complex binds to mRNA, and the large ribosomal subunit becomes attached and the initiation complex is completed. In the elongation phase, the ribosome moves along the mRNA transcript a distance that corresponds to the three nucleotides. An incoming tRNA places a new amino

Fig. 8-53. Activation of amino acid (*AA*) by activating enzyme (*AE*). ~ = energy bond.

$$AA + AE \longrightarrow AE - AA \sim Pi \xrightarrow{+ RNA} AE \genfrac{}{}{0pt}{}{AA \sim Pi}{tRNA} \xrightarrow{- AE} t\text{-}RNA \sim AA$$

acid on the growing chain. In the termination phase, a stop signal terminates the protein formation. The tRNA ~ amino acid dissociates from the enzyme and moves to a specific position on the large subunit. Another position on the large subunit is occupied by the last tRNA to attach and which binds the carboxyl end of the growing peptide chain. The tRNA molecule has at least three recognition regions, one for the activating enzyme and, hence, for the amino acid, one for the ribosome, and a sequence of three nucleotides called the **anticodon**, which pairs (hydrogen bonds) with the codon of the mRNA. Therefore, the anticodon of tRNA pairs with the codon of mRNA, and the next amino acid is in position for peptide bond formation, causing a transfer of the growing peptide to the new tRNA. After the peptide bond is formed, a translocation occurs, moving the newly attached tRNA peptide into the position previously occupied by the old tRNA-peptide. This latter tRNA is then displaced. A new codon is exposed on the mRNA for another tRNA amino acid to attach, and the process is repeated. The protein is made from the free amino end to the free carboxyl end. More than one ribosome may "read" an mRNA at a time—this creates polyribosomes (polysomes). Synthesis stops when one of the punctuation mark codons is reached. A gene (three nucleotides in this case) is on DNA, a codon is on mRNA, and an anticodon is on tRNA.

APPLIED CONCEPTS

Read laboratory reports, research findings, and current literature in addition to your college textbooks in this field. Genetic engineering is an ever-changing field with new findings emerging almost every day.

- Study the major differences between highly and moderately repetitive DNA.
- Understand DNA replication (biosynthesis) connected to DNA gyrase, ligase, polymerase, and topoisomerase—review terminology.
- Study fundamental research methods in modifications and repair of DNA as applied to genetic engineering and gene splicing.
- Apply Chargaff's rules to the genetic code including biochemical genetics and viral genetics.
- Understand viral mutations related to the functions and structural compositions of DNA and RNA.
- Read about current designs, methods, and evaluation of various genetic tests and special medical instruments to obtain electron micrographs, x-ray diffraction, nuclear magnetic resonance techniques, ultracentrifugation, autoradiographs.
- Understand denaturing and renaturing of DNA.
- Visit a clinical or molecular genetics laboratory; understand the working of a fully automated DNA synthesizer or gene machine, the chemicals that are used, and the organic reactions that take place.
- Compare the Watson-Crick model (traditionally proposed as a right-handed double helix) for DNA, which was challenged, and a new Z-DNA model (considered as a left-handed double helix) with special focus on assumptions (given and implied), molecular biology applications, and current research trends.
- Understand terms such as target and vehicle DNA, plasmids, genomes, modern DNA cloning techniques, and genetic repair.
- Use the genetic code dictionary as a guideline, study the definitions and usage of introns, exons, operons, template binding, supercoiled DNA, RNA polymerase, mutagen chemistry, nonsense suppressions as tRNA mutations.
- Understand the organic structure and function of various antibiotics such as tetracycline and streptomycin and how one molecule of these antibiotics suppresses the protein synthesis process.
- Read research reports and journals related to protein biosynthesis, molecular biology, and the relationship of protein biosynthesis to cytology for advanced terminology resources.

DNA AND RNA, PROTEIN SYNTHESIS: REVIEW QUESTIONS

1. Which of the pairs do not normally form hydrogen bonds in nucleic acids?

   A. Adenine-thymine
   B. Adenine-guanine
   C. Guanine-cytosine
   D. Adenine-uracil

2. Both DNA and RNA contain all the nitrogen bases except:

   A. guanine.
   B. adenine.

C. cytosine.

D. thymine.

3. The sugar found in DNA is:

   A. deoxyribose.

   B. ribose.

   C. dextrose.

   D. deoxyglucose.

4. Nucleic acids are composed of repeating units of:

   A. nucleotides.

   B. nucleosides.

   C. nitrogen bases.

   D. adenines.

5. Which is not a pyrimidine?

   A. Guanine

   B. Thymine

   C. Cytosine

   D. Uracil

6. DNA always differs from RNA by:

   A. forming hydrogen bonds between strands.

   B. having thymine and not uracil.

   C. being found only in the nucleus.

   D. having a sugar-phosphate backbone.

7. The following is one strand of a double helix of DNA (showing only nitrogen bases). What is the structure of its complementary strand? (A = adenine, G = guanine, T = thymine, C = cytosine, U = uracil)

A.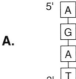

B.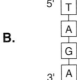

C.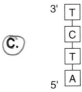

D.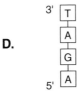

8. Given the following data, which organism probably has the most heat stable DNA?

Organism	(A + T)/(G + C) ratio
Mycobacterium phlei	0.49
Escherichia coli	1.02
Calf thymus	1.29
Bacteriophage T2	1.90

- **A.** *Mycobacterium phlei*
- **B.** *Escherichia coli*
- **C.** Calf thymus
- **D.** Bacteriophage T2

9. Methods to differentiate between DNA and RNA might involve all of the following except:

- **A.** reaction of ribose with orcinol under suitable conditions.
- **B.** ultraviolet absorption by nitrogen bases at 260 nm.
- **C.** chromatography to separate the different nitrogen bases.
- **D.** ^{14}C labeled uracil.

10. The genetic code is composed of sequences of:

- **A.** three nucleotides.
- **B.** three nucleosides.
- **C.** three amino acids.
- **D.** two amino acids.

11. The genetic code (triplet code) consists of 64 sets of three nucleotides each. Which statement is incorrect concerning the triplet code?

- **A.** The code is universal (i.e., all living organisms have the same code).
- **B.** All 64 triplets code for amino acids.
- **C.** More than one triplet can code for the same amino acid.
- **D.** A triplet may code for only one amino acid or termination codon.

12. Select the correct association.

- **A.** Duplication—synthesis of DNA using DNA as a template
- **B.** Transcription—synthesis of RNA using DNA as a template
- **C.** Translation—synthesis of proteins using information on RNA
- **D.** All of the above

13. Translation of the genetic code does not directly require:

- **A.** activated tRNA ~ amino acid.
- **B.** ribosomes.
- **C.** mRNA.
- **D.** DNA.

14. Select the incorrect association.

- **A.** DNA — codon
- **B.** mRNA — anticodon
- **C.** tRNA — gene
- **D.** All of the above

15. Translation is the synthesis of proteins using mRNA as a guide. All of the following statements are correct concerning translation except:

- **A.** mRNA initially binds to the small ribosomal subunit.
- **B.** the codon of tRNA pairs with the anticodon of mRNA.
- **C.** protein synthesis is from the free amino to the free carboxyl end of the protein chain.
- **D.** more than one ribosome may read a given mRNA at a time.

16. All of the following processes occur on the ribosome except:

- **A.** binding of mRNA to be "read" by tRNAs.
- **B.** activation of tRNA and its amino acid.
- **C.** peptide bond formation.
- **D.** binding of AUG codon with formyl methionine tRNA.

1–6. 1-B, 2-D, 3-A, 4-A, 5-A, 6-B. See text for explanation.

7. C The complementary DNA strand is the opposite of the given strand and must be $3' \rightarrow 5'$.

8. A The higher the percentage of G + C pairs, the higher is the heat stability because more hydrogen bonds (three per G + C pair vs. two per A + T pair) are present, making it more difficult to disrupt the double helix. This means that when the ratio $\dfrac{A + T}{G + C}$ is smaller, G + C is larger.

9. B The chemical differences between DNA and RNA must be sought and exploited. Answer A uses the fact that RNA contains ribose and DNA contains deoxyribose. Answers C and D use the fact that RNA contains uracil and DNA does not. Answer B measures nitrogen bases, in general, and does not distinguish between them and, therefore, could not distinguish between RNA and DNA. This method does distinguish between proteins and nucleic acids.

10–16. 10-A, 11-B, 12-D, 13-D, 14-D, 15-B, 16-B. See text for explanation.

Generalized Eukaryotic Cells

Self-Managed Learning Questions

1. How does molecular biology link with eukaryotic cell biology? Examine physics and chemistry of eukaryotes.
2. How is the cell membrane held together? Focus on dispersal of proteins among phospholipids. How do polar molecules pass through the cell membrane?
3. Why do substances need to move across the cell membrane? What functions do the cell membrane perform?
4. Do you understand the role of each organelle inside the cell? What happens to the eukaryote if ribosomes are missing, cytoplasm is missing, Golgi apparatus is missing, and so on?
5. What are the characteristics of polar, nonpolar, and amphipathic molecules? (Amphipathic molecules are slightly soluble in oil and water and highly soluble in ethanol.)
6. What is fluorescent antibody tagging? Review "The Rapid Intermixing of Cell Surface Antigens After Formation of Mouse-Human Heterokaryons" by D. L. Frye and M. Edidin (1970), published in *Journal of Cell Science*. What are the major assumptions, hypotheses, and conclusions of this research study? What are the limitations of the research study?
7. How can autoradiology be used to determine the structure of a replicating DNA molecule?
8. Design an experiment that would allow you to determine the rate at which the insulin receptor forms patches on the cell membrane.
9. How many chromosomes are present in a rat, crayfish, elephant, and pigeon.
10. Why do eukaryotic cells in animals not have cell walls? (Animal locomotion requires flexibility.)

INTRODUCTION

Learn the detailed structure and functions of eukaryotic cells (Table 8-2 and Figure 8-54). Connect the study of generalized eukaryotic cells to specialized eukaryotic cells such as neural cells (neurons), contractile cells (sarcomeres), epithelial cells, and connective cells. Evaluate the physical and chemical aspects of cell membrane transport models, ion channels, chromosome movement mechanics, cellular adhesion, and membrane receptors.

NUCLEUS: STRUCTURE AND FUNCTIONS

The nucleus is the largest organelle in the eukaryotic cell, and it functions as the control center of the cell (Figure 8-55). It is a large, round structure that is surrounded by the nuclear membrane and contains the nucleolus and chromosomes.

The nucleolus can be found within the nucleus; it consists of approximately 10% to 20% of the RNA and protein of the cell. There usually is only one nucleolus, but there may be several (the exact number of nucleoli is characteristic of a species). The nucleolus is composed of a meshwork of microfilaments and granules, and its primary function is to assemble ribosomes, although it may have other functions. During nuclear division, the nucleolus disperses and then reorganizes after division is completed.

There are two membranes that surround the nucleus of a cell, collectively called the **nuclear envelope**. The nuclear envelope regulates the flow of materials, mainly RNA and water-soluble molecules, into and out of the nucleus through nuclear pores, which are

TABLE 8-2. Anatomy and Physiology of Eukaryotic Cell Organelles

Name of Organelle	Structure (Physical and Chemical)	Function of Organelle
Cell membrane	Lipid bilayer with proteins distributed in mosaic pattern.	Protection; regulates passage of materials; maintains cell shape; communicates
Centrioles	Pair of hollow cylinders inside the centrosome; each consists of nine triple microtubules	Spindle formed between these structures during nuclear division
Chromosomes	Long thread-like structures comprised of DNA and proteins.	Contain genes that direct the structure and activity of the cell
Cilia	Surface specializations which project from the cell surface comprised of smaller microtubules.	Movement of cell and material outside of cell; ciliated cells lining respiratory tract keep mucus away from lungs; not present in all cells
Endoplasmic reticulum	Network of internal membranes that extend through cytoplasm	Transports materials between cells
Smooth	Outer surfaces lack ribisomes.	Produces steroids, lipid metabolism, detoxified drugs
Rough	Outer surfaces contain ribosomes.	Manufactures and transports proteins
Flagella	Hollow tubes that project from cell surface comprised of smaller microtubules.	Helps cellular locomotion; found only in spermatozoa in humans
Golgi complex	Layers of flattened membrane sacs.	Packages secretions and manufactures lysosomes
Lysosomes	Membranous sacs that contain digestive enzymes.	Release enzymes that break down worn parts
Microfilaments	Rod-like; consists of contractile protein.	Provide structural support; assist in cell movement
Microtrabecular lattice	Network of thin protein strands that form the cell framework.	Connects microtubules, organelles, and microfilaments into a unit; positions organelles
Microtubules	Hollow tubes constructed of tubulin protein.	Provide structural support; assist in cell movement; present in centrioles, cilia, and flagella
Mitochondria	Sacs comprised of two membranes. The inner membrane folds to form cristae.	Plays role in cell respiration; energy source for the cell.
Nucleolus	Nonmembranous, spherical body located inside nucleus and contains RNA and protein.	Assembles ribosomes and may have other purposes
Nucleus	Round structure surrounded by a nuclear membrane and located inside a cell. Contains nucleolus and chromosomes.	Main control center of the cell
Ribosomes	Particles composed of RNA and protein. Some are attached to the endoplasmic reticulum and some float freely in the cytoplasm.	Manufacture protein

channels used by the interior of the nucleus to communicate with the cytoplasm. At times, the outer membrane of the nuclear envelope folds outward into the cytoplasm and becomes part of the network of the **endoplasmic reticulum** (ER).

MEMBRANE-BOUND ORGANELLES: STRUCTURES AND FUNCTIONS

Cytoplasm is a watery milieu containing membrane-bound organelles, centrioles, and storage molecules (e.g., lipid droplets and glycogen). Enzymatic activity, or glycolysis, takes place in the cytoplasm.

Mitochondria are double-membraned organelles that produce ATP. The inner membrane is folded into cristae that contain the enzyme systems of electron transport and oxidative phosphorylation. The matrix contains a circular DNA molecule, prokaryotic type ribosomes, elementary bodies (ionic crystals), and enzymes of the Krebs cycle. Mitochondria replicate independently of the cell.

Lysosomes are single-membraned organelles containing acid hydrolases (digestive enzymes). Functions of lysosomes include digestion of the cell at death (autolysis), digestion of substances within the cell, and digestion of substances taken in by phagocytosis (heterolysis). Storage diseases result when one or more of the hydrolytic enzymes are absent or defective. Lysosomes are produced in the rough (granular) ER and packaged in the Golgi apparatus.

ER is a double-membrane system running throughout the cell. It probably breaks up and reforms and is continuous with the cell membrane and nuclear envelope. In this way, it is probably a precursor for other membrane systems and peroxisomes. Rough ER contains ribosomes on its surface and is involved in protein synthesis. Smooth ER (SER) is devoid of ribosomes and may serve several functions, a primary one being steroid synthesis. In the liver, SER plays an important role in the metabolism of endogenous small organic molecules, exogenous drugs, and toxins. In muscle, SER is called the **sarcoplasmic reticulum** and plays a role in impulse conduction and muscle contraction via calcium regulation. It may also have a storage function, storing starch in plants and glycogen in animals.

The **Golgi complex** is a collection of smooth membranes probably continuous with the

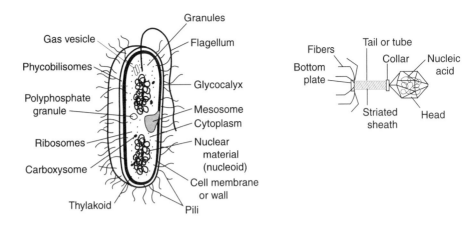

Prokaryotic cell

Bacteriophage

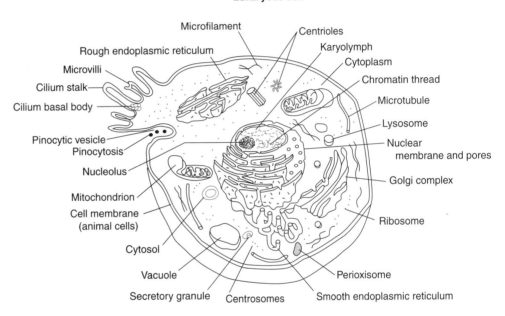

Eukaryotic cell

Fig. 8-54. Typical prokaryotic and eukaryotic cells and bacteriophage. (Adapted with permission from Bresnick SD: *Columbia Review Intensive Preparation for the MCAT.* Baltimore, Williams & Wilkins, 1996, p 374.)

SER. Its primary function is in packaging and secretion of proteins and polysaccharides. It also plays a role in synthesis of complex polysaccharides attached to proteins in the ER by the trimming and elongation of polysaccharides. All eukaryotic cells have one or more Golgi bodies. The Golgi body complex usually appears as a side view of a stack of pancakes.

Ribosomes are important in protein synthesis. They are composed of rRNA and protein, and are divisible into a large subunit and a small subunit. Cells are held together in tissues by junctional complexes. There are several types, but the most important are the tight junction (zonula occludens), desmosome (macula adherens, or spot weld), and gap junction (electronic couple). The tight junction is a zone of fusion between adjacent cells and precludes the passage of most molecules between cells (e.g., in the lining of the gut or kidney tubule cells). The desmosome is a small point of contact; there may be numerous desmosomes joining two adjacent cells (e.g., in a spinous layer of skin). Gap junctions are microchannels between adjacent cells that provide passage of ions and small molecules (e.g., in smooth muscle liver cells).

Peroxisomes have single membranes and are part of a group of organelles formerly called **microbodies**. They contain enzymes for the metabolism of oxygen or hydrogen peroxide. Peroxisomes are found in large numbers in the liver.

PLASMA MEMBRANE: STRUCTURE AND FUNCTION

Cell membranes are composed of lipids (e.g., cholesterol, phospholipids) and many types of proteins with distinctive functions (e.g., receptors, ion transporters, second messengers, enzymes, cell coat). Cell membranes vary greatly in composition depending on the cell type and their function. In general, the lipids form a bilayer (two molecules thick)

Nucleus

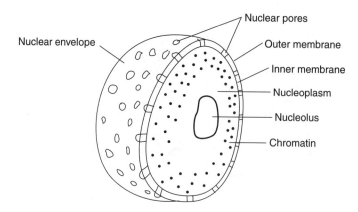

Fig. 8-55. Eukaryotic nucleus.

Close-up of nuclear pores

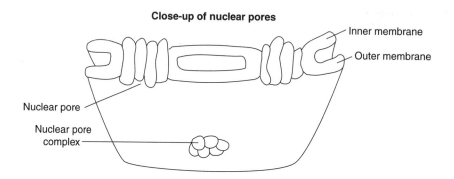

in which the polar ends of the lipid molecules (particularly phospholipids) extend outward and the nonpolar extend inward, adjoining each other (Figure 8-56). The lipid bilayer is interrupted by integral proteins that penetrate the width of the lipid bilayer. Smaller protein molecules may decorate the outer and inner sides of the lipid bilayer in very large numbers (e.g., molecules and enzymes of the electron transport chain in mitochondria) or relatively small numbers (e.g., membrane receptors and antigen recognition molecules on white blood cells).

Cell membranes may be quite fluid (membrane molecules readily flow—fluid mosaic model) or relatively rigid. The membrane becomes more rigid when cholesterol is substituted for phospholipids, when fatty acid chains of lipid molecules are saturated, or when there is a large number of protein molecules present on the inner and outer surface of the lipid bilayer. Even greater rigidity is possible when closely packed sheets of cells are held together by junctional complexes, microfilaments, or microtubules (Figures 8-57 and 8-58). Surface membrane coats such as the basal lamina further restrict membrane movement. Membrane proteins that contribute to membrane traffic include channel proteins and transport proteins.

Substances move through the membrane by diffusion, osmosis, facilitated diffusion, active transport, endocytosis, or exocytosis. **Diffusion** is the random movement of free

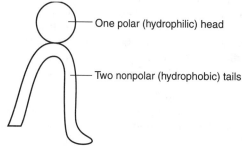

Fig. 8-56. Typical phospholipid
molecule.

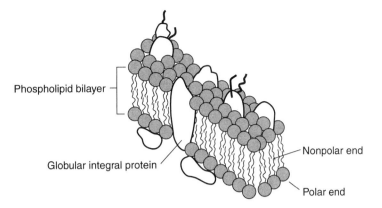

Fig. 8-57. Fluid mosaic membrane model.

Phospholipid bilayer

Globular integral protein

Nonpolar end

Polar end

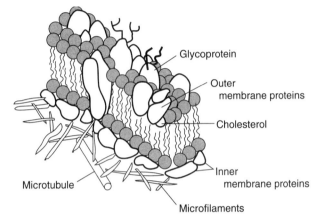

Fig. 8-58. Rigid membrane model.

Glycoprotein

Outer membrane proteins

Cholesterol

Inner membrane proteins

Microtubule

Microfilaments

molecules or ions or particles in solution or suspension under the influence of thermal motion toward a uniform distribution throughout the available volume. This can occur through cell membranes if the substance diffuses through the cell "pores." In diffusion, the net movement of solute is from the region of higher concentration to that of lower concentration. Small organic molecules (ethanol, glycerol), some ions (Cl^-), and H_2O are moved by diffusion.

Osmosis is diffusion through a semipermeable membrane. In osmosis, a solute cannot cross the membrane to equalize its concentration on both sides. This then creates a concentration difference for water across the membrane and the water diffuses in response to this to the side with the lower concentration of water (which is the side with the highest concentration of solute). Tonicity refers to relative concentrations of solute in two solutions. Isotonic means the two are equal. A hypertonic solution has more solute per unit volume than the reference. Osmosis (flow of solvent) occurs from hypotonic to hypertonic solution. If a red blood cell is placed in a solution less concentrated than itself (i.e., it is hypertonic), it swells until it hemolyzes (bursts). If the red blood cell is placed in a solution more concentrated than itself, it crenates (shrinks). **Osmotic pressure** is the hydrostatic pressure needed to oppose the movement of the solvent.

Facilitated diffusion is a process by which substances insoluble in a membrane are carried across the membrane with the concentration gradient by means of a carrier substance. Saturation kinetics are observed; that is, as the substrate concentration rises relative to the number of carrier molecules, the rate of transport levels off. Some sugars and amino acids are transported in this fashion.

Active transport is the process of moving molecules uphill against an electrochemical gradient; a carrier molecule is involved as well as the expenditure of energy (ATP). This system exhibits saturation kinetics and inhibition by inhibitors of energy production (e.g., cyanide or 2,4-DNP). An important active transport system is the Na^+–K^+ pump, which is responsible for maintaining the electric gradient of various membranes and neurons.

Other locations of active transport include the gut (for sugars and amino acids) and the kidney tubules (for secretion and reabsorption of ions and small molecules).

Endocytosis is a process by which large molecules are surrounded by plasma membrane and brought into the cell. Exocytosis is a reverse process whereby molecules are exported out of the cell. Endocytosis occurs as phagocytosis, pinocytosis, or receptor-mediated endocytosis.

Phagocytosis, also called "**cell eating**," is a process by which large particulate matter, bacteria, or even cells are engulfed by the cell membrane through invagination, forming a vesicle that is internalized. The vesicle then may combine with a primary lysosome to become a secondary lysosome (phagosome). The enzymes digest its contents. This is an energy-requiring process.

Pinocytosis is similar to phagocytosis but on a smaller scale. It occurs in response to proteins or strong solutions of electrolytes. It involves the uptake of liquids and is called "**cell drinking.**" This is an energy-requiring process.

Receptor-mediated endocytosis is carried out by the plasma membrane containing protein receptors that have ligand binding sites. Vesicles are formed between receptors and ligands, which, in turn, form endosomes. Ligands separate from the receptors and move to various points in the cell.

Plasma Membrane

In the plasma membrane, membrane channels are ion channels and pores that are formed by proteins in the lipid bilayer. Membrane channels allow the passage of ions, but they are selective, meaning that they may allow only one certain type of ion to pass through. Ions can move in either direction through a membrane channel. Examples of the types of membrane channels are potassium, sodium, chloride, and calcium channels. Membrane channels can be (1) voltage-gated, meaning they open or close depending on the voltage across the membrane; (2) chemically gated, wherein they open or close in response to the presence or absence of a specific chemical; and (3) nongated, meaning they are always open.

The **sodium-potassium pump** is found in all animal cells. It is a membrane glycoprotein. Its function is to repeatedly break down one molecule of ATP to ADP, bring two K^+ ions into the cell, and export three Na^+ ions. It also serves as an antiport, where two coupled solutes are transported in opposite directions. In step 1 of Figure 8-59, three Na^+ ions and one ATP bind to the protein pump. In step 2, ADP is released, causing a change in the conformation of the pump. In step 3, the three Na^+ ions are released and two K^+ ions bind to the pump. In step 4, Pi is released, which causes a change in the conformation of the pump, releasing the two K^+ ions. Then the process is repeated.

When cells have too much negative charge within them and the inside of the cell is more negative than the outside of the cell, the difference between the charges is called the **membrane potential.**

Membrane receptors are a site on the cell surface that is specialized to combine with a specific substance, such as a transmitter substance or a hormone. Receptor proteins work like switches (on–off) when particular substances bind to them. The receptors usually are arrayed at the plasma membrane, and some are located inside the cell. Receptors for a hormone called **somatotropin** switch the enzymes that crank up metabolic machinery for growth and division. Receptor malfunctions may contribute to forms of cancer and diabetes.

Cell adhesion molecules, which are membrane proteins, are essential to the formation of an adult organism. The function of these molecules is to help organize the cells into tissues. In an embryo, groups of cells that are about to migrate lose their specific adhesion molecules, but gain them again when they reach their new location. This way, the cells can move throughout the embryo and then reorganize into tissue.

CYTOSKELETON: STRUCTURE AND FUNCTION

Microfilaments are aggregated proteins with no lumen and may be important for maintenance of cell structure and cytoplasmic streaming. Microtubules are aggregated proteins with a lumen, may be important for intracellular transport and structure, and are inhibited by colchicine.

Cilia (see Figure 8-54) are long extensions of the plasma membrane that contain a highly ordered and coordinated set of microtubules. The cilia move mucus and debris from passageways (e.g., the trachea) in humans and provide locomotion in protozoans. At the cell surface, cilia are bound to the cell by centrioles (basal body or kinetosome).

Microvilli, which increase the surface area of the cells, are shorter, more numerous extensions of the plasma membrane found primarily in absorptive cells.

Flagella are longer than cilia, are used for locomotion, and are composed of a cylinder of nine paired microtubules with two unpaired centrally. They contain ATPase.

Centrioles are organelles that are used in cell (the nuclear membrane disappears)

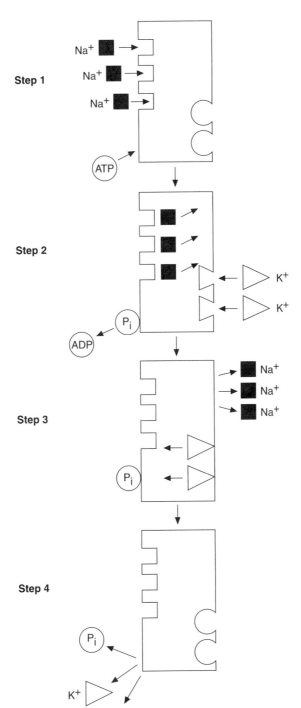

Fig. 8-59. Sodium-potassium pump. *ADP* = adenosine diphosphate; *ATP* = adenosine triphosphate.

division. They are found in all eukaryotic cells, including those cells that do not produce cells with cilia or flagella. Centrioles are hollow cylinders containing nine sets of triple-fused microtubules. They are located in a dense area of the cytoplasm known as the **centrosome** near the nucleus.

Mitosis

Mitosis occurs to maintain an optimal nucleus-to-cytoplasm volume ratio and to allow growth, cell replacement, differentiation, and specialization of cells in a multicellular organism. All human somatic cells are diploid and 2n. They contain twice as many chromosomes (46) and twice (2n) the haploid amount of DNA (n) to express the entire genome (i.e., 23 chromosomes—a set from each parent gamete).

Cell division involves the processes of cytokinesis (division of the cytoplasm, not discussed) and karyokinesis (division of the nucleus). The cell cycle is divided into four

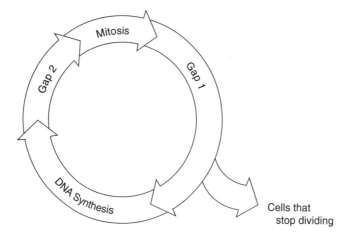

Fig. 8-60. Eukaryotic cell cycle.

phases (Figure 8-60). G₁ (Gap) is the first period of cell growth. It immediately follows cell division and precedes DNA replication (synthesis phase). G₂ follows DNA replication and precedes the M phase. M (mitosis) is the period of separation of the chromatids. Before each mitosis, the DNA is replicated (phase S) so that, when mitosis occurs, the daughter cells each retain twice the number of chromosomes as in the parent cell (e.g., 46 chromosomes in humans).

Interphase comprises G₁, S, and G₂. Prophase, metaphase, anaphase, and telophase are part of the M phase (Figure 8-61). In **prophase**, the DNA coils tightly and becomes visible as chromosomes. The nuclear envelope may disappear. The centrioles consist of a cylinder of nine sets of three tubules each, found near the nucleus in a region called the **centrosome**. The centrosome contains two copies of a pair of centrioles at right angles to each other. A pair of centrioles move to opposite poles of the nucleus and spindle fibers (microtubule structure) are formed from a region near them. In **metaphase**, the

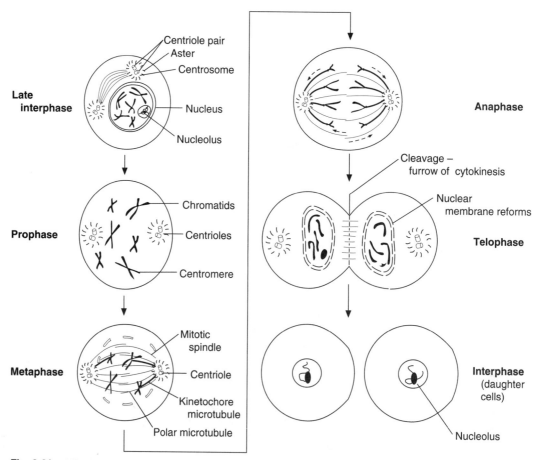

Fig. 8-61. Mitosis.

chromosomes arrange radially along the equatorial plane of the cell and the spindle fibers are attached to the centromeres of each chromosome (composed of two chromatids, each of which becomes a new chromosome after the centromere uncouples). In **anaphase**, individual chromosomes divide at their centromeres and each new resulting chromosome migrates to the opposite pole, being guided by the spindle fibers. Each chromatid of the chromosome at metaphase gives rise to a complete new chromosome after the centromeres uncouple. In **telophase**, the chromosomes uncoil, the nuclear envelope reforms, cytokinesis occurs, and the centrioles replicate themselves. The cell enters interphase.

Centrioles, as discussed previously, are hollow cylinders consisting of nine triple-fused microtubules. Early in prophase, the membranes of two pairs of centrioles separate and migrate toward opposite poles of the cell. Asters are star-like groupings of microtubules, composed mostly of protein, that extend outward in all directions from the centrioles. The microtubules that extend from the region surrounding the centrioles form mitotic spindles. These occur only in animal cells.

Chromatids are chromosomes that have not yet separated from their duplicates. The basic unit of a chromosome is a single double-stranded molecule of DNA that is complexed with numerous proteins. When this molecule doubles, the chromosome is then made up of two joined chromosomes, each containing one DNA molecule that is complexed with proteins. These twin chromatids are attached to each other at their centromere, a small circular zone that directs the movement of a chromosome during cell division. Telomeres can be found at the ends of chromosomes and contain moderately repetitive DNA. Kinetochores are three-layered structures that develop in the centromere late in prophase, one on each chromatid (Figures 8-62 and 8-63).

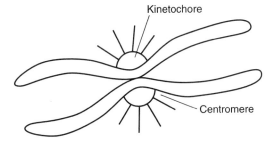

Fig. 8-62. Chromosome.

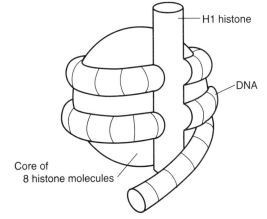

Fig. 8-63. Nucleosome.

During prophase, the nuclear membrane breaks down and allows the contents of the nucleus to blend with the cytoplasm. The nucleolus becomes disorganized and it is believed that the ribosomes that were contained in the nucleolus are released into the cytoplasm at this time. In telophase, a new nuclear membrane formed around each set of chromosomes is produced in part from the lipid components of the old nuclear membrane. Each centrosome serves as a mitotic center that organizes microtubules. Some microtubules, called **polar microtubules**, run between mitotic centers and lead to the developed spindle. Polar microtubules are unstable. Chromatin changes rapidly during prophase as a result of coiling, super coiling, and compacting. The later stages of prophase include development of kinetochores in the centromere region.

The condensed chromosomes start to move at the start of prometaphase. The nuclear envelope suddenly disintegrates into membranous sacs. The quick disintegration is activated by maturation–promoting factor (MPF) during mitosis. Clusters of microtubules called **kinetochore microtubules** associate with the kinetochores. The polar microtubules break down, and others from the same or the opposite pole attach to the kinetochore microtubules.

The chromosome is pulled around randomly until the kinetochore of one chromatid is connected to microtubules from one pole, while the kinetochore of the second chromatid is connected to microtubules from falling apart. The polar microtubules pull until the kinetochores approach a region halfway between the ends of the mitotic spindle. The cell reaches metaphase when all the kinetochores arrive at the equatorial plate. The arms of chromosomes drag along passively as the kinetochores are pulled apart. During anaphase, the poles of the mitotic spindle are pushed farther apart by some polar microtubules. This leads to the separation of daughter chromosomes. It takes approximately the energy for hydrolysis of 20 ATP molecules to move a chromosome from the equatorial plate to the pole.

Meiosis

Meiosis has two phases (Figure 8-64). The first, a reductional division, is different from mitosis. In prophase I, the replicated DNA coils to become the chromosome, and there is exact pairing (synapsis) of the pairs of homologous chromosomes, allowing crossing over to occur. The nuclear envelope disintegrates, and the centrioles migrate to opposite poles of the nucleus. In metaphase I, the two members of the homologous pair align along the equatorial plane. The disposition of the maternal and paternal members of the pair toward either pole is random. The spindle fibers attach to the centromere of only one member of each homologous pair. In anaphase I, chromosomes of each homologous pair separate by moving toward opposite poles, and the centromeres do not uncouple. In telophase I, cytokinesis occurs. In spermatocytes, the distribution of the cytoplasm is equitable, giving two cells of equal size. In oocytes, the division is unequal, giving one secondary oocyte and one polar body. In interphase I, there is a short period in which chromosomes may uncoil somewhat and the nuclear membrane may be partially reconsti-

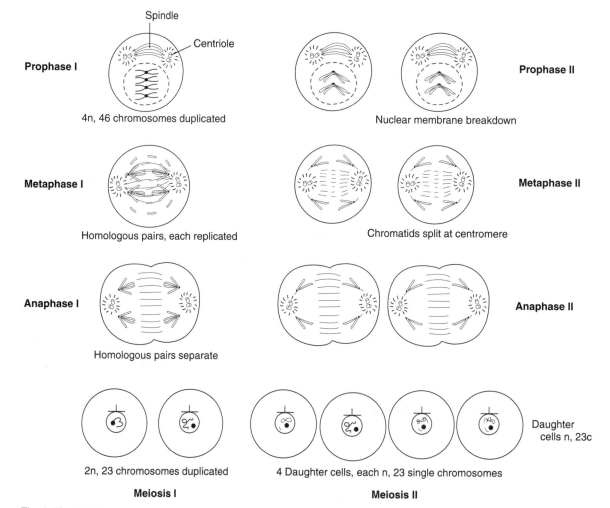

Fig. 8-64. Meiosis.

tuted. The daughter cells then contain the haploid number of chromosomes, each composed of two daughter chromatids. Prophase II, metaphase II, and anaphase II are all like the corresponding mitosis phases. Telophase II is like mitosis but with haploid cells.

APPLIED CONCEPTS

- Recognize and understand the following terms:
  - —specificity, saturation, and competition in mediated transport
  - —cell inclusions, e.g., glycogen, melanin pigment, and hemoglobin
  - —problems in basic physiology related to tonicity (isotonic, hypotonic, hypertonic) and calculation of osmolarity and osmolality
  - —integral and peripheral proteins (compare and contrast), cristae, cisternae (*trans*, medial, and *cis*), nucleosome, microtrabeculae, autophagy, hyaluronic acid, metastasis, autocrine motility factor (AMF), megakaryocytes, macrophages, polypeptide growth factor, interleukin, fibrils, and connective tissue (embryonic, adipose, reticular, vascular)
  - —random growth of cancer cells, malignant tumors, chemotherapy procedures
- Learn the definitions (including structure and function) of the following mitotic and meiotic terminology: mitotic spindle, cleavage furrow, astril fibrils, asters, telomeres, kinetochores, and nuclear membrane breakdown.
- Learn mechanistic differences between mitosis (somatic cell division) and meiosis (reproductive cell division), e.g., stages in prophase, which are leptonema, zygonema, pachynema, diplonema, and diakinesis.

GENERALIZED EUKARYOTIC CELLS: REVIEW QUESTIONS

1. Eukaryotes are characterized by all of the following except:
   A. genetic material within a nuclear envelope.
   B. organelles bound within membranes.
   C. presence of cell walls made of murein.
   D. subcellular structural units to carry out specific functions.

2. "Contains DNA or RNA, no means of energy production, cannot reproduce self directly" would be a description of:
   A. an animal cell.
   B. a plant cell.
   C. a bacteria.
   D. virus.

3. Which is not a feature of the unit membrane model of the cell membrane?
   A. Continuous lipid bilayer present
   B. Globular proteins floating in lipids
   C. Hydrophobic ends of lipids not in contact with water
   D. Continuous protein bilayers outside lipid layer

4. The concept of "cell drinking" refers to:
   A. phagocytosis.
   B. pinocytosis.
   C. both phagocytosis and pinocytosis.
   D. neither phagocytosis nor pinocytosis.

5. The substance(s) not ordinarily found in cell membranes is(are):
   A. globular proteins.
   B. phospholipids.
   C. DNA.
   D. cholesterol.

6. Active transport is due to:
   A. thermal diffusion.
   B. concentration gradient variations.
   C. phagocytosis.
   D. Na^+–K^+–ATPase pump.

7. Which of the following is not a function of smooth endoplasmic reticulum?
   A. Metabolism of drugs and toxins in the liver
   B. Synthesis of proteins

    C. Conduction of impulses in muscle

    D. Synthesis of steroids

8. Chloroplasts are:

    A. found only in prokaryotes.

    B. vestigial structures in animal cells.

    C. responsible in producing negative ions.

    D. used during photosynthesis.

9. Mitochondria are responsible for:

    A. transport of molecules.

    B. protein synthesis.

    C. cell replication.

    D. energy production.

10. Synthesis of proteins occurs in the:

    A. lysosomes.

    B. Golgi bodies.

    C. mitochondria.

    D. rough endoplasmic reticulum.

11. Centrioles:

    A. exist in the nucleus.

    B. constitute chromosomes.

    C. make microvilli.

    D. form spindle fibers during cell division.

12. Facilitated diffusion:

    A. enables carrier substances to carry molecules across the membrane.

    B. can go against a concentration gradient.

    C. requires energy.

    D. is a result of saturation kinetics.

13. If container A has a higher concentration of a solute than container B and they are separated by a semipermeable (to solute) membrane, then:

    A. nothing happens because the membrane is only semipermeable.

    B. solute particles move from B to A.

    C. solvent moves from B to A.

    D. solvent moves from A to B.

14. What probably limits the size that a cell may attain?

    A. Surface area

    B. Volume of a cell

    C. Balance of surface area and volume

    D. Specialization of the cell

15. Which structure is found in eukaryotes but not prokaryotes?

    A. Ribosomes

    B. Mesosomes

    C. Cell walls

    D. Mitochondria

16. Which structure or molecule is not found or made in the nucleus of eukaryotes?

    A. Nucleolus

    B. Microsomes

    C. tRNA

    D. Chromatin

17. If red blood cells are put into a hypertonic solution, they will:

    A. remain the same size.

    B. hemolyze.

    C. swell up.

    D. shrink.

18. Which structure does not play a part in motion of cells?

    A. Microvilli
    B. Cilia
    C. Flagella
    D. Pseudopods

19. Which of the following substances probably would not cross a membrane by simple diffusion?

    A. Ethanol
    B. Chloride ion
    C. Glucose
    D. Water

20. Synapsis and crossing over of chromosomes occur in which phase of meiosis?

    A. Interphase I
    B. Prophase I
    C. Prophase II
    D. Metaphase I

21. When do the centromeres divide in meiosis?

    A. Anaphase I
    B. Anaphase II
    C. Telophase I
    D. Telophase II

22. The correct sequence of steps in mitosis is:

    A. prophase, metaphase, interphase, anaphase, telophase
    B. interphase, anaphase, metaphase, prophase, telophase
    C. interphase, prophase, metaphase, anaphase, telophase
    D. anaphase, prophase, interphase, metaphase, telophase

23. Which is not true about the cell cycle?

    A. There are typically four phases, G1, G2, S, and M.
    B. Interphase corresponds with the M phase.
    C. S is the phase of DNA synthesis.
    D. M is the phase of cell division.

24. Which is not true about mitosis?

    A. It can maintain an optimal nucleus to cytoplasm volume ratio.
    B. It can allow growth of organisms.
    C. It has phases of karyokinesis and cytokinesis.
    D. It results in haploid daughter cells when the parent cells are diploid.

25. The chromosomes become coiled and visible and the nuclear membrane disintegrates. This is what phase of mitosis?

    A. Interphase
    B. Prophase
    C. Metaphase
    D. Telophase

26. The key difference in anaphase I of meiosis and anaphase of mitosis is:

    A. crossing over occurs in anaphase I of meiosis.
    B. centromeres divide in anaphase I of meiosis.
    C. homologous chromosomes move to opposite poles in anaphase I of meiosis.
    D. all of the above.

27. A key difference in the mechanism of mitosis and meiosis is that:

    A. mitosis has crossing over of homologous chromosomes during prophase.
    B. meiosis has a second duplication of DNA during interphase I.
    C. meiosis has alignment of homologous chromosomes in metaphase I and separation of homologous chromosomes in anaphase I.
    D. mitosis has a reductional division.

28. The main difference in the outcome of mitosis versus meiosis is that:

    A. meiosis produces identical daughter cells and mitosis produces different daughter cells.
    B. mitosis occurs only in vertebrates.
    C. meiosis produces somatic cells.
    D. meiosis results in haploid cells and mitosis results in diploid cells when the parent cells are diploid.

29. The primary oocyte remains arrested in what phase of meiosis from birth to puberty?

    A. Prophase I
    B. Prophase II
    C. Metaphase I
    D. Metaphase II

1–12. 1-C, 2-D, 3-B, 4-B, 5-C, 6-D, 7-B, 8-D, 9-D, 10-D, 11-D, 12-A. See text for explanation.

13. C The solvent moves across the semipermeable membrane from the side where it is more concentrated and the solute is less concentrated (side B) to the side where it is less concentrated and the solute is more concentrated (side A). This is osmosis.

14. C The nutritional and energy requirements and waste production of a cell are proportional to the volume of the cell. The volume of a cell is proportional to a linear dimension (l = length) cubed, i.e., l^3. The flux (i.e., the exchange rates) of materials in (nutrients) and out (wastes) is proportional to the surface area of a cell. The surface area is proportional to a linear dimension squared, i.e., l^2. As the cell increases in size (as volume increases), the requirements, given by l^3, increase much more rapidly than supply and waste removal, given by l^2. Hence, a balance between surface area and volume is required such that supply (and waste removal) can keep in balance with cell requirements.

15. D Membrane-bound organelles are not found in prokaryotes (e.g., the mitochondrion). The cell walls (also in plants) and mesosomes (invaginations of cell membrane) are found in prokaryotes. Ribosomes are found in both, although the structures are different.

16. B Microsomes are artifacts produced from the endoplasmic reticulum during cell homogenization and centrifugation. Nucleolus and chromatin are parts of DNA. All RNA, including tRNA, are made from the DNA template in the nucleus.

17. D The solvent (water) flows from the hypotonic (red cells) to the hypertonic solution by osmosis.

18. A Pseudopods are cytoplasmic extensions that aid in motion as found in the amoeba. Microvilli are evaginations (outpouches) of the cell membrane that increase its surface area and function to permit more area for flux of materials in and out of cells, as is necessary in the gut.

19. C Some ions, lipid soluble substances, and very small molecules (such as ethanol, glycerol, and urea) can diffuse through membranes. Polar molecules, ions (especially cations), and larger molecules must enter by other processes.

20–29. 20-B, 21-B, 22-C, 23-B, 24-D, 25-B, 26-C, 27-C, 28-D, 29-A. See text for explanation.

Specialized Eukaryotic Cells

Self-Managed Learning Questions

1. Draw a chart highlighting the major similarities and differences among neural cells, contractile cells, epithelial cells, and connective cells.
2. Explain the advantages and disadvantages of freeze-fracture and freeze-etch techniques used to analyze cell organelles.
3. What are gap junctions? How do they hold epithelial cells together. What role do tight junctions play in this respect?
4. Is the neuromuscular junction a chemical synapse? Why? Can you demonstrate it using a conceptual model and hypothesis?
5. What are excitatory and inhibitory synapses?
6. What are glial cells? List several functions of glial cells.

NEURAL CELLS AND TISSUE

Histologically, the nervous system is composed of neurons and glial cells. Neurons conduct impulses, and glial cells provide some sort of supportive function. There are many kinds of neurons and glial cells—only a typical neuron is discussed here. A neuron has

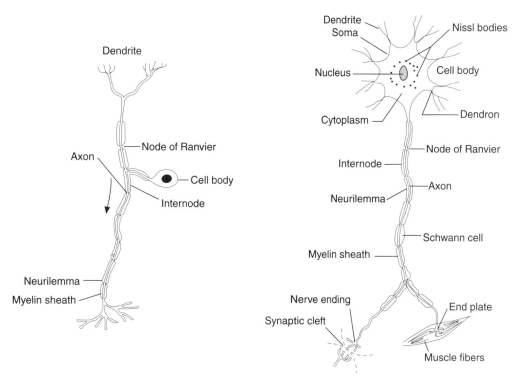

A   B

Fig. 8-65. (A) Neuron, type I. (B) Neuron, type II.

a cell body or soma that is characterized by having Nissl bodies (ribosomes), one or more short branched projections of the body called **dendrites**, and, usually, one long projection called an **axon** (Figure 8-65).

There are three special types of **neurons:** sensory, motor, and association. Sensory neurons transfer impulses from the various sense organs to the spinal cord or brain, such as happens when a person picks up a hot frying pan. Association neurons transfer and connect the messages between the sensory neurons and the motor neurons. They are located in the brain and spinal cord. Association neurons transfer impulses similar to a switching station at a telephone exchange. In the case of the hot frying pan, the impulse travels from the spinal cord to motor neurons, with the help of association neurons. Motor neurons transfer impulses to various muscles and glands. Again, in the case of the hot frying pan, the impulse travels along motor neurons to muscles in the arm. This causes the muscles in the arm to retract and the frying pan to be dropped. The brain then receives the impulse, causing the person to feel pain.

Myelin sheaths (tightly wrapped insulators made of cell membranes of glial cells) around axons increase the speed of conduction (saltatory conduction). Schwann cells are found outside the central nervous system; they are specialized glial cells that form sheaths around some neurons. On some axons, Schwann cells form the cellular sheath and the myelin sheath.

The myelin sheath of an axon is not continuous; between Schwann cells are gaps called **nodes of Ranvier**. An axon can fire action potentials at the nodes of Ranvier, but, in the areas of the myelin sheath where there are no nodes of Ranvier, the electric charges cannot cross the membrane. Therefore, the current flows to the next node of Ranvier and is depolarized; it is thus conducted down the axon by flowing from node to node.

Synapse

Impulses can travel in either direction in a dendrite or an axon; dendrites usually convey impulses toward the soma, and axons usually convey impulses away from the soma. Do not confuse impulse travel direction with ion transport direction. The nervous system contains approximately 150 billion neurons. Direction is achieved by the presence of **synapses** between adjacent neurons or a neuron and an effector (muscle or gland). Synapses typically include an axon ending with a transmitter substance, a synaptic cleft, and a dendrite, muscle, or gland with receptors for the transmitter substance.

Resting Potential, Action Potential

An impulse causes the axon to release the chemical transmitter, which diffuses across the cleft to the receptors and induces an impulse there, which is then transmitted. An impulse or action potential is set up in a neuron when the **potential difference** (voltage) across its membrane reaches a threshold potential. The resting potential of a neuron is determined by the balance of Na^+ (most outside) and K^+ (most inside) on each side of the cell membrane—the outside is positive relative to the inside. An impulse or transmitter substance can disturb the ionic balance in such a way that Na^+ moves inside and K^+ moves outside (only Na^+ moves in the early phase of the action potential). This causes the cell potential to move toward the threshold potential. Once the threshold potential is reached, the action potential is initiated and moves down the neuron to the axon end, releases the transmitter, and the process repeats in the next neuron. The refractory period is that time during which the nerve cannot respond to a stimulus. An Na-K-ATPase maintains the concentration across the nerve membrane by active transport of the ions. See Figures 8-66 and 8-67.

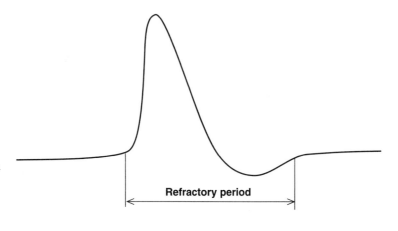

Fig. 8-66. Various potentials of a nerve.

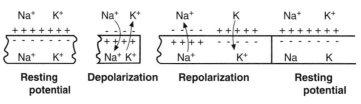

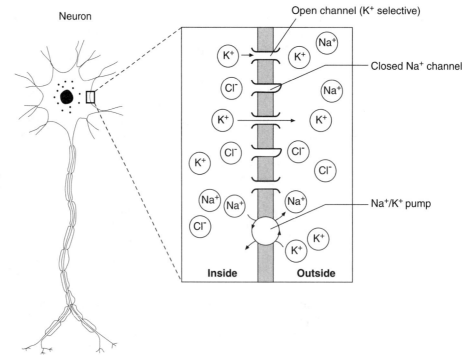

Fig. 8-67. Ineractive ion pumps and channels.

CONTRACTILE CELLS AND TISSUES

Striated, Smooth, and Cardiac Muscle

Skeletal muscle consists of multinucleated cells (striated) fused together to form a single cell called a **syncytium**. Smooth muscle is composed of distinct spindle-shaped uninucleated cells. Cardiac muscle is composed of uninucleated cells joined together by a sawtoothed array of junctional complexes (including extensive gap junctions), termed the intercalated disc, which speeds impulse conduction.

Sarcomere

A **sarcomere**, the functional unit, is limited by regions that anchor the actin (thin filaments) called the **Z-lines**. Myosin (thick filaments) alternate with the actin and are not anchored. Bands are labeled as shown in Figure 8-68.

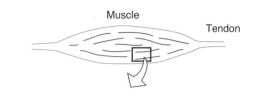

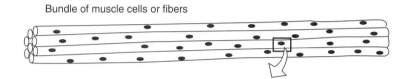

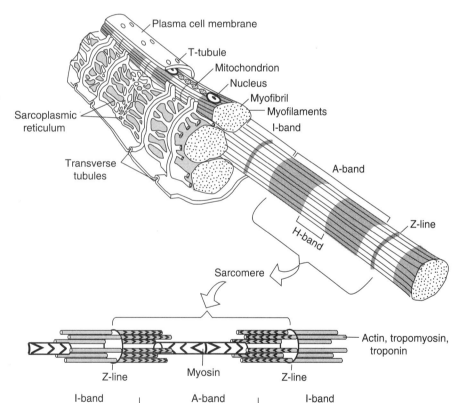

Fig. 8-68. Components of a sarcomere (skeletal muscle).

Calcium Regulation of Contraction

Calcium is important for muscle contraction. When the muscle contracts, the Z-lines move together, the I- and H-bands decrease in size, and the A-band remains the same size. The actin complex is composed of actin, tropomyosin, and troponin. Actin has sites that bind to heavy meromyosin when contraction occurs. Tropomyosin is an α-helical protein wound around the actin (which is two intertwined α-helical chains) and blocks the myosin binding site. Troponin is a regulator protein bound to tropomyosin and has a site for binding Ca^{2+} and a site that inhibits myosin from binding to actin. When there is no Ca^{2+} present, the troponin and tropomyosin prevent myosin binding and, hence, contraction. When Ca^{2+} is present, the Ca^{2+} binds to troponin, causing a conformational change, which, in turn, causes tropomyosin to shift, uncovering the actin binding region for myosin, and contraction proceeds. Myosin is composed of light meromyosin (the tail) and heavy meromyosin (the head). The head binds to actin and contains an ATPase to break the bonds to actin. Contraction is caused by the alternating action of the heads of myosin binding and releasing actin in a ratchet-like fashion. The sarcolemma (cell membrane of muscle) sends a system of membranes (T-tubules) into the muscle. When an impulse from a nerve reaches the sarcolemma, it is transmitted down the T-tubules, which release Ca^{2+} into the sarcoplasm (muscle cell interior) for contraction. The sarcoplasmic reticulum (specialized smooth endoplasmic reticulum), which abuts upon the T-tubules, removes the Ca^{2+} from the sarcoplasm.

EPITHELIAL CELLS AND TISSUES

Simple Epithelium and Stratified Epithelium

Epithelial cells line a body cavity or an exterior body surface. They fit tightly together and form a continuous layer, barring the movement of dissolved materials through the space between the cells. Examples of epithelial tissue are the outer layer of the skin, the linings of the digestive and respiratory tracts, and the lining of kidney tubules. A simple epithelium consists of a single layer of cells, such as the lining of the stomach. A stratified epithelium consists of many layers of cells, such as the outer layer of the skin.

CONNECTIVE CELLS AND TISSUES

Major Cell and Fiber Types

Tendons, ligaments, cartilage, vertebral discs, tooth dentin, the dermis of the skin, and the mesentery of the gut are all **connective tissues**. Most connective tissues consist of cells embedded in an extracellular matrix. Bone is considered a special connective tissue because the extracellular matrix has been hardened by mineral deposits (calcium). Connective tissue differs from the other three basic kinds of tissue (nervous, muscle, and epithelium) in that connective tissue is largely secretory material. The secreted molecules are extremely diverse. Collagen is the most prevalent molecule in connective tissue (basically three peptides wrapped around each other like a rope). There are at least 12 different kinds of collagen (types I to XII). Other major components of connective tissue are chondroitin sulfate proteoglycan, heparan sulfate proteoglycan, hyaluronic acid, lipoproteins, glycoproteins, and phosphoproteins. In all but special connective tissues, the cell that synthesizes and secretes all these molecules is termed a fibroblast (*fibro* = fiber, *blast* = former). Other cells present in connective tissue are the endothelial cells of blood vessels, macrophages (histiocytes), lymphocytes, and mast cells.

Loose Versus Dense Connective Tissue

Loose connective tissue is the most common. It consists of fibers strewn randomly through a semifluid matrix. Its flexibility allows the parts that it connects to move. Dense connective tissue is strong and less flexible than loose connective tissue. Dense connective tissue is mainly made up of collagen fibers. In regular dense tissue, the collagen fibers have a definite pattern. In irregular dense tissue, the collagen fibers are arranged in bundles that are distributed randomly throughout the tissue.

Cartilage

Cartilage cells construct a mineralized cartilage matrix scaffolding and then die. The scaffolding is partially removed by multinucleated cells, or **osteoclasts**. Bone-forming cells (**osteoblasts**) accompanied by capillaries invade the remainder of the mineralized scaffolding and begin to secrete bone. Some osteoblasts become osteocytes (bone maintenance cells) when, in the process of bone formation, they become totally surrounded by secreted bone matrix. Osteoblasts and osteocytes are tethered together through gap junctions that form between their numerous cell processes.

Extracellular Matrix

The **extracellular matrix** that surrounds animal cells consists of a meshwork of polysaccharides that are permeated by fibrous proteins. Collagen is the most common protein in the extracellular matrix. This matrix holds the cells together as tissues, and, in turn, the cells secrete the extracellular matrix and establish its orientation.

APPLIED CONCEPTS

- Understand the biochemistry of multiple sclerosis with emphasis on the deterioration of myelin sheaths at irregular intervals along the axon.
- What is "sprouting" and how does it help in regeneration of an injured neuron?
- What is the serum myoglobin test and the urine myoglobin test? Review the structure of myoglobin found in skeletal and cardiac muscle cells. Is myoglobin released into the bloodstream after a muscle tissue injury? Usually, the reference normal values are 12–90 ng/mL for serum myoglobin in an adult.

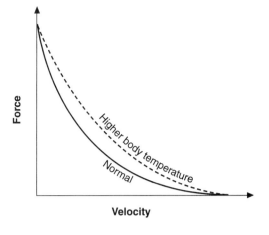

Fig. 8-69. Muscle force versus velocity.

Force

Higher body temperature

Normal

Velocity

- Analyze the muscle force versus velocity graph (Figure 8-69) based on temperature increase between a normal and an exercising muscle (neuronal functions similar to muscle functions).

SPECIALIZED EUKARYOTIC CELLS: REVIEW QUESTIONS

1. All of the following are specifically associated with a neuron except:

    A. lack of a nucleus.
    B. Nissl bodies.
    C. dendrites.
    D. axons.

2. What entity of neurons allows for one-way conduction of impulses in the nervous system?

    A. Axons
    B. Dendrites
    C. Synapses
    D. Somas

3. Which of the following can usually conduct impulses away from the neuron cell body or toward it?

    A. Axon
    B. Dendrite
    C. Both
    D. Neither

4. When the potential difference across a nerve membrane equals the threshold, what results?

    A. An action potential
    B. Synthesis of transmitter substances
    C. Destruction of transmitter substances
    D. Nothing until the resting potential is exceeded

5. What ion(s) determine the resting potential of a nerve cell?

    A. Sodium
    B. Potassium
    C. Calcium
    D. Both **A** and **B**

6. The concentrations of ions across the cell membrane is maintained by:

    A. Diffusion.
    B. Active transport.
    C. Osmosis.
    D. Facilitated transport.

7. Myelin sheaths are found:

    A. Surrounding tendons.
    B. Covering the brain.

C. Covering muscles.
D. Around axons of neurons.

8. During the early phase of the action potential:

   A. only Na^+ moves.
   B. only K^+ moves.
   C. Na^+ moves into the cell and K^+ moves out.
   D. Na^+ moves out of the cell and K^+ moves in.

9. The refractory period occurs:

   A. before threshold is exceeded.
   B. before the action potential.
   C. after the action potential.
   D. roughly during the action potential.

10. Select the muscle type composed of distinct cells.

    A. Smooth
    B. Skeletal
    C. Cardiac
    D. Both **A** and **C**

11. The A-band of striated muscle represents:

    A. myosin only.
    B. actin only.
    C. both **A** and **B**.
    D. neither **A** nor **B**.

12. The Z-line as seen in striated muscle anchors:

    A. both actin and myosin.
    B. neither actin nor myosin.
    C. actin.
    D. myosin.

13. During muscle contraction, all of the following occur except that:

    A. Z-lines move together.
    B. A-band decreases in size.
    C. I-band decreases in size.
    D. H-band decreases in size.

14. Which of the following ions is of most importance in the mechanical contraction of muscle?

    A. Na^+
    B. Ca^{2+}
    C. K^+
    D. Cl^-

15. Troponin:

    A. binds Ca^{2+}.
    B. binds to tropomyosin.
    C. inhibits binding of myosin to actin.
    D. performs all of the above functions.

ANSWERS AND EXPLANATIONS

1–9. 1-A, 2-C, 3-C, 4-A, 5-D, 6-B, 7-D, 8-A, 9-D. See text for explanation.

11. C Technically, the band is visible as such because of the myosin, but within the limits of the band, actin is also present.

12-15. 12-C, 13-B, 14-B, 15-D. See text for explanation.

Microbiology

Self-Managed Learning Questions

1. Review the Gram stain experiment and what the hypotheses and assumptions are behind the laboratory procedure of Gram-positive and Gram-negative bacteria. What are the chemical compounds used in the staining procedure? Understand

the chemistry of peptic-doglycan and how the plasma membrane is covered by peptidoglycan.

2. Review how physicians or clinical scientists test antibiotic susceptibility using the tube dilution method and the disk diffusion method. Compare and contrast the hypotheses, assumptions, conclusions, and observational errors of both methods.
3. Visit a clinic to enhance understanding of the scientific principles in obtaining cultures of blood, stool, throat, sputum, urine, and some wounds. Understand the physical design and working of a syringe and how much sample is drawn in different patients. Analyze and assess contamination of specimens and how they cause inaccurate results.
4. Read about the basic differences among the following: (1) Eastern equine encephalitis virus, (2) California equine encephalitis virus, (3) Venezuelan equine encephalitis virus, (4) Western equine encephalitis virus. Name the diseases caused by each of these viruses.

VIRAL STRUCTURE AND LIFE HISTORY

Learn the structures, life history, and sources of disease for bacteria, bacteriophage, virus, and fungus. Viruses are usually called **"nonliving"** and differ from bacterial and other "living" organisms because they (1) do not contain both DNA and RNA, (2) have no metabolic machinery for energy production or protein synthesis, (3) do not develop from other viruses but depend on the host's metabolic machinery to synthesize them, and (4) have no membranes to regulate exit and entry of substances. A **virion** is the form of a virus existing outside of a host cell. A **viroid**, similar to a virus, infects plants, and contains only a single strand of RNA and no protein coat. The process by which a virus causes disease is **pathogenesis** and its capacity to produce illness or death is known as **virulence**. **Tropism** is the capacity of a virus to selectively enter and infect cells.

Nucleic Acid (DNA and RNA) and Protein Components

Structurally, most viruses consist of a protein coat (**capsid**) surrounding a core (center) of nucleic acids, which are encoded with genetic information and composed of either DNA or RNA.

Typical Bacteriophage Structure and Function

Some viruses specifically attack bacteria and are called **bacteriophages** (Figure 8-70). Bacteriophages, in general, consist of a head made of a protein coat and a core (as discussed), as well as a tail made of protein, which is specialized for attaching to bacteria. A bacteriophage attaches to the surface of a bacteria, the core of RNA or DNA is injected into the bacteria, and the protein coat remains on the surface. The cycle then may proceed as described for viruses and is called **lytic** or **virulent**.

The bacteriophage nucleic acid may become combined with the bacterial nucleic acid, however, and remain as such for long periods before new bacteriophages are produced and cell rupture occurs. In this case, the bacteriophage is called **lysogenic** or **temperate**. The nucleic acid from the bacteriophage is called a **prophage**. Newly released bacteriophages may contain some bacterial nucleic acid, which may be passed on to other bacteria when they are attacked by these bacteriophages. This is the mechanism of transduction.

Rickettsiae multiply by binary fission, contain both RNA and DNA, and have both synthetic and energy-producing enzyme systems; they are classified as bacteria.

Size Relative to Bacterial and Eukaryotic Cells

Viruses are simpler in structure than bacteria; they are so simple that they cannot be called cells. Viruses are specific, with each type attacking only one or a limited number of host species and causing a definite disease with characteristic symptoms. Most viruses are antigenic, causing animal hosts to produce antibodies that aid in recovery and protect

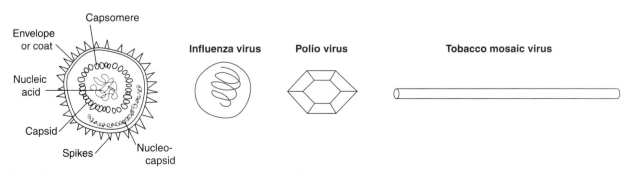

Fig. 8-70. Typical virus and several common viruses (about 100 nanometers in diameter).

against later attacks. Viruses are also particulate. In other words, as extracted for study, viruses consist of a liquid in which ultramicroscopic particles are suspended. These particles range in size from 10 to approximately 300 nm. Most viruses that cause animal infections are spherical. Viruses are more resistant to injurious conditions, such as heat, dryness, and disinfectants, than are the vegetative cells of bacteria, but they are less resistant than bacterial spores.

Generalized Phage and Animal Virus Life Cycles

There are many variations of the basic life cycle of a virus. A cell may have a special receptor or region that is recognized by the virus and to which the virus attaches. Although receptor binding of virus to cell may be exhibited, subsequent steps in the viral life cycle also must be successful for infection to occur. The virus may enter the cell via a process similar to phagocytosis (steps 1 and 2 on Figure 8-71). In the cell, the central core of DNA or RNA and occasionally special enzymes or proteins take over the host's metabolic machinery to produce new coat proteins and new viral DNA or RNA. This may occur in the nucleus, the cytoplasm, or both (see step 3 on Figure 8-71). The viral coat and viral core (DNA or RNA) then combine to form complete viral particles (see step 4 on Figure 8-71). At a certain point, the host cell lyses (bursts) and releases the new viral particles as well as uncombined viral coats and viral cores (see step 5 on Figure 8-71). Sometimes, the viral particles exit by a process similar to reverse phagocytosis and incorporate part

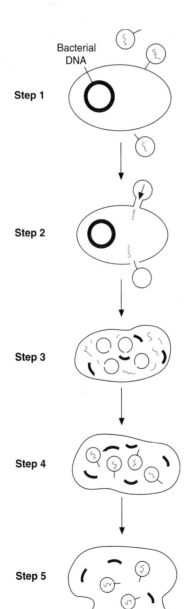

Fig. 8-71. Sequence of viral infection of a cell.

of the host's cell membrane onto their protein coat in doing so. This is typical of a virus that attacks an animal or plant cell. Once inside the animal host, the primary methods by which viruses reach target organs are via the lymphatic system, the bloodstream, or the nerves. The presence of the virus in the blood is called **viremia**. Continued viral infection depends on the balance between ongoing viral replication and host defense mechanisms (i.e., viral clearance and neutralizing antibodies). Antiviral treatment in humans is designed to disrupt viral binding or entry into the cell or to interfere with DNA or RNA replication.

PROKARYOTIC CELLS

Eukaryotes differ from prokaryotes in that eukaryotes have membrane-bound structures. The eukaryote is, thus, divided into a cell membrane, cytoplasmic region, and nuclear region.

Cell Structure and Physiology

Prokaryotes differ from eukaryotes in that eukaryotes have (1) genetic material in a nucleus and DNA conjugated with proteins, (2) organelles bound within membranes, (3) subcellular structural units to carry out specific functions (e.g., ATP production, photosynthesis), and (4) cell walls made of cellulose or chitin rather than murein (amino sugars and amino acids) as in prokaryotes. The DNA of prokaryotes is found in a nonmembrane region called the **nucleoid**. Enzymes for metabolism and energy production are either free in the cytoplasm or bound to the cell membrane, and the ribosomes are smaller than in eukaryotes. Viruses are neither prokaryotes nor eukaryotes but constitute a group unto themselves. Prokaryotic cells have no well-defined nucleus. Examples are bacteria and cyanobacteria (blue-green algae). They are subdivided into four groups: (1) **Gracilicutes** (gram-negative bacteria), (2) **Firmicutes** (gram-positive bacteria), (3) **Tenericutes** (mycoplasmas), and (4) **Mendosicutes** (Archaeobacteria).

Bacterial Life History

The general characteristics of bacterial structure are discussed under prokaryotes. More specifically, from outside in, a bacterium may have a capsule, which is usually made of a polysaccharide mucoid material and protects the bacterium from phagocytosis. Inside the capsule is the cell wall, which prevents a hypertonic bacterium from bursting. Inside the cell wall is the cell membrane, which may contain invaginations called **mesosomes**, where localization of enzymes concerned with similar functions may be found. The cytoplasm and nucleoid are as previously described. The DNA is circular and haploid. Some bacteria contain flagella for locomotion—these are structurally different from their eukaryotic counterparts.

Bacteria have three common shapes: cocci (spherical or ovoid), bacilli (cylindrical or rod-like), and spirilla (helically coiled). The cocci are often found in clusters: diplococci (two bacteria together), streptococci (linear chains of cocci), or staphylococci (grape-like clusters of cocci). All of these are made up of individual bacteria with distinct cell walls.

Metabolically, bacteria are aerobic or anaerobic. Anaerobic bacteria may use fermentation (in which an organic molecule such as pyruvate or lactate is the final electron acceptor) or inorganic substances as final electron receptors (such as $S \rightarrow H_2S$). An **obligate anaerobe** is one that is killed if exposed to oxygen, usually because it cannot handle the highly toxic peroxides produced in oxidative metabolism. A **facultative anaerobe** can survive in the presence or absence of oxygen. Bacteria may use a variety of molecules as nutrients. Some are photosynthetic, others are heterotrophic (using organic molecules made by other organisms), still others are chemosynthetic (making organic molecules and energy from inorganic precursors). The last group is important in fixation of nitrogen for use by all organisms. The variety of metabolic nutrients required and products produced is extremely important in studying basic genetics and biochemistry, as well as in differentiating among the different types of bacteria.

Most bacteria reproduce asexually by binary fission, which produces two identical haploid daughter cells by the simple process of mitosis. Genetic recombination (e.g., transfer and rearrangement of genetic information) may occur by three distinct means: transformation, transduction, and conjugation. **Transformation** involves a bacterium picking up free DNA from a medium, the free DNA being from a different bacterium. **Transduction** is the transfer of parts of DNA between bacteria by bacteriophages. In **conjugation**, there is pairing of "male" and "female" forms. DNA is passed sequentially between them via structures called **pili**. All or a fraction of the DNA may be passed in this way. These three genetic mechanisms allow extraordinary adaptability and variability of bacteria. Because bacteria can reproduce in as little as 20 minutes, a new trait, such as drug resistance, can spread rapidly in a given population.

FUNGI

Fungi are composed of eukaryotic cells, are plant-like, but contain no chlorophyll. They are unicellular (e.g., yeast) or multicellular (e.g., molds, mushrooms) with little differentiation into tissue types. They are parasitic (survive upon living organisms) or saprophytic (survive upon dead organic matter), and they can digest food extracellularly by the excretion of digestive enzymes before absorbing them or can absorb already digested foods. Multicellular fungi tend to be filamentous with individual filaments called **hyphae**. Masses of hyphae are called **mycelia**. Fungi are important as causes of disease, in spoilage of food and materials, as decomposers of dead organic matter, as sources of food (mushrooms), in food production (bread yeast, cheese molds), and in alcohol production.

Life History and Physiology

Reproduction is by sexual or asexual means (or both) with the latter predominating. The specific cycles vary among the different groups of fungi. Various sexual stages include ascus formation (has haploid spores), basidium (2n) formation, or fusion of special cells to form zygotes (2n). Asexual structures or stages include the spores (n), the sporangium (n), and the conidia (n). These are either spores or give rise to spores. The sporangium and conidia arise from specialized hyphae. A general scheme for the life cycle of a typical fungus is shown in Figure 8-72. Spores can result from sexual or asexual reproduction.

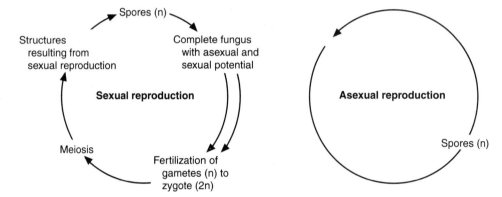

Fig. 8-72. Life cycle of a typical fungus.

APPLIED CONCEPTS

- Understand the significance of bacteria in medicine (size of bacteria, distinction as gram-positive or gram-negative, and multiplying ratio and rate) such as for Pseudomonadales, Eubacteriales, Spirochaetales, Actinomycetales, Rickettsiales, and Mycoplasmatales.
- Recognize and understand the following terms: bacterial cytoplasm, movement of bacterial DNA (intercellular movement by conjugation, transduction, and transformation), endospores, auxotrophs, bacterial surface analysis (study of extracellular gels and slimes causing stickiness to surfaces), bacterial infections (laboratory procedures such as incubation and basic treatment methods of salmonellosis, shigellosis, and staphylococcal and streptococcal infections).
- Understand the medical usage of terms such as specific immunity; cellular immunity (T lymphocytes) and humoral immunity (B lymphocytes); cytotoxic T cells; heterophilic antigens; agglutination (Weil-Felix test); opsonization; IgA, IgD, IgE, IgG, IgM; allergies and hypersensitivities; Coombs test; immunohematology Ouchterlony test; radial immunodiffusion procedure; viroids, prions, and virusoids.
- Study to conceptualize energy, T cells, and how two signals are used before they attack an invading virus (e.g., applications in renal transplants, hay fever); also study hybridomas (i.e., how cells are created in the laboratory).
- Compare and contrast DNA viruses (herpesviruses, poxviruses, rhabdoviridae, togaviridae). Review the laboratory cultivation and analysis techniques (e.g., inoculation techniques, electron microscope analysis of biopsies, and darkfield microscope analysis).
- Study the life cycles and current research papers on viral cancer, Epstein-Barr virus, papilloma virus, human T-cell leukemia-lymphoma-virus-1, and life history of fungi to substantiate blastomycosis, histoplasmosis, and rhinosporidiosis.
- Identify the basic sterilization and disinfection tests, such as the phenol coefficient test, tissue toxicity test, and use-dilution test, as well as air and liquid filtration systems and ultraviolet radiation sterilization and physical sterilization (ultra-high heat) methods.

Read the following information as comprehension of text (information presentation passage):

The **acquired immune deficiency syndrome** (AIDS) is transmitted by the **human immunodeficiency virus** (HIV). Two forms of HIV have been identified, HIV-1 and HIV-2. HIV-1 is the more common form. The primary modes of transmission include sexual transmission, parenteral exposure, and perinatal transmission. Individuals at highest risk for HIV infection include homosexual and bisexual men, persons with hemophilia, blood transfusion recipients, intravenous drug abusers, sex partners of individuals carrying the virus, and children born to mothers with HIV. Not all patients with HIV have AIDS. According to the Centers for Disease Control (CDC) definition, a person is characterized as having AIDS if that person has the HIV virus and exhibits one of 23 specific symptoms, such as specific types of pneumonia, cancer, or fungal or parasitic infections. This definition is disease based, whereas a new definition, which is undergoing a period of public comment, is laboratory based. Under the new definition, patients would be considered to have AIDS if their T4 lymphocytes (white blood cells whose levels are reflective of immune system function) are less than 200 (normal levels are approximately 1000). The acute stage of infection with HIV may be associated with a mononucleosis-like illness (fever, lymphadenopathy, sweats, myalgia, rash, sore throat, nausea, headache). Symptoms are generally nonspecific, however, causing little discomfort and passing unnoticed. T4 levels are normal at the time of infection. During the early stage, the patient may be asymptomatic, having persistent generalized lymphadenopathy (enlargement of the lymph nodes), aseptic meningitis, dermatologic manifestations, and T4 levels greater than 400. During the middle stage, the patient may continue to be asymptomatic, having persistent generalized lymphadenopathy, thrush, hairy leukoplakia, or idiopathic thrombocytopenic purpura. At this stage, T4 levels range from 200 to 400. During the late stage, **opportunistic infections** (infections seen primarily in individuals with an impaired immune system) develop, as do malignancy (e.g., Kaposi's sarcoma), wasting, and dementia; T4 levels are below 200.

The HIV is an RNA retrovirus in the lentivirus family. Lentiviruses are characterized by slow progression of infection and persistence of the virus despite the host's immune response. They frequently have a lengthy incubation period before symptoms develop. The interval from the time of infection with HIV to development of the clinical disease averages approximately 10 years. The HIV antigen (foreign material to which the body's immune system reacts), however, can be detected within 1 to 4 weeks and HIV antibodies (molecules formed to fight specific antigens) can be detected within 3 to 12 weeks after infection.

Structurally, the HIV has a dense cylindrical core that encases two molecules of the viral RNA. The core is surrounded by a spherical lipid envelope that is acquired as the virion buds from the surface of an infected cell. HIV contains three structural genes—one for the viral core, one for the enzymes involved in viral replication, and one for the envelope proteins. The outer envelope of the HIV binds to the CD4 molecule, which is expressed on the surface of T4 cells and monocyte-macrophages (these cells are essential components of the human immune system; T4 cells activate other T cells, natural killer cells, macrophages, and B cells, which produce antibodies). When the virus invades a human cell, it makes copies of its genes and splices them into the genes of the cell. The infection may enter a latent phase until cellular activation occurs. Upon activation, the genes force the cell to complete the formation of a new HIV and to release a mature virion from the surface of the cell via budding. The ultimate result of HIV infection is a profound immunosuppression caused by depletion and functional abnormalities of the CD4+ T cell, which leads to the development of opportunistic infections. The immune system normally responds to a viral infection by sensing the protein coat of an invading virus and attacking the invader. In the case of AIDS, the immune system successfully controls the infection for years but, for unknown reasons, is unable to clear it. Over time, there is a progressive decline in the quality and function of the CD4+ population, and the infection ultimately progresses. As a result, immunity cannot be generated against opportunistic pathogens to which the patient ultimately succumbs. Therapy for AIDS includes antiretroviral agents that inhibit HIV replication (e.g., zidovudine [AZT], ddI, ddC) or interfere with the binding of HIV to CD4+ cells. But, it is unlikely that antiretroviral treatment will eradicate the virus in an infected person because the virus exists in a dormant state for an indefinite period. Therefore, vaccines may be the best approach to preventing HIV transmission, infection, and disease progression. Vaccines that stimulate the immune system after infection with HIV but before the development of AIDS are under evaluation, as are vaccines for administration to patients at high risk of exposure to HIV.

1. Bacteriophages:

   A. cause disease in humans.
   B. are viruses.
   C. are bacteria.
   D. can reproduce by binary fission.

2. Select the substance not ordinarily found in viruses:

   A. Carbohydrates
   B. Proteins
   C. RNA
   D. DNA

3. Viruses:

   A. are considered to be living organisms.
   B. consist of protein, lipids, and carbohydrates only.
   C. do not arise from other viruses directly.
   D. have an incomplete metabolic machinery for energy production.

4. In the replication of a virus in a host cell:

   A. the virus directs the metabolic machinery of the host.
   B. the host directs synthesis of new viral particles.
   C. viral particles are made as a single unit (i.e., coat and core).
   D. coat and core structures are released from the host and then combined.

5. Structurally, bacteriophages differ from the usual virus by:

   A. having a protein coat.
   B. having a core of DNA or RNA.
   C. being able to replicate independently of a host cell.
   D. having a tail region made of protein for attaching to cells.

6. The part of the cycle of a bacteriophage that may be different from that of a typical virus is:

   A. the taking over of the host cell's metabolic machinery.
   B. incorporation of its nucleic acid into the host cell's nucleic acid.
   C. lysis of the host cell.
   D. synthesis by the host cell of coat and core separately and then combining to form a complete particle.

7. Which structure may protect a bacteria from phagocytosis by white blood cells?

   A. Mesosome
   B. Capsule
   C. Nucleoid
   D. Cell wall

8. Select the incorrect association.

   A. cocci—spherical
   B. bacilli—rod-like
   C. diplococci—two cocci
   D. staphylococci—linear combinations of cocci

9. The process whereby a bacterium picks up DNA from a medium and incorporates it into its own DNA is called:

   A. binary fission.
   B. conjugation.
   C. transformation.
   D. transduction.

10. Bacteria transfer (exchange) genetic information among themselves by all methods except:

    A. transformation.
    B. transduction.
    C. budding.
    D. conjugation.

11. Methods used to distinguish among various bacteria types may include all of the following except:

    A. shape.
    B. nutrient requirements.
    C. products of metabolism.
    D. antiseptic surgery.

12. A form of hepatitis (inflammation of the liver) is caused by a virus. The serum of patients with hepatitis may contain antigens from the virus, HBsAg (hepatitis B surface antigen) and HBcAg (hepatitis B core antigen). (An antigen is a substance foreign to the body capable of eliciting an immune response.) Select the correct statement.

    A. This information is inconsistent with what is known about modes of viral replication.
    B. The HBcAg is probably a lipid.
    C. The HBsAg is probably a protein.
    D. Enzymes found in liver cells probably do not increase in the serum during the acute disease.

13. Which of the following agents would block the replication of a virus? Assume all agents can only affect the host cell and its contents.

    A. An agent that blocks synthesis of lipids
    B. An agent that blocks synthesis of carbohydrates
    C. An agent that blocks synthesis of proteins
    D. An agent that blocks synthesis of bioorganic molecules

14. In the treatment of viral infections, a drug is discovered that directly blocks the synthesis of the viral protein coat. This drug:

    A. probably adversely affects protein synthesis by the host cell and hence may cause side effects in the host.
    B. probably does not affect host protein synthesis.
    C. probably causes naked virions to fall off because they are not slightly bound to the surface of the cell.
    D. probably allows coronaviruses, picornaviruses, and sometimes togaviruses to function as non-mRNA molecules.

15. Given a bacterial population without resistance to a certain drug, all of the following may cause introduction of bacterial resistance (excluding mutations) except:

    A. transformation.
    B. binary fission.
    C. transduction.
    D. conjugation.

ANSWERS AND EXPLANATIONS

1–11. 1-B, 2-A, 3-C, 4-A, 5-D, 6-B, 7-B, 8-D, 9-C, 10-C, 11-D. See text for explanation.

12. **C** From the knowledge about viral replication, the coat (protein) and core (nucleic acid) are synthesized separately and then combined. When cell lysis occurs, complete viral particles as well as coat (e.g., HBsAg) and core (HBcAg) may be released. Because the cells do lyse, their contents would also appear (e.g., the liver enzymes). And, because the antigens are found in the serum, it is not unreasonable to expect the liver enzymes to be there also. Indeed, an increase in certain liver enzymes is key to the diagnosis of hepatitis. Also, because incomplete viral particles are liberated into the serum, it might be expected that other viral products might also appear as antigens. Some do, for example, the "e"-antigen and viral DNA-polymerase.

13. **C** Viruses need the synthesis of proteins by the host cell machinery to make their protein coats and the enzymes necessary to make nucleic acids.

14. **A** It is the host's metabolic machinery that makes viral protein. Therefore, if the synthesis of viral coat protein is blocked, it is likely, although not necessary, that this is due to a blockage of host protein synthesis.

15. **B** Without new mutations, binary fission can produce only identical nonresistant daughter cells. The other mechanisms allow the introduction of new nucleic acid, which may contain drug-resistant genes.

Enzymes

1. Understand the reaction classes of oxidoreductases, transferases, hydrolases, lyases, ligases, and isomerases.
2. Relate the effect of pH on reaction velocity and discuss why enzymes are usually assayed at pH with maximum activity.
3. Compare and contrast apoenzymes, holoenzymes, and isoenzymes (enzymes having different molecular structures and catalyzing the same reaction).
4. Compare and evaluate enzyme assay methods: fixed time or end point method, kinetic or continuous monitoring, and immunoassay methods. Understand the limitations and experimental errors for these methods.

ENZYMES AND CELLULAR METABOLISM

Focus on the molecular structure and functions of enzymes for the human body. Understand that enzymes are chiral molecules and behave as stereospecific or geometry-specific biochemicals. Enzymes are classified as isomerases, ligases, oxidoreductases, transferases, hydrolases, and lyases. Review the molecular structure and special functions of elastase, plasmin, trypsin, urease, α-amylase, enterokinase, and bovine pancreatic ribonuclease. Recognize allosteric effectors and the role they play in enzymology. Identify important coenzymes such as biotin, nicotinamide, and lipoic acid.

STRUCTURE AND FUNCTION

Enzymes are the agents by which organisms make (anabolism) needed molecules or are involved in biosynthesis. Enzymes are usually named for the reaction they cause or for their substrate. A substrate is the substance upon which the enzyme acts. Most enzyme names end in the letters *-ase*. The enzyme sucrase is named for the substrate sucrose. Some enzymes are named for the reaction they cause and their substrate, such as the enzyme DNA polymerase, which helps make the molecules of DNA. Enzymes also break down complex molecules (catabolism) into simpler ones, thus producing energy, and, in general, maintaining homeostasis (e.g., by regulating entry and exit of molecules and ions). A key aspect of their function is that they can be regulated to function as needed.

The total enzyme (holoenzyme) may be composed of a protein (apoenzyme) part with or without an associated molecule called a **prosthetic group** (nonprotein organic molecule), also called a **cofactor** or **coenzyme** or a **metal ion**. The enzyme molecule catalyzes (by lowering the activation energy) chemical reactions at the conditions found in living organisms—conditions under which these reactions would not ordinarily occur. The protein part passes through the reaction unchanged (like a true catalyst), but the other groups (e.g., prosthetic group), which function as donors or acceptors of chemical groups, may or may not pass through the reaction unchanged. Some enzymes exist as zymogens and are activated by the cleaving of certain peptide bonds. A portion of the molecule may or may not be lost, but a conformational change usually occurs to expose the active site of the enzyme. An example is the conversion of trypsinogen to trypsin by enterokinase.

A key feature of enzyme function is its specificity. This means that enzymes are able to recognize certain molecules and not others due to minor chemical differences between them. A microenvironment is created by the tertiary structure of the protein, creating distinctive requirements of spatial and electric organization (distribution of positive-negative charges or polar groups) that a molecule must possess in order to be bound by the molecule. This microenvironment need not be rigid as in the lock (enzyme) and key (molecule or substrate) idea, but may be inducible in the enzyme by the substrate as in the "induced fit" hypothesis. Specificity may be absolute (only one molecule acceptable to the enzyme) or relative (a series of molecules acceptable, but some more than others). Because enzyme reactions are reversible, an enzyme can still have absolute specificity by reacting with one molecule in one direction and with another molecule in the opposite direction. The bonding is of a noncovalent type (hydrogen, ionic, van der Waals, hydrophobic).

Another key aspect of enzyme function is the **active site** idea. The substrate (molecule) is bound as discussed for specificity. The appropriate chemical reaction is then catalyzed by structures in this active site. For a reaction to occur, the bound molecule must be able to undergo the reaction that is catalyzable by the enzyme. It is doubtful that the active site functions by causing mechanical bond strain in appropriate bonds in which the bonds are broken and new ones are made. Rather, the active site has the appropriate groupings (e.g., side groups of the amino acids, appropriate prosthetic groups) and a microenvironment conducive to lowering the activation energy of the reaction. The combination required varies with the type of reaction being catalyzed. For example, a reaction that involves a hydrolysis reaction of an ester may have serine (with its OH group) to displace

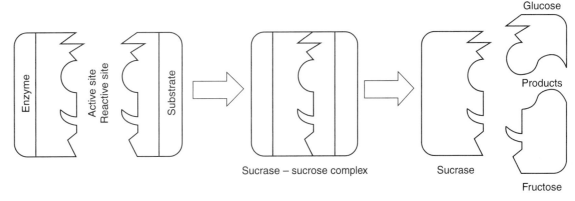

Fig. 8-73. Enzyme and substrate model (two parts of a jigsaw puzzle).

the alcoholic part of the ester, aspartic acid (with its CO_2H) or histidine (acts as acid or base) for acid-base catalysis, and a hydrophilic microenvironment (versus a hydrophobic one) because ions are produced during the reaction (Figure 8-73).

In 1958, the induced fit theory was introduced. This theory states that the active site of an enzyme must adjust to fit the reactive site of the substrate. As the enzyme and the substrate join, the enzyme may change slightly in shape to fit the substrate better. In both the lock and key hypothesis and the induced fit theory, a specific interaction occurs between the active site of the enzyme and the reactive site of the substrate. During the interaction, the enzyme and the substrate are joined by weak chemical bonds that are made and broken easily. The following equation shows the breakdown of sucrose by sucrase:

sucrase + sucrose $\rightarrow$ sucrase—sucrose complex $\rightarrow$ sucrase + glucose + fructose

enzyme + substrate $\rightarrow$ enzyme—substrate complex $\rightarrow$ enzyme + product

The lock and key model provides a rigid conformation of the enzyme, whereas the induced fit model provides a flexible configuration. In addition, the lock and key model does not account for the effects of allosteric ligands (molecules that bind to the enzyme at a place other than the active site to cause a conformational change in the enzyme).

Control of Enzyme Activity and Feedback Inhibition

Enzymes are controlled in a number of ways. Feedback inhibition (FI) is a basic and effective method of enzyme control (Figure 8-74). In FI, the product of the enzyme reaction feeds back and blocks the enzyme from converting more substrate to product. In this manner, excessive product is not produced. Similarly, when the product is present in low amounts, there is no enzyme inhibition and the enzyme converts substrate to product.

Enzyme Reaction: $$\text{Substrate (S)} \xrightarrow{\text{Enzyme (E)}} \text{Product (P)}$$

Excess Product:

(1) Excess product present: $S \xrightarrow{E} P$

(2) Enzyme binds product: $E \cdots P$

(3) Reaction is blocked: $S \xrightarrow[\;/\!/\;]{E \cdots P}$

Insufficient Product:

(1) Low amounts of product: $S \xrightarrow{E} P$

(2) Enzyme does not bind product

(3) Reaction proceeds: $S \xrightarrow{E} P$

Enzyme Cofactors or Coenzymes

Many enzymes are made up of protein and a nonprotein part. A nonprotein molecule found in some enzymes is called a **coenzyme**. Coenzymes are organic molecules that work with enzymes. A coenzyme binds weakly to the protein part of an enzyme and can join and leave it easily. Coenzymes are needed for certain chemical reactions to take place.

Some coenzymes are made of vitamins or their parts. Organisms cannot make most

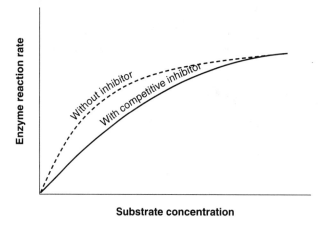

Fig. 8-74. Competitive inhibition.

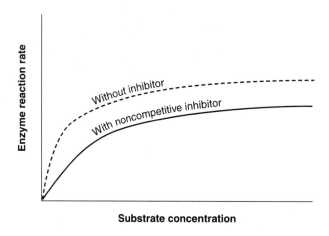

vitamins and must take them in as part of their food. If vitamins are lacking, certain coenzymes cannot be made and the metabolism of the organism does not function normally.

Cellular metabolism consists of a series of complex biochemical reactions. These reactions are of four types: (1) carbon bond reactions (making and breaking of C bonds), (2) isomerization, substitution, and reorganizing reactions, (3) oxidation and reduction reactions, and (4) electrophilic group-transfer reactions (nucleophile to nucleophile). Learn to apply and integrate these four reactions with the four major biochemical processes of glycolysis, citric acid cycle, electron transport chain, and oxidative phosphorylation. Understand various mechanisms that determine and control biochemical synthesis of lipids, fatty acids, lipoproteins, amino acids, and urea. Relate biochemical synthesis to basal metabolic rate. Carefully review Gibbs free energy linked to cellular metabolism. In doing so, compare and contrast exergonic, isogonic, and endergonic reactions related to $\Delta G = \Delta G° + RT (\ln[P_1][P_2]/[R_1][R_2])$. P_1 and P_2 are the biochemical products and R_1, R_2 are the biochemical reactants. Understand Lipmann's law as it applies to eukaryotes and prokaryotes. Lipmann's law states that the ADP-ATP coupling is the receptor and distributor of biochemical energy in all living organisms (or more complex systems).

Biochemical Energy Production

Energy production involves the stepwise degradation of organic molecules from more reduced to more oxidized states (reduced means abundance of hydrogen atoms and lack of, or few, oxygen atoms). The process may be aerobic (in the presence of oxygen) or anaerobic (without the presence of oxygen). Fermentation is a type of anaerobic respiration in which the final acceptor of electrons is an organic molecule. In aerobic respiration, O_2 is the final acceptor of electrons, producing H_2O (the fate of hydrogens in organic molecules being oxidized), and CO_2 is also produced (the fate of carbon).

Key organic molecules in energy production are as follows:

1. ATP. The bonds between the inorganic orthophosphates (P_i) are high energy (P ~ P) and, when hydrolyzed (split by adding water), this energy (approximately

7–8 kcal/mole) is released. ATP is the main short-term energy storage molecule. ADP and P_i combine to form ATP.

2. NAD^+ and $NADP^+$ (nicotinamide adenine dinucleotide and nicotinamide adenine dinucleotide phosphate). These carry two electrons and one hydrogen to form, respectively, NADH and NADPH (reduced forms of coenzymes NAD and NADP, respectively). NADH transfers its electrons to the electron transport system. NADPH is used for synthetic purposes and is the major product of the pentose shunt in which glucose-6-phosphate dehydrogenase is a key enzyme. ($NADH_2$ is also a reduced form of the coenzyme NADP.) Niacin is a part of NAD^+ and $NADP^+$.

3. FAD (flavin adenine dinucleotide). FAD carries two electrons and two hydrogens as $FADH_2$ (reduced form of coenzyme FAD) to the electron transport chain. Its most important role is in the breakdown of fatty acids. Riboflavin is a component of FAD.

4. Cytochromes (b, c, a). Cytochromes transfer electrons (which are attached to iron) and they are part of the electron transport chain. The iron is in a porphyrin ring (together called heme), which is bound by a protein.

Biochemical Processes

The four key processes of energy production are glycolysis, the citric acid cycle (Krebs cycle), or tricarboxylic acid cycle (TCA cycle), the electron transport system (ETS), and oxidative phosphorylation. Gluconeogenesis and glycogen synthesis should be studied after glycolysis to understand the differences.

In animals, the primary site for **gluconeogenesis**, or formation of glucose, is the liver. The involvement of oxaloacetate in the initial steps of gluconeogenesis provides a connection between this process and the Krebs cycle. All of the intermediates of the Krebs cycle may thus serve as precursors of glucose.

Gluconeogenesis requires a supply of pyruvate. In animals, the primary source is the lactate and pyruvate produced by the glycolysis occurring in active skeletal muscle. Lactate and pyruvate can easily penetrate cell membranes and enter the bloodstream for transport

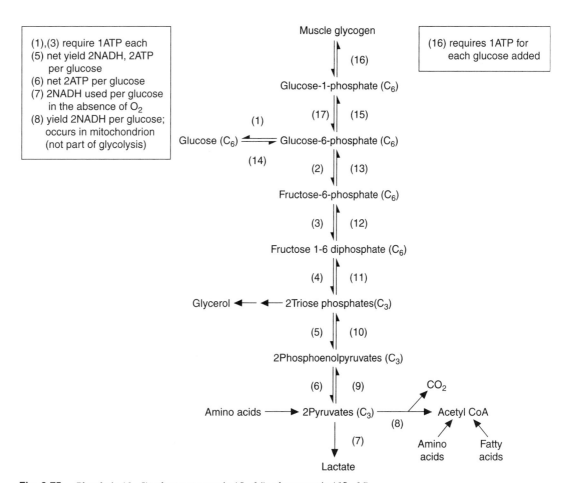

Fig. 8-75. Glycolysis (1–8); gluconeogenesis (9–14); glycogenesis (15–16).

Fig. 8-76. Glycolysis.

	Glycogen	
	Glycogenolysis ↓ ↑ Glycogenesis glucose	
	Glycolysis ↓ ↑ Gluconeogenesis lactate	

Step	Molecules produced	ATP yield
Glycolysis	2ATP 2NADH	2ATP 4ATP + 2ATP*
Pyruvate to acetyl CoA	2NADH	6ATP
	2ATP 6NADH 2FADH$_2$	2ATP 18ATP 4ATP
* These 2ATPs are used up in transporting the electrons across the mitochondrial membranes.		38ATP

to the liver. Glycogen, a glucose polymer and storage form of glucose in animals, is required for the expenditure of energy (UTP, or uridine triphosphate) in animals (Figure 8-75).

Glycolysis

Glycolysis (Figure 8-76) converts glucose (C_6) to two pyruvates (C_3), producing two ATPs and two NADHs. If there is no oxygen, the NADH converts pyruvate to lactic acid (as during exercise), which may be converted to alcohol (as in a type of fermentation). The latter process is anaerobic glycolysis. In the presence of oxygen, the pyruvate (C_3) is converted to acetyl CoA (C_2) and CO_2 with two NADHs produced per original glucose. CoA (coenzyme A) is an acyl carrier for which the vitamin pantothenic acid is a key component. Acetyl CoA may also arise from fatty acid and amino acid breakdown. Anaerobic glycolysis yields a net of two ATPs per glucose. Aerobic glycolysis (because it proceeds to the citric acid cycle and ETS) yields a total of 38 ATPs per glucose. Of the 686 kcal (for glucose → CO2 + H_2O), aerobic processes store 308 kcal (for 45% efficiency) as ATP; anaerobic efficiency is much less. Fats store the most energy (9.1 kcal/g), whereas proteins (which store approximately 4.1) and carbohydrates (which store approximately 4) are about the same.

Krebs (Citric Acid) Cycle

The acetyl CoA (C_2) enters the **citric acid cycle** (Figure 8-77) by combining with oxaloacetic acid (C_4) to form citrate (C_6). This is degraded stepwise to oxaloacetic acid again, producing three NADHs, one FADH$_2$, and one ATP (from GTP, or guanosine triphosphate) for each cycle (the cycle must double to get production per original glucose), as well as CO_2 and H_2O. The NADH and FADH$_2$ enter the ETS in the following sequence:

$$\text{NAD} \xrightarrow{(1)} \text{FAD} \to \text{Ubiquinone (CoQ)} \xrightarrow{(2)} \text{Cyt } b \to \text{Cyt } c \to \text{Cyt } a \xrightarrow{(3)} O_2$$

Each intermediate is first reduced (receives electrons from) by the preceding intermediate and oxidized (gives electrons to) by the following intermediate, with oxygen as the final acceptor being converted to water.

Electron Transport Chain and Oxidative Phosphorylation (Figures 8-78 and 8-79)

Adenosine triphosphates are produced at 1, 2, and 3 by the process called **oxidative phosphorylation**. Each NADH produces three ATPs and each FADH$_2$ produces two ATPs. Malonate is a potent inhibitor of the citric acid cycle. Cyanide is a potent inhibitor of the ETS at Cyt a. An exception is the NADH produced outside the mitochondria from glycolysis. The electrons of NADH are transported by a shuttle to ubiquinone and only two ATPs per NADH (of glycolysis) are produced.

Glycolysis occurs in the cell cytoplasm. The citric acid cycle occurs in the matrix of the mitochondrion. Electron transport and oxidative phosphorylation occur on the inner membrane of the mitochondrion. The transfer of electrons down the respiratory chain

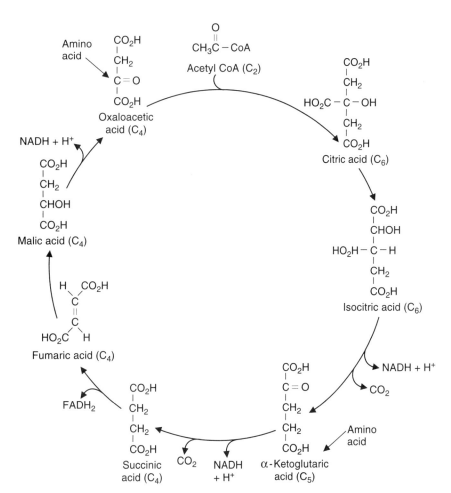

Fig. 8-77. Citric acid cycle.

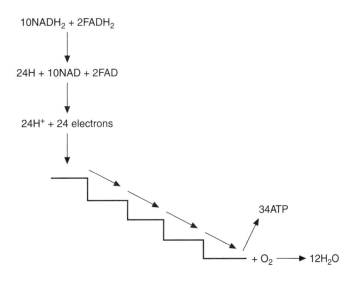

Fig. 8-78. Electron transport chain.

from NADH to molecular oxygen is the primary source of the energy used for the formation of ATP by the coupling of ADP phosphorylation.

The net product in the linking of electron transport and oxidative phosphorylation can be expressed as follows: $NADH + H^+ + 3ADP + 3P_i + \frac{1}{2} O_2 \rightarrow NAD^+ + 3ATP + 4H_2O$.

APPLIED CONCEPTS

- Identify basic comparative relationships among catalytic mechanisms (cationic, acid-base, electrostatic, nucleophilic covalent, and electrophilic covalent).
- Describe the structure and functions of digestive enzymes such as carboxypeptidase, aminopeptidase, pepsin, maltase, and sucrase.

Problem Solving in the Biological Sciences 459

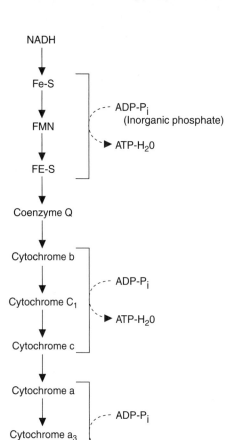

Fig. 8-79. Oxidative phosphorylation.

- Familiarize yourself with enzyme kinetics, emphasizing the following: assumptions in various models, Michaelis-Menten equation forms and how to graph them, catalytic efficiency, competitive and noncompetitive inhibitors, pH effect on rate of enzymatic reaction, and Bi Bi reactions (bisubstrate reactions such as Ping Pong Bi Bi reactions and rapid equilibrium random Bi Bi reactions).
- Learn various applications of biocatalyst electrodes such as biofueling of cells, bioreaction, clinical integrated microbiosensing (amperometric), and the electropolymerization process.
- Learn usage and application of terms such as metabolites, catabolism, anabolism, amphibolism, Mitchell's chemiosmotic theory (proton gradient and proton motive force similar to electromotive force), phototrophs, chemotrophs, metabolic inhibitors, zymase, enolase, and irreversibility of metabolic pathways.
- Understand the causes and effects for the following diseases: Cori's, Andersen's, McArdle's, Krabbe's, Tay-Sachs (enzyme deficiency), and beriberi.
- Develop a more in-depth understanding of glycolysis, especially glucose catabolism or the Embden-Meyerhof glycolytic pathway, and of the pentose phosphate pathway, muscle glycolysis, and glycogen metabolism in maintaining blood glucose levels through glucagon production.
- Review discussion of concentration cells and electrochemical cells with application to the Nernst equation for aerobic metabolism, both for prokaryotes and eukaryotes.
- Identify experimental methods and techniques used in metabolite pathways research such as isotopic labeling of metabolites, nuclear magnetic resonance and mass spectrometer techniques, measurement with Geiger counters and liquid scintillation counters, autoradiography, cell storing, organ perfusion techniques, and tissue slice techniques. Review papers in mitochondrial research using freeze-fracture and freeze-etch micrographs.
- Compare and contrast glycolysis, gluconeogenesis, glycogenesis, and glycogenolysis for muscle glycogen and liver glycogen.

1. Enzymes probably play a direct role in all of the following except:

    A. maintenance of resting membrane potential by extrusion of Na^+ from cells.
    B. synthesis of mRNA from DNA.
    C. storage of hereditary information.
    D. production of ATP.

2. Because enzymes are proteins, they are affected by the same factors that affect proteins. An enzyme is "designed" to function under a certain set of conditions. Which of the following conditions would be most conducive to the normal function of a human cellular enzyme?

    A. Temperature = 25°C
    B. Temperature = 37°C
    C. pH = 1.0
    D. pH = 10.0

3. NAD^+ is a noncovalently bound coenzyme for the enzyme α-glycerol-phosphate dehydrogenase. NAD^+ picks up an H^{-1} (hydride) and becomes NADH; the enzyme is not affected by the reaction. The activation energy was lowered by the system.

    A. This is not true catalysis because the NAD^+ was changed in the reaction.
    B. This is true catalysis because the NAD^+ was not covalently bound to the enzyme.
    C. This is true catalysis because the activation energy of the reaction was lowered by the enzyme, which was unchanged in the reaction.
    D. None of the above is correct.

4. Succinate dehydrogenase catalyzes the following reaction: succinate $\rightleftharpoons$ fumarate. The specificity of the enzyme is:

    A. relative because it binds more than one substrate.
    B. absolute because it catalyzes only one reaction of one pair of substrates.
    C. absolute because it has only one substrate, succinate.
    D. none of the above.

5. D-amino acid oxidase catalyzes the following reaction:

$$
\begin{matrix} (1) & (2) \\ R-CH-CO_2H & + & \tfrac{1}{2}O_2 \end{matrix} \longrightarrow R-C-CO_2H \ + \ R'NH_2.
$$

(with HNR' below the CH and O below the second carbon)

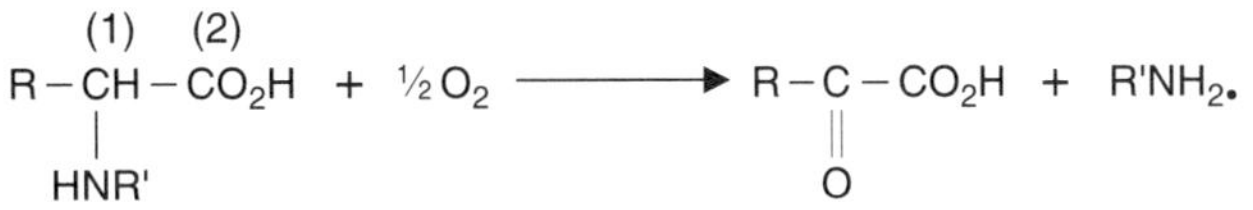

Following are some relative rates of reaction of various substrates with this enzyme.

Substrate	Relative rate	R	R'
D-Tyrosine	13.6	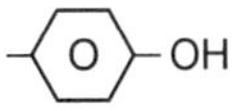 —⟨O⟩—OH	H
D-Alanine	4.6	—CH_3	H
D-Isoleucine	1.6	—C(—CH_3)—CH_2—CH_3	H
D-Leucine	1.0	—CH_2—CH(—CH_3)(CH_3)	H
L-Tyrosine	0	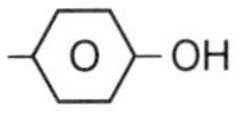 —⟨O⟩—OH	H
L-Leucine	0	—CH_2—CH(—CH_3)(CH_3)	H
D-Leucylalanyltyrosine	0	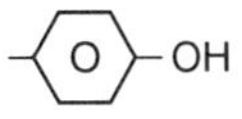 —⟨O⟩—OH	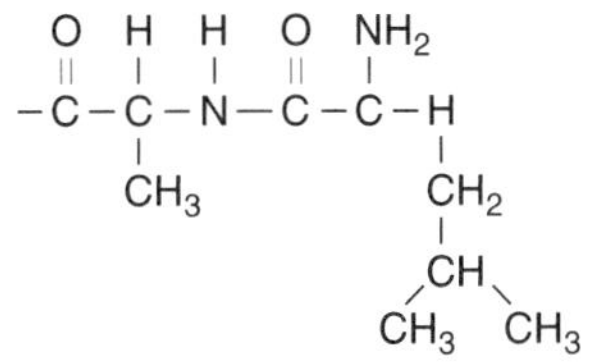 —C(=O)—C(—CH_3)—N(H)—C(=O)—C(—NH_2)(—CH_2—CH(—CH_3)(CH_3))—H

The figure implies that:

A. the specificity of D-amino acid oxidase is absolute because D-tyrosine has a much higher rate of reaction than other substrates.

B. the configuration of carbon number 1 is not important for the reaction to occur.

C. from the data given, the group at **R** has more effect on the outcome of the reaction than the group at **R'**.

D. the specificity of the enzyme is relative because several molecules may react with the enzyme.

6. Enzymes usually combine readily with substrates in order for a reaction to occur. When the reaction is over, despite only minor changes in the substrate, the product (derived from the substrate) usually readily dissociates from the enzyme. The best reason for this might be that:

A. although the site of attachment for the substrate has not changed, the overall conformation of the enzyme may be made unfavorable to the product by the reaction.

B. minor differences in spatial or electric organization of a molecule are all that are required to make a molecule unacceptable to the enzyme.

C. the enzyme is forced into an unnatural conformation, causing it to forcibly expel the product.

D. the substrate is covalently bound to the enzyme because of the specificity of the enzyme, whereas the product is not.

7. Malonate blocks (inhibits) the catalysis of the following reaction by succinate dehydrogenase:

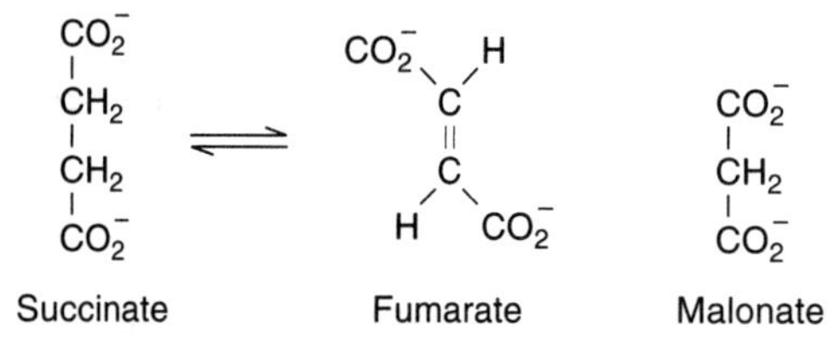

Succinate   Fumarate   Malonate

Diethyl malonate will not block the reaction nor will the diethyl esters of succinate or fumarate undergo the reaction. The information implies that:

I. Inhibition of the enzyme may be brought about by molecules that resemble the substrate but cannot undergo the reaction.

II. The active site of the enzyme may contain positive ions or at least require the presence of $-CO_2^-$ on the substrate.

III. Monoethyl malonate will not inhibit the reaction.

A. I only
B. II and III only
C. I and II only
D. I, II, and III

8. Which substance has the highest energy content per gram?

A. Proteins
B. Fats
C. Carbohydrates
D. Phospholipids

9. The cytochromes are part of the:

A. citric acid cycle.
B. oxidative phosphorylation.
C. glycolysis.
D. electron transport system.

10. In the biological production of energy from chemical molecules, the stepwise degradation is:

A. by addition of hydrogens to molecules.
B. by removal of oxygen from molecules.

    C. from more oxidized to more reduced states.

    D. from more reduced to more oxidized states.

11. Select the substance which is not an electron carrier in cellular energy production:

    A. NAD^+

    B. ATP

    C. FAD

    D. ubiquinone

12. Select the incorrect association.

    A. ATP — adenine

    B. NAD — nicotinamide or niacin

    C. FAD — folic acid

    D. Cytochromes — porphyrin ring

13. Select the incorrect statement concerning glycolysis.

    A. End product may be lactate.

    B. If anaerobic, no ATPs are produced.

    C. If aerobic, the ATP yield can be 36 ATPs because its products enter the citric acid cycle and electron transport system.

    D. It occurs in the cytoplasm.

14. Select the incorrect statement regarding the citric acid cycle.

    A. The first step is the combination of acetyl CoA and oxaloacetate to form citrate.

    B. It is not a true cycle because CO_2 and H_2O are its net products.

    C. Each turn of the cycle yields three NADHs, one $FADH_2$, and one ATP (from guanosine triphosphate, or GTP).

    D. It occurs in the mitochondrion.

15. Select the incorrect statement.

    A. The final receptor of electrons in the electron transport system is oxygen.

    B. Oxidative phosphorylation (production of ATPs) occurs only at certain steps in the electron transport system.

    C. The electron transport system can produce ATPs without oxidative phosphorylation occurring.

    D. Both electron transport and oxidative phosphorylation occur on the inner membrane of the mitochondrion.

16. At which stage does cyanide block cellular production of energy?

    A. Glycolysis

    B. Citric acid cycle

    C. Electron transport system

    D. Oxidative phosphorylation

17. The following are structures of a typical fatty acid and a hexose:

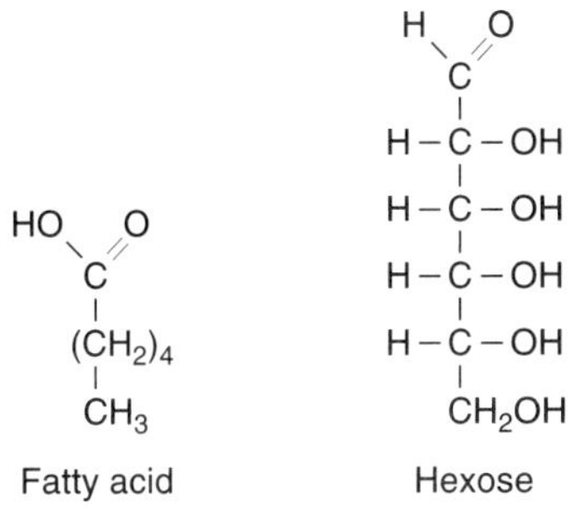

Fatty acid   Hexose

If equal weights of both were degraded bioenergetically to CO^2 and H^2O, the fatty acid would yield:

    A. more energy because it is more reduced than the hexose.

    B. less energy because it is more oxidized than the hexose.

    C. less energy because it is more reduced than the hexose.

    D. more energy because it is more oxidized than the hexose.

1. **C** The storage of hereditary information is a function of DNA. Enzymes play no direct role in this. All of the other processes require direct involvement of enzymes.

2. **B** The function of a cellular enzyme should be maximal at those conditions found in the internal milieu of a cell or a particular compartment of a cell. These conditions would generally be similar to the condition of the whole organism. The temperature of 37°C is the normal body temperature and the normal pH of blood is 7.40. The other conditions are extreme, but there are enzymes that can function at or near most of these—some in humans and some not.

3. **C** True catalysis occurs when the activation energy is lowered by the active site environment of the enzyme. Coenzymes serve the accessory function of transferring chemical groups.

4. **B** Nearly all enzymatic reactions are truly reversible. The product occupies the same site occupied by the substrate, so the enzyme can recognize it, and the substrate–product can be considered as a pair.

5. **D** The relative specificity of the enzyme should be clear from the several different substrates undergoing the reaction. A case might be made for the "absolute" specificity for D-amino acids, which is supported by the data. The configuration of carbon number 1 is essential to the reactivity of the substrate because this is the carbon about which the D or L configuration is determined. The **R** group represents the side chains of the various amino acids; if the configuration is D at the α-carbon (1 in diagram), the reaction can still occur, although it is variable. The **R′** could represent a second (or more) amino acid, as in D-leucylalanyltyrosine, which does not react at all. Hence, with the limited information given, the presence of a group (other than H) appears critical in the reaction.

6. **B** Although the other options may seem reasonable, the simplest answer is **B**, which emphasizes that only small differences in substrate structures can affect enzyme recognition and reaction.

7. **C** The structures not given are shown.

Diethyl malonate

Monoethyl malonate

Diethyl succinate

Diethyl fumarate

Statement I is reasonable in that malonate and succinate are similar and specificity is based on similarity in structure. Also, this reaction requires the group shown for the reaction to occur and malonate does not have this.

Even though malonate will bind at the active site and block succinate, it will not react. It appears that only molecules with one or two $-CO_2^-$ (which is negative) are attracted to the active site. There is no evidence regarding a molecule with one $-CO_2^-$ and one $-CO_2CH_2CH_3$.

8-16. **8-B, 9-D, 10-D, 11-B, 12-C, 13-B, 14-B, 15-C, 16-C.** See text for explanation.

17. **A** A reduced compound has all (or mostly) hydrogens and not oxygens. The fatty acid has many more hydrogens and fewer oxygens so it is more reduced. The more reduced a compound, the higher the energy that can be released when it

is oxidized to CO_2 and H_2O. The factor of the number of atoms in each molecule is eliminated by considering the substances on a weight basis.

Reproductive System

Self-Managed Learning Questions

1. Get more information on aminoscopy and review the basic concepts in biology, chemistry, and physics by answering the following questions:
   - How does a fiber optic lighted instrument work?
   - What are the special characteristics of the amniotic fluid and what is their significance? (The color of the amniotic fluid can indicate fetal hypoxia.)
   - What is the chemical composition of the amniotic fluid? What are the organic chemical structure and reaction mechanisms for bilirubin, creatinine, glucose, and lipids in the amniotic fluid.
   - How are chromosomal abnormalities detected in amniotic fluid? What errors can be made in amniotic fluid analysis? How long does the procedure take? What is the volume of sample collected?
   - Are there any risk factors involved? What special precautions should be taken?
   - Should ultrasound be used to locate the placenta and fetal positions?
2. Understand the physics of the diagnostic ultrasound examination by answering the following questions:
   - Can an ultrasound beam penetrate air? Why or why not?
   - Why is it difficult for sound waves to pass through fat layers?
   - What are the differences between radiographic mammography and breast ultrasound?
   - How can Doppler ultrasound determine blood flow and blood flow direction, and how is it used in fetal monitoring?
   - Construct a basic diagram of an ultrasound machine to understand the design, mechanics, and errors made in using this instrument.
3. Analyze, evaluate, and find credible research articles to answer the following questions:
   - What are imaginal discs in insects and how are they formed?
   - Is differentiation irreversible? Give supporting examples.
4. Review reproductive system essentials as links to the endocrine system and mendelian genetics (sex-linked characteristics) and review major differences and similarities between embryogenesis and gametogenesis.
5. Visit a hospital or clinic; talk to nurses or doctors in the obstetrics and gynecological wards. Observe and analyze sonograms, rooms where newborns are kept, and special infant instrumentation.
6. Familiarize yourself with current issues and problems related to the reproductive systems of females and males (e.g., in vitro fertilization and embryo transfer technology).

REPRODUCTION

Male and Female Gonads and Genitalia

Female Anatomy

The labia are composed of the major folds, or labia majora, and the minor folds, or labia minora (Figure 8-80). The clitoris (located between the minor folds ventrally) is sensitive. The vagina, the passage from the external genital opening, terminates in the cervix (part of the uterus), which has an os (opening) to the uterine cavity (where the fertilized egg implants). The placenta derives from the uterus and the developing embryo. Connected

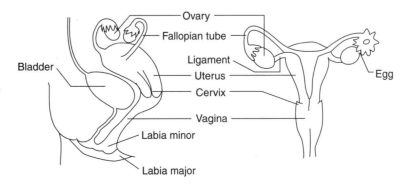

Fig. 8-80. Female reproductive system.

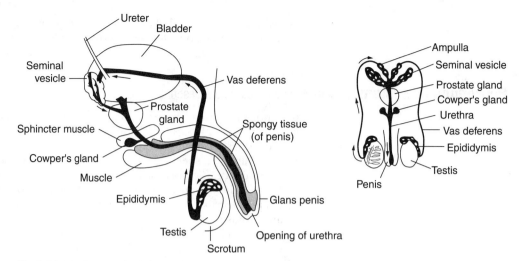

Fig. 8-81. Male reproductive system.

to the uterus are the fallopian tubes that lead to the ovaries (but are not connected to them).

The female gonads, the ovaries, lie behind (retroperitoneally to) the abdominal cavity. They produce female hormones. They also produce the female gametes. Each female gamete is called an **egg**, or **ovum**. An ovum is huge compared to a spermatozoon. Ova are produced by meiosis. Even before a female is born, egg-producing cells in the ovary have developed into primary oocytes. At the baby girl's birth, all the primary oocytes for a lifetime are present. Primary oocytes are diploid.

Male Anatomy

The testicles are located outside the body because spermatogenesis requires a temperature lower than body temperature (Figure 8-81). The scrotum is the sac that contains the testicles. Spermatozoa travel from the testis to the epididymis (where spermatozoa maturation is completed) to the vas deferens to the ejaculatory duct to the penile urethra to the exterior. The seminal vesicles and prostate gland contribute fluid to the ejaculate (which averages 1–2 ml). The penis consists of a glans penis (which is sensitive) and a shaft (consisting of cavernous tissue for blood engorgement). Penile erection (due mostly to parasympathetic stimulation) results from veins of the penis clamping down and, hence, holding blood in the penis. Ejaculation is a reflex mediated by the sympathetic nervous system. Males continue to produce spermatozoa from puberty onward.

The spermatozoa is produced by meiosis, which results in production of haploid gametes. Gametes have only half the number of chromosomes contained in the body cells. Human body cells contain 46 chromosomes, and gametes contain only 23 chromosomes. Before a male is born, the testes develop retroperitoneally to the abdominal cavity.

Gametogenesis by Meiosis

Gametogenesis in Females

The ovary contains oogonia (2n), which replicate their DNA and differentiate (before birth) into primary oocytes (46 chromosomes each made up of two chromatids, DNA = 2n), which become surrounded by follicular cells (from the mesenchymal stroma), and together constitute the primordial follicle (Figure 8-82). The primary oocytes are arrested

DNA replication

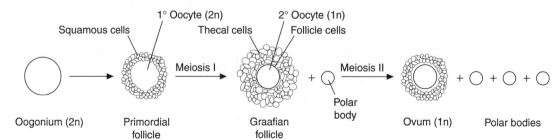

Fig. 8-82. Gametogenesis in females.

DNA replication

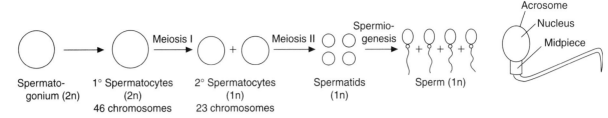

Fig. 8-83. Gametogenesis in males.

in the prophase of the first meiotic division, and they may remain as such from birth to menopause. There are approximately 5 million oogonia, but only 1 million primary oocytes at birth and about 40,000 at puberty—the remainder degenerate (become atretic follicles). Beginning at puberty, a group of primordial follicles begins differentiation to graafian follicles. The primary oocyte divides unevenly to form the secondary oocyte and a polar body, each cell having the haploid number of chromosomes (23) but containing DNA in their duplicated (daughter) chromatids. The secondary oocyte is surrounded by the zona pellucida (a gel-like substance), which is surrounded by follicular cells. These are surrounded by thecal cells, which secrete estrogens. Ovulation occurs by expelling the secondary oocyte and zona pellucida plus some follicular cells (corona radiata) into the fallopian tubes. If fertilization occurs in the fallopian tubes (the usual location), the secondary oocyte completes meiosis to become an ovum and a polar body (both 1n—the replicated chromatids uncouple at their centromeres). The ovum fuses with the spermatozoon. If the ovum is not fertilized, it degenerates. The follicular and thecal cells left behind become the corpus luteum, a main source of progesterone, which maintains pregnancy. The other follicles that began to develop degenerate because only one follicle completes development and is ovulated from one ovary during each cycle. The polar bodies that result from the division of the primary oocyte, the secondary oocyte, and possibly the first polar body are nonfunctional. Polar bodies have nuclear material but no cytoplasm. Hence, each primary oocyte (2n) produces only one gamete (1n).

Gametogenesis in Males

The first step in gametogenesis in males is a differentiation of spermatogonia (2n), which includes DNA replication into primary spermatocytes (2n) [Figure 8-83]. Primary spermatocytes divide reductionally to form two secondary spermatocytes, both functional haploid cells (23 chromosomes) having duplicated chromosomes (daughter chromatids) and DNA. Secondary spermatocytes divide equally and at the centromeres of their duplicated chromosomes to form spermatids (1n and 23 individual chromosomes). The second step is spermiogenesis, in which spermatids (1n) are transformed into spermatozoa (1n). A spermatozoon consists of a head, a middle part, and a tail. The head contains an acrosome (contains digestive enzymes to penetrate the egg, derived from the Golgi apparatus) and nuclear material (DNA) surrounded by little cytoplasm. The midpiece contains mitochondria for power. The tail has the structure of a centriole and provides locomotion. Leydig or interstitial cells (which produce testosterone) and Sertoli cells (which support spermatozoa development) are also in the testis. Spermatozoa deposited in the vagina by the penis reach the cervix within 90 seconds and migrate up the fallopian tubes to fertilize the ovum there.

Reproductive Sequence

The female menstrual cycle is typically 28 days and consists of a menstrual flow (menses), a follicular (ovary) and proliferative phase (uterus), ovulation, and a luteal (ovary) and secretory phase (uterus). The first day of menses is the first day of the cycle. Shedding of the uterine lining occurs during the menstrual flow. Development of the follicle under the stimulation of follicle stimulating hormone (FSH) and proliferation of the cells of the uterine lining under the stimulation of estrogen (from the ovary) occur in the follicular and proliferative phase (Figure 8-84). A rapid increase of estrogen triggers a surge of luteinizing hormone (LH) at midcycle, which causes ovulation to occur (at approximately 14 days before the first day of menses). Just before ovulation, there is a slight decrease in body temperature, which then increases with ovulation—the progesterone causes the temperature increase. During the luteal and secretive phase, the corpus luteum

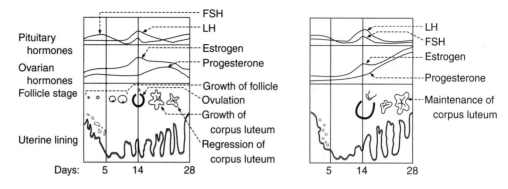

Fig. 8-84. Menstrual cycle. (*A*) Without pregnancy (*B*) With pregnancy.

secretes progesterone, which, with estrogen, readies the uterine wall for the acceptance of the fertilized egg. If fertilization and implantation occur, the corpus luteum continues to secrete progesterone under the stimulation of human chorionic gonadotropin (HCG) released from the placenta. If implantation does not occur, the corpus luteum degenerates and menses (shedding of the uterine lining) occurs. The cycle repeats itself as FSH and estrogen concentrations increase. Menstrual cycles occur until nearly all the oocytes are depleted, resulting in menopause.

Structure and Function of the Placenta

The placenta is the organ that exchanges nutrients and waste products between the mother and the developing fetus. The placenta develops when the blastocyst attaches itself to the uterine lining. The chorion creates responses in the endometrium, and the endometrium proliferates and develops more blood vessels. This interaction is the beginning of the placenta, which grows as the fetus develops.

The main function of the placenta is to bring nutrients to the fetus from the mother and to take wastes away. This is done through the blood, but the circulatory systems of the mother and fetus are separate. Oxygen and nutrients pass from the mother's blood through the placental tissue to be diffused into the fetus's blood. Wastes from the fetus are transported through the placental tissue to the mother's blood, where it is then transported to the mother's kidney for disposal. The placenta also produces HCG, without which the luteum would degenerate and the fetus would be aborted.

Extraembryonic Membranes

Allantois is formed from endoderm and mesoderm, amnion is a growth of ectoderm and mesoderm, and the full growth of ectoderm and mesoderm becomes chorion. Mammals, birds, and reptiles all have extraembryonic membranes (Figure 8-85).

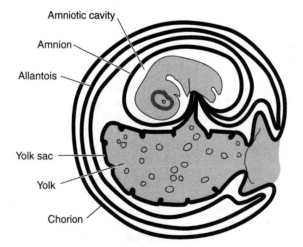

Fig. 8-85. Anatomy of an embryo.

DEVELOPMENTAL MECHANISMS

How a single egg develops into a complex organism is not completely understood. The concepts of differentiation, determination, and induction are integral to understanding the changes that occur.

Cell Specialization

When a cell becomes specialized, it generally loses its ability to divide or reproduce itself (e.g., nerve cells, muscle cells, red blood cells). Therefore, most cell division occurs in **stem cells,** which are highly undifferentiated, multipotential cells with a high rate of cell division (e.g., bone marrow stem cells and crypt cells of the gut).

The concept of **determination** is related to that of differentiation in that, as a cell differentiates, fewer options become available. That is, at certain points, a cell or tissue may be "determined" to become one of a certain set of cells and not others. For example, the surface cells of the gastrula are "determined" to become ectodermal structures and not endodermal or mesodermal structures. So, although in the blastula all the cells were surface cells and, apparently, had the option of becoming ectodermal cells, only those that did not invaginate became so. The mechanism of determination is probably also related to the environmental differences of cells and their interaction with preset sequences of gene activation and inactivation. Occasionally, the cells resulting from cleavage of a zygote are not determined until after three divisions (eight cells). Up to this point, each cell can develop into a complete organism. After this point, only incomplete organisms would develop from each cell. Cleavages up to this point are called indeterminate because each cell has all the options available. The next cleavage is called determinate because the daughter cells no longer have all options available. In some instances, the first cleavage may be determinate.

Differentiation is the process whereby a cell can change into more specialized cells to become a tissue. A tissue is a set of similar cells that carries out a specific function, such as muscle. All the varied cells of the human body (e.g., muscle, bone, skin, and nerve) arise from the same zygote. What is it about the zygote that allows this differentiation to occur? It is generally accepted that all cells in an organism contain the same genetic information (sequences of genes on DNA). What probably makes one cell different from another is which of these genes is activated. The set of activated genes is responsible for the characteristics of each cell—the structural components, metabolic machinery, and general composition of the cell. Therefore, after gastrulation, different tissues must have different sets of genes activated. No activation of genes occurs in blastula or late gastrula. Induction turns on protein synthesis.

In general, differentiation is not brought about by the daughter cells having different genes (i.e., different sets of genetic material). If the cytoplasm of the zygote was totally homogeneous, then each daughter cell, resulting from the cleavage, would be identical with regard to the nucleus and the cytoplasm and would remain undifferentiated. But, if there was an asymmetric distribution of cytoplasmic constituents and the cleavage resulted in daughter cells with different distributions of these constituents, then the daughter cells would be different; that is, a small amount of cytoplasmic differentiation would have occurred. If these cytoplasmic differences led to the activation of different sets of genes in their respective nuclei, differences between the cells would be perpetuated in their daughter cells, and some degree of true differentiation (production of daughters different from parent cells) will have occurred. Therefore, asymmetric distribution of cytoplasmic constituents is one way that differentiation may be brought about. Then, in general, if a factor can affect the cytoplasmic composition of a cell (which can affect the set of activated genes) or if it can affect the nucleus directly to activate (or inactivate) genes, and if this effect is unevenly distributed among the cells, then differentiation of the cells along different lines can be brought about.

Other factors that cause cells to differentiate are (1) neighboring cells and physical environment. Neighboring cells may affect cell growth by secreting a diffusible chemical that stimulates or inhibits the cytoplasm or nucleus. An example is tissue induction in which a given tissue can induce cells in contact with it to develop along a certain line. For example, the dorsal lip of the blastopore induces the overlying ectoderm to become neural tissue. The physical environment influences cell development by differences in light, temperature, pressure, humidity, pH, and so on. As the embryo develops, some cells are internal, some are on the surface, some have lots of yolk, and some have a little yolk, so there are more opportunities for agents to act on cells in a differential manner. In general, the more specialized a cell becomes (i.e., the more differentiated), the less likely it is to differentiate to perform other functions or even to divide. Certain cells remain at low levels of differentiation so that they may differentiate as they are needed. Examples are the mesenchymal cell found throughout the body and the bone marrow stem cell, which can give rise to all the blood elements. Occasionally, a cell may dedifferentiate (i.e., revert to a less differentiated form), and, thus, its potential to divide increases. This happens in many cancer cases.

Induction

Induction occurs when one tissue causes an adjacent tissue to develop in a different manner than it was originally. Induction usually happens only to embryonic tissue, but it also occurs in the production of certain white blood cells in the adult immune system. The process takes place by triggering a sequence of gene expression in the responding cells. A tissue cannot induce itself; rather, different tissues interact and induce each other. One of the challenges researchers in developmental biology are facing is determining the chemical nature of specific inducers. In some cases, diffusible proteins may be involved; in other cases, extracellular materials (such as collagen) may be involved. Anchor cells give rise to primary and secondary inducers that activate genes 1 and 2 (Figure 8-86).

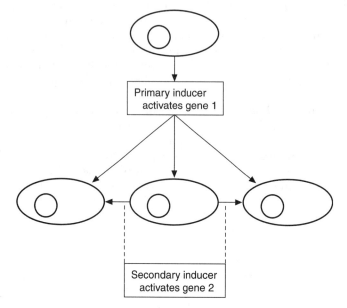

Fig. 8-86. Induction at microscopic level.

APPLIED CONCEPTS

- Focus on the functions of various parts of the reproductive systems in females and males. Understand the cellular and molecular physiology of each gland or organ (e.g., development of follicles in the ovary, function of spermatocytes) and the physics of ultrasound tests in a pregnant woman.
- Understand the chemical and endocrinal relationship among FSH, LH, and gonadotropin releasing hormone (GnRH) as released in the female and inhibition by male hormones such as testosterone and inhibin.
- Distinguish among terms such as spermatogenesis, spermatids, spermatocytes, spermiogenesis, progesterone, follicular fluid, testosterone (interstitial Leydig cells), amniotic fluid, teratogen, oocytes, oogonia, syncytiotrophoblasts, osteoblasts, and allantois.
- Determine the fundamental causes and effects of the following: vasectomy, episiotomy, oophorectomy, lumpectomy, mastectomy, cryptorchidism, mittelschmerz, endometriosis, amenorrhea, and dysmenorrhea.
- Understand various factors linked to parturition, including uterine contraction frequency and the role of oxytocin during labor.
- Understand the instrumentation and objectives of various tests such as Papanicolaou smear test, semen analysis (pH, volume, count, fertility), colposcopy, dilation and curettage, computed tomography and mammography, ultrasound cancer test, prostate gland cancer test, ectopic pregnancy test, tubal ligation sonograms (to determine fetal position and development), and amniocentesis.
- Recognize the chemicals used and functions of birth control pills, intrauterine contraceptive devices, condoms, diaphragms, contraceptive sponges, and tampons. Which of these devices cause the toxic shock syndrome and how can it be prevented?
- Investigate and understand the technology behind induced abortion techniques such as use of suction, saline solution, and basic scraping.
- Most home pregnancy tests are inaccurate tools to predict pregnancy. The basic test tube is used to test HCG in urine. Particle clumping in a ring-like form indicates positive testing of HCG and no clumping or no ring indicates negative testing of HCG. Understand why these tests are not reliable depending on type and stage of pregnancy. Blood tests are more accurate.

- Understand the concept of natural titrants such as semen (alkaline with a pH of 7.5) and vaginal secretions (acidic with a pH of approximately 3.5–4.0) and how various hormonal releases affect their biochemical nature.
- Recognize modern fetal surgery techniques (done on unusual tissues or organs), development of graafian follicles, new fetal ultrasonography tests, artificial insemination methods (in vitro and embryo transfer), and karyotyping.
- Understand the abnormal inheritance traits and diseases: sickle-cell anemia, Huntington's chorea, Turner's syndrome, Klinefelter's syndrome, and Down's syndrome. Determine the specific chromosomal abnormality causing the abnormal traits and learn the use of karyotyping techniques to photograph chromosomes. (Birth defects are usually caused by various factors related to centromeres, such as their shape and size.)

REPRODUCTIVE SYSTEM: REVIEW QUESTIONS

1. The testicles are located outside the body because:
   A. that is the normal embryologic location.
   B. there is direct connection from the epididymis to the penile urethra.
   C. there is a need for automatic peripheral nerves.
   D. spermatogenesis requires a temperature lower than body temperature.

2. Spermatozoa travel through all of the following structures except the:
   A. ureter.
   B. urethra.
   C. vas deferens.
   D. epididymis.

3. What structure is directly attached to the ovary?
   A. Vagina
   B. Uterus
   C. Fallopian tubes
   D. None of the above

4. The placenta of humans is composed of tissue derived from the:
   A. uterus and developing embryo.
   B. uterus only.
   C. developing embryo only.
   D. fallopian tubes.

5. The menstrual period (total cycle) is typically closest to:
   A. 2 weeks.
   B. 4 weeks.
   C. 2 months.
   D. 1 year.

6. The sequence of stages (F = follicular phase, L = luteal phase, O = ovulation) of the menstrual cycle (in reference to the ovary) following the menstrual flow is:
   A. F, O, L
   B. L, O, F
   C. O, F, L
   D. F, L, O

7. Ovulation usually occurs:
   A. 1–3 days after menses (blood flow).
   B. 14 days before menses.
   C. 1–3 days before menses.
   D. during menses.

8. The corpus luteum secretes:
   A. progesterone.
   B. LH.
   C. FSH.
   D. HCG.

9. The organ in the female analogous to the glans penis in the male is the:

    A. vagina.
    B. labia minora.
    C. labia majora.
    D. clitoris.

10. Which hormone is found primarily during the first half (follicular and proliferative phase) of the menstrual cycle?

    A. FSH
    B. Progesterone
    C. Prolactin
    D. HCG

11. Which substance is not secreted by the ovary or uterus in a pregnant woman?

    A. FSH
    B. HCG
    C. Progesterone
    D. Estrogen

12. In males, gametes are formed in the:

    A. vas deferens.
    B. Leydig cells.
    C. epididymis.
    D. seminiferous tubules.

13. Polar bodies:

    A. are the poles of magnets.
    B. result from gametogenesis in the male.
    C. result from gametogenesis in the female.
    D. form dipoles.

14. Fertilization of the ovum by the spermatozoon usually occurs in the:

    A. ovary.
    B. fallopian tubes.
    C. uterus.
    D. vagina.

15. Select the incorrect association.

    A. Oogonium—1n
    B. Primary oocyte—2n
    C. Secondary oocyte—1n
    D. Ova—1n

16. Corpus luteum:

    A. results from mature ovum.
    B. contains no hormones.
    C. degenerates before ovulation.
    D. degenerates after ovulation.

17. Tissue or cells not found in the testis are:

    A. seminiferous tubules.
    B. Leydig cells.
    C. spermatogonia.
    D. seminal vesicles.

18. Which of the following contains no developing ovum?

    A. Graafian follicle
    B. Primordial follicle
    C. Corpus luteum
    D. Oocytes

19. Select the incorrect association.

    A. Spermatogonia—2n
    B. Primary spermatocytes—2n

C. Secondary spermatocytes—1n
D. Spermatozoa—2n

20. Which is not associated with the male reproductive system?

    A. Epididymis
    B. Leydig cells
    C. Thecal cells
    D. Sertoli cells

21. The number of mature gametes resulting from meiosis of the primary oocyte in the female is:

    A. 1
    B. 2
    C. 3
    D. 4

22. The number of mature gametes resulting from meiosis in the male is:

    A. 1
    B. 2
    C. 3
    D. 4

23. Factors important in the differentiation of cells include:

    A. cytoplasmic composition and distribution of constituents.
    B. characteristics of neighboring cells.
    C. physical environmental agents.
    D. all of the above.

24. As a cell becomes more specialized for a particular function, the opportunity for it to become specialized for other functions:

    A. decreases.
    B. increases.
    C. remains the same.
    D. increases steadily and decreases exponentially.

25. A cell found in the middle layer of the three-layered gastrula has probably lost the option to become:

    A. epidermis.
    B. kidney.
    C. muscle.
    D. blood.

26. Select the following situation(s) that have the best likelihood of leading to differentiated daughter cells after a cleavage occurs:

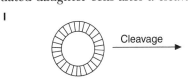

Blastula (all cells similar)
pH or medium = 7.4

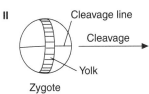

Zygote

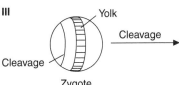

Zygote

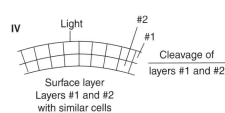

Surface layer
Layers #1 and #2
with similar cells

Rim of similar cells

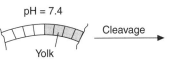

A. III, IV, VI

B. II, IV, V, VI

C. II, III, IV, V, VI

D. I–VI

27. Which of the following cells or cell types is the most differentiated?

    A. Mesenchymal cell

    B. Nerve cell

    C. Cancer cell

    D. Bone marrow stem cell

ANSWERS AND EXPLANATIONS

1-25. 1-D, 2-A, 3-D, 4-A, 5-B, 6-A, 7-B, 8-A, 9-D, 10-A, 11-A, 12-D, 13-C, 14-B, 15-A, 16-D, 17-D, 18-C, 19-D, 20-C, 21-A, 22-D, 23-D, 24-A, 25-A. See text for explanation.

26. A Differentiation is possible if a factor can affect a group of similar cells in an unsymmetric or unequal manner. In I, the pH affects all the similar cells equally. In II, the cleavage results in two cells with similar yolk distributions. In III, the cleavage results in different yolk distributions so the daughter cells are different cytoplasmically, which can lead to differentiation. In IV, the light may either affect the surface layer only or affect the surface layer more strongly than the underlying layer. This can potentially affect gene activation and can lead to differentiation between the cell layers. In V, the rim of similar cells is probably affected similarly by the symmetrically diffusing chemicals, and the daughter cells will probably be similar. In VI, although the pH is constant, this can have different effects on cells with and without yolks, and, hence, result in potentially differentiated daughter cells.

27. 27-B. See text for explanation.

Developmental Embryology

Self-Managed Learning Questions

1. Understand the differences between animal and vegetable poles, superficial and complete cleavage; draw diagrams to explain these concepts.
2. Define and distinguish the several steps leading to regulative development and mosaic development.
3. Compare gastrulation between mammals and birds (e.g., between a cat and a chicken).

EMBRYOGENESIS

Fertilization

Embryogenesis can be broken down into fertilization, cleavage, blastulation, gastrulation, and neurulation. **Fusion** of the gametes produced by meiosis involves first the penetration of the ovum by the spermatozoon. The acrosome (part of sperm that contains hydrolytic enzymes) dissolves the corona radiata (collection of follicle cells) and zona pellucida around ovulated ovum, and only the head of the spermatozoon (contains the DNA) penetrates the ovum. Upon such penetration, a reaction in the ovum occurs, preventing additional spermatozoa from entering. After the ovum completes meiosis II, the male (n) and female (n) pronuclei fuse, and cleavage of the fertilized egg (zygote = 2n) begins.

Cleavage

Growth, differentiation, and morphogenesis occur together after the first few cleavages. The amount of yolk in the egg is an important determinant of the cleavage pattern. In humans, there is very little yolk. Cleavage is complete and regular. The egg has polarity (i.e., is asymmetrical) by virtue of the yolk distribution in some vertebrates. The first few cleavages (4–5) result in a grape-like cluster of cells called the **morula**. These divisions occur without cell growth; hence, the morula is not much larger than the zygote.

Blastulation

The morula develops into the blastula, a single-layer hollow sphere of cells with a cavity called the blastocoel. In mammals, this superficial layer of cells is called the trophoblast and is important in implanting the blastula into the uterine wall. The trophoblast layer covers an inner cell mass, which develops into the embryo. From this point, morphogenesis (i.e., movement of cells to delineate shape and function) begins.

Gastrulation

Gastrulation results first in the positioning of two, then three, germ layers. In amphibians, it begins with invagination of the sphere at the blastopore. A two-layered structure with a new cavity, the archenteron, results and opens to the outside via the blastopore (site

19 days

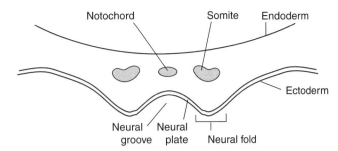

Fig. 8-87. Ectoderm of human embryo.

20 days

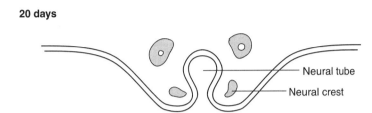

of invagination). Cells from the lip of the blastopore migrate between the two layers of cells to form a third layer. In mammals, the three layers develop from the inner cell mass, now called the embryonic disk. The three germ layers—ectoderm, mesoderm, and endoderm—differentiate into defined tissues and organs (Figure 8-87).

Neurulation

The neural groove forms the neural tube. At the margins of the neural tube detachment are a group of cells called the neural crest cells, which form the adrenal medulla, melanocytes, and myelin sheaths, among other tissues. The neural tube develops into the central nervous system (spinal cord and brain). Ventral to the neural tube, mesodermal tissue forms somites, which gives rise to the vertebral column (formed on, but not from, the notochord) and associated muscles.

Major Structures Arising Out of Primary Germ Layers

The ectoderm develops into the nervous system, the epidermis of the skin and its derivatives, the lens of the eye, and the linings of the mouth and nasal canal. The endoderm develops into the inner linings of the gut (esophagus, stomach, intestines), associated organs (liver, gallbladder, pancreas), the lung, the thyroid gland, and the urinary bladder. The mesoderm develops into the skeletal system (bones, cartilage, notochord), muscles, kidney, circulatory system (heart, blood cells, vessels), dermis of skin, and outer coverings of internal organs. Figure 8-88 is a schematic summary of this sequence.

APPLIED CONCEPTS

- Understand the precursors (radioactive) to analyze haploid cell mutations. What graphical plots would you except?
- Which hormones play an important role in embryogenesis? Discuss them in relation to several phases, such as gastrulation, cleavage, and neurulation.
- What is Coombs direct antiglobulin test? What does it detect? Are there any errors associated with this test for early diagnosis of erythroblastosis fetalis in newborns?

DEVELOPMENTAL EMBRYOLOGY: REVIEW QUESTIONS

1. The blastula is generally preceded by the:

    A. gastrula.
    B. morula.
    C. neurula.
    D. gastrula and morula.

2. The three germ layers—the ectoderm, the mesoderm, and the endoderm—are found at which stage?

    A. Morula
    B. Gastrula
    C. Blastula
    D. Neurula

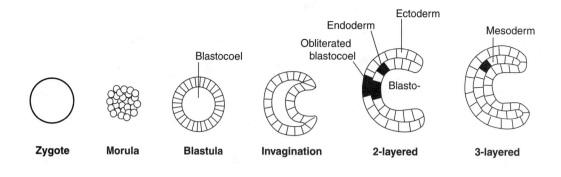

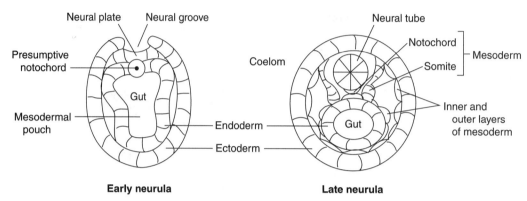

Fig. 8-88. Early development of frog embryo (embryogenesis).

3. Select the one item that is not derived from the ectoderm germinal layer.

   A. Nerve
   B. Muscle
   C. Lens of eye
   D. Epidermis of skin

4. Select the organ or tissue that is not derived from the mesodermal germinal layer.

   A. Muscle
   B. Kidney
   C. Intestines
   D. Bones

5. Select the organ or tissue that is derived from the endodermal germinal layer.

   A. Muscle
   B. Kidney
   C. Intestines
   D. Bones

6. The individual cells resulting from the cleavage of a fertilized egg may occasionally give rise to complete organisms up to the third cleavage. Select the correct statement.

   A. Cleavages before the third cleavage were determinate cleavages.
   B. The number of cells resulting from the third cleavage is 16.
   C. Determinate cleavages cannot occur, in general, before the third cleavage.
   D. The cells resulting after the next cleavage are probably different in cytoplasmic composition.

7. Once the spermatozoon head penetrates the _____, a reaction ensues that _____.

   A. corona radiata; causes the pronuclei to fuse.
   B. corona radiata; prevents penetration by additional spermatozoa.
   C. ovum; causes the pronuclei to fuse.
   D. ovum; prevents penetration by additional spermatozoa.

8. All of the following processes occur during the process of fertilization of the egg by the spermatozoon except that:

   A. the acrosome dissolves the corona radiata.
   B. only the head of the spermatozoon enters the ovum.
   C. the spermatozoon nucleus completes its second meiotic division.
   D. the ovum nucleus completes its second meiotic division.

9. The correct sequence of the early states of development is:

   A. morula, gastrula, blastula, neurula
   B. morula, blastula, gastrula, neurula
   C. blastula, morula, gastrula, neurula
   D. neurula, blastula, gastrula, morula

10. Which of the following stages is essentially the same size as the zygote?

   A. Gastrula
   B. Blastula
   C. Morula
   D. None of the above

11. The first stage of development in which a cavity appears is the:

   A. neurula.
   B. morula.
   C. gastrula.
   D. blastula.

12. Morphogenesis begins at which stage?

   A. Morula
   B. Blastula
   C. Gastrula
   D. Neurula

ANSWERS AND EXPLANATIONS

1–5. 1-B, 2-B, 3-B, 4-C, 5-A. See text for explanation.
6. D The implication of the question is that the divisions after the third division are determinate and result in cells that have different cytoplasmic components. The number of cells resulting from the nth cleavage is 2n, assuming that at each cleavage all cells divide. Then $2^3 = 8$, not 16.
7–12. 7-D, 8-C, 9-B, 10-C, 11-D, 12-B. See text for explanation.

Genetics and Evolution

Self-Managed Learning Questions

1. Read the following information critically and evaluate actual validity from examples seen in biology and physiology laboratories:
   • Heredity is transmitted by genes that exist in pairs.
   • The two genes of each pair separate from one another, and each gamete receives only one gene of each pair when gametes are formed (law of segregation).
   • When two alternate forms of the same gene are present in a human, only one of the alternatives is usually expressed (law of dominance).
   • If two or more independent characteristics in a genetic cross are considered, each characteristic is inherited without relation to other traits (law of independent assortment).

2. Examine the laws stated and identify key words, implied and stated assumptions, and how current genetic research supports or contradicts each law. Identify evidence related to those laws.

3. Prove mathematically and with examples that meiosis accounts for the segregation of alleles and that incomplete dominance follows Mendel's laws.

4. Analyze and evaluate the paradox that life was generated from nonliving molecules or by abiogenesis. Research the apparatus designed by Stanley Miller and Harold Urey in analyzing origin of organic molecules. Compare and validate the underlying assumptions with the biosphere studies being carried out in Arizona. What experimental errors have been identified by scientists?

GENETICS

Molecular genetics, mutations, and comparative chordate anatomy should be studied as parts of the large-scale evolution process. The history and mechanisms controlling evolution (for various organisms) should be directly applied to problem solving in gene flow, genetic drift, and genetic (chromosomal) mapping. Recognize and appraise this section as a series of hypotheses, explanations, and conclusions and determine how current information is used to solve special mathematical problems in genetics.

Mendelian Laws of Inheritance and Their Application

Gametes (haploid) are formed during meiosis by the separation of homologous chromosomes (diploid state). This results in the separation of each of the alleles of a homolog into a different gamete. This is Mendel's First Law of Segregation (of alleles of the same trait). Different traits (i.e., loci) may be on the same chromosome or on different chromosomes. If the traits are on different chromosomes, the alleles of these different traits should separate independently of each other into gametes. This is Mendel's Second Law of Independent Assortment (of alleles of different traits). But, if different traits are on the same chromosome, they may be far apart or close together. Traits far apart on the same chromosome separate into gametes as if they were on separate chromosomes. This is possible because of crossing-over (reciprocal exchange of parts of homologous chromosomes) during synapsis in the first meiotic prophase. The farther apart two different traits are on a chromosome, the easier it is for crossing-over to occur. Alleles of traits that are close together do not separate frequently by the mechanism of crossing-over into different gametes because they tend to remain on the same chromosome, so they cannot independently (of each other) assort, do not follow Mendel's second law, and are called **linked traits** (or genes) [Figure 8-89].

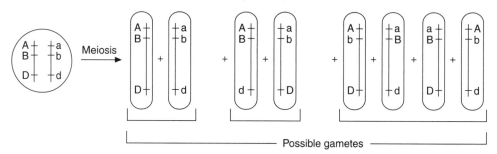

Possible gametes

Fig. 8-89. Mendel's law, crossing-over, recombination, and gamete formation. A diploid (2n) cell shows a pair of homologous chromosomes with loci for three different traits with alleles A,a; B,b; and D,d. Traits A,a and B,b are linked. Traits A,a and D,d and traits B,b and D,d are not linked. According to Mendel's first law, each allele of a given trait (A versus a, B versus b, and D versus d) segregate independently of each other. In Mendel's second law, alleles of different traits (e.g., A,a and D,d) assort independently. This is not true for A,a and B,b because they are linked. In recombination of the linked genes A,a versus B,b, A,a and B,b do not assort independently of each other because they are so close together. It would normally be expected that A and B or a and b would be together in gametes, but, by crossing over, Ab and aB also are possible (but at less than expected frequencies).

Recombination is the process of separating alleles of linked traits into different gametes, that is, onto different homologous chromosomes. Linkage (recombination) studies and cytogenetics (study of markings, e.g., bands on chromosomes) are used to map chromosomes as to the loci of traits. Another of Mendel's contributions to genetics was his recognition that genes are particulate (i.e., not indivisible or blendable). Mendel's mechanisms of assortment and segregation and the later discovered ideas of recombination illustrate mechanisms of **genetic variability** that can be viewed as the passage to offspring, via gametes, of different combinations of alleles than existed in the parent.

Hardy-Weinberg Principle

The Hardy-Weinberg law states that, under the following conditions, gene and genotypic frequencies remain constant from generation to generation in sexually reproducing populations in which (1) there is a large population, (2) there are no mutations or there is mutation equilibrium, (3) there is no immigration or emigration of the population, and (4) there is random reproduction. Large populations are required because gene frequencies undergo random fluctuations called **genetic drift**. In a small population, these random changes may cause an increase in certain alleles, leading to homozygosity. This effect is small in large populations (e.g., greater than 10,000 breeding individuals). Mutations always occur, so there would never be a time of mutation equilibrium. Immigration or emigration leads to loss or gain of certain alleles that change gene frequencies. Reproduction includes all the steps from mate selection through mating and development of the embryo to growth of the young to reproductive maturity. All of these conditions, and all in between, must be random for gene frequencies to remain constant (or for there to be random reproduction). But, in all populations, nonrandom reproduction exists, and this nonrandom reproduction is called **natural selection** as set forth by Darwin. Reproduction is nonrandom because phenotypes vary, and different phenotypes result in differences in reproductive capabilities. Natural selection does change gene frequencies by causing new combinations of genes, which results in new phenotypes. Additionally, recombination and gene mutation, if left alone, can destroy favorable gene combinations and substitute unfavorable combinations for them. Natural selection also serves a conservative function by eliminating these unfavorable combinations. Natural selection can act on gene frequencies only when the genetic variation is expressed as phenotypic variation, and that phenotypic variation can lead to changes in gene frequencies only when it reflects underlying genetic variation.

The Hardy-Weinberg principle states that under certain random mating conditions, gene frequencies will remain constant from generation to generation. This principle is useful in population genetics. Gene frequencies may be expressed as a decimal or as a percent. Under the Hardy-Weinberg principle, the gene frequency of dominant and recessive alleles remains the same from generation to generation. In other words, the sum of all the allele frequencies for a gene within a population is equal to 1.0, or 100%. Each genotype is made of two alleles. The chance of getting a particular genotype is the product of the probabilities of the two alleles.

The Hardy-Weinberg equation states, $p^2 + 2pq + q^2 = 1$, where p = frequency of dominant allele, q = frequency of recessive allele.

For example, in a population of dogs, 16% are white. The gene for white is recessive. To find the frequency of the dominant gene (dominant = W, recessive = w), apply the Hardy-Weinberg principle as shown in Figure 8-90.

p + q

	p	q
p	WW	Ww
q	Ww	ww

WW = homozygous dominant
2Ww = heterozygous dominant
ww = homozygous recessive

Fig. 8-90.

p + q

	p	q
p	p^2	pq
q	pq	q^2

$(p + q)(p + q) = 1$
$p^2 + 2pq + q^2 = 1$
$p + q = 1$

In the population of dogs, the 16% that are white are the homozygous recessive dogs. Hence, $q^2 = 0.16$, $q = 0.4$, $p = 1 - 0.4 = 0.6$. The frequency of the dominant gene W = p = 0.6.

To determine the frequency of heterozygosity for whiteness and nonwhiteness for the dog population, determine $2pq = 2(0.6)(0.4) = 0.48$.

Finally, p = 0.6 = 60%
q = 0.4 = 40%
2pq = 0.48 = 48%

$p^2 = (0.6)2 = 0.36 = 36\%$

$q^2 = (0.4)2 = 0.16 = 16\%$

$p^2 + 2pq + q^2 = 36\% + 48\% + 16\% = 100\%$

The examples cited should be studied and applied to various population genetics problems.

Gene Mapping

Simple **gene mapping** is done using recombinant techniques with viral and bacterial DNA. The map is a linear, one-dimensional structure. The map units indirectly represent the percent recombination between various traits (genetic loci). The traits must be measurable in some manner (e.g., nutrient use, products produced, temperature dependence). The combination of traits in the offspring, as compared with the parents, helps determine the recombinant frequencies (percentages) that help determine the gene map. An example of a two-factor (trait) cross is shown in Figure 8-91.

A series of two-factor crosses may be used to sequence the gene loci. The maximal possible frequency of any recombinant is 50%. If the frequency of recombination between the loci is near 50%, then there is no linkage. The smaller the recombination frequency between the two loci, the stronger the linkage (i.e., the closer together the traits). Triple

Fig. 8-91. The original genotypes are in the highest frequency. The larger the percentage of recombinants, the farther apart are the traits on the map. Consequently, the traits are linked less tightly. The trait loci (a or a^+ and b or b^+) are linked.

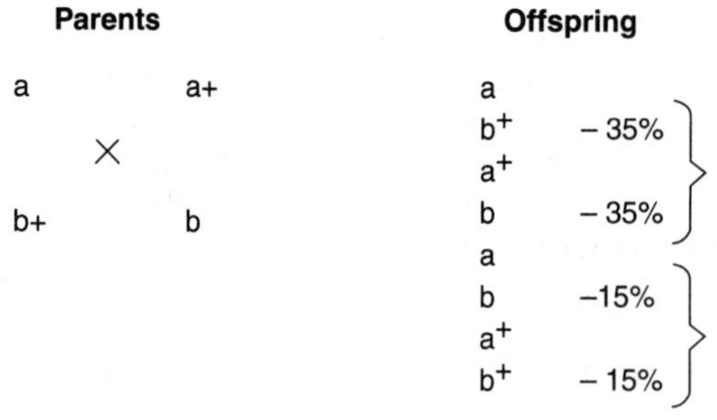

Parents		Offspring	
a	a+	a	
		b^+	− 35%
×		a^+	
		b	− 35%
b+	b	a	
		b	−15%
		a^+	
		b^+	− 15%

Offspring (8 genotypic classes result)	Genotype frequency	Recombination frequency	Recombination status
x y z	30%	60%	No recombination.
x^+ y^+ z^+	30%		
x^+ y^+ z	10%	20%	Recombination between central locus *and* z. Single recombination.
x y z^+	10%		
x^+ y z	7%	14%	Recombination between central locus *and* x. Single recombination.
x y^+ z^+	7%		
x^+ y z^+	3%	6%	y is now identified as central locus. This is lowest frequency cross and the y factors are out of place with the others. Double recombination.
x y^+ z	3%		

Fig. 8-92

factor (i.e., three traits at three loci) is used to order gene loci. The (original) parental genotypes appear in the highest frequency, single recombinants next, and double recombinants in the lowest frequency. The probability of the central locus recombining with both outside loci (double recombination) is equal to the products of the probability of it combining with each one individually (single recombination). In Figure 8-92, y is closer to x than to z, that is, it has a lower recombination frequency for x than for z.

Factors that modify the percentage distributions of the offspring may affect the analysis. Besides the probability factor (i.e., each cross does not lead to exact ratios, just as in mendelian crosses), conditional lethal mutations may occur and cause some genotypes not to survive, and, therefore, not to be counted.

Population Growth

Although many factors affect the ultimate growth of a population (species), four factors can be used to describe the growth rate (R). These are the birth rate (B), the death rate (D), the carrying capacity (C), and the number of individuals in the population (N). B is the rate of live births per unit population (e.g., $5/1000$ means 5 live births per 1000 individuals). D is similarly defined. Both are dependent on the age of the population and the reproductive capacity of the population. Very old or young populations have a high D. C represents the number of individuals that the environment is able to support. C is independent of the R of the population, but, over time, the total N can affect its value (e.g., by using up the food supply). The maximum growth rate may vary as the C of particular environments varies. The equation linking these four factors follows:

$$R = (B - D) \times \left(\frac{C - N}{C}\right) \times N$$

Note that B − D is the intrinsic growth rate (IGR) of the population. The key points to remember are as follows:

1. R is directly proportional to IGR.
2. R is directly proportional to N.
3. When N is small, the term $(C - N)/C$ is approximately 1, and growth is exponential.
4. When N approaches and equals C, the term $(C - N)/C$ is 0, and the population is in zero growth (mild fluctuations may occur).
5. The $(C - N)/C$ factor results in the S-shaped growth curve for populations.

Population growth curves are shown in Figure 8-93.

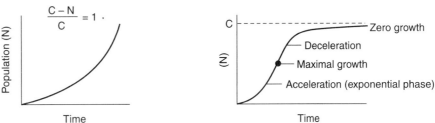

Fig. 8-93. Population growth.

Age distributions of populations are important in understanding and predicting changes in population growth. Age distribution curves may be drawn in many ways; Figure 8-94 is one example (with different distributions). Survivorship of the population may also be graphically represented as shown in Figure 8-95.

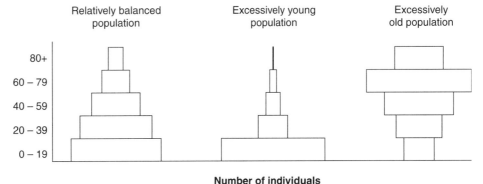

Fig. 8-94. Age distribution.

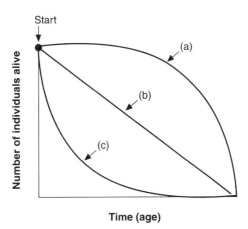

Fig. 8-95. Survivorship of the population. (*a*) Individuals live to older ages, many younger and older. (*b*) Death rates are the same at all ages, and there is equal representation of all ages. (*c*) Younger die at high rates, with few older in the population.

Meiosis and Genetic Variability

For a discussion of meiosis, see Generalized Eukaryotic Cells. Each organism has a set of chromosomes. Chromosomes of eukaryotes are a complex of DNA, histone (basic protein), and nonhistone protein. The normal complement of chromosomes is diploid (2n) as occurs in somatic cells. Gametes (male and female) are **haploid** (1n). Gametes combine to form the diploid cell. The complement of chromosomes may be divided into autosomes and sex chromosomes (having to do with sex determination). Humans have 22 pairs of autosomes and one pair of sex chromosomes (X, Y) for a total of 46. The female is XX, and the male is XY. Either the whole set of chromosomes can be in some multiple of n, which is called **polyploidy** (e.g., 4n = tetraploidy), or one or more chromosomes may be missing or in excess, which is called **aneuploidy** (e.g., monosomy, in which only one of a chromosome type is present, or trisomy, in which three representatives of a given chromosome are present). Down's syndrome (mongolism) is caused by trisomy 21 (i.e., there are three of the chromosomes numbered 21).

On each chromosome there is a sequence of genes. In this discussion, a gene is a specific trait. Hence, each locus (or position) on a chromosome is for a specific trait. In the **diploid** (2n) cell, there is a pair of homologous chromosomes, which pair in meiosis. Homologous chromosomes are similar by having the same sequence of trait loci (except the pair X and Y); hence they are the same size. For any given general trait (e.g., eye color), there are many alternative genes (e.g., blue, brown) for its determination. The alternative genes for a general trait constitute a set of **alleles** for that trait. Because there is only one locus (usually) for a simple trait on a chromosome, there can be only one allele of that trait per homologous chromosome. Then, for any given trait, there is a maximum of two alleles per diploid cell (one on each homologous chromosome). But the total number of different alleles for a given trait can be greater than two (e.g., there are many different alleles for types of hemoglobin, such as normal adult, fetal, sickle, hemoglobin C, and hemoglobin Milwaukee). For an individual, the specific alleles present are called the genotype. If the alleles for a given trait on each homologous chromosome are identical, the genotype is called **homozygous**. If the alleles for a given trait on each homologous chromosome are different, the genotype is called **heterozygous**. The term genotype can refer to the alleles of a specific trait or the total genetic makeup (all of the alleles) of an individual. Each of the alleles (genes) of a given trait attempts to express itself via its protein product. If one allele of a pair expresses itself over another (e.g., eye color with brown over blue), then that allele is dominant and the other recessive. (These terms go together like "oxidation and reduction" in chemistry.) If both alleles express themselves, they are called codominant. The expression (what is seen as the trait of the individual) of the genotype is called the **phenotype**.

Sex-linked Characteristics

In the sex chromosomes, the X is larger than the Y (i.e., has more loci for traits); hence, traits on the X may not appear on the Y. Traits of this type are called **sex-linked traits**. Examples in humans are hemophilia, color blindness, and glucose-6-phosphate dehydrogenase deficiency. The X and Y chromosomes are homologous because they can pair (synapse) in meiosis. Sex-linked traits are unique in their inheritance because the male (with only one X chromosome) can express recessive alleles (phenotypes) because there is only one allele present. The female requires both recessive alleles to be present for expression of the recessive trait. Furthermore, transmission to the male occurs usually only from the mother. Whereas, if the daughter is diseased, both mother and father must have passed on the allele (Figure 8-96). (Barr bodies are inactivated "excess" X chromosomes in which only one X remains active. This phenomenon is referred to as the Lyon or Lyon-Russel hypothesis.)

Cytoplasmic inheritance is the determination of genetic traits by constituents of the

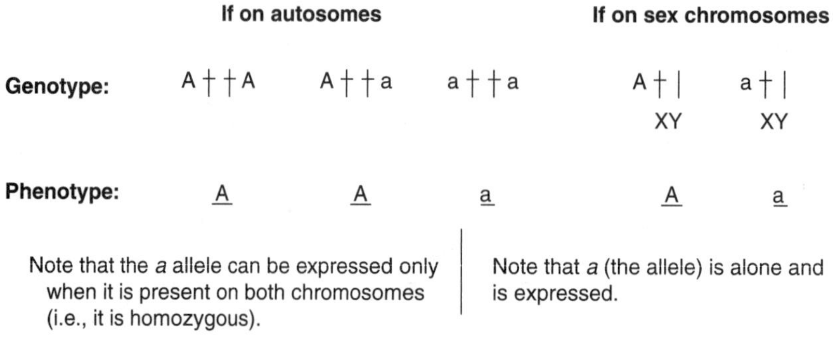

	If on autosomes			If on sex chromosomes	
Genotype:	A ┆┆A	A ┆┆a	a ┆┆a	A ┆│ XY	a ┆│ XY
Phenotype:	<u>A</u>	<u>A</u>	<u>a</u>	<u>A</u>	<u>a</u>

Note that the *a* allele can be expressed only when it is present on both chromosomes (i.e., it is homozygous). | Note that *a* (the allele) is alone and is expressed.

Fig. 8-96. Autosomal and sex chromosomes: phenotype expressions given a trait with alleles *A* = dominant, *a* = recessive, and phenotypes *A* and *a*.

cytoplasm rather than the nucleus. This inheritance does not follow mendelian laws. The mother (most of the cytoplasm of the zygote comes from the ovum) plays the major role in this type of inheritance. Chloroplasts (contain DNA), mitochondria (contain DNA), centrioles, and basal bodies of flagella and cilia are examples of structures that replicate without input from the nucleus.

Pedigree Charts

Pedigrees are diagrams that show phenotypic appearance of traits in a family. The basic nomenclature is shown in Figure 8-97. A dominant autosomal trait with complete **penetrance** (i.e., the trait appears in all persons with the allele) has a pedigree that shows both sexes affected, many individuals affected, and passage of the trait from affected parent to children, even if they are heterozygous (Figure 8-98).

Case *(1)* is probably heterozygous for the trait because, if it is homozygous, then all offspring would be affected.

An autosomal recessive trait also shows both sexes affected, but fewer individuals are affected and passage may be from an unaffected parent (because the parent is heterozygous) to an affected offspring (Figure 8-99).

A sex-linked recessive trait usually shows only males affected and passage of the trait from an unaffected mother to a son. The trait affects a daughter only if the father has it and the mother is, at least, heterozygous (Figure 8-100).

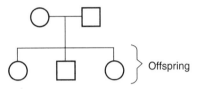

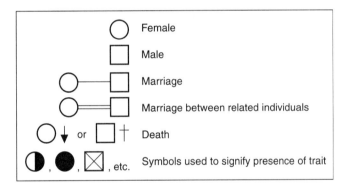

Fig. 8-97. Pedigree terminology.

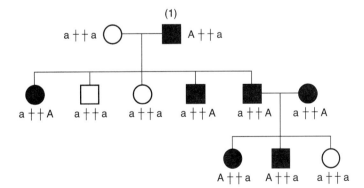

Fig. 8-98. Dominant pedigree.

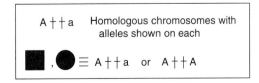

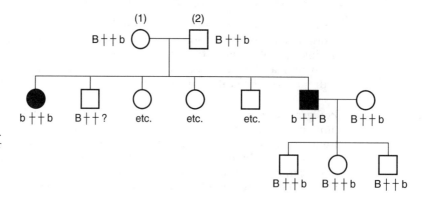

Fig. 8-99. Recessive pedigree. Both parents are heterozygous for the recessive allele.

† ? ≡   ? = B or b without affecting phenotype

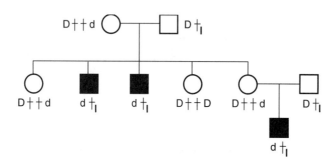

Fig. 8-100. Sex-linked pedigree.

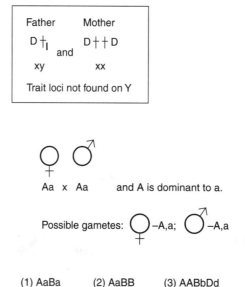

Father	Mother
D †₁	D † † D
and	
xy	xx
Trait loci not found on Y	

Aa   x   Aa   and A is dominant to a.

Possible gametes: ♀ –A,a; ♂ –A,a

Genotype (Diploid):	(1) AaBa	(2) AaBB	(3) AABbDd	(4)AaBbDd
Possible gametes (Haploid):	AB,Ab,aB,ab	AB,aB	ABD,ABd,AbD,Abd	ABD,ABd,AbD,Abd,aBD,aBd,abD,abd
	(1)	(2)	(3)	(4)

Fig. 8-101. Gamete formation by example.

Punnett Squares

Punnett squares are useful ways of determining the genotypes possible from the mating of two individuals with known genotypes. First, the possible gametes are determined (Figure 8-101); then these are combined in all possible ways. By knowing dominant-recessive relationships, the frequency of phenotypes can be ascertained. The Punnett square gives expected ratios only; Figures 8-102 and 8-103 are examples.

Mutations produce a small but important change in the gene frequencies of the gene

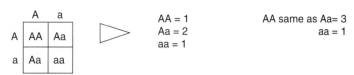

Fig. 8-102. Punnett square with one trait.

Punnett square	Genotype frequency	Phenotype frequency
	AA = 1 Aa = 2 aa = 1	AA same as Aa= 3 aa = 1

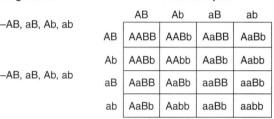

AaBb x AaBb

Possible gametes

♀ –AB, aB, Ab, ab

♂ –AB, aB, Ab, ab

Punnett square

	AB	Ab	aB	ab
AB	AABB	AABb	AaBB	AaBb
Ab	AABb	AAbb	AaBb	Aabb
aB	AaBB	AaBb	aaBB	aaBb
ab	AaBb	Aabb	aaBb	aabb

A dominant to a
B dominant to b

Genotype frequency

AABB = 1   aaBb = 2
AABb = 2   AAbb = 1
AaBb = 4   aaBB = 1
AaBB = 2   aabb = 1
Aabb = 2

Phenotype frequency

A – B – (AABB,AABb,AaBb,AaBB) = 1 +
aaB – (aaBb,aaBB) = 2 + 1 = 3
A–bb (Aabb,AAbb) = 2 + 1 = 3
aabb (aabb) = 1

Fig. 8-103. Punnett square with two traits.

pool of a population. These gene frequencies determine the genotypic ratios that determine the distribution of phenotypes in the population. Genotypic ratios (i.e., numbers and types of genotypes) can be determined from the gene frequencies and the Punnett square method as shown in Figure 8-104, in which allele B = 0.8 and allele b = 0.2 as frequencies in the population and genotypic frequencies are BB = 0.64, Bb = 2(0.16) = 0.32, and bb = 0.04.

Fig. 8-104. Genotypic frequencies.

	B (0.8)	b (0.2)
B (0.8)	BB (0.64)	Bb (0.16)
b (0.2)	Bb (0.16)	bb (0.04)

Mutations

Another set of mechanisms responsible for genetic variability is **mutations**. A mutation may be considered a stable heritable change in genetic material (DNA). Changes or structural changes in chromosomes called **chromosomal aberrations** that may occur at the level of the chromosome (Figure 8-105) are as follows:

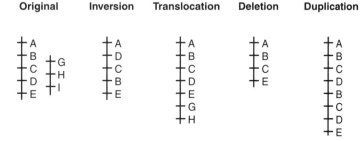

Fig. 8-105. Chromosomal aberrations.

Original	Inversion	Translocation	Deletion	Duplication
A	A	A	A	A
B	D	B	B	B
C G	C	C	C	C
D H	B	D	E	D
E I	E	E		B
		G		C
		H		D
				E

1. Inversion—sequence of genes on the chromosomes is reversed.
2. Translocation—a part of one chromosome attaches to another.
3. Deletion—a part of the chromosome is missing.
4. Duplication—part of the chromosome is repeated.

Mutations are the ultimate source of all new genes in the population, and, as such, they are the raw material for all evolutionary changes. Genes mutate forward to new genes and backward to the old gene. The mutation pressure is the net change of these two processes. Genes arising by mutation tend to be recessive, and because they are rarely homozygous, they tend to be carried silently, or not expressed, in the population for long periods of time. Stable alleles are those with low mutation rates; they tend to increase in frequency. This contrasts with unstable alleles, which have high mutation rates and tend to decrease in frequency. This process results in a slow shift in gene frequencies in the population. It seems reasonable that mutation alone could cause evolutionary change. The major reason that mutation alone does not cause evolutionary change is that mutation is random and, consequently, usually is in a direction away from the evolutionary trend of the organism. Therefore, mutation alone has a slow and nondirectional effect on evolution, except in polyploidy. Polyploidy is the doubling of the set of chromosomes (e.g., 2n 1A 4n), usually by nondisjunction during meiosis. What results is an organism with a larger set of chromosomes with phenotypic differences among them. Mutations in somatic cells have no effect on evolution because they are not passed on to the offspring.

EVOLUTION

Natural Selection

Evolution is the study of the changes that occur in organisms, how the changes occur, and the results of the changes. These changes may be minor and lead to better adaptation to an environment, or they may be major and lead to a totally different species. Changes come about when organisms are "selected" to survive on the basis of phenotypic differences. These phenotypic differences must be based on underlying genetic differences, as found in the germ cells, to lead to evolutionary change. The survival of selected organisms leads to changes in the gene frequencies and gene combinations in the population, which, in turn, leads to changes in phenotypic characteristics and, hence, evolution.

Taxonomy

A hierarchical classification that exists for organisms has been attributed primarily to Linnaeus. Organisms are grouped at each level on the basis of similarities. As the hierarchy is ascended (shown below), the similarities become more general. A well-known mnemonic is given with the hierarchy:

Kings Kingdom	Fine Family
Play Phylum	Grain Genus
Chess Class	Sand Species
On Order	

All organisms are given a two-component Latin name. The first is the genus (capitalized) and the second is the species (not capitalized) [e.g., *Homo sapiens*].

Phenotypic differences are in a distribution in any population, and this distribution is often an approximation of the bell-shaped curve (Figure 8-106). An example is the distribution of height in humans. Environmental factors (meteorologic, geographic, physical, or biological) also vary greatly. It is a small step to infer that certain characteristics are better suited for certain environments. Or, to look at it differently, environments may select organisms with certain phenotypic characteristics that are most likely to survive in them. As discussed, if these phenotypic characteristics reflect genetic differences, then a change in gene frequencies and evolution can occur. Environmental factors and reproductive factors (i.e., natural selection) interact with each other. In summary, mutations provide the raw material for evolution, but it is the selection pressure for certain pheno-

Fig. 8-106. Distribution of phenotypic differences.

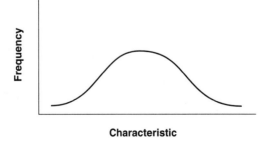

types exerted by natural selection and environmental factors that determines the course of evolution.

The fitness of a genotype refers to its reproductive contribution to subsequent generations relative to the contribution of other genotypes of phenotypes. In other words, if a "fit" animal survives its environment and competition for reproduction, then that individual passes its genes along. An animal that is not fit does not reproduce and its genes are not passed on. An individual can influence its fitness by producing its own offspring and by helping the survival of relatives that have the same genes from a common ancestor.

Species Concept and Speciation

The consequences of evolution are seen in the changes that may occur in a given species. These changes can be minor and be reflected as clines. Clines are gradual variations in a species due to geographic (environmental) variations such as altitude or latitude. Subspecies (races) result when an abrupt environmental change is associated with an abrupt change in characteristics. Finally, the evolutionary changes may be so great as to result in a totally new species—a process called **speciation**.

A species is viewed as a set of genetically distinct organisms that share a common gene pool (i.e., gene flow is possible between them) and are reproductively isolated from all other such groups. The first step in speciation is usually geographic isolation of two populations of the same species. A barrier (e.g., rivers, oceans, canyons, mountains) prevents the populations from coming together to mate. The two separate populations will tend to differ because (1) gene frequencies usually differ, (2) each population experiences different mutations, and (3) the different environments exert different selection pressures. The second factor in speciation then comes into play; it is reproductive isolation. The two populations begin to differ such that gene flow between them is no longer possible even if they are brought together. This is brought about by intrinsic reproductive isolating mechanisms that act at all the steps of reproduction. These are (1) ecogeographic isolation (organisms can no longer survive in each other's environment), (2) habitat isolation (organisms may occupy only certain, but different, habitats within the same range), (3) seasonal isolation (the breeding periods may be at different times of the year), (4) behavioral isolation (mating rituals differ), (5) mechanical isolation (nonfitting of genitals), (6) gametic isolation (fertilization cannot occur), (7) hybrid nonviability (the offspring cannot reproduce), and (8) developmental isolation (fertilization can occur, but the embryo dies). Consequently, geographic isolation followed by reproductive isolation leads to new species.

General patterns of evolution are divergent (moving from one species to different species, the usual pattern), convergent (moving from separate species to common species), or parallel (two species resulting from one species but evolving in a parallel fashion). Adaptive radiation is the gradual divergent differentiation of a species, usually as a response to environmental variations. Homologous structures are those that arise from a common structure even though functions may be different. Analogous structures have common functions but arise from different structures.

Origin of Life

Most scientists believe that the primitive atmosphere on Earth millions of years ago contained nitrogen, carbon dioxide, methane, ammonia, hydrogen, and water vapor. These elements could have acted together as a result of volcanic heat, lightning, or ultraviolet light to produce amino acids, carbohydrates, and nucleic acid, the building blocks of life. According to the fossil record, the very oldest fossils contain microfossils, or prokaryote and unicellular eukaryote organisms. In this evolutionary theory, the simplest plants and simple invertebrate animals evolved next, then jawless fish and more complex invertebrates (such as trilobites), then jawed vertebrates, insects, and vascular plants. Next came reptiles, early mammals, and seed plants. When dinosaurs became extinct, the dominant vertebrate organisms were mammals and birds (Table 8-3).

Comparative Anatomy

The major adaptive evolutionary changes are discussed for chordates. **Chordates** are distinguished by (1) a dorsal, hollow nerve cord, (2) gill slits in the throat region, and (3) a notochord. Chordates are divided into invertebrate chordates (tunicates, acorn worms, cephalochordates, or Amphioxus) and vertebrates. **Vertebrates** have a vertebral column, closed circulatory system (enabling large growth), a better developed nervous system, and improved sensory apparatus. Fish include the Agnatha (jawless fish, e.g., lampreys), Chondrichthyes (fish with cartilaginous skeletons, e.g., sharks), and Osteichthyes (bony fish). The pectoral fins, pelvic fins, and lateral line system are important for balance. Lobe fin fish (or crossopterygians, e.g., latimeria) invaded land, had lungs, and had stubby fins (bones into fins—a crucial step for land invasion) and, in the evolution

TABLE 8-3. Evolutionary Timetable

Geologic Era	Period	Time	Features (in millions of years ago)
Precambrian	—	2700	Marine invertebrates; protozoans
Paleozoic	Cambrian	600	Trilobites; brachiopods
	Ordovician	500	First fish
	Silurian	430	First air-breathing animals; first insects
	Devonian	410	First amphibians; sharks; sea lilies
	Carboniferous	350	First reptiles; insects
	Permian	275	Mammal-like reptiles; emergence of modern insects
Mesozoic	Triassic	225	First dinosaurs
	Jurassic	175	First birds, flying reptiles; dinosaurs; first mammals
	Cretaceous	130	Primitive mammals; first modern birds; dinosaurs become extinct
Cenozoic	Tertiary	60	Rapid development of higher mammals and birds
	Quaternary	2	Appearance of modern humans; extinction of giant mammals

theory, gave rise to the amphibians. Amphibians (frogs, toads, salamanders) are still dependent on the water because their eggs are easily desiccated. Reptiles (snakes, turtles, lizards, crocodiles, and alligators) arose from amphibians. Total land life was possible because of the amniotic egg, which would not desiccate and which had a sufficient food supply. Reptiles are also advanced beyond amphibians by (1) internal fertilization by copulation, (2) a partly divided ventricle of the heart to separate oxygenated and deoxygenated blood, (3) ribs to aid in respiration, and (4) a brain with small cerebral hemispheres. The pterosaurs (extinct) gave rise to the birds. Aves (birds) can fly because of special feathers (modified reptile scales, large quills for flying surface, fan-like tail feathers for stabilization, contour and down feathers for insulation), a light skeleton and a special breastbone to accommodate flight muscles, warm-blooded, efficient respiration with the four-chambered heart, and advanced sight and muscular coordination by the brain.

In the evolution theory, mammals arose from a different type of reptile than did the birds. Key distinguishing features of mammals are (1) internal development of young and nutrition by mammary glands, (2) a strengthened jaw and differentiated teeth, (3) a diaphragm to separate thorax and abdomen and to be used in breathing, (4) legs swung underneath the body, and (5) a greatly enlarged brain.

APPLIED CONCEPTS

- Review evolution and genetics—especially the weaker points in scientific hypotheses and theories. Identify possible assumptions (implicit and explicit) in current research methodology.
- Conceptualize the following terms as related to genetics: molecular genetics using replica plating or enrichment techniques (limited, penicillin or delayed); episomes; merozygotes; interrupted bacterial mapping; transductional bacteriophage mapping; cis-trans test; transfection; cytogenetics and chromosome mapping; pleiotropic effects; mutant types (sterile, semilethal, or lethal); epistatic and nonepistatic genetic interaction.
- Understand the following evolution-related terms: fossils (trilobite); comparative anatomy genetics (comparing structural similarities and differences among closely related animals, e.g., fish, amphibians, reptiles, and birds); homology and homologous structures; natural selection; isolating mechanisms (e.g., Galapagos islands); polyploidy; Oparin's hypothesis; Miller's amino acid apparatus; genetic drift using the Hardy-Weinberg principle (e.g., Founder principle); splitting evolution and phyletic evolution.
- Review the sex chromatin test (to detect the absence or presence of Barr chromatin body—an inactivated X chromosome in a spot at the periphery of the cell nucleus). What are normal and abnormal values of Barr body analysis and how does it help in detecting Turner's syndrome?

GENETICS AND EVOLUTION: REVIEW QUESTIONS

1. Which of the following is correct for gene mapping?
   A. Only three-factor crosses may be used to sequence gene loci.
   B. The recombination frequencies are always representative of the recombination rates of the gene loci.

C. The recombination frequency is equal to the map units.
D. Viral DNAs are used for gene mapping.

2. Which statement is incorrect concerning X and Y chromosomes?

   A. X is larger than Y.
   B. X and Y are not homologous.
   C. XY is a genotypic male.
   D. Traits appearing on X but not on Y are called sex-linked traits.

3. Which of the following is an example of aneuploidy?

   A. 4n
   B. Trisomy 21
   C. XO (no Y chromosome)
   D. Both **B** and **C**

4. Select the incorrect statement about the number and type of chromosomes in the normal human male.

   A. There are 44 autosomal chromosomes
   B. There are 46 chromosomes total
   C. There are two X chromosomes
   D. There is one Y chromosome

5. In the typical somatic cell, the number of chromosomes is symbolized as:

   A. 1n.
   B. 2n.
   C. 3n.
   D. 4n.

6. Chromosomes (eukaryotes) are composed of all of the following except:

   A. histones.
   B. nonhistone protein.
   C. DNA.
   D. RNA.

7. Select the incorrect statement:

   A. A recessive allele is only expressed when it is homozygous.
   B. A dominant allele can be expressed when heterozygous.
   C. A codominant allele may express itself completely or partially when homozygous or heterozygous, respectively.
   D. Dominant alleles may not be expressed.

8. Mendel's first law states that:

   A. alleles of the same trait segregate (separate on homologous chromosomes) in the formation of gametes.
   B. alleles of different traits separate independently of each other in the formation of gametes.
   C. genes are particulate in nature.
   D. genes are indivisible (i.e., cannot be subdivided and yet produce a given trait).

9. If the genotype for a trait is Aa (A dominant to a), possible gametes are:

   A. Aa only.
   B. AA and aa.
   C. A and a.
   D. Aa, A, and a.

10. Given the following representative pedigree, select the most likely pattern of inheritance.

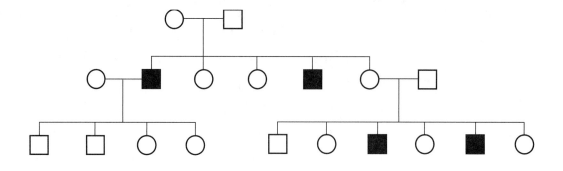

A. Autosomal dominant
B. Autosomal recessive
C. Sex-linked dominant
D. Sex-linked recessive

11. Given the following representative pedigree, select the most likely pattern of inheritance.

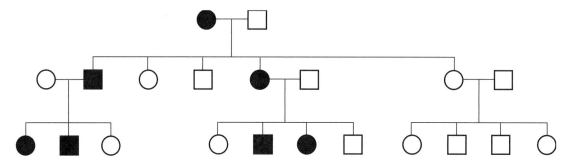

A. Autosomal dominant
B. Autosomal recessive
C. Sex-linked dominant
D. Sex-linked recessive

12. Suppose round peas (R) are dominant to wrinkled peas (r) and green peas (G) are dominant to yellow peas (g). The following cross is made: RrGg × RrGg. What are the expected phenotypes and their frequencies in the offspring (assume the traits are not linked)?

A. 3 Round, green; 1 wrinkled, yellow
B. 2 Round, green; 1 round, yellow; 1 wrinkled, green
C. 9 Round, green; 3 wrinkled, green; 3 round, yellow; 1 wrinkled, yellow
D. All round, green

13. If the genotype for two traits is AaBB, the possible gametes are:

A. Aa, BB.
B. AB, aB.
C. A, a, B, B.
D. Ab, ab, AB, aB.

14. Mendel's second law states that:

A. alleles of the same trait segregate (separate on homologous chromosomes) in the formation of gametes.
B. alleles of different traits separate independently of each other in the formation of gametes.
C. genes are particulate in nature.
D. genes are indivisible.

15. Suppose the only alleles that determine blood type are A and B, and that they are codominant. If both parents are type AB, what are the expected ratios of their children's blood types? Type A = AA, type B = BB, type AB = AB (genotypes of each type).

A. 1 Type A; 2 type AB; 1 type B
B. 1 Type A; 1 type B
C. 3 Type AB; 1 type A; 1 type B
D. All type AB

16. Select the correct statement.

    A. Phenotypic differences alone serve as a basis for evolution.
    B. Phenotypic differences serve as a basis for evolution when they reflect somatic cell genetic differences.
    C. Phenotypic differences serve as a basis for evolution when they reflect germ cell genetic differences.
    D. None of the above.

17. The ultimate source of all new genes in a population is due to:

    A. mitosis.
    B. mating.
    C. meiosis.
    D. mutation.

18. Mutations do not affect evolutionary change primarily because they are:

    A. expressed.
    B. recessive.
    C. too rare.
    D. random.

19. All of the following are conditions under which evolution would not occur except:

    A. large populations.
    B. nonrandom reproduction.
    C. no mutations.
    D. no immigration or emigration.

20. Genetic drift may lead to evolution in populations that are:

    A. any size.
    B. large.
    C. small.
    D. divergent.

21. Which is not considered as part of the evolutionary concept of the reproductive process?

    A. Mate selection and mating behavior
    B. Embryo development
    C. Growth of young to reproductive maturity
    D. All of the above are part of the reproductive process

22. Darwin's idea of natural selection is the same as:

    A. polyploidy.
    B. mutation pressure.
    C. genetic drift.
    D. nonrandom reproduction.

23. Populations that are separated by geographic barriers tend to differ because:

    A. gene frequencies usually differ among them.
    B. mutations vary among populations.
    C. there are different environmental pressures.
    D. of all of the above factors.

24. Structures that have different functions but arise from a common structure are called:

    A. convergent.
    B. divergent.
    C. analogous.
    D. homologous.

25. Assuming all other factors are constant, which situation does not result in an increase in the population growth rate?

   A. Increase in the total individuals in the population near the carrying capacity
   B. Decrease in the death rate
   C. Increase in the birth rate
   D. Increase in the intrinsic growth rate

26. A factor that would be detrimental to the flight of birds is:

   A. a light skeleton.
   B. advanced sight and muscle coordination.
   C. a three-chambered heart.
   D. large quill feathers or fan-like tail feathers.

27. The primary reason amphibians are still dependent on the water is that:

   A. their lungs are inadequate.
   B. they are cold blooded.
   C. their eggs are easily desiccated.
   D. they need to breathe through moist skin.

28. A wildlife resources manager wants to increase the productivity of a lake. He desires greater catches of fish and larger-size fish maintained over a long period of time. This increase is accomplished best by:

   A. increasing the amount of food available to the fish.
   B. keeping the fish population near the maximal growth rate point.
   C. restricting the number of fish caught for several years.
   D. stocking the lake with reproductive-sized fish the first year.

29. Which type of heart can separate oxygenated and deoxygenated blood completely?

   A. Two chambered.
   B. Three chambered.
   C. Four chambered.
   D. Five chambered.

30. What is the correct hierarchy (from highest to lowest) of the given levels of taxonomy?

   A. Class, order, family, genus
   B. Order, family, genus, class
   C. Family, genus, class, order
   D. Family, class, order, genus

31. Organisms are given a two-component scientific name. The first part is the:

   A. class.
   B. order.
   C. species.
   D. genus.

ANSWERS AND EXPLANATIONS

1–2. 1-D, 2-B. See text for explanation.

3. D   Aneuploidy is the loss (Y is lost in XO) or addition (an extra 21 is added in trisomy 21) of one or more individual chromosomes. Polyploidy means a multiplication of the whole set of chromosomes as in 4n.

4. C   The normal male has 44 autosomes, one X and one Y chromosome. The normal female has 44 autosomes and two X chromosomes.

5. B   2n = diploid. Gametes are haploid (1n). Occasionally, somatic cells are triploid (3n) or tetraploid (4n).

6. D   RNA is made using the DNA of chromosomes as a template; it is not an integral part of a chromosome.

7. A   Recessive alleles may be expressed when sex linked. Dominant alleles may not have penetrance.

8. A   See text for explanation.

9. C   The genotype Aa produces the gametes with A and a separately by Mendel's First Law of Segregation of alleles of the same trait. Note that A and a are on different but homologous chromosomes.

10. **D** The trait appears only in males, can be carried by females, and the males apparently inherit it only from their mothers.

11. **A** There is no sex preference and no skipped generations. The trait is only passed from those parents expressing the disease, and many individuals are affected. This is characteristic of a highly penetrated autosomal dominant allele. The initial mother *(1)* is heterozygous for the allele; if she were homozygous, every one of her children would have the trait.

12. **C** Use the Punnett square in the following figure to derive genotypic frequencies (gametes are RG, Rg, rG, rg for each parent).

	RG	Rg	rG	rg
RG	RRGG	RRGg	RrGG	RrGg
Rg	RRGg	RRgg	RrGg	Rrgg
rG	RrGG	RrGg	rrGG	rrGg
rg	RrGg	Rrgg	rrGg	rrgg

Then, based on the dominance-recessive relationships given, the phenotypes and their ratios are as follows:

All R-G- are round, green (RRGG-1, RRGg-2, RrGG-2, RrGg-4) = 9
All rrG- are wrinkled, green (rrGG-1, rrGg-2) = 3
All R-gg are wrinkled, yellow (RRgg-1, Rrgg-2) = 3
rrgg is wrinkled, yellow (rrgg-1) = 1

13. **B** Each gamete will contain one allele of each trait in all possible combinations. Each gamete can have an A or a, and it must have a B, giving AB and aB combinations.

14. **B** See text for explanation.

15. **A** Use the Punnett square shown in the following figure to determine the genotypes (gametes of each parent are A,B).

	A	B
A	AA	AB
B	AB	BB

Using the information, relate phenotypes to genotypes given in the question as follows:

Type A: (AA = 1) = 1
Type B: (BB = 1) = 1
Type AB: (AB = 2) = 2

16–27. 16-C, 17-D, 18-D, 19-B, 20-C, 21-D, 22-D, 23-D, 24-D, 25-A, 26-C, 27-C. See text for explanation.

28. **B** The point of optimal yield is at the maximum growth rate (MGR). If the MGR can be determined and the population kept at this level, the lake will produce the greatest yield. Increasing the food (that is, the carrying capacity) will not increase the yields per se. If the amount of fish caught is restricted, the lake will approach the carrying capacity and zero growth rate, and the yield will decrease. Adding more fish may overload the carrying capacity, and, of itself, may not increase the yield. Arguments for each choice may be made; the best answer is **B**.

29–31. 29-C, 30-A, 31-D. See text for explanation.

Nervous System

Self-Managed Learning Questions

1. Compare the functions and distributions of rods and cones in the visual system.
2. What causes the blind spot on the retina and what causes afterimages?

3. Compare the perception of sound when a vibrating tuning fork is held close to the ear and when it touches the skull. Compare the amplitude and frequency.
4. Test the primary taste buds by preparing equal volumes of the following solutions (varying concentrations) to understand temperature effects on taste: salt solution (NaCl), sugar solution, lemon juice solution, and quinine solution.
5. Analyze several types of sensors used by animals such as snakes, bats, rats, cats, and turtles.

The complexity of this system is partly due to current and ongoing research efforts linking it to the enormous details associated with sensory reception and processing. Review the four major parts of the nervous system, that is, the **central nervous system** (CNS), **peripheral nervous system**, and **autonomic nervous system**, or ANS (sympathetic and parasympathetic), and the sense organs (eyes, nose, ears, tongue, and skin). The CNS is the command center (messages or impulses arrive there and are sent to various glands, organs, and muscles). Understand the similarities and differences between the motor (efferent) and the sensory (afferent) systems. The efferent system is divided into the autonomic and somatic nervous systems. The most efficient way to review the nervous system is to understand the biological aspects of the four major parts, that is, to understand the structural or anatomic functions of each part and the physiologic role of each part, including dimensions and equations related to optics, sound, and fluids. Understand the concepts behind the labeled-line law, which states that each type of sensory nerve fiber transmits only one modality of sensation.

NERVOUS SYSTEM STRUCTURE AND FUNCTION

The nervous system is divided into the CNS, consisting of the brain and spinal cord, and the peripheral nervous system (PNS), consisting of the cranial nerves (CNS) and peripheral nerves (PNs).

In the CNS, the hindbrain (rhombencephalon), midbrain (mesencephalon), and forebrain (prosencephalon) are the gross divisions of the brain, and most are bilateral. The hindbrain consists of the myelencephalon (medulla) and metencephalon (pons). The midbrain is not further divided. The forebrain consists of the diencephalon (hypothalamus and thalamus) and the telencephalon (the cerebral hemispheres). The cerebellum is a derivative of the metencephalon. Respiratory and circulatory regulation, coughing, and vomiting reflexes are functions of the medulla. These are functions basic to life. The cerebellum is concerned with muscle coordination (e.g., balance). No general functions are localized in the midbrain or pons; they serve important relay functions. The hypothalamus is the important regulator of the internal environment; it controls hormones of the pituitary via releasing factors, thirst and hunger centers, water balance, and temperature regulation, and it controls behavior (e.g., sexual behavior and aggression). The thalamus is the relay center for nearly all sensory input. The cerebrum (especially the cerebral cortex, i.e., surface) is the integrating and interpretation center for all sensory input and voluntary motor activity. In addition, memory, learning, and emotions are located there (Figure 8-107).

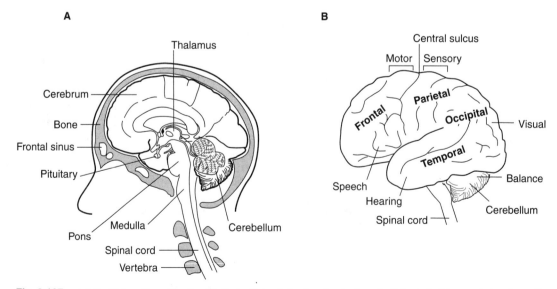

Fig. 8-107. (*a*) Sagittal section of brain. (*b*) Brain (lateral view) and spinal cord. (Adapted with permission from Fix JD: *High-Yield Neuroanatomy.* Baltimore, Williams & Wilkins, 1995, p 102.)

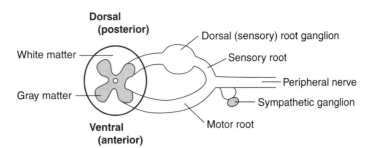

Fig. 8-108. Spinal cord.

The spinal cord (SC) has an interior of gray matter (neuron cell bodies) surrounded by white matter (myelinated axons). Serving as a path between the brain and the periphery (senses and muscles or glands) is the primary function of the SC. Descending tracts (from the brain to the SC) and ascending tracts (from the SC to the brain) are in the white matter. Sensory nerves (afferent—toward the CNS) enter dorsally and motor nerves (efferent—away from the CNS) exit ventrally. Several reflexes, such as the knee jerk, are at the SC level (Figure 8-108).

The PNS consists of the ANS and the somatic nervous system (SNS). The ANS is entirely motor, consisting of two motor neurons fastened together. The cell body of the first neuron is located in the CNS (SC or brain stem) and the second neuron cell body is clustered with other similar neuron cell bodies into ganglia. The ANS is divided into the sympathetic system (arising from the thoracolumbar levels of the SC) and the parasympathetic system (PS), originating at the craniosacral levels of the CNS.

Sensor and Effector Neurons

The simplest functional organization of the nervous system is the **reflex arc**. The basic structure consists of a sensory neuron, which detects a stimulus and transmits it to the spinal cord, where a motor neuron is stimulated that transmits the impulse to an effector (gland or muscle), which causes the organism to respond (Figure 8-109).

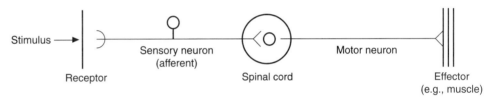

Fig. 8-109

Not all neurons stimulate other neurons. Some inhibit other neurons. This adds another level of functional complexity. In the example, the afferent neuron could have also stimulated an interneuron (in the spinal cord), which could have inhibited the motor neuron of the antagonist of the muscle that contracted (Figure 8-110). This can be magnified many times, thereby affording numerous possibilities for antagonistic or synergistic actions in the nervous system.

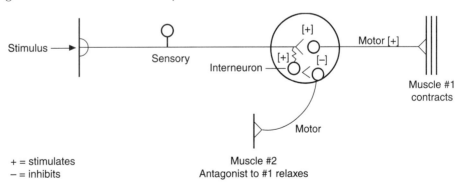

+ = stimulates
− = inhibits

Fig. 8-110

Sympathetic and Parasympathetic Nervous System

The sympathetic system (SS) peripherally consists of a chain of ganglia called the sympathetic chain, which is parallel to and adjacent to the spinal cord. These ganglia receive axons from the neurons located in the CNS and themselves send out much longer axons to many organs and tissues. The SS may affect all organs they innervate simultaneously (i.e., in a diffuse manner). In general, the SS moves the organism away from homeostasis

TABLE 8-4. Classification Chart of Cranial Nerves

Memorizing Symbol*	Name of Nerve (Connection)	Type of Nerve	Medical Dysfunctions and Disorders
Oh	Olfactory I (smell)	Sensory	Anosmia (loss of smelling sensation)
Oh	Optic II or Ocular II (sight)	Sensory	Anopsia (loss of visual acuity)
Oh	Oculomotor III (proprioceptive)	Motor	Diplopia (double vision) and squinting (strabismus)
To	Trochlear IV (proprioceptive)	Motor	Diplopia (double vision) and squinting (strabismus)
Touch	Trigeminal V (proprioceptive)	Sensory (face and head), motor (mastication muscles)	Trigeminal neuralgia (muscle paralysis)
And	Abducens VI (starts in pons)	Motor	Eyeball movements affected
Feel	Facial VII motor (facial expression and salivation)	Sensory (taste), control	Bell's palsy (loss of taste) and facial muscles affected
Very	Vestibulocochlear VIII (organ of Corti, medulla)	Sensory	Vertigo (rotational balance) and tinnitus (ringing of ears)
Green	Glossopharyngeal IX (connected to medulla and taste buds in tongue)	Sensory (taste), motor (swallowing and salivation)	Loss of taste and loss of saliva secretion
Vegetables	Vagus X (connected to medulla and jugular foramen)	Sensory (larynx), motor (voice, swallowing, slowing of heart, peristalsis of upper gastrointestinal tract and stimulating endocrine glands, e.g., pancreas)	Interrupts sensations from many organs. More research papers should be read to keep current
A	Spinal accessory XI (cranial and spinal connections)	Motor	Swallowing actions, head rotations, and shoulder movements are prevented
H	Hypoglossal XII (connected to medulla and tongue muscles)	Motor	Swallowing and speech control by tongue movements affected

* The 12 cranial nerves can be either sensory or motor or both. They can be memorized by an acronym: Oh, Oh, Oh, to touch and feel very green vegetables—AH! (this order is followed around the ventral surface of the brain).

as in the "fight or flight" phenomenon. Sympathetic discharges cause the heart rate to increase, digestive process to stop, circulation to the skin to decrease, and blood flow to the heart and muscles to increase. The ganglia of the parasympathetic system (PS) are located near the end-organ and receive long axons from the first neuron whose cell body is in the CNS. The ganglia of the PS generally exert specific effects directed at one organ or tissue. The PS tends to maintain homeostasis and, in general, opposes actions of the SS. Actions of the PS include slowing of the heart rate and increasing the digestive processes. The vagus nerve is an important parasympathetic nerve to the heart and abdominal viscera. Acetylcholine is the postganglionic (after the synapses in the ganglia) transmitter in the PS. Norepinephrine is the postganglionic transmitter for the SS.

There are 31 spinal nerves (SNs). They are classified according to the level of their connection with the spinal cord—8 cervical, 12 thoracic, 5 lumbar, 5 sacral, 1 coccygeal. Each nerve contains motor and sensory components. The motor neurons are located in the ventral portion of the cord and the sensory neurons in ganglia (dorsal root ganglia) immediately adjacent to the SC. The peripheral nerves are myelinated for most of their length by the Schwann cell.

There are 12 cranial nerves (CNS). Some are sensory only, some are motor only, and some carry both. In addition, motor neurons of the parasympathetic system may also be present. The medical functions and related disorders for the 12 nerves are listed in Table 8-4. The brain and spinal cord are covered by meninges. These are, from the outside in, the dura mater (tough fibrous layer), the arachnoid (vascular and nutrient layer), and the pia mater (fragile layer directly attached to nervous tissue). See Figure 8-111.

SENSORY RECEPTION AND PROCESSING

Sensors are the cells of the nervous system that convert stimuli (either physical or chemical) into signals. These signals are then transmitted to other parts of the nervous system where they are then processed and interpreted. Most sensors are simply modified neurons, but a few are other types of cells closely associated with neurons.

Skin, Proprioceptive, and Somatic Sensors

The skin is one of the largest sensory organs. Thousands of tiny touch receptors are located in the skin. These receptors are specialized for specific sensations, such as pain, temperature, or pressure. A **proprioceptor** is one of a variety of sensory end organs (such as the muscle spindle or Golgi tendon organ). Proprioceptors are found in muscles, tendons, and joint capsules. Their function is to sense position and movement. There are several types of sensors: chemical sensors, electric sensors, mechanical sensors, optical

Divisions of the Nervous System

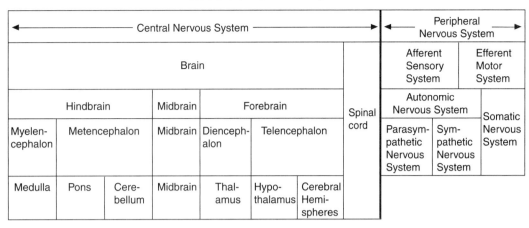

Central Nervous System							Peripheral Nervous System		
Brain						Spinal cord	Afferent Sensory System		Efferent Motor System
Hindbrain			Midbrain	Forebrain			Autonomic Nervous System		Somatic Nervous System
Myelen-cephalon	Metencephalon		Midbrain	Dienceph-alon	Telencephalon		Parasym-pathetic Nervous System	Sym-pathetic Nervous System	
Medulla	Pons	Cere-bellum	Midbrain	Thal-amus	Hypo-thalamus	Cerebral Hemi-spheres			

Fig. 8-111. Divisions of the nervous system.

sensors, and temperature sensors. Somatic sensors of several types can be related to stimulus generated. Physical and chemical stimuli can be analyzed. Sensors are usually connected with the eyes, ears, nose, and they transmit stimuli at several levels.

The relationship between variation in the density of touch receptors in the skin and the sensory cortex can be experimentally verified. The somatosensory system can be explored by the two-point discrimination test. Two points on the skin are stimulated simultaneously using a pair of calipers or forceps to understand the working of the somato-sensory homunculus of the left cortex. Fingers and lips are the most sensitive parts of the body and have the greatest density of receptors.

Olfaction and Taste

Olfaction is the sense of smell. The olfaction sensors are neurons embedded in a layer of epithelial cells at the top of the nasal cavity. When an odorant molecule enters the nose, it binds to receptors located on olfactory hairs of the sensors. These receptors can react to as many as 50 odors. A G-protein is then activated, which, in turn, activates an enzyme that causes an increase of a second messenger in the cytoplasm of the sensor. This second messenger binds with sodium channel proteins and opens them, causing an influx of Na^+. The sensor depolarizes and fires action potentials, which are interpreted by the brain as a specific smell.

Taste, or gustation, is closely related to smell. Taste also depends on chemoreceptors that respond to certain chemicals. The tongue and roof of the mouth contain approxi-mately 10,000 clusters of sensors called taste buds, which last only a few days before they are replaced. A taste bud is made up of many taste sensors that are not neurons and do not fire action potentials. Instead, these taste sensors release neurotransmitters onto the dendrites of the sensory neurons, which then fire action potentials that are transported to the CNS. Particular regions of the tongue have specialized taste buds for certain tastes, such as sweet, sour, salty, and bitter, but there is some overlap with other regions of the tongue.

APPLIED CONCEPTS

- Identify the following technical terms, learn their definitions (both structural and functional), and apply them to study the nervous system: soma of neuron, stretch reflex, reverberating circuit, somesthetic area, enterioceptive and proprioceptive systems, cochlear biosensors, Meissner's corpuscle, Wernicke's area (impulse veloci-ties are approximately 300 fps), cholinergic nerves, brain microphages, astrocytes, voltage-sensitive Na^+ and K^+ channels, spinal tap (to extract cerebrospinal fluid), and ependymocytes.
- Distinguish between excitatory (epinephrine, enkephalin, norepinephrine) and in-hibitory (dopamine, glycine, and gamma aminobutyric acid—GABA) transmitters, excitatory postsynaptic potential (EPSP) receptor sites, and preganglionic fiber and postganglionic fiber.
- Understand the major (different) receptor sites such as kinesthetic receptors, mus-carinic (cholinergic) receptors, nicotinic (cholinergic) receptors, dopaminergic receptors, adrenergic receptors, opiate receptors, and other neuronal receptors.
- Understand light receptors in the eye such as iodopsin, lumirhodopsin, metarho-

dopsin, parathodopsin, photopsin, rhodopsin, luminous-rhodopsin, and scotopsin (to see images).

- Recognize the scope, design, and relevance of the following procedures and instruments: tonometry, ophthalmoscopy, myelography, cavitron ultrasonic surgical aspirator (to shatter brain tumors), positron emission tomography (PET), electroencephalogram, audiometer (if 0–25 dB can be heard easily, probably no hearing loss has occurred), and artificial ear implants and thin filament biosensor technology.
- Recognize the effects and causes for diseases such as cataracts, glaucoma, deafness, trachoma, shingles, sciatica, and cerebral diseases (epilepsy, dyslexia, Tay-Sachs disease, Alzheimer's disease, Parkinson's disease).

NERVOUS SYSTEM:
REVIEW QUESTIONS

1. Which of the following statements about the spinal cord is incorrect?

    A. Gray matter is central.
    B. White matter is peripheral.
    C. Sensory nerves enter ventrally.
    D. Motor nerves exit ventrally.

2. Which of the following is not part of the central nervous system?

    A. Thalamus
    B. Hypothalamus
    C. Spinal cord
    D. Cranial nerves

3. Glial cells are found in the:

    A. muscular system.
    B. endocrine system.
    C. nervous system.
    D. skeletal system.

4. The peripheral nervous system includes:

    A. spinal nerves.
    B. cranial nerves.
    C. the spinal cord.
    D. both A and B.

5. The autonomic nervous system includes:

    A. the sympathetic system.
    B. the parasympathetic system.
    C. the somatic nervous system.
    D. both A and B.

6. The hindbrain contains the:

    A. thalamus.
    B. medulla.
    C. cerebrum.
    D. spinal cord.

7. All of the following are associated with the forebrain except the:

    A. diencephalon.
    B. telencephalon.
    C. myelencephalon.
    D. hypothalamus.

8. All of the following are functions of the medulla except:

    A. voluntary movements.
    B. respiratory regulation.
    C. circulatory regulation.
    D. cough reflex.

9. The cerebellum:

    A. regulates respiration.
    B. is the site of memory.

C. coordinates motor activity.
D. is the site of behavior.

10. Select the incorrect statement concerning the sympathetic nervous system (SNS).

A. Sympathetic ganglia are near the spinal cord.
B. The SNS causes the heart rate to increase.
C. The SNS increases blood flow in certain tissues.
D. The SNS moves the organism toward homeostasis.

11. Select the incorrect statement concerning the parasympathetic nervous system (PNS).

A. Ganglia are located near the end-organ.
B. The PNS increases the heart rate.
C. The PNS maintains homeostasis.
D. The PNS increases digestive actions.

12. The vagus nerve:

A. is linked heterogeneously to the parasympathetic system.
B. is linked to the gut and the heart through specialized skeletal muscles.
C. is not a cranial nerve.
D. has afferent fibers that transmit information from receptors in the thorax.

13. Select the correct sequence of the meninges from outside inward (A = arachnoid, D = dura, P = pia):

A. A, D, P
B. D, P, A
C. P, A, D
D. D, A, P

ANSWERS AND EXPLANATIONS

1–17. 1-C, 2-D, 3-C, 4-D, 5-D, 6-B, 7-C, 8-A, 9-C, 10-D, 11-B, 12-D, 13-D. See text for explanation.

Endocrine System

Self-Managed Learning Questions

1. Visit a health food store and examine the labels and pamphlets describing anabolic steroids. Review the credibility of information, the arguments presented to sell such body-building chemicals, and their side effects. In men, anabolic steroids cause hair loss, breast enlargement, and testes shrinkage; in women, they cause breast and uterus shrinkage, facial and bodily hair growth, and irregular menstrual cycles.

2. Analyze the composition of blood. There are 30 to 40 hormones present in blood in concentrations of as little as 1 picogram (10^{-6} mg)/ml. What instruments are used to detect hormonal changes in babies, adults, and elderly people?

3. Radionuclides are used to determine the size, structure, and position of the thyroid gland. Sodium iodide labeled with ^{131}I is given in both liquid and capsule form. Examine the records of an older patient and the special precautions taken to avoid incorrect waiting periods and incorrect patient preparation. How is the radionuclide detected and why is ^{131}I NaI used for this experimental procedure?

4. Compare the reliability, convenience, and validity of serum aldosterone and urine aldosterone tests.

ENDOCRINE SYSTEMS: HORMONES AND THEIR SOURCES

Learn the cellular mechanisms of hormone action to understand specificity and target tissues connected to release and transport each hormone. Review and memorize the organic structure and the physical and chemical properties (molecular weight, density, melting and boiling point, interaction with other body hormones or chemicals) of various hormones. The chemical structures of a few hormones are shown in Figure 8-112.

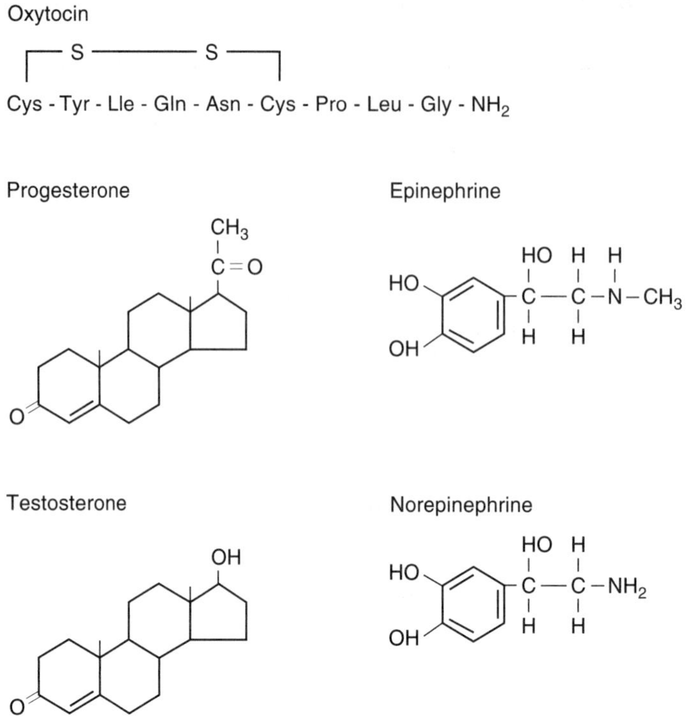

Oxytocin

Cys - Tyr - Lle - Gln - Asn - Cys - Pro - Leu - Gly - NH$_2$

Progesterone

Epinephrine

Testosterone

Norepinephrine

Fig. 8-112. Chemical structure of hormones.

FUNCTION OF THE ENDOCRINE SYSTEM

The **endocrine system** is a diverse collection of glands and tissues. It controls the functions of organs and its messages are mainly distributed through the blood to the entire body by chemical signals called hormones. Hormones are also secreted into the surrounding tissue fluid. There are strong interactions between the nervous system and the endocrine system.

A **hormone** is a chemical message between the cells of a multicellular organism (Figure 8-113). A chemical communication system that uses a hormone is usually made up of at

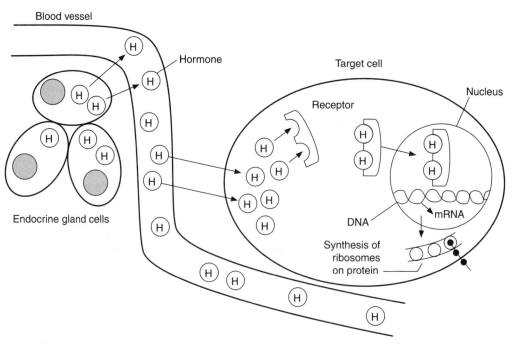

Fig. 8-113. Gene activation by steroid hormones.

least two cells; one produces the hormone and the other receives it. The receiving cell is called the **target cell**. The target cell interprets the message and responds developmentally, physiologically, or behaviorally. Hormones exert their actions in many ways (some still unknown). Some protein hormones seem to act via cyclic adenosine monophosphate (cAMP) by combining with specific receptors on the target cell membrane. Some steroids exert their effect by combining with receptors in the target cell cytoplasm (they diffuse through the lipid cell membrane). They then move into the nucleus to interact with DNA to cause synthesis of mRNA, which makes specific proteins (usually enzymes).

In recent years, scientists have discovered that specialized cells in the digestive tract and some other organs, such as the kidney, also release hormones. Therefore, the scope of the field of endocrinology has been broadened to include the study of chemical messengers that are produced by cells found throughout the body rather than by single, discrete organs.

Major Endocrine Glands

Hormones are substances released from special secretory tissues, called endocrine glands, into the blood. From there they circulate to their target tissues, combine with the target receptor, and exert their effect. Hormones are regulators, not catalysts (as enzymes are), of organism homeostasis. The major glands and organs are the hypothalamus gland, pituitary gland, thyroid gland, parathyroid gland, adrenal gland, pancreas, gut, ovaries, testis, liver, kidney, pineal gland, thymus gland, skin, and placenta. Gut hormones (gastrin, secretin, cholecystokinin-pancreozymin) are discussed under Digestive System; ovarian, placental, and testicular hormones and follicle stimulating hormone (FSH), luteinizing hormone (LH), and prolactin are discussed under Reproductive System.

The hypothalamus synthesizes releasing factors (RF), inhibiting factors (IF), vasopressin (antidiuretic hormone, or ADH), and oxytocin. Vasopressin causes the kidney to retain water; that is, it makes the urine more concentrated. Oxytocin causes contraction of certain smooth muscles and plays a role in the uterine contractions of labor and milk ejection in lactation. Oxytocin and vasopressin are stored in the posterior pituitary until released. RFs and IFs act on the anterior pituitary (AP). RFs cause the corresponding hormones of the AP to be synthesized and released from it. IFs inhibit release of the corresponding hormones. All of the hormones of the hypothalamus are peptides or proteins. Examples are thyroid stimulating hormone (TSH)-releasing factor (TRF) and prolactin inhibiting factor (PIF).

The anterior pituitary (AP) synthesizes and releases several trophic (growth stimulating and supporting) hormones, among others. Hormones secreted are TSH, adrenocorticotropic hormone (ACTH), FSH, and LH, which are all trophic hormones to the glands indicated by their names. The AP also secretes growth hormone (GH) and prolactin (also called lactogenic hormone). GH functions via somatomedins (produced in the liver) to stimulate the growth of many tissues in the body. Oversecretion of GH results in giantism (if before adolescence) or acromegaly (if as an adult). All of the AP hormones are proteins or glycoproteins. Melanocyte stimulating hormone (MSH) is secreted by the intermediate lobe of the pituitary gland.

The thyroid gland produces thyroxin and calcitonin. Thyroxine, which is a modified tyrosine with iodine attached, works by increasing the rate of metabolism. Calcitonin decreases the calcium in the blood by causing it to move into the bones.

The four pea-sized parathyroid glands are located on the thyroid gland, but are not part of it; they secrete parathyroid hormone (PTH, a protein), which regulates calcium and phosphorus metabolism. Calcium and phosphate are resorbed from bone under the influence of PTH.

The adrenal gland is composed of a cortex and medulla. The cortex is stimulated by ACTH to synthesize glucocorticoids (the primary one being cortisol), which perform many functions including regulation of blood sugar and fighting stress (e.g., infections). Mineralocorticoids (the primary one being aldosterone) are also synthesized by the cortex but usually as a result of stimulation by angiotensin II. Aldosterone causes the kidney to retain sodium (and hence water) and secrete potassium. The medulla synthesizes epinephrine, which is a sympathetic stimulant (see Muscle System). The cortical hormones are steroids. The medullary hormones are modified tyrosines.

The islet cells of the pancreas secrete insulin from β-cells and glucagon from α-cells. Insulin lowers blood glucose concentration by causing cells to take up glucose; it also causes amino acid and fatty acid uptake. Glucagon increases blood glucose concentration by stimulating glycogenolysis (glycogen breakdown) and gluconeogenesis (synthesis of glucose from amino acids) by the liver. Insulin and glucagon are both proteins. Diabetes mellitus is due to a deficiency of insulin.

Vitamin D is taken in as a nutrient, then goes through a series of activation steps. First, it is activated by ultraviolet light in the skin; then, it is hydroxylated successively in the liver and kidney and becomes a true hormone. Its main role is to increase absorption of calcium by the gut through the stimulation of the synthesis of a calcium-binding protein. Vitamin D is a steroid.

The kidney secretes renin and erythropoietin, and helps in the synthesis of active vitamin D. Renin is an enzyme molecule that splits a small peptide called angiotensin I off the renin substrate (produced in the liver). Angiotensin I is further split by enzymes in the lung or blood to yield angiotensin II, which is a potent constrictor of blood vessels and which stimulates synthesis and release of aldosterone from the adrenal. Erythropoietin is a protein hormone that stimulates the bone marrow to synthesize more red blood cells.

The pineal gland probably produces a host of hormones, but the best known is melatonin, which is a modified tryptophan. The pineal gland suppresses pituitary, gonadal (ovary and testis), adrenal, and thyroid function. These effects may be mediated via the hypothalamus.

Thymosin is produced by the thymus gland and plays a role in the immunologic system.

MAJOR HORMONES OF ENDOCRINE GLANDS

Memorize Table 8-5 in the order presented. Understand the major functions and actions of each hormone mechanistically (i.e., visualize and analyze mechanics of hormone production in a gland and observe the chemical structure of the hormone). What possible factors determine functions and actions of a specific hormone? Be prepared to address some minor functions as well. On the MCAT, analyze each question and response for correctness and validity according to experimental information provided in the passage. Do not expect to find minor functions or actions in classic biology or physiology textbooks. Try recognizing new hormonal actions or functions by reading research journals and reports (as additional material).

CELLULAR MECHANISMS OF HORMONE ACTION

Hormones regulate themselves by means of a process called feedback inhibition. A gland produces a hormone and this hormone, or a product, feeds back at some level to shut off its synthesis (Figure 8-114). On the figure, the long loop shows the specific hormone feeding back on the hypothalamus to inhibit release of the RF. This then prevents release of the trophic hormone, which prevents the synthesis of the specific hormone. As this decreases, its inhibition on the hypothalamus decreases and more of the RF is released, which causes more trophic hormone to be released, and so on. This cycle can continue as such or be modified positively or negatively by factors outside of the hypothalamus-pituitary-gland axis. The short loops show mechanisms that are the same as for the long loop, but the hormones feed back on the gland that stimulated their synthesis (i.e., the pituitary) instead of on a point farther removed (i.e., the hypothalamus). For a given hormone all combinations discussed may exist.

TRANSPORT OF HORMONES

There are two groups of hormones, determined according to where the hormones bind their receptors. Water-soluble hormones do not cross cell membranes easily and their receptors are membrane proteins with binding regions that project from the surface of the cell. Lipid-soluble hormones pass easily through cell membranes and their receptors are located in the cytoplasm or in the nucleus of a cell. A hormone can pass unnoticed through many tissues until it reaches the target tissue. The receptor sites in the target tissue are specialized and are similar to locks; only a specific hormone "key" will fit the lock and therefore influence the cell.

APPLIED CONCEPTS

- Learn important terms such as intracellular mediators (cyclic AMP and GMP), neurosecretory cells, and somatomedins and learn the major differences between stimulatory and inhibitory hormones.
- Understand the basic hormonal disorders (causes and effects) such as adrenal disorders (Cushing's syndrome, Addison's disease), pituitary disorders (gonadal failure in both males and females), thyroid disorders (hypothyroidism and hyperthyroidism), parathyroid disorders (hypoparathyroidism and hyperparathyroidism), and pancreatic disorders (diabetes mellitus).
- Learn the fundamental structure and functions of new growth factors such as tumor angiogenesis factors, platelet-derived growth factors, epidermal growth factors, nerve growth factors, and lymphokines and fibroblast growth factors. Relate these to distress and resistance as it links to the immune system inhibition.

TABLE 8-5. Hormones and Their Functions

Hormone-Secreting Gland	Hormone (Biological Name)	Chemical Structure or Functional Group	Major Functions
Pituitary (anterior) or adenohypophysis	Prolactin (PRL)	Protein	Stimulates secretion of milk by the mammary glands
	Growth hormone (GH)	Protein (hypothalamic)	Regulates growth of bones
	Adrenocorticotropin (ACTH)	Polypeptide (hypothalamic)	Stimulates secretion of adrenal cortex hormones, e.g., glucocorticoids
	Thyroid-stimulating hormone (TSH)	Glycoprotein (hypothalamic)	Stimulates activity of thyroid gland to release hormones
	Follicle-stimulating hormone (FSH)	Glycoprotein (hypothalamic)	Stimulates ovarian follicle maturity and spermatogenesis
	Luteinizing hormone (LH)	Glycoprotein (hypothalamic)	Stimulates ovulation and corpus luteum formation
Pituitary (posterior) or neurohypophysis	Oxytocin (OT)	Peptide (neurosecretory, hypothalamic)	Stimulates uterine contractions (muscular) and milk secretion by mammary glands
	Antidiuretic hormone or vasopressin (ADH)	Peptide (hypothalamic) in neurosecretory	Regulates water reabsorption by kidneys and raises blood pressure by constricting arterioles
Thyroid	Thyroxine and triiodothyronine (T_4 and T_3)	Amino acids (TSH)	Increase in thyroxine and production increases metabolic rate
	Calcitonin	Peptide (calcium in blood)	Retains calcium in the bones, lowers blood calcium levels
Parathyroid	Parathyroid hormone	Peptide (calcium in blood)	Increases release of calcium from bone, raises blood calcium levels
Adrenal cortex	Glucocorticoids	Steroids (ACTH)	Multiple carbohydrate metabolism causes increase in blood sugar, anti-inflammatory
	Mineralocorticoids (aldosterone)	Steroids (potassium in blood)	Reabsorption of Na^+ and excretion of K^+ in kidneys
	Gonadocorticoids	Steroids	Maintain male sexual characteristics
Adrenal medulla	Epinephrine or adrenaline (EP)	Catecholamine (autonomic nervous system)	Glycogen to glucose conversion, increases blood sugar and blood vessel constriction
	Norepinephrine or noradrenaline (NP)	Catecholamine (autonomic nervous system)	Cardiac muscle contraction, blood vessel constriction, increases heart rate
Pancreas	Glucagon	Polypeptide (blood glucose and amino acids)	Glycogen to glucose conversion in liver
	Insulin	Polypeptide (blood glucose)	Lowers blood sugar, leads to hypoglycemia
	Somatostatin	Peptide (growth hormone feedback)	Inhibits release of insulin and glucagon
Ovaries (follicles and corpus luteum)	Estrogen	Steroid (FSH and LH)	Enhances female sexual characteristics
	Progesterone	Steroid (FSH and LH)	Growth of uterine lining
	Inhibin	FSH and LH	Inhibits secretion of FSH
Testes	Testosterone (androgen)	Steroid (FSH and LH)	Enhances male sexual characteristics
	Inhibin	FSH and LH	Inhibits secretion of FSH
Thymus	Thymosin and thymopoietin	Peptide	Stimulates growth of T cells
Pineal	Melatonin	Catecholamine	Inhibits reproductive activities (is produced in darkness, not produced with light)

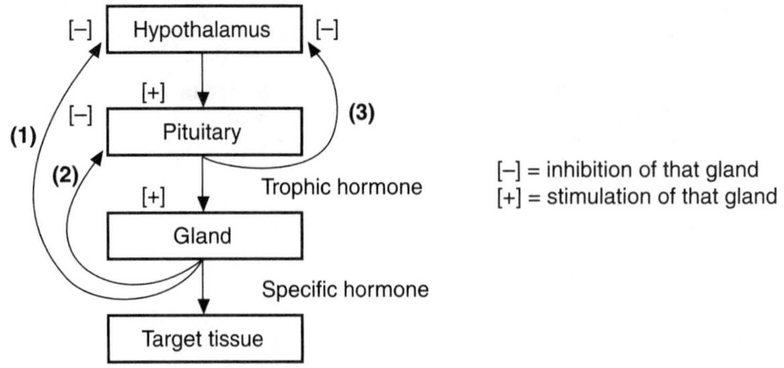

Fig. 8-114. Feedback loops.

[−] = inhibition of that gland
[+] = stimulation of that gland

- Learn major differences between autocrine, endocrine, and paracrine hormones; learn functional aspects of pheromones and identify probable causes for their action.
- Understand experimental design of radioimmunoassays to measure hormone molarities.

ENDOCRINE SYSTEM: REVIEW QUESTIONS

1. Insulin is:

   A. secreted by the pancreas.
   B. a protein.
   C. involved in the metabolism of glucose, amino acids, fats.
   D. all of the above.

2. Vitamin D:

   A. is actually a hormone after modification in the body.
   B. increases absorption of calcium from the gut.
   C. requires metabolic changes in the skin, liver, and kidney to function.
   D. is all of the above.

3. Select the incorrectly paired hormone and disease or deranged process associated with an excess or deficiency of it.

   A. Growth hormone—acromegaly
   B. Insulin—diabetes mellitus
   C. Cortisol—enhanced inflammation
   D. Thyroxine—altered metabolic rate

4. All of the following hormones are correctly paired with one of its major functions except:

   A. thyroxine—increases metabolic rate.
   B. glucocorticoids—increases blood sugar levels.
   C. aldosterone—role in "fight or flight" sympathetic response.
   D. parathyroid hormone—regulation of calcium-phosphorous metabolism.

5. Select the endocrine gland that is incorrectly paired with its hormone product.

   A. Adrenal cortex—cortisol
   B. Adrenal medulla—aldosterone
   C. Adrenal medulla—epinephrine
   D. Adrenal cortex—mineralocorticoids

6. Select the hormone incorrectly paired with its target tissue.

   A. Thyroid stimulating hormone (TSH)—thyroid glands
   B. Adrenocorticotropic hormone (ACTH)—anterior pituitary
   C. Luteinizing hormone (LH)—ovary or testis
   D. Melanocyte stimulating hormone (MSH)—melanocytes

7. Which hormones are synthesized by the hypothalamus?

   A. Releasing factors
   B. Vasopressin
   C. Oxytocin
   D. All of the above

8. The hormone synthesized and released by the anterior pituitary is:

    A. thyroid stimulating hormone (TSH).
    B. follicle stimulating hormone (FSH).
    C. growth hormone (GH).
    D. all of the above.

9. Which of the following tissues secrete hormones?

    A. Pancreas
    B. Ovaries
    C. Gastrointestinal tract
    D. All of the above

10. All of the following are general characteristics of hormones except that:

    A. hormones are secreted into the blood.
    B. hormones are regulators, not initiators of homeostatic processes.
    C. hormones are all proteins.
    D. hormones do not function like enzymes.

11. All of the following are general characteristics of hormones except that:

    A. hormones regulate themselves by feedback inhibition.
    B. hormones may be proteins, peptides, steroids, or modified amino acids.
    C. some protein hormones act via cyclic adenosine monophosphate (cAMP).
    D. most steroid hormones act via cAMP.

12. Melatonin is produced by the:

    A. pineal gland.
    B. skin.
    C. liver.
    D. pituitary gland.

13. Thymosin is concerned with:

    A. metabolic rate.
    B. immunologic competence.
    C. calcium-phosphate.
    D. none of the above.

14. Calcitonin:

    A. decreases serum calcium.
    B. has no effect on serum calcium.
    C. is made in the parathyroid gland.
    D. is a steroid.

15. All of the following are true about glucagon except that it:

    A. causes glycogenolysis.
    B. is a steroid.
    C. causes gluconeogenesis.
    D. is made in the pancreas.

16. In the hypothalamic-pituitary-adrenal axis, if the long feedback loop holds, then:

    A. ACTH inhibits the production of ACTH-releasing factor (RF) by the hypothalamus.
    B. cortisol inhibits the production of ACTH by the pituitary.
    C. cortisol inhibits the ACTH-RF produced by the hypothalamus.
    D. none of the above are correct.

ANSWERS AND EXPLANATIONS

1–5. 1-D, 2-D, 3-C, 4-C, 5-B. See text for explanation.

    6. C In the long feedback loop, the specific hormone (cortisol) of the gland (adrenal) feeds back past the pituitary to the hypothalamus.

7–16. 7-D, 8-D, 9-D, 10-C, 11-D, 12-A, 13-B, 14-A, 15-B, 16-C. See text for explanation.

1. What happens during a heart attack or stroke? How does an artificial pacemaker work?
2. What is colloid osmotic pressure? What causes this pressure to develop in seeping plasma?
3. Trace the circulation of blood through the following vertebrate hearts:
   - Fish heart (1 atrium, 1 ventricle)
   - Frog heart (2 atria, 1 ventricle)
   - Reptile heart (2 atria, 2 ventricles with incomplete partition)
   - Bird heart (2 atria, 2 ventricles completely separated)
4. Visit a Red Cross clinic and learn the basic mechanics of cardiopulmonary resuscitation, and how blood donations are obtained for patients at different age groups.
5. What is cryogenics of blood banks? What is the temperature and time that blood can be stored? What malfunctions or errors can be detected in blood bank storage units?

Identify the complex structure and working of contractile cells and tissues with emphasis on the cardiac muscle. Identify the thermoregulatory function of the cardiovascular system and its components: the heart, blood, and arterial-venous systems. Visit a hospital or clinic if possible to study heart transplant operations, artificial heart machines, and blood bank operations. Learn the following laws and their limitations, why these laws are true, and under what conditions they are valid; there are both stated and unstated assumptions associated with these laws: (a) Marey's law—if blood pressure decreases, the heart beats faster in an inversely proportional relationship, (b) Starling's law—relates length of stretched cardiac muscle fibers to strength of contraction in a directly proportional relationship (the longer the stretched fiber, the stronger the contraction), and (c) Frank-Starling law—the heart automatically adjusts its pumping capability depending on the blood volume to be pumped by it in a directly proportional relationship (the more the blood volume to be pumped, the higher the pumping capability). Cardiac muscle is not plastic; the tone of the heart makes it contract continuously. Heart rate and cardiac output are listed in Table 8-6.

TABLE 8-6. Heart Rate and Cardiac Output

Normal heart beat	$\approx$ 70 beats/minute
Normal volume of blood pumped by one ventricle	= 5 L/minute
Vigorous exercise heart beat	$\approx$ 200 beats/minute
Vigorous exercise blood volume	= 28 L/minute by one ventricle

FUNCTIONS

The function of the circulatory system is to maintain tissue oxygenation, supply nutrients, and remove wastes. This function is compromised when the heart, blood vessels, or blood fail to perform as intended. The lungs are critical in O_2 and CO_2 homeostasis. Malfunction in these systems can lead to a decreased flow of suitable blood (e.g., blood with enough O_2) to tissues, which can lead to their death. A decline in blood pressure or loss of blood volume can have similar effects.

As shown in Figure 8-115, generally the velocity of blood flow in any segment of the cardiovascular system is inversely proportional to the total cross-sectional area of the vessels of the segment. Efficient circulation requires an adequate volume of circulating blood. Blood encounters resistance as it flows through blood vessels. Resistance to blood flow is affected by physical and biological variables such as viscosity, temperature, and diameter. Four equations are provided for studying the relationships among various circulation variables.

1. By using **thermoregulation**, organisms can alter the rate of heat exchange between their bodies and the environment by controlling the flow of blood to the skin. If an organism is too warm, the blood vessels increase the flow to the skin, where the heat escapes. If the organism is too cold, the blood vessels constrict, decreasing blood flow to the skin and reducing heat loss.

$$\text{Resistance (R)} = \frac{\text{Pressure gradient } (\Delta P)}{\text{Flowrate (Q)}}$$

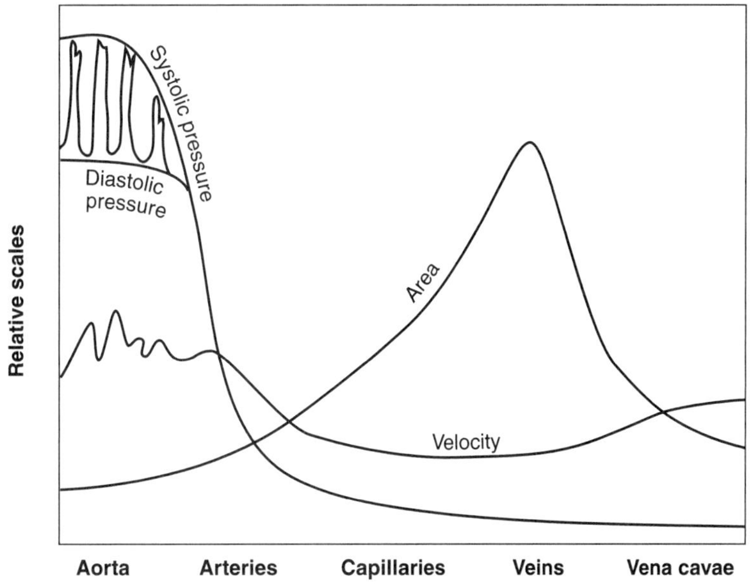

Fig. 8-115. Fundamental principles of blood circulation.

This equation is analogous to Ohm's law in electric circuits:

$$R = \frac{V}{I} = \frac{Voltage}{Current}$$

2. The ventricles eject only a portion of their contained blood with each beat. The ejection fraction (EF) is that fraction of the end-diastolic volume that is ejected during systole. Normally, EF > 0.5.

$$Ejection\ fraction\ (EF) = \frac{Stroke\ volume\ (SV)}{End\text{-}diastolic\ volume\ (EDV)}$$

3. The following equation is used to study heart murmurs (vibrations set up within the heart and great vessels by turbulent blood flow):

$$Critical\ velocity\ (v_c) = \frac{R\eta}{\rho r},\ where$$

R = Reynolds number, η = blood viscosity, ρ = blood density,

r = tube or vessel radius

4. Cardiac output (CO) is measured as follows:

$$Cardiac\ output\ (CO) = \frac{60I}{Ct},\ where$$

I = indicator or dye in mg,

$C = \dfrac{I}{V}$ the mean concentration in mg/l

V = Volume of liquid in which dye is injected in liters, and

t = Time in seconds

FOUR-CHAMBERED HEART: PULMONARY AND SYSTEMIC CIRCULATION

The elements of the circulatory system in humans are the heart, the blood vessels, the blood, and the lymphatics. The heart consists of two atria (left—LA and right—RA) and two ventricles (left—LV and right—RV). Between the RA and RV is the tricuspid valve (TV, three leaflets). Between the RV and the pulmonary artery (PA) is the pulmonary valve (PV). Between the LA and LV is the mitral (bicuspid) valve (MV, two leaflets). Between the LV and the aorta is the aortic valve (AV). The PV and AV valves are called semilunar valves (three half-moon-shaped leaflets) that prevent reflux of blood back into their respective ventricles during diastole. The TV and MV are attached via chordae tendineae to papillary muscles on their respective ventricles to prevent reflux into the corresponding atria during systole. Improper functioning of the valves, particularly in

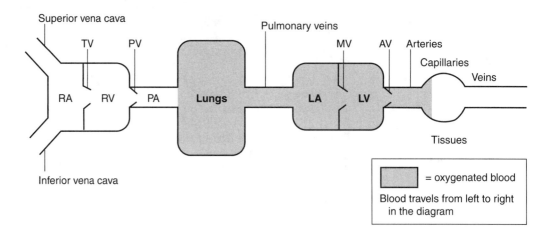

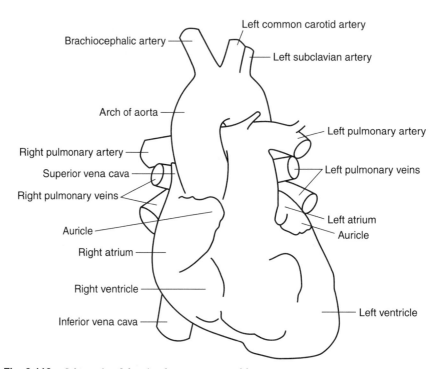

Fig. 8-116. Schematic of the circulatory system and heart.

the mitral valve, is one of the causes of heart murmurs. A schematic of the heart and circulation is shown in Figure 8-116.

The heart is made of cardiac muscle, which differs from skeletal muscle (see Muscle System) by (1) being made of branching, uninuclear cells, (2) having specializations of cell membranes called intercalated discs that both join cells together and decrease resistance to impulse conduction, (3) being able to initiate beats without the need of a nerve impulse, and (4) being largely involuntary. The microscopic structures are similar.

The circulatory system can be subdivided into three types based on the anatomy of the blood vessels. These are (1) the systemic circulation, which supplies blood to the head, extremities, and trunk (the main artery is the aorta and the main veins—including lymphatic drainage—are the inferior and superior vena cava), (2) the pulmonary circulation, which supplies blood to the lungs, and (3) the coronary circulation, which supplies blood to the heart. The coronary arteries arise at the base of the aorta at the aortic valve. The arteries give rise to the coronary veins that enter the coronary sinus (on the atria), which empties into the RA.

BLOOD VESSELS

Blood vessels consist of arteries, arterioles, capillaries, and veins. Vessels are made of (to different degrees), from the inside out, an intima (endothelial cell lining), a media (consisting of muscle and elastic tissue), and an adventitia (connective tissue covering).

Arteries contain a lot of smooth muscle or elastic tissue and carry blood from the heart (not always oxygenated blood). The contraction of the ventricles in systole imparts energy and pressure to the blood as it enters the arteries. This causes expansion (elastic nature) of the arteries during systole, which stores the energy part. During diastole the elastic recoil converts the stored energy to pressure and maintains the pressure. The blood pressure is higher during systole than diastole in the arteries. But, because of the recoil of the arteries and the effect of the arterioles, the diastolic blood pressure remains well above zero in the arteries. An average blood pressure is $^{120}/_{80}$ (systolic/diastolic) measured in mm Hg. Arterioles connect arteries and capillaries and are the location of the greatest resistance to blood flow. Blood pressure varies directly as the flow of blood (amount of blood pumped by the heart) and directly as the resistance to flow: blood pressure $\propto$ (heart output) $\times$ (resistance). Resistance to flow varies inversely as the fourth power of the radius (r) of the vessel: resistance $\propto 1/r^4$.

Arterioles can change their radii greatly and are important determinants of blood pressure. Sympathetic nerves stimulate smooth muscle cells in the walls of the arterioles; that is, they make the radius smaller. Capillaries contain only endothelial cells, which allow transport of substances across them. Nearly all the transfers of substances between the blood and the tissues occur across the capillaries or the small venules. The hydrostatic pressure, generated by the heartbeat, tends to push fluid and molecules (not cells) out of the capillary. The oncotic pressure, due primarily to the presence of proteins such as albumin in the blood, tends to pull fluid and molecules into the capillary. Hence, the net transfer of fluid depends on the balance of hydrostatic pressure and oncotic pressure. On the arterial side of the capillary, the hydrostatic pressure dominates, and fluid leaves the capillary and enters the tissue space (not the cells directly). At the venule end of the capillary and within the venule itself, the oncotic pressure dominates and draws fluid (containing different substances than those that exited) back into the bloodstream (Figure 8-117). Not all the fluid and proteins are pulled back in; some are returned to the blood vessels via the lymphatics (see Lymphatic and Immune Systems).

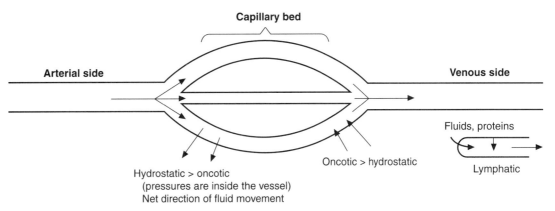

Fig. 8-117. Capillary fluid exchange.

Veins have less muscle and elastin than arteries, some have valves to prevent backward flow of blood, and they carry blood to the heart (heart valves also prevent backward movement). Veins can contain a lot of blood under low pressure; that is, they have a high capacitance and can act as a reservoir. Veins are assisted by skeletal muscle contractions to move blood forward. The lymphatic vessel system is an auxiliary system of vessels that carries both white blood cells and extracellular fluids (including blood proteins) back into the general circulation. The two largest lymph vessels, the right lymphatic duct and the thoracic duct, empty into the venous system (generally into the subclavian veins) in the root of the neck. Inflammation of the lymphatic vessels can cause severe retention of fluids, particularly in the extremities, as is seen in elephantitis.

Flow of molecules and cells into and out of the vascular system is aided by the structure and activity of endothelial cells that make up the walls of capillaries. Three types of capillaries—closed, fenestrated, and discontinuous—handle molecules and cells in three distinctive ways (Figure 8-118). Closed capillaries transport molecules to and from the bloodstream by using pinocytotic vesicles (e.g., muscle). Fenestrated capillaries have circular openings that facilitate transport of larger molecules (e.g., in the kidney glomeruli, hormonal glands), and discontinuous capillaries, including venules (e.g., in bone marrow, liver, spleen), facilitate the movement of cells in addition to molecules. The basal lamina, a secreted connective tissue membrane on which the endothelial cells rest and

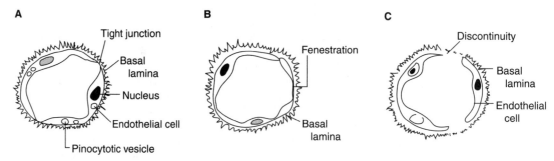

Fig. 8-118. (*A*) Closed capillary. (*B*) Fenestrated capillary. (*C*) Discontinuous capillary.

to which they are attached, also facilitates or diminishes transport depending on its thickness. In uncontrolled diabetes mellitus, the basal lamina increases, slowing transport. In the kidney, the basal lamina is the primary filter of the blood in that the glomerular capillaries are fenestrated.

SYSTOLIC AND DIASTOLIC PRESSURE

Heartbeats are divided into systole (contraction) and diastole (relaxation) on the basis of the state of the ventricles. Beats originate in the sinus node, which is considered the pacemaker of the heart. Impulses activate the atria to contract (diastole), then pass to the atrioventricular node. From this point, impulses pass down the bundle of His to the left and right branch bundles to the Purkinje fibers, which activate the left and right ventricles, causing them to contract (systole). Beats can originate in other parts of the heart if the sinus node fails. Furthermore, some of the bundles or fibers may become injured so that they cannot conduct impulses—then the impulses find alternative paths. Sympathetic nerves increase the heart rate and force of contraction. Parasympathetic nerves (e.g., the vagus nerve) decrease the heart rate. During systole, the ventricles are ejecting blood into the large vessels (PA, aorta); during diastole, the ventricles are being filled with blood from the atria. The RV pumps blood to the lungs and the LV pumps blood to the rest of the body.

COMPOSITION OF BLOOD

Principle and Concepts

Blood consists of formed elements: red blood cells (RBCs, or erythrocytes), white blood cells (WBCs), and platelets. Blood also consists of many nonformed elements, such as proteins, lipids, hormones, dissolved gases, ions, and carbohydrates. RBCs contain hemoglobin, which is made of four polypeptide chains called globin; four hemes, which are porphyrin rings; and four irons; they are biconcave discs (Figure 8-119).

Fig. 8-119

The hematocrit is the percentage of whole blood that is RBCs. The plasma is whole blood minus the formed elements. Serum is plasma after clotting has occurred.

WBCs are mostly neutrophils (a type of granulocyte) and lymphocytes. Eosinophils, basophils, and monocytes are also found in the blood. Neutrophils are involved in inflammatory reactions and are responsible for pus formation. They can phagocytize bacteria and other foreign substances. Lymphocytes are the key elements in the immunologic response system. Platelets are fragments of cells called megakaryocytes (located in the bone marrow). They play a part in the clotting of blood. All of the formed elements arise from precursor cells in the bone marrow. Proteins in the blood are albumin (maintains oncotic pressure and acts as a nonspecific carrier protein) and globulins. Globulins include the immunoglobulins, which are antibodies, carrier proteins, and the coagulation factors (e.g., fibrinogen, prothrombin). Calcium is also required for clotting; agents such as ethylenediaminetetraacetic acid and oxalate complex calcium may prevent clotting. Vitamin K is responsible for formation of some of the clotting factors, and, thus, the clotting of blood.

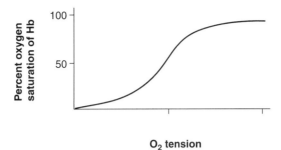

Fig. 8-120. Hemoglobin-oxygen saturation curve.

Percent oxygen saturation of Hb

100

50

O$_2$ tension

Role of Hemoglobin in Oxygen Transport

Hemoglobin (Hb) carries oxygen (O$_2$) attached to iron (Fe). O$_2$ is picked up slowly by Hb at low O$_2$ tension, but this rapidly accelerates as O$_2$ tension increases, and it eventually levels off at high O$_2$ tension (Figure 8-120). (The tension of a gas is the pressure of the gas.) The percent of oxygen saturation of Hb is due to the allosteric nature of the Hb molecule. The first subunit binds O$_2$ slowly, but once bound, the bound O$_2$ causes a conformational change in the second subunit, which causes it to pick up the next O$_2$ faster. This is repeated in the third and fourth subunits until the Hb is saturated. Hb releases O$_2$ more readily at low pH than at high pH; this is called the **Bohr effect**. Hb picks up O$_2$ in the lung and releases it in the tissues. Release and uptake is primarily a function of O$_2$ tension (pressure) gradients, but pH and other factors play a role. Carbon dioxide, dissolved in blood as bicarbonate, is transported from the tissues to the lungs and is bound to Hb and some other proteins. Its uptake (at tissues) by blood and release (in the lungs) by blood is also a function of CO$_2$ pressure gradients. Gases diffuse from regions of higher pressure to regions of lower pressure.

APPLIED CONCEPTS

- Recognize the following concepts and terms with a definition, basic sketch, and current medical usage: erythrocyte sedimentation rate, reticulocyte count, prothrombin time, partial thromboplastin time, vasomotion, blood osmotic pressure, filtration and reabsorption pressure in capillaries, platelet plug, pressure curves for the atria and ventricles, 14 blood clotting factors (e.g., Stuart-Prower factor, Hageman factor), metarteriole, baroreceptors and chemoreceptors, circulation time, neurogenic and hypovolemic shock, capillary beds and plasma analysis.
- Understand the physical mechanisms and other causes leading to the following circulatory system disorders and diseases: induced erythrocythemia in athletes; edema; congenital defects (e.g., dextrorotation of the heart, tetralogy of Fallot, pulmonary and aortic stenosis); Buerger's or Raynaud's disease; coarctation; aneurysm or cerebral hemorrhage; aplastic anemia; atrial fibrillation; toxoplasmosis; histiocytosis; malaria; plague; and HIV infection through blood. Understand also the techniques of human leukocyte antigen typing or tissue typing for transplant procedures and the differences between etiology and pathogenesis of atherosclerosis.
- Identify equipment, instruments, and measurement units to determine various cardiovascular and blood-related factors such as reticulocyte count, blood osmotic pressure, and pressure curves for atria and ventricles.
- Review the design and the working and modern research techniques associated with electrocardiograms (ambulatory, resting, or stress), Holter monitor, artificial pacemaker, ultrasonic cardiogram, artificial heart monitor, cold spot myocardial imaging, angiography, cardiac catheterization, heart-lung machine, laser angioplasty, balloon-laser welding, catheter arthrectomy, balloon valvuloplasty, sphygmomanometer, and construction of a blood pressure monitor.
- Determine the molecular structure and side effects (in biochemical terms) of anticoagulants, antihypertensive medication, inotropic medication, antiarrhythmic medication, fibrinolytic drugs, debriding and antiplatelet drugs, and Fluosol-DA (blood substitute) drugs.
- Learn the comparative relationships between Virchow's lipid infiltration theory and Rokitansky's encrustation theory.

CIRCULATORY SYSTEM: REVIEW QUESTIONS

1. Which statement or statements are correct?

   A. Veins and arteries carry both oxygenated and deoxygenated blood.
   B. Veins carry only deoxygenated blood.
   C. Arteries carry only oxygenated blood.
   D. Both **B** and **C** are correct.

2. Which of the following is not part of the conduction system of the heart?

   A. Atrioventricular node
   B. Chordae tendineae
   C. Bundle of His
   D. Purkinje fibers

3. Cells in the blood are normally derived from precursor cells in the:

   A. liver.
   B. spleen.
   C. bone marrow.
   D. connective tissue.

4. All are types of white blood cells except:

   A. megakaryocytes.
   B. neutrophils.
   C. eosinophils.
   D. lymphocytes.

5. The mitral valve is located between the:

   A. left atrium and left ventricle.
   B. left and right ventricles.
   C. left and right atria.
   D. superior vena cava and the heart.

6. Which agent chelates calcium and may prevent clotting of blood?

   A. Vitamin D
   B. Ethylenediaminetetraacetic acid
   C. Vitamin K
   D. NH_3

7. All of the following are true about albumin except that it:

   A. is found in the plasma.
   B. plays a role in immunologic reactions.
   C. is made in the liver.
   D. plays a role in maintaining the colloid oncotic pressure of the blood.

8. The beats of the heart are initiated by:

   A. the brain.
   B. the sympathetic nerves.
   C. the parasympathetic nerves.
   D. the sinoatrial node.

9. The Bohr effect on hemoglobin function:

   A. makes electrons in the hemoglobin easier to ionize.
   B. is to make it a CO_2 carrier.
   C. is to increase the affinity of hemoglobin for oxygen at higher altitudes.
   D. causes it to release oxygen more readily at lower pH values.

10. Which statement is correct concerning the heart?

   A. The right ventricle pumps blood to the body excluding the lung.
   B. The right ventricle pumps blood to the lung.
   C. The left ventricle pumps blood to the lung.
   D. The left ventricle pumps blood to the body including the lung.

11. Which is the correct sequence of blood passing through the heart? (R = right, L = left, A = atrium, V = ventricle, SVC = superior vena cava, IVC = inferior vena cava)

   A. RA to RV to SVC/IVC to LA to LV to lungs to aorta to RA
   B. SVC/IVC to LA to LV to lungs to RA to RV to aorta to SVC/IVC
   C. SVC/IVC to RA to RV to lungs to LA to LV to aorta to SVC/IVC
   D. RA to RV to LA to LV to lungs to aorta to IVC/SVC to RA

12. Heart muscle differs from skeletal muscle in all of the following except:

    A. having striations.
    B. being made of distinct cells.
    C. having intercalated discs.
    D. having the capacity to originate beats without nervous impulses.

13. Layers of blood vessels include all of the following except:

    A. tendineae.
    B. media.
    C. adventitia.
    D. intima.

14. The greatest resistance to blood flow is in the:

    A. capillaries.
    B. veins.
    C. arteries.
    D. arterioles.

15. All of the following might increase blood pressure except an:

    A. increase in sympathetic tone of vessels.
    B. increase in the radius of a vessel.
    C. increase in blood output by the heart.
    D. increase in resistance of vessels.

16. The oncotic pressure of blood:

    A. has no effect on the movement of fluid.
    B. causes fluid to move into the tissues from the blood vessels.
    C. causes fluid to move into the blood vessels from the tissues.
    D. causes fluid to move from higher pressure to lower pressure.

17. On the venous side of the capillary:

    A. hydrostatic pressure exceeds oncotic pressure and causes fluid to move into the tissues.
    B. oncotic pressure exceeds hydrostatic pressure and causes fluid to move into the tissues.
    C. hydrostatic pressure exceeds oncotic pressure and causes fluid to move into the blood vessel.
    D. oncotic pressure exceeds hydrostatic pressure and causes fluid to move into the blood vessel.

18. Regarding the fluid that escapes from the blood on the arterial side of the capillaries:

    A. some of the fluid and proteins are carried off by lymphatics.
    B. all of the fluid is returned to the blood at the venous end of the capillary.
    C. the fluid normally contains red blood cells.
    D. none of the above are correct.

19. Select the item that is most likely a red blood cell:

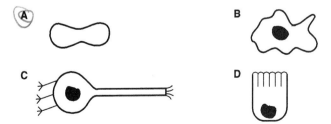

20. Which of the following is involved in the immune response?

    A. Neutrophils
    B. Lymphocytes
    C. Platelets
    D. Basophils

1–14. 1-A, 2-B, 3-C, 4-A, 5-A, 6-B, 7-B, 8-D, 9-D, 10-B, 11-C, 12-A, 13-A, 14-D. See text for explanation.

15. **B** Sympathetic tone means there is a decrease in the radius of the vessels. A decrease in the radius of the vessels means an increase in resistance (resistance $\propto 1/r^4$). This means that the pressure increases (pressure $\propto$ resistance). An increase in radius causes a decrease in blood pressure. Therefore, as radius increases, the resistance decreases (resistance $\propto 1/r^4$), and as resistance decreases, the pressure decreases (pressure $\propto$ resistance). Options **C** and **D** are discussed in the text.

16–20. 16-C, 17-D, 18-A, 19-A, 20-B. See text for explanation.

Lymphatic and Immune Systems

Self-Managed Learning Questions

1. Study the definitions of and illustrate the following terms: agranular leukocytes, hemolytic anemia, endogenous pyrogens, bursa of Fabricius, antigenic determinant, systemic anaphylaxis.
2. Review the research done on verification of the "theory of immunosurveillance" and identify what assumptions are not applicable to some pathogens. Understand the experimental techniques and limitations in production of monoclonal antibodies.
3. Understand the basic concepts related to the science of transplanting organs. Understand the limitations, claims, and challenges of organ and tissue transplantation. Learn the definitions of autograft, homograft, and graft rejection. Review the chemical structure of the antibiotic cyclosporin and how it is used to suppress T cells. Perform critical analysis of the "Uniform Anatomical Gift Act" for organ donation by reviewing the claims and assumptions presented.

Review the basic structures and functions of these systems. Understand the mechanisms that work in these systems to regulate various processes in the human body. Examine the composition of blood on both a physical and chemical basis and the mechanisms that control flow of lymph at various lymph nodes. Review the physical structure, physical properties, chemical properties, and stereochemistry of helper T cells, killer T cells, suppressor T cells, and T-cell receptors. Place emphasis on autoimmunity, active immunity, and passive immunity in studying publications on immunology and current medical literature. Examine and recognize current research involving bone marrow transplants, and spleen and thymus surgical procedures. Associate your knowledge of microbiology (especially virus and bacteria life history) with immune system response time.

STRUCTURE AND FUNCTION

The lymphatic and immune system is the surveillance system of the body against foreign invaders; it distinguishes between self and nonself. When properly functioning, it protects against bacteria, viruses, fungi, and parasites. When it encounters foreign (nonself) material (called an **antigen**), the immune system becomes activated. An antigen is recognized by characteristic shapes (epitopes) on its surface to which antibodies are formed in an attempt to neutralize the antigen. The organs of the immune system are called **lymphoid organs** and include the bone marrow, thymus, lymph nodes, spleen, tonsils, adenoids, appendix, and Peyer's patches (lymphoid tissues in the small intestine).

Lymphatic vessels are widely dispersed peripherally within the connective tissues supporting the epithelium of all potential portals into the body (e.g., skin, oral cavity, urinary tract, genital tract, digestive tract, and respiratory tree). Individual cells or diffuse aggregations of cells (as large as the tonsils) can be found. Lymphatic capillaries flow into lymph nodes (regionally positioned fluid filters found in the neck, armpits, abdomen, and groin) and larger lymphatic vessels (an auxiliary drainage network to veins that interconnect the lymph nodes). Lymphatic vessels are generally one cell thick and are made of endothelial cells (similar to the cells lining blood vessels). These vessels begin as blind pouches in all tissues of the body (Figure 8-121). They remove fluid, proteins, and particulate

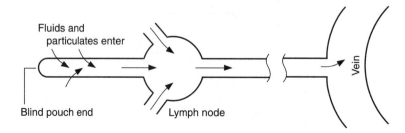

Fig. 8-121. Lymphatics.

matter that arise in tissues directly or by extravasation from the blood vessels. Once in the lymphatics, the lymph (or removed materials) is "filtered" at the lymph nodes and eventually reenters the circulatory system by flowing into the large veins in the thorax (chest cavity) via the thoracic duct or right lymphatic duct. Lymph flow is passive and requires muscle action (acting as a pump) to move lymph along the vessels. If lymph vessels are destroyed, lymph nodes are blocked, or there is no muscle action, then the lymph does not flow and the fluid remains in the tissues. That tissue swells and becomes edematous. Gravity tends to retard the flow of lymph back into the blood vessels. The key functions of the lymphatic system are the return of fluid and proteins to the circulation from the tissues and protection against foreign materials.

IMMUNE SYSTEM

Cells

The cells of the immune system include **lymphocytes** and **phagocytes** (macrophages, neutrophils), which are produced in the bone marrow. Phagocytes are white blood cells that devour (phagocytize) foreign matter such as bacteria and dead cells to clear them from the system. In addition, they mediate the presentation of antigens to lymphocytes and secrete factors that activate T cells. Lymphocytes are classified as **B cells** or **T cells.** B cells are produced continuously and mature in the bone marrow, whereas T cells mature in the thymus, which is located behind the breast bone. T cells differ from other cells of the immune system in that their pool is established during the fetal and early postnatal period and is maintained throughout life by expansion of T cells that are located peripherally. Both B cells and T cells can distinguish between self and nonself and initiate an immune reaction in the presence of foreign material (antigens). The immune cells circulate throughout the body via the blood or lymphatic vessels.

Tissues

Bone marrow, which is found inside bones, manufactures B cells, which are important to the immune system. Approximately 2.4 million red blood cells are destroyed (recycled) each minute and are immediately replaced by new ones that are made in the bone marrow.

The **spleen** is the major lymphoid organ of the general circulation and, as such, is a key organ in fighting systemic infections. It is located in the abdominal cavity behind the stomach and is the size of a small fist. The spleen also doubles as a destruction and storage center for red blood cells.

The **thymus gland** functions as part of the lymphatic system and is necessary for the proper development of the immune system. Its two main functions are to activate the immune responses of T cells, which then can differentiate into cells that respond to certain antigens, and to function as an endocrine gland by secreting hormones, including thymosin.

Lymph nodes contain lymphocytes and macrophages. Lymphocytes are involved in the antibody response to antigens (foreign materials). Removing particulate matter (e.g., bacteria and dead cells) by phagocytosis and helping lymphocytes in the immune response are functions of the macrophage, which performs a similar function all over the body (especially in the lung, liver, and spleen). Lymph nodes often swell and become tender (**lymphadenopathy**) during infection or inflammation due to this function. There are more cells, both macrophages and lymphocytes, in a swollen lymph node. Although the lymph node has some capacity for cell division, large influxes of cells occurring during periods of inflammation are transported into the lymph nodes through the vascular system and exit into the nodule through the walls of the venules (Figure 8-122). The location of the swollen node (e.g., at the angle of the jaw) is important in localizing the infection (e.g., the throat or tooth) or even a cancer (i.e., metastasis from the primary cancer) because nodes drain lymphatic vessels from given regions of the body.

Antigens, Antibodies, and Antigen-Antibody Reactions

B cells control **humoral immunity** by secreting antibodies. Antibodies interact with antigens such as bacteria or viruses, but cannot penetrate living cells. Each B cell makes an antibody that is specific for a given antigen, just as keys are made to open specific locks. When a B cell interacts with its antigen, plasma cells are formed that manufacture and release the specific antibody. Antibodies belong to one of several classes of **immunoglobulins** (Ig): IgG, IgA, IgM, IgE, or IgD. Each Ig class has unique characteristics. All immunoglobulins are made up of two heavy and two light chains that form the shape of a Y (Figure 8-123). The ends of the Y contain the epitopes to which the antigen binds and are known as the variable (V) region. The stem end of the Y is called the constant (C) region and is the same in all antibodies of the same class. As a result of antigen-antibody binding, the antibody may disable the antigen, coat (**opsonize**) the antigen (e.g., bacteria), cause the release of complement, or block virus entry into cells. **Comple-**

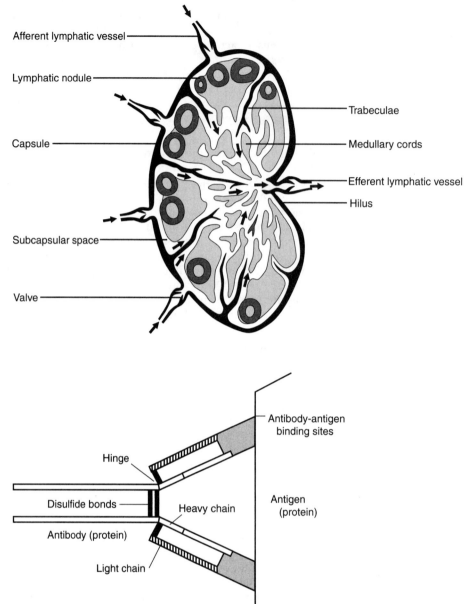

Fig. 8-122. Lymph node (enlarged).

Afferent lymphatic vessel

Lymphatic nodule

Capsule

Subcapsular space

Valve

Trabeculae

Medullary cords

Efferent lymphatic vessel

Hilus

Fig. 8-123. Basic structure of an antibody molecule.

Hinge

Disulfide bonds

Antibody (protein)

Light chain

Heavy chain

Antibody-antigen binding sites

Antigen (protein)

ment consists of a series of proteins that assist antibodies in attacking antigens. T cells control **cellular immunity.** Cytotoxic T cells attack host cells that have been invaded by bacteria or malignancy. Helper, or inducer, T cells (identified by the T4 marker) regulate other T cells, natural killer cells, macrophages, and B cells (without T cell intervention, B cells cannot form antibodies). T cells work by secreting cytokines (e.g., interferon, tumor necrosis factor, and interleukin), which are powerful chemical messengers. Cytokines initiate a wide variety of protective responses, including the inflammatory response.

APPLIED CONCEPTS

Review newspaper articles, research reports, and current periodicals to understand research trends, new instrumentation, and experimentation techniques in immunology. The following tasks are to be emphasized:

- From your knowledge in inorganic chemistry and biology, determine the structures and mechanisms associated with immunoglobulin homology units (IgA, IgD, IgE, IgG, and IgM) and develop visual understanding of Fab and Fc fragments of IgG molecules (linked to the stereochemistry of heavy and light chains).
- Identify the following terms with definitions and sketches: Hassall's corpuscles, mal-

pighian corpuscles, Billroth's cords, wandering macrophages, tonsils, hyaluronic acid, phagocytic margination, spleen, and thymus glands.

- Review background information and arguments on the strength, applications, and soundness (based on credibility of scientific analysis) of antibody diversity hypotheses, both on somatic mutation and somatic recombination. Review hypothesis concerning membrane attack complex in the immune system.
- Understand the causes, research experimentation, and basic medical techniques related to Hodgkin's disease, leukocytosis, blood transfusion problems, lymphangiography (to detect lymphomas and various lymphatic tissue tumors), and experimental procedure to produce the hypoxanthine, amethopterin, thymine (HAT) medium used for producing antibodies against antigens.

LYMPHATIC AND IMMUNE SYSTEMS: REVIEW QUESTIONS

1. The lymphatic system:

   A. returns fluid and proteins to blood vessels.
   B. has a direct connection to the heart.
   C. consists of vessels only.
   D. is not integral to the function of the body.

2. Lymph nodes:

   A. are found in veins.
   B. contain lymphocytes only.
   C. may contain lymphocytes and macrophages.
   D. are not directly important in protecting the body against disease.

3. Macrophages:

   A. are found in lymph nodes only.
   B. are phagocytic cells.
   C. are the lining cells of lymphatic vessels.
   D. are all of the above.

4. An enlarged lymph node may mean:

   A. infection.
   B. inflammation.
   C. cancer.
   D. all of the above.

5. Lymph moves toward the veins due to:

   A. tissue pressure.
   B. muscle action.
   C. pumping action of heart.
   D. gravity.

6. T lymphocytes are found in all of the following except:

   A. lymphoid tissues.
   B. the spleen.
   C. the thymus gland.
   D. bone marrow.

ANSWERS AND EXPLANATIONS

1–6. 1-A, 2-C, 3-B, 4-D, 5-B, 6-B. See text for explanation.

Digestive System

Self-Managed Learning Questions

1. Review the biochemistry of pepsin, pepsinogen, and gastric juice reactions. Understand the anatomic and functional differences between chief cells and parietal cells.
2. Draw a basic diagram of the stomach lining and the location of gastric glands. Explain why the gastric juice does not digest the walls of the stomach (each epithelial cell of the stomach lining has a life span of approximately 3 days).
3. Understand experimental procedures to determine cause of heartburn (pyrosis) and difficulty in swallowing (dysphagia). What are the special instruments and mechanisms used to detect esophageal problems? (The manometric catheter with

a pressure transducer is inserted through the nostril into the esophagus, and the pH electrode with catheter determines esophageal acidity.)

Understand the histology and mechanisms associated with the digestive system. The gastrointestinal tract has the peritoneum and other muscular control layers such as tunica serosa, tunica muscularis, tunica submucosa, and tunica mucosa. Review the microscopic structure of muscularis mucosae and the lamina propria, and the circular and longitudinal muscle to understand the role and mechanisms of the digestive process. Review histology of the digestive system integrated with the biochemical and muscular actions within the system.

INGESTION: STRUCTURES AND THEIR FUNCTIONS

The structure and function of the digestive system are discussed in relation to the path of a bolus (Figure 8-124).

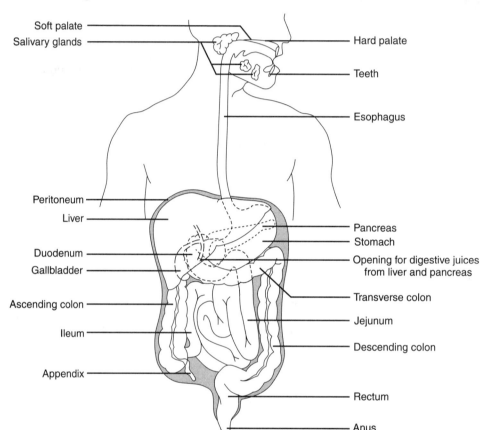

Fig. 8-124. The digestive system. (Adapted with permission from Bresnick SD: *Columbia Review Intensive Preparation for the MCAT.* Baltimore, Williams & Wilkins, 1996, p 434.)

Teeth and Tongue

The **teeth** and the **tongue** are responsible for breaking food down into swallowable chunks (called boluses). Adults have 32 teeth; children have 20 (called deciduous teeth). Each quadrant (quarter) contains two incisors (for cutting), one canine (for tearing), two premolars (for crushing), and three molars (for grinding). Salivary glands secrete alkaline saliva to moisten food for swallowing, protect against bacteria, and begin digestion of starch. Swallowing is initiated voluntarily but becomes involuntary as food enters the pharynx. The swallowing center is located in the medulla, and the hypoglossal (XII) and glossopharyngeal (IX) nerves are responsible for the esophageal phase after the bolus passes from the pharynx.

Stomach

The bolus enters the **stomach** from the esophagus where it may be stored for several hours. Grinding and liquefying the food are the main functions of the stomach, which is accomplished by its strong muscle. Hydrochloric acid and intrinsic factor (for absorption of vitamin B_{12}) are secreted by parietal cells, and the hydrolytic enzyme pepsin (digests proteins) is secreted by the chief cells of the stomach. Mucus is secreted by goblet cells to protect the stomach from the acid. The acid kills many bacteria and its secretion is controlled by the vagus nerve and the hormone gastrin.

Digestive Glands

Food (now chyme) is propelled to the **duodenum** by peristalsis (propulsive contractions in the gut) through a relaxed pyloric sphincter. Most chemical digestion takes place in the duodenum, not the stomach. Chyme entering the duodenum causes the release of secretin (which stimulates the pancreas to release bicarbonate and fluid) and cholecysto-kinin-pancreozymin (which stimulates the pancreas to release primarily enzymes and water and the liver to release bile). The pancreas secretes inactive enzymes called zymogens. One of them, trypsinogen, is converted to trypsin by the enterokinase, an activating enzyme located in the duodenal mucosa. Other enzymes, chymotrypsin, lipases, and amylases, are also secreted. Bile is secreted by the liver and stored in and released from the gallbladder. Bile salts in bile emulsify lipids to make them more available for digestion. The duodenum has an alkaline pH. Chyme passes into the jejunum where the mucosa contains disaccharidases and peptidases for the final breakdown of nutrients before they are absorbed by active transport.

The **liver** is a vital organ with numerous functions. The major functions are as follows:

1. Synthesis and storage of glycogen to be converted to glucose under the stimulation of epinephrine or glucagon
2. Gluconeogenesis—the synthesis of glucose from amino acids stimulated by glucagon and epinephrine via cyclic adenosine monophosphate (by gluconeogenesis and removal of storage glycogen, the liver plays an important role in regulation of blood glucose)
3. Production of proteins by synthesizing coagulation factors and albumin, among others
4. Production of bile and cholesterol
5. Defense against foreign materials (e.g., bacteria) by macrophages (called Kupffer cells)
6. Detoxification and degradation of toxins, drugs, and normal metabolites
7. Packaging of fats for transport and oxidization of fatty acids to ketone bodies for use by other tissues
8. Deamination using amino acids (removal of nitrogen) and production of urea
9. Interconversion of fats, carbohydrates, and amino acids
10. Storage of substances such as iron and vitamins A, D, and B_{12}
11. Production of red blood cells in cases of severe anemia in the adult and at the site of destruction of old red blood cells

Small and Large Intestines

The **small intestine** is composed of the duodenum, jejunum, and ileum, in that order. The duodenum is important for absorption of Ca^{2+} and Fe^{3+}, the jejunum for most sugars, amino acids, and fats, and the ileum for vitamin B_{12} (complexed to intrinsic factor) and bile salts. In the **colon (large intestine)**, the remaining water from the small intestine is largely absorbed, as are most ions, compacting the chyme into feces. Feces are stored in the sigmoid colon and rectum until they are defecated. The **appendix** is a vestigial appendage of the cecum (first segment of the colon).

The small intestine has mucosal projections called **villi**. Crypts are regions at the base of villi where new cells are generated and digestive enzymes are synthesized by glandular cells. The simple columnar epithelium lines the intestinal tract and consists mainly of absorptive cells and goblet cells. Absorptive cells have thousands of microvilli, extensions of the plasma membrane, to increase the surface area of the cell. Absorbed products are transported through them and released basolaterally. The microvilli are bathed by mucus (secreted by neighboring goblet cells) to aid in trapping digested food. The basal plasma membrane is infolded to facilitate active transport. Like all epithelial cells, absorptive and goblet cells rest on the basal lamina that separates them from the blood capillaries located in the connective tissue beneath. The connective tissue (lamina propria) surrounding the blood capillaries is secreted by fibroblasts (Figures 8-125 and 8-126).

Once the products of digestion (molecules and ions) are transported across the absorptive cells, they are transported into the general circulation through the small lymphatic channels, the lacteals, as well as the small veins that coalesce to form the hepatic portal system. The connective tissue of the ileum houses lymphatic nodules (**Peyer's patches**), which are colonies of lymphocytes that provide a first line of defense against bacterial infection.

Muscular Control of Digestion

Food is pushed through the pharynx by **peristalsis**, a wave of involuntary smooth muscle contractions that moves food progressively down from the pharynx toward the anus (Figure 8-127). Peristalsis is started by the stretching from a bolus of food. It can also work in the opposite direction (vomiting). When the body is upright, gravity also helps move the food through the esophagus, but it is not necessary. Astronauts can eat without the

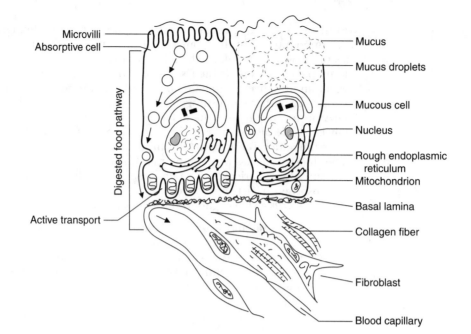

Fig. 8-125. Intestinal lining.

Microvilli
Absorptive cell
Digested food pathway
Active transport

Mucus
Mucus droplets
Mucous cell
Nucleus
Rough endoplasmic reticulum
Mitochondrion
Basal lamina
Collagen fiber
Fibroblast
Blood capillary

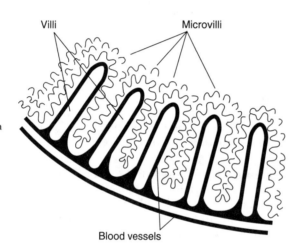

Fig. 8-126. Microvilli and villi in the folds of the intestinal wall.

Villi
Microvilli
Blood vessels

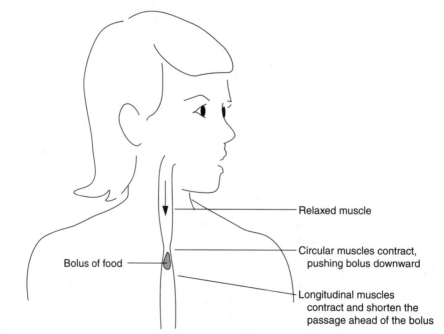

Fig. 8-127. Peristalsis.

Relaxed muscle
Circular muscles contract, pushing bolus downward
Bolus of food
Longitudinal muscles contract and shorten the passage ahead of the bolus

aid of gravity. The entrance to the stomach normally is closed by the sphincter, a thick ring of smooth muscle at the junction of the esophagus and the stomach. Peristalsis causes the sphincter to relax enough to allow the food into the stomach. After approximately 3 or 4 hours, peristaltic waves propel the chyme through the stomach exit and into the duodenum, where more peristaltic waves move it through the intestines toward the anus.

APPLIED CONCEPTS

- Understand causes, effects, and research related to digestive disorders such as peptic ulcer, gallstone, pancreatitis, hepatitis, cirrhosis, appendicitis, porphyria, regional ileitis, and Crohn's disease.
- Review the histology of pancreas and liver with emphasis on differences between falciform and round ligaments in the pancreas and liver.
- Learn the chemical composition, pH value, and average daily secretions of saliva, gastric juice, pancreatic juice, and bile.
- Diagnostic tests concerning esophageal acidity, manometry, and acid perfusion should be carefully analyzed. Antacids and anticholinergics increase pH-reducing ability. Review the experimental equipment design and a complete working model of equipment used.
- Review the nature of the following diagnostic tests: esophagogastroduodenoscopy and endoscopic retrograde cholangiopancreatography.

DIGESTIVE SYSTEM: REVIEW QUESTIONS

1. In the normal adult with a full set of teeth, which type of tooth has the incorrect maximum number in parentheses?

   A. Incisors (4)
   B. Canines (4)
   C. Premolars (8)
   D. Molars (12)

2. All of the following are functions of saliva except:

   A. digestion of starch.
   B. digestion of protein.
   C. lubrication of food.
   D. protection against bacteria.

3. Select the incorrect association.

   A. Stomach—grinds and liquefies food
   B. Pancreas—digestive enzymes
   C. Small intestine—absorption of fluid and food
   D. Colon (large intestine)—absorption of food

4. The correct sequence of structures in the gut is:

   A. stomach, esophagus, small intestine, large intestine.
   B. esophagus, stomach, large intestine, small intestine.
   C. esophagus, stomach, small intestine, large intestine.
   D. esophagus, small intestine, stomach, large intestine.

5. Which of the following is not a function of the liver?

   A. Synthesis of insulin
   B. Synthesis of carbohydrates, proteins, fats
   C. Detoxification of drugs
   D. Synthesis of bile

6. Most nutrients are absorbed in the:

   A. esophagus.
   B. stomach.
   C. small intestine.
   D. large intestine.

7. Digestion of carbohydrates occurs mostly by enzymes from the:

   A. pancreas.
   B. liver.
   C. stomach.
   D. salivary glands.

8. Monosaccharides cross the intestinal wall mainly by:

   A. active transport.
   B. diffusion.
   C. facilitated transport.
   D. both **A** and **C**.

9. Swallowing is:

   A. voluntary.
   B. involuntary.
   C. both voluntary and involuntary.
   D. caused by gustatory receptors.

10. Secretion of bicarbonate and fluid from the pancreas is stimulated by:

    A. secretin.
    B. cholecystokinin.
    C. enterokinase.
    D. gastrin.

11. Acid secretion from the stomach may be stimulated by:

    A. gastrin.
    B. vagus nerve.
    C. neither **A** nor **B**.
    D. both **A** and **B**.

12. Select the enzyme not made in the pancreas.

    A. Trypsin
    B. Lipase
    C. Amylase
    D. Pepsin

13. Vitamin B_{12} is absorbed in the:

    A. ileum.
    B. jejunum.
    C. duodenum.
    D. stomach.

14. Iron is absorbed in the:

    A. stomach.
    B. jejunum.
    C. ileum.
    D. duodenum.

15. The absorptive area of the small intestine is increased by structures called:

    A. crypts.
    B. villi.
    C. microvilli.
    D. villi and microvilli.

16. The liver does not play a role in the metabolism of:

    A. fats.
    B. carbohydrates.
    C. proteins.
    D. carboxylic acids.

17. The digestion of starch by amylase produces:

    A. galactose.
    B. glucose.
    C. maltose.
    D. both **B** and **C**.

18. The digestion of small peptides and disaccharides occurs:

    A. in the stomach lumen.
    B. in the lumen of the bowels.

C. on the mucosal cell surface.
D. inside the mucosal cell.

ANSWERS AND EXPLANATIONS

1–20. 1-A, 2-B, 3-D, 4-C, 5-A, 6-C, 7-A, 8-D, 9-C, 10-A, 11-D, 12-D, 13-A, 14-D, 15-D, 16-D, 17-D, 18-C. See text for explanation.

Excretory System

Self-Managed Learning Questions

1. Review the mechanisms of waste disposal for worms, insects, birds, sponges, and other sea creatures.
2. How do fish survive in saltwater and how is osmoregulation carried out by marine fish and freshwater fish? Do fish drink or absorb saltwater? Do they get dehydrated? What are osmoconformers?
3. What is estivation? How do frogs and other amphibians control water intake in very dry environments?
4. What is the anion gap? How can metabolic acidosis be monitored with the anion gap? What laboratory errors can result in an anion gap?

CHEMISTRY OF BODY FLUIDS

Focus on the functional unit of a kidney—the nephron. There are 1 million nephrons per kidney. Each nephron is made up of glomerulus and the tubule (made up of renal corpuscles, podocytes, and distal and proximal tubules). Understand the histology of podocytes and examine sample electron micrographs. Identify various types of nephrons, such as juxtamedullary nephrons and cortical nephrons, and their special functions (e.g., body fluid transport). Review the mechanics of tubular reabsorption (both active and passive), the definition and use of milliosmol as a concentration unit, and the workings of various hydrostatic forces involved in effective filtration. Work with numerical problems to apply various concepts to experimental data on kidneys and filtration rates of body fluids.

Body Fluid Composition

Human body fluids divide into an **intracellular** (IC) compartment and an **extracellular** (EC) compartment. The EC compartment is further divided into an **interstitial** (I) compartment (outside of cells and outside of the circulation) and a **plasma** (P) compartment (circulatory component). Each compartment has a particular substance that tends to maintain its volume. Potassium (K^+) ion is the main molecule of the IC compartment. Sodium (Na^+) ion is the main molecule of the EC compartment. Protein, in addition to Na^+, is important in the P compartment.

In the plasma there are **cations**, primarily Na^+ and K^+, balanced by **anions**, primarily chloride (Cl^-) and bicarbonate (HCO_3^-). There are also many small organic molecules, such as glucose and amino acids. Larger organic molecules, such as proteins and fat complexes, are also present.

The acidity, measured by the pH, is relatively constant at pH $\approx$ 7.40 for the plasma. The major sources of acidity are the CO_2 (produced in tissues) and acids from the oxidation of glucose, fats, and amino acids such as pyruvate, lactate, or sulfur (from sulfur-containing amino acids). Bicarbonate (basic) is produced by the kidney to balance these acids. The ratio of dissolved CO_2 and HCO_3^- is the determinator of the pH. As CO_2 increases, the pH decreases, and as HCO_3^- increases, the pH increases:

$$pH \propto \frac{[HCO_3^-]}{P_{CO_2}}$$

where P_{CO_2} is the partial pressure of CO_2

CO_2 undergoes this reaction with water as follows:

$$CO_2 + H_2O \rightleftharpoons H_2CO_3$$

And, carbonic acid dissociates to give H^+, $H_2CO_2 \rightleftharpoons H^+ + HCO_3^-$ (remember H^+ is measured by the pH.

Physiologic Buffers in Body Fluids

The main buffer in the extracellular fluid (ECF) is bicarbonate. To use the Henderson-Hasselbalch equation,

$$pH = pK + \log \frac{base}{acid}$$

use actual experimental values of an average person: pK = 6.1 for the ECF.

Example: Add 10 mmol/L of hydrochloric acid to 1 L of water and to 1 L of ECF. Assume that the ECF $[HCO_3^-]$ is 20 mmol/L and the $[H_2CO_3]$ is 1.2 mmol. Study pH changes.

Solution: For water, 10 mmol HCl contains 10 mmol = $^{10}/_{1000}$ = 0.010 mol hydrogen ion. Therefore, by definition, pH = $-\log [H^+]$ = $-\log [.010]$ = 2.00.

For ECF, 10 HCl + 20 NaHCO$_3$ → 10 NaCl + 10 NaHCO$_3$ + 10 H$_2$CO$_3$. Bicarbonate reduces the change in pH caused by addition of H^+. Using the Henderson-Hasselbalch equation and noting that there is already 1.2 mmol H$_2$CO$_3$ in the fluid,

$$pH = 6.1 + \log \frac{10}{10 + 1.2}$$

$$= 6.1 + \log \frac{10}{11.2} = 6.99$$

HCO_3^- is the most important physiologic buffer because its two components can be regulated by the kidneys and the lung.

ROLE OF THE EXCRETORY SYSTEM IN BODY HOMEOSTASIS

The body regulates the composition of its body fluids within fairly narrow limits because too much or too little of most substances is toxic to cells. The kidney is the central regulator. In general, substances taken into the body (by the gastrointestinal tract, lungs, skin or directly into vessels) and substances made in the tissues are in balance with substances used by the tissues and excreted by the body (in the lungs, gastrointestinal tract, skin, and kidneys). That is, input equals output. This results in fairly constant levels of most substances in the blood. Changes in the function or amount of the load can destroy homeostasis and cause changes in body fluid composition.

The heart and blood vessels keep blood flowing to all the organs and tissues, allowing a constant exchange between the tissues and the blood. If cardiovascular function decreases, fluid nutrients cannot get to tissues and wastes accumulate in tissues and the blood. If the heart output decreases too much, the kidney cannot function. The lymphatic vessels return fluid and protein to the cardiovascular system to help maintain its function. When lymphatic function decreases, fluid accumulates in the tissues, and the heart has less blood to pump, which compromises its function. The lungs remove CO_2 from the body and supply the O_2 needed. If lung function is affected, the acidity of blood is affected as is the production of energy (which requires O_2). The skin plays a role in the passage of water and ions (Na^+, K^+, Cl^-) in the form of sweat. If sweating is excessive, water and ion loss can compromise the circulation. The gastrointestinal tract is responsible for the intake of nutrients and excretion of certain wastes and ions (Na^+, K^+, Cl^-, HCO_3^-) and water. Therefore, malfunctions (e.g., diarrhea) can lead to body fluid abnormalities.

Finally, the kidney fine-tunes the body fluids. After the other systems have upset or tried to correct the homeostasis, the kidney can return the body fluids to a new (not necessarily the same) homeostasis. When kidneys malfunction, substances (e.g., urea) collect in the blood or substances that would ordinarily not be retained or excreted (e.g., sugar, excess Na^+) are excreted.

Kidney: Structure and Function

The structure and function of the **kidney** is described in association with the path of blood through the kidney and the formation of urine by the kidney (Figures 8-128 and 8-129).

Blood from the renal artery enters the center of the kidney (**hilus**) and divides into hundreds of branches as it radiates outward into the cortex. At a million locations within the cortex of each kidney, the smallest of arteries, the arterioles, branch into a knotted cluster of capillaries termed the **glomerulus**, then fuse together again into an arteriole before breaking finally into the vast capillary beds of the kidney. The capillary loops of the glomerulus have small holes called fenestrae that readily allow passage of much of the watery ions and smaller molecules, but retain the larger blood proteins, blood cells, and platelets within the capillary. The actual filter of the kidney is a slightly thickened basal lamina of the capillary endothelial cells. The knotted glomerulus is housed in the first segment of the nephron, a long, folded tubule capped by a cellular funnel, termed **Bowman's capsule**, which wraps around the glomerulus and aids in the filtration and directs the filtrate toward the cellular tubule. In the proximal convoluted tubule (PCT), proteins, amino acids, sugars, and other nutrients are reabsorbed by active transport by the tubular cells. Most of the cells of the tubular nephron are cuboidal epithelial cells and, like those absorptive cells of the small intestine, possess both microvilli and modifications of the basal plasma membrane to aid in active transport. They rest on a basal lamina.

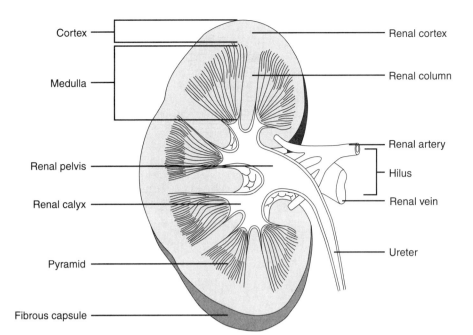

Fig. 8-128. Kidney.

Cortex — Renal cortex

Medulla — Renal column

Renal artery

Hilus

Renal pelvis — Renal vein

Renal calyx — Ureter

Pyramid

Fibrous capsule

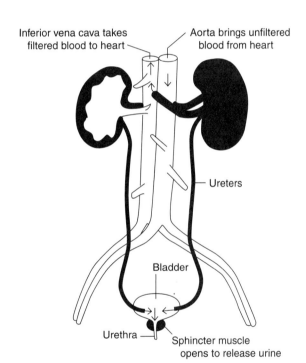

Fig. 8-129. Excretory system.

Inferior vena cava takes filtered blood to heart

Aorta brings unfiltered blood from heart

Ureters

Bladder

Urethra — Sphincter muscle opens to release urine

Nephron: Structure and Function

The **nephron** is the functional unit of the kidney; there are approximately 1 million nephrons in each kidney (Figures 8-130 and 8-131). Each nephron contains a Bowman's capsule that is connected to a long renal tube that is partially coiled. Within the Bowman's capsule is a cluster of capillaries called the **glomerulus**. The glomerulus filters blood and produces a fluid that is absent of cells and large molecules. The force that drives the filtration is the pressure of arterial blood.

Formation of Urine

Plasma contains waste products of the tissues, one of the most important being **urea**. Urea, is the result of the breakdown of nitrogen-containing organic molecules, especially amino acids (Figure 8-132). Creatinine is a product of muscle metabolism and is also continuously released into the plasma. Both are excreted by the kidneys.

Sodium, potassium, and bicarbonate are reabsorbed in the kidney, as is most of the water. Hydrogen ion and ammonium ions are secreted into the tubular lumen by the PCT cells. Toxic substances and waste molecules are also secreted into the lumen by the PCT cells. The fluid remaining in the lumen continues into the descending limb of the

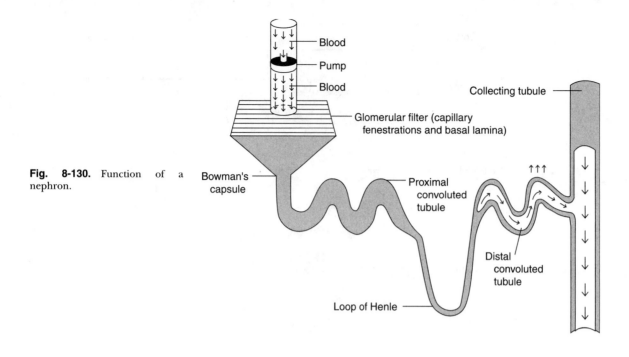

Fig. 8-130. Function of a nephron.

Blood
Pump
Blood
Glomerular filter (capillary fenestrations and basal lamina)
Collecting tubule
Bowman's capsule
Proximal convoluted tubule
Distal convoluted tubule
Loop of Henle

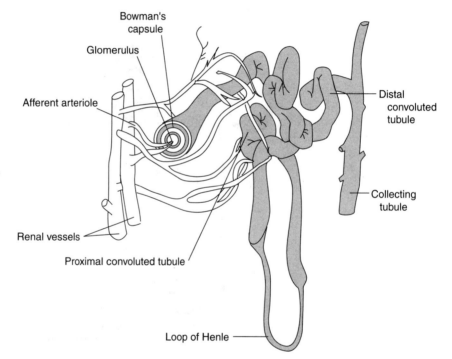

Fig. 8-131. Microscopic view of the nephron.

Bowman's capsule
Glomerulus
Afferent arteriole
Distal convoluted tubule
Collecting tubule
Renal vessels
Proximal convoluted tubule
Loop of Henle

Fig. 8-132. Urea molecule.

Urea molecule

loop of Henle (LOH) where Na^+ is picked up from the medulla (inside of kidney) interstitium. The filtrate continues around the LOH to the ascending limb of the LOH where Cl^- is actively extruded into the medulla and Na^+ passively follows. A Cl^- pump that requires energy as ATP is responsible for this extrusion against the concentration gradient. This countercurrent multiplier system between the limbs of the LOH maintains a high concentration of Na^+ in the medulla. The filtrate (urine) passes on to the distal convoluted tubule (DCT) where Na^+ in the lumen is exchanged for K^+ (and H^+) in the cells stimulated by aldosterone (from the adrenal gland). The filtrate (now urine) continues to the collecting tubule (CT), which dips into the medulla with its large Na^+ concentration. The Na^+ in the medulla draws most of the water out of the CT into the medulla, where the water is picked up by a system of blood vessels called the **vasa rectae**. Antidiuretic hormone (ADH, or vasopressin) is synthesized in the hypothalamus and stored in and released from the posterior pituitary. **ADH** acts on the CT to increase water resorption and results in a more concentrated urine.

Storage and Elimination of Wastes

Urine passes, in order, through the calyces, the pelvices, the ureter, the urinary bladder, and the urethra to the outside of the body. When the urinary bladder, which can hold up to 1½ pints, is full, it activates stretch senses in its wall and a spinal reflex relaxes its sphincter. Two additional sphincter muscles located at the base of the urethra control the timing of urination. In males, the urethra is long and passes through the penis; in females, the urethra is short and opens just above the opening of the vagina. The short length of the urethra is the reason why bladder infections are more common in females than in males because bacteria have less distance to travel up the urethra of a female to reach the bladder.

APPLIED CONCEPTS

- Understand the basic differences between nephrology and urology and obtain a basic recognition of kidney stones and methods to remove them, prostate hypertrophy in males, glomerulonephritis, cystitis, nephrosis, and nephrectomy. Understand the physics of various instruments used to correct the above renal disorders.
- Understand the design, construction, and working of an artificial kidney and dialysis machine. Recognize the symptoms of a complete renal failure and know the pathological studies done to correct the failure or to make histological recommendations to a specialist.
- Understand several types of acid-base disturbances (e.g., metabolic acidosis and metabolic alkalosis). What experiments are done to identify causes for each and what toxins contribute to acidosis and alkalosis?

EXCRETORY SYSTEM: REVIEW QUESTIONS

1. Functions of the kidneys include all of the following except:

    A. excretion of NH_3 from protein oxidation as urea.
    B. regulation of fluids and electrolytes.
    C. elimination of toxic substances.
    D. elimination of carbon dioxide directly.

2. All of the following are part of the human kidney except the:

    A. glomerulus.
    B. loop of Henle.
    C. malpighian tubules.
    D. collecting ducts.

3. Filtration of blood occurs at which structure in the kidney?

    A. Loop of Henle
    B. Collecting ducts
    C. Tubules
    D. Glomerulus

4. Select the correct statement concerning the antidiuretic hormone (ADH).

    A. ADH is synthesized in the posterior pituitary gland.
    B. ADH acts on the collecting duct of the kidney.
    C. ADH is also called aldosterone.
    D. All of the above are correct.

5. Select the correct sequence of filtered blood through the kidney.

    A. Bowman's capsule, glomerulus, tubules, collecting duct
    B. Glomerulus, Bowman's capsule, collecting ducts, tubules
    C. Bowman's capsule, collecting ducts, glomerulus, tubules
    D. Glomerulus, Bowman's capsule, tubules, collecting duct

6. The volume of fluid in the plasma is maintained by:

 A. protein.
 B. Na^+.
 C. Na^+ and protein.
 D. K^+.

7. The cations of Na^+ and K^+ are balanced in the plasma by:

 A. Cl^-.
 B. HCO_3^-.
 C. Cl^- and HCO_3^-.
 D. proteins.

8. The acidity of the plasma is caused by:

 A. oxidation of glucose and fats.
 B. metabolism of sulfur-containing amino acids.
 C. production of CO_2 by the tissues.
 D. all of the above.

9. Carbon dioxide when dissolved in water:

 A. has base properties.
 B. has acid properties.
 C. is neutral.
 D. behaves as a ketone.

10. Urea:

 A. is a product of protein metabolism.
 B. contains only carbon, hydrogen, and oxygen.
 C. is excreted by the lungs.
 D. is a product of protein regeneration.

11. The _____ is part of the circulatory system.

 A. Bowman's capsule
 B. loop of Henle
 C. medulla
 D. glomerulus

12. All of the following substances are filtered at the glomerulus except:

 A. platelets.
 B. proteins.
 C. glucose.
 D. sodium.

13. Reabsorption of most of the water, glucose, amino acids, sodium, and other nutrients occurs at the:

 A. loop of Henle.
 B. collecting duct.
 C. proximal convoluted tubule.
 D. distal convoluted tubule.

14. The high concentration of sodium in the medulla is maintained by the:

 A. proximal convoluted tubule.
 B. distal convoluted tubule.
 C. loop of Henle.
 D. collecting duct.

15. The movement of Cl^- out of the ascending limb of the loop of Henle occurs by:

 A. diffusion.
 B. active transport.
 C. osmosis.
 D. facilitated diffusion.

16. In the distal convoluted tubule:

 A. K^+ moves into the lumen.
 B. H^+ moves into the tubular cells.

C. Na$^+$ moves into the lumen.

D. Na$^+$ is actively extruded into the medulla.

17. Malfunction in which of the following systems might result in body fluid disturbances?

A. Heart

B. Skin

C. Lung

D. All of the above

ANSWERS AND EXPLANATIONS

1–17. **1-D, 2-C, 3-D, 4-B, 5-D, 6-C, 7-C, 8-D, 9-B, 10-A, 11-D, 12-A, 13-C, 14-C, 15-B, 16-A, 17-D.** See text for explanation.

Muscle System

Self-Managed Learning Questions

1. Describe the relationship of muscles with bones, ligaments, and tendons. Draw diagrams to illustrate anatomic and physiologic connections (e.g., skeletal muscle is attached to the bones and contracts voluntarily, allowing humans to walk, run, or move their hands to draw).

2. Draw a table showing the differences among smooth, skeletal, and cardiac muscle, highlighting the speed of contraction, striations or intercalated discs, shape and size of fibers, and number of nuclei per fiber.

3. Visit a laboratory or clinic to help you understand the physical working of a nerve box. (The sciatic nerve from the hind leg of a frog can be tested to measure the strength of the stimulus or stimulus artifact.) The nerve box consists of stimulation electrodes, recording electrodes, and several wires. Understand the use of the several dials and knobs on the box (e.g., frequency knob, voltage knob, and time duration knob).

Learn about nervous control of muscles. Compare and contrast characteristics of motor and sensory control. Distinguish between the control mechanisms for voluntary and involuntary muscles. Develop a detailed understanding of the sliding filament theory and mechanisms of muscular contractions (emphasize myosin binding mechanism in contractile process). Review the differences between isotonic and isometric contractions. Focus on the location, shape, and size of the 700 skeletal muscles, but do not memorize them.

FUNCTIONS

Muscles work in pairs (or in more complex arrangements). For a muscle that moves a joint in one direction, there is an **antagonistic muscle** that moves the joint in the opposite direction (i.e., undoes that motion). There are also **synergistic muscles** that aid in the motion caused by a given muscle. At the elbow, the triceps (extension) and biceps (flexion) are examples of antagonistic muscles (Figure 8-133). At the shoulder, the deltoid

Fig. 8-133. Attachments of a muscle. (Reproduced with permission from Bresnick SD: *Columbia Review Intensive Preparation for the MCAT.* Baltimore, Williams & Wilkins, 1996, p 446.)

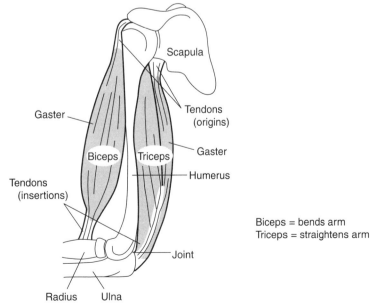

Biceps = bends arm
Triceps = straightens arm

(raises arm) and supraspinatous (raises arm) are examples of synergistic muscles. Complex neural pathways ensure coordination of the muscle groups. A **flexor** decreases the angle of a joint. An **extensor** increases the angle of a joint. An **abductor** moves a limb away from the midline. An **adductor** moves a limb toward the midline.

Muscle tone differs from tetanus in that groups of muscle fibers alternatingly contract and relax allowing form and position (at rest) to be maintained.

Skeletal muscle uses O_2 in aerobic metabolism when it is available. In the absence of O_2, the production of energy requires that there be a final electron acceptor. This electron acceptor becomes pyruvate, which is converted to lactate (Figure 8-134).

Fig. 8-134. Formation of lactate.

NADH could transfer an H:⁻ and H⁺ is picked up from solution.

The amount of lactate formed becomes a measure of the lack of O_2 (the usual electron acceptor). This is a partial measure of the **oxygen debt** that muscles incur during exercise when their rate of O_2 demand exceeds that supplied. After exercise, the lactate is converted back to pyruvate, and the electrons are passed to O_2 as O_2 is supplied to the muscles and the oxygen debt is repaid. In summary, during exercise, the energy metabolism of muscle switches from aerobic to anaerobic and an oxygen debt is incurred, which is repaid when the exercise ends.

The skeletal muscles act across joints to move body parts. Each muscle has an origin and an **insertion**. In general, the origin is stationary, and, when the muscle contracts, the insertion (and the bone it is attached to) moves toward the origin (see Figure 8-133). The functioning unit of the striated muscle is the **myofibril** (muscle fibers or cells are composed of myofibrils). Myofibrils are composed of linearly arranged sarcomeres.

During intense physical activity, oxidative metabolism cannot supply all the ATP that muscles require. As soon as intense muscular activity ceases, aerobic processes must provide ATP for the resynthesis of creatine phosphate. These aerobic activities account for the deep, rapid breathing that continues after muscular activity has ceased. The elevated rate of respiration provides the oxygen required to produce ATP for the resynthesis of creatine phosphate and to convert lactic acid back to glucose and glycogen.

When skeletal muscles are not used, the muscle fibers diminish in size. Regular exercise, on the other hand, can produce increases in muscle size, endurance, and strength. Endurance exercises, such as running, produce cardiovascular and pulmonary changes, causing the muscles to be better supplied with materials such as oxygen and carbohydrates. **Muscle cramps** are involuntary muscle contractions that are painful. Their precise cause is unknown—possibly a low oxygen supply causes them.

BASIC MUSCLE TYPES AND LOCATIONS

The three types of muscles are smooth, cardiac, and striated, or skeletal (Figure 8-135). The cytoplasm of all three muscle types is filled with contractile proteins.

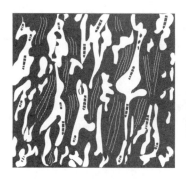
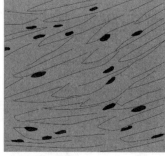
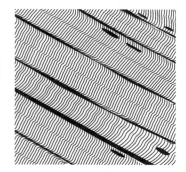

Cardiac muscle tissue   Smooth muscle tissue   Skeletal muscle tissue

Fig. 8-135. Three types of muscle tissue: cardiac, smooth, and skeletal.

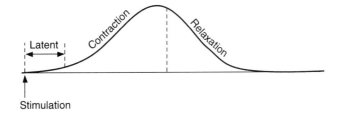

Fig. 8-136. Phases of muscle contraction.

Latent

Contraction

Relaxation

Stimulation

Smooth muscle is so named because its contractile protein is so organized that it lacks microscopic striations; smooth muscle is composed of distinct spindle-shaped, uninucleated cells. They are innervated by the autonomic nervous system and are largely involuntary, but not every muscle cell is innervated. Therefore, smooth muscle cells are interconnected by gap junctions that propagate a wave of contraction. They can contract slowly and maintain contractions for long periods of time. This feature is useful for their function in organs where they are found, including the gut (for peristalsis and churning of food), blood vessels (for regulation of blood pressure), and many ducts (e.g., the ureter for peristalsis).

Cardiac muscle is composed of uninucleated cells joined together by a saw-toothed array of junctional complexes (including extensive gap junctions) termed the **intercalated disc** to speed impulse conduction. Microscopically, cardiac muscle appears striated. The muscle fibers are highly branched, probably adding to their strength.

Skeletal muscle consists of multinucleated cells fused together to form a single cell called a **syncytium**. Skeletal muscle is distinctly striated microscopically. Skeletal muscles contract rapidly but tire easily. A simple twitch of a muscle involves the following steps: (1) impulse from a nerve stimulates the muscle, (2) a brief latent period lapses, (3) the phase of contraction begins, and (4) a phase of relaxation occurs (Figure 8-136). If the muscle is stimulated during the relaxation phase, it can be made to contract again. If these stimuli are in rapid succession, the contractions can be made to summate to a sustained contraction called **tetanus**.

NERVOUS CONTROL OF MUSCLES

Smooth muscle is under the control of the nervous system. Nervous tissue receives stimuli and transmits information, controlling the actions of muscle and glands. Nerve action potential causes muscles to contract at the neuromuscular junction. Depolarized skeletal muscle cells open their Na^+ channels, and their plasma membranes generate action potentials. Neurotransmitters from the motor neurons bind to receptors in the postsynaptic membrane. Ion channels for Na^+ and K^+ are hence opened. The postsynaptic membrane is then depolarized and transmitted to the muscle fiber, which contains voltage-controlled ion channels. This generates an action potential that is transmitted to several sites on the muscle tissue. There is a high Ca^{2+} concentration in the sarcoplasmic reticulum and a low Ca^{2+} concentration in the sarcoplasm.

Smooth muscle is involuntary and provides contractile forces for most internal organs. Skeletal muscles are voluntary and carry out all movements; they also generate the movement of breathing. Cardiac muscle is involuntary, and the contractions are generated from the muscle itself, not from the nervous system. Innervation is by the autonomic nervous system but beats are originated by specialized muscle cells. Skeletal muscles are innervated by the somatic nervous system and are voluntary. The control of voluntary movements originates in a portion of the cerebral cortex (surface of cerebrum) and is coordinated by impulses from the cerebellum.

APPLIED CONCEPTS

- Develop basic recognition of muscle twitch (slow and fast), tetanus, treppe, tic, and tremor.
- Understand the mechanisms associated with muscular dystrophy, cramps, and muscular atrophy.
- Acquaint yourself with electromyogram and the instruments used to obtain it. Learn the design and working of these instruments.
- Understand the glycogen-lactic acid system, smooth muscle contractions, and the role played by calmodulin. Understand the chemical process and reactions underlying glycogen-lactic acid systems.
- Visit a pathologist's or a coroner's laboratory or a hospital if possible to examine the stiffness of muscles of a corpse and how the time of death is related to stiffness.

Ask questions about ATP replenishment after animals or humans die and observe the myosin-actin bridges under a microscope.

- Review the assumptions, hypotheses, and experimental validity of the sliding filament theory by Huxley and Huxley. Why do actin and myosin filaments slide past each other as the muscle contracts? How much sliding force is exerted and is it true that the filaments can slide up to 10 nanometers?

MUSCLE SYSTEM: REVIEW QUESTIONS

1. All of the following are muscle proteins except:

   A. actin.
   B. myosin.
   C. fibrinogen.
   D. troponin.

2. One of the histology muscle types has striated fibers and is involuntary. It is:

   A. smooth muscle.
   B. skeletal muscle.
   C. cardiac muscle.
   D. none of the above.

3. Intercalated discs are found in which type of muscle?

   A. Skeletal
   B. Cardiac
   C. Smooth
   D. All types

4. Which type of muscle is a syncytium?

   A. Skeletal
   B. Cardiac
   C. Smooth
   D. All types

5. All are true concerning smooth muscle except they:

   A. are composed of distinct spindle cells.
   B. are largely involuntary.
   C. have intercalated discs.
   D. are found in the gut.

6. All are true concerning cardiac muscle except:

   A. it is a syncytium.
   B. it is striated.
   C. it is involuntary.
   D. gap junctions speed conduction.

7. All are true concerning skeletal muscles except:

   A. they are a syncytium.
   B. they are involuntary.
   C. they are responsible for locomotion.
   D. they contract rapidly but tire readily.

8. Select the incorrect statement concerning muscles.

   A. Ligaments attach bone to bone.
   B. Flexors decrease the angle at a joint.
   C. Adductors move a limb away from the midline.
   D. Tendons attach muscle to bone.

9. Muscle tone depends on:

   A. continual low-level contraction of all fibers in the muscles.
   B. summation of twitches to a plateau.
   C. presence of short fibers that constantly appear contracted.
   D. alternating contractions of different fiber groups in a muscle.

10. During exercise:

   A. muscles depend on the Krebs cycle for energy.
   B. O_2 becomes the electron acceptor.
   C. lactate levels decrease.
   D. energy metabolism changes from aerobic to anaerobic.

11. The phase of contraction of a muscle occurs when:

   A. tropomyosin binds and releases actin.
   B. myosin alternately binds and releases actin.
   C. actin alternately binds and releases myosin.
   D. none of the above biochemical reactions occur.

ANSWERS AND EXPLANATION

1–11. **1-C, 2-C, 3-B, 4-A, 5-C, 6-A, 7-B, 8-C, 9-D, 10-D, 11-B.** See text for explanation.

Skeletal System

Self-Managed Learning Questions

1. Visit a zoological laboratory or museum and observe different types of bones (such as dinosaur bones). Construct a table listing the shape, size, color, and any other special characteristics, such as density, special lines or bumps, or holes. Compare these bones to the exoskeleton of insects and how cuticles and joints are arranged.
2. Visit a seafood restaurant or a seafood market and observe skeletons and bones of crabs, lobsters, fish, and clams. Analyze and read about the chemical structure of the exoskeleton and what elements and compounds are common among several classes of organisms.
3. Learn about the tensile strength, compressive strength, and other elastic properties of compact bones, eggshells, human teeth, and fingernails. (The tensile strength of human hair is 20×10^7 N/m^2 and the compressive strength of dentin in teeth is 18×10^7 N/m^2. Review the structure of hydroxyapatite crystals and how they bind collagen fibers. What crystal size and type do hydroxyapatite salts form?

FUNCTIONS

Review the skeletal system with focus on the axial skeleton, appendicular skeleton, and articulations (arthrology is a medical specialty). Understand the six types of synovial joints (ball-and-socket, ellipsoidal, gliding, hinged, pivot, and saddle).

BONE STRUCTURE

Bones in the human are of two types: flat and long. **Flat bones** include the skull bones, ribs, and vertebrae and contain red marrow (for blood cell production). They are found where little movement is required, and they perform protective functions in general. **Long bones** (Figure 8-137) include the bones of the hands, feet, arms, and legs, contain yellow marrow, and are involved primarily in locomotion and motion.

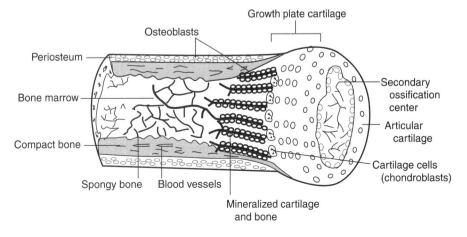

Fig. 8-137. Long bone.

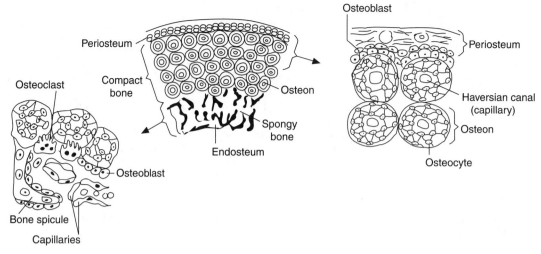

Fig. 8-138. Bone cross section.

When bone (Figure 8-138) is laid down, it may be spongy or compact. **Spongy bone** is porous like a sponge with the bone present as spicules and the spaces filled with either red or yellow bone marrow. **Compact bone** is densely packed but richly vascularized. It is very strong and found where great strength is required, such as in the cortex of long bones.

Bone is composed of a crystal part (65% hydroxyapatite, which is a complex of Ca^{++} and PO_4^- as well as Na^+, K, Mg^{2+}, and other anions) and an organic part (35% type I collagen and other noncollagenous proteins and growth factors). Collagen molecules are arranged end-to-end and are quarter staggered side-to-side to form a collagen fibril. Collagen fibrils are coated with noncollagenous proteins that aid in the alignment and deposition of the hydroxyapatite crystals along the collagen.

Cartilage cells construct a mineralized **cartilage matrix** scaffolding, then die. The scaffolding is partially removed by multinucleated cells, or **osteoclasts**. Bone-forming cells **(osteoblasts)**, accompanied by capillaries, invade the remainder of the mineralized scaffolding and begin to secrete bone. Some osteoblasts become **osteocytes** (bone maintenance cells). During the process of bone formation, osteocytes become totally surrounded by secreted bone matrix. Osteoblasts and osteocytes are tethered together through gap junctions that form between their numerous cell processes. Compact bones are made of smaller units called **osteons**, which have central microscopic channels called **Haversian canals** (Figure 8-139).

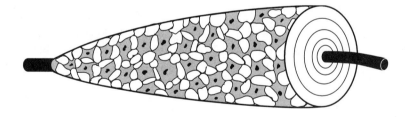

Fig. 8-139. Osteon.

Osteon

SKELETAL STRUCTURE

Bone can be formed directly within primitive connective tissue (intramembranous bones such as skull bones) or can be formed from a cartilaginous model (endochondral bone formation, such as long bones). The basic functional unit in mature bone is the osteon (Haversian system) found in both compact bone and bony spicules. Periodically, old osteons are replaced by new bone (bone turnover) throughout the lifetime of the human. Osteoclasts destroy old bone and osteoblasts replace old bone with new. Approximately 5%–10% of compact bone is replaced yearly.

A **joint** is where two ore more bones come together. The human skeleton has a wide variety of joints allowing a range of different movements. The contacting and mobile surfaces between bones are covered by cartilage. Joints are enclosed in joint capsules full

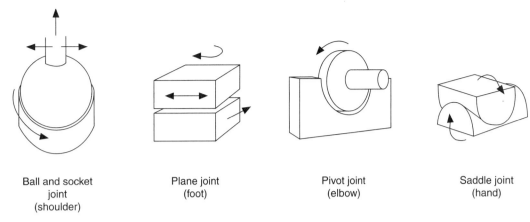

Ball and socket
joint
(shoulder)

Plane joint
(foot)

Pivot joint
(elbow)

Saddle joint
(hand)

Fig. 8-140. Types of joints.

of a lubricant called **synovial fluid**. Types of joints include the knee joint, which is a **hinge**; shoulder and hip joints, which are **ball-and-socket** joints; and the elbow, which is a **pivotal** joint (Figure 8-140).

CARTILAGE STRUCTURE AND FUNCTION

Ligaments help hold bones together at the joint; that is, they are attached bone to bone. **Tendons** connect muscles to bones; they also help hold bones together at joints.

Parathyroid hormone (PTH) causes Ca^{2+} (and phosphate) to be removed from the bony matrix, causing demineralization of bone. The Ca^{2+} appears in the serum. The bone matrix serves as a storage depot for many cations (Ca^{2+}, K^+, Mg^{2+}, Na^+) and serves to buffer (help control the levels of) these in the blood (as well as being an H^+ buffer). PTH is stimulated by low serum calcium. **Calcitonin** is secreted from special cells in the thyroid gland. It is stimulated by high serum calcium and causes Ca^{2+}, among other cations, to be deposited in bone. Figure 8-141 is a schematized drawing of some of the bones of the human body.

APPLIED CONCEPTS

- Understand the mechanisms behind athletic injuries, such as pulled hamstring, runner's knee, shin splint syndrome, and Achilles tendonitis.
- Understand the organic structure of polyactic acid (plastic) used for artificial ligaments.
- Differentiate among gomphosis, symphysis, synchondrosis, and syndesmosis in joints.
- Understand the nature of the following skeletal disorders and medical procedures: bone scintigraphy, hypertrophic osteoarthropathy, osteoporosis, spondylitis, collagen disease, bone fracture types (e.g., closed, open, greenstick), rheumatoid arthritis, Paget's disease, and piezoelectric effect in bone caused by mechanical and physical stress.
- Understand the laboratory methods to produce hydroxyapatite crystals (Ca_{10} $(PO_4)_6$ $(OH)_2$) and how the fluoride ion can change it to fluroapatitel.
- Visit a clinical or biotechnology laboratory to understand how bone research and surgical experiments are done for bone replacements and to produce new bone-like materials. Review and understand the working of equipment and procedures used in bone technology research.
- Review the physiology of bones under zero gravity conditions that lead to increased fluidity or thinning of bones. What chemical and physical factors control the bone density change?

SKELETAL SYSTEM: REVIEW QUESTIONS

1. All bone is formed:
   - A. from a cartilage model.
   - B. without a cartilage model.
   - C. within 1 to 2 hours.
   - D. without the use of osteoblasts.

2. Parathyroid hormone:
   - A. helps in demineralization of bone.
   - B. helps in mineralization of bone.

Problem Solving in the Biological Sciences   535

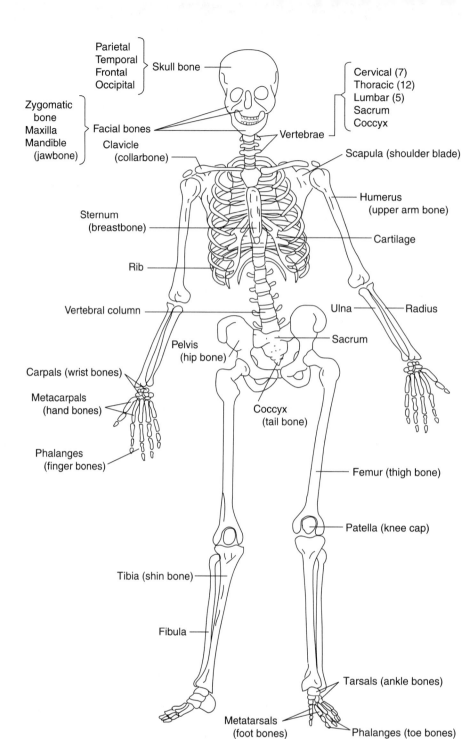

Fig. 8-141. Human skeleton.

Parietal
Temporal
Frontal
Occipital } Skull bone

Cervical (7)
Thoracic (12)
Lumbar (5)
Sacrum
Coccyx

Zygomatic
bone
Maxilla
Mandible
(jawbone) } Facial bones

Clavicle
(collarbone)

Vertebrae

Scapula (shoulder blade)

Humerus
(upper arm bone)

Sternum
(breastbone)

Cartilage

Rib

Vertebral column

Ulna — Radius

Sacrum

Pelvis
(hip bone)

Carpals (wrist bones)

Metacarpals
(hand bones)

Coccyx
(tail bone)

Phalanges
(finger bones)

Femur (thigh bone)

Patella (knee cap)

Tibia (shin bone)

Fibula

Tarsals (ankle bones)

Metatarsals
(foot bones)

Phalanges (toe bones)

C. increases basal metabolic rate.
D. leads to Graves' disease when in excess.

3. Which cell makes bone?

A. Osteoblast
B. Osteocyte
C. Osteoclast
D. All of the above

4. Haversian canals are:

A. markings seen on Mars.
B. nutrient systems of bone.
C. found in the inner ear.
D. communication between the left and right cerebral hemispheres.

5. Components of a mature Haversian canal system would include all except:

   A. osteoblasts.
   B. lacunae.
   C. canaliculi.
   D. blood vessels.

6. Components of the human axial skeleton include all except the:

   A. sternum.
   B. vertebral column.
   C. hips.
   D. skull.

7. Components of the appendicular human skeleton include all the following except the:

   A. shoulder girdle.
   B. arm bones.
   C. ribs.
   D. leg bones.

8. The humerus, radius, and ulna are found in the:

   A. vertebral column.
   B. shoulder girdle.
   C. arm.
   D. leg.

9. All the following are parts of the vertebral column except the:

   A. cervical spine
   B. thoracic spine
   C. caudal spine
   D. lumbar spine

10. The parietal and occipital bones are found in the:

    A. vertebral column.
    B. skull.
    C. hip girdle.
    D. foot.

11. The bones of the wrist are called:

    A. carpals.
    B. metacarpals.
    C. tarsals.
    D. metatarsals.

12. The hip bone connects the _____ to the _____.

    A. femur; sternum
    B. humerus; sacrum
    C. femur; sacrum
    D. humerus; sternum

13. Phalanges are found in the:

    A. fingers.
    B. toes.
    C. fingers and toes.
    D. Nissl bodies inside a neuron.

14. Bone is composed of _____ and _____.

    A. calcium; phosphate
    B. globular proteins; ions
    C. collagen; hydroxyapatite
    D. enzymes; calcium

15. _____ serves as the focus of the deposition of the crystal matrix.

    A. Collagen
    B. Osteocyte
    C. Hydroxyapatite
    D. Cartilage

16. The hormone that mobilizes Ca^{2+} from bone is:

    A. thyroxine.
    B. parathyroid hormone.
    C. calcitonin.
    D. vitamin D

ANSWERS AND EXPLANATIONS

1 – 16. 1-C, 2-A, 3-A, 4-B, 5-A, 6-C, 7-C, 8-C, 9-C, 10-B, 11-A, 12-C, 13-C, 14-C, 15-A, 16-B. See text for explanation.

Respiratory and Skin Systems

Self-Managed Learning Questions

1. Using the different shapes and sizes of rubber balloons, try to inflate them with air and release air by pinching the neck or opening of each balloon. Construct a clear model highlighting differences between the rubber balloon wall and the actual lung tissue. Understand the concept of dead space or volume and how the elasticity of the wall is related to the pressure in the balloon. Review assumptions and faults in the model of a balloon representing human lungs.

2. Explain to a study partner or another student how gas laws such as Boyle's law, Charles' law, and the real gas equation apply to inhaling and exhaling air from the lungs. Understand the limitations of each law and the approximations needed.

3. Determine your tidal volume, expiratory and inspiratory reserve volume, and vital capacity using a spirometer. Obtain data on three students or friends with different body weights and ages and analyze the observations.

4. Carefully examine the different parts of a spirometer and the pneumograph equipment and determine what errors can arise if they are used incorrectly.

5. Analyze breathing mechanisms underwater and in space. Understand the physical principles controlling decompression sickness (divers and pilots experience this sickness) or nitrogen bubbles.

RESPIRATORY SYSTEM

The respiratory and skin systems are both subjected to external environmental factors. Pollution and ozone layer depletion lead to various breathing and skin problems. The health sections of newspapers and magazines are good sources for new techniques and problems as they are discovered. Students should review racing, running, and other exercises that affect ventilation of lungs and sweating. Students should also review the mechanisms controlling inspiration and expiration and the protective actions of the skin. Memorize the basic volumes and capacities shown in spirograms (total lung capacity is approximately 5000 ml and anatomic dead space is approximately 100 ml). Review the design construction and working of a spirometer and a bronchoscope.

Function

The respiratory system moves air in and out of the lungs (highest O_2 and lowest CO_2 tension) and allows diffusion of gases in and out of the body. Oxygen moves into the blood (lower O_2 tension and highest CO_2 tension) where it is taken up and used. In the tissues, CO_2 is produced by oxidation of nutrients. The CO_2 then diffuses into the blood where it dissolves in the serum, is converted to carbonic acid ($CO_2 + H_2O \rightarrow H_2CO_3$) and then to bicarbonate (HCO_3^-), or combines with hemoglobin. Next, it circulates to the lungs where the stated reactions are reversed and the CO_2 is expired. In all cases, the gases go from higher tensions (pressures) to lower tensions. By regulating the amount of carbonic acid and bicarbonate in the serum, the lungs are important in the regulation of acid-base balance in the body.

Tracking Air Flow Through the Respiratory System

Functions of lungs are summarized as (1) **gas exchange**, (2) **thermoregulation**, and (3) **protection** against disease and particulate matter. In humans, air enters through the mouth or nose where it is cleaned, warmed, and moistened. It then passes down the trachea to two main bronchi, then to bronchioles, and then to alveoli (Figures 8-142 and

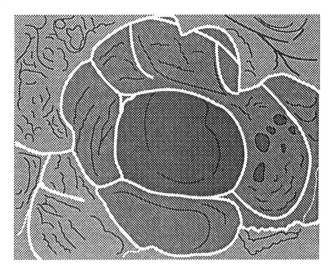

Fig. 8-142. A cluster of alveoli viewed through the smallest respiratory duct, the terminal portion of a bronchiole.

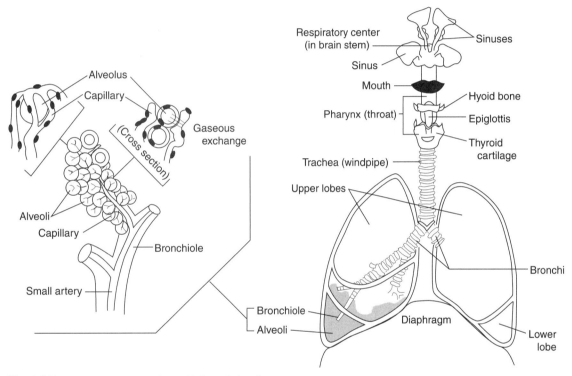

Fig. 8-143. Respiratory system; bronchiole and alveoli.

8-143). Gas exchange occurs in the alveoli. Incomplete cartilage rings hold the trachea, bronchi, and bronchioles open. Mucus (secreted by mucous cells) traps ingested particles, which are then moved out of the respiratory tract by ciliary action (ciliated epithelial cells) of the lining cells (respiratory epithelium). This epithelium is classified as pseudostratified ciliated columnar epithelium and has basic features of epithelium (i.e., it is avascular with basal lamina and junctional complexes to maintain the sheet of cells). Connective tissue beneath the basal lamina supplies the cells through its microvascular supply (Figure 8-144). **Coughing** is a reflex action mediated by the medulla (glossopharyngeal and vagus nerves). The reflex is initiated by a stimulation (e.g., by particles) of the tracheobronchial tree, followed by expulsion of these particles and mucus as sputum (or phlegm). **Sneezing** is a reflex mediated by the medulla also, but the initial stimulation is in the nose, followed by forceful expulsion of the irritating substance and naso-oral secretions.

Effects of Smoking

Tobacco smoke consists of gases such as CO_2 and tiny unburned carbon particles. These substances harm the cilia and mucous membranes that line the breathing passages. Many

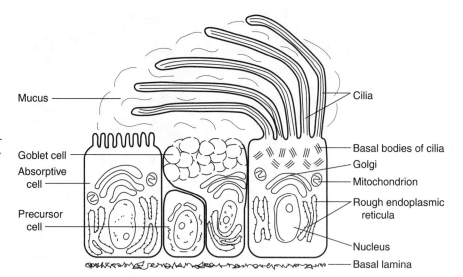

Fig. 8-144. Respiratory epithelium (specialized eukaryotic cells).

Mucus

Goblet cell

Absorptive cell

Precursor cell

Cilia

Basal bodies of cilia

Golgi

Mitochondrion

Rough endoplasmic reticula

Nucleus

Basal lamina

smokers cough frequently. The cough is the effort of the body to clear the breathing passages. Healthy cilia and mucous membranes accomplish the cleaning process automatically. Smoke also damages the lungs. Long-term smoking can cause the walls of the alveoli to rupture, or break. As a result, the surface area for gas exchange decreases considerably. This condition, called **emphysema**, interferes with oxygen intake.

Breathing Structures and Mechanisms

Inspiration is accomplished by the contraction of the **diaphragm** (via impulses from the phrenic nerve), which moves downward or by action of certain rib muscles that lift up the rib cage. These mechanisms create a negative pressure inside the chest cavity, which causes the lungs to expand and pull in air. Expiration is a passive process caused by the elastic recoil of the chest wall and lung tissue itself. Respiration is largely involuntary, but some voluntary control is possible over the rate and depth of respiration. The control center of respiration is in the medulla of the brainstem. It causes an increase in the rate of respiration when there is a decrease in pH (e.g., more acidic), an increase in CO_2 tension (which causes a drop in pH), or a decrease in oxygen tension in the blood. Also, impulses from the cerebrum can affect ventilatory rate, such as occurs with anxiety, causing the rate to increase.

A key substance for the function of lungs is **surfactant** (dipalmitoyllecithin—a phospholipid). This substance coats the alveoli and creates a variable surface tension in them. As the alveoli get smaller, the surfactant decreases the surface tension. This prevents the alveoli from collapsing during expiration, because high surface tension would cause alveoli to collapse. In the absence of surfactant, collapsed alveoli require fairly high inspiratory forces to re-expand them. This is what happens in respiratory distress syndrome of the newborn in whom there is an absence of surfactant. The infant is not strong enough to re-expand the collapsed alveoli.

SKIN SYSTEM

Function

Functions of the skin system include (1) protection from physical agents (e.g., wind and water)—afforded by the stratum corneum and melanocytes (protection from radiation), (2) protection from microbial agents, especially bacteria—afforded by the stratum corneum and some secretions of the sebaceous glands, (3) thermoregulation, (4) waste removal (e.g., excess water, salts, and urea)—via the sweat glands, (5) first activation of vitamin D—by ultraviolet light, and (6) providing sensation—by the many nerve endings.

Homeostasis occurs when the systems of the body keep the internal environment of the body at a steady state. **Osmoregulation** is the regulation of the chemical composition of the body fluids. The skin functions to some extent in helping to maintain homeostasis. The skin, lungs, and digestive systems maintain a part of fluid balance and help in eliminating wastes. Blood is filtered nonselectively and then glucose and amino acids are reabsorbed into the blood by the kidneys. Marine vertebrates usually retain water and excrete salt by the action of specialized cells in their gills. Aquatic vertebrates have problems of osmoregulation.

Thermoregulation is the regulation of the internal body temperature between the narrow limits necessary for life. Too high or low a temperature can cause proteins (enzymes especially) to become less effective or totally inactive (denatured) and cause the protoplasm to gel (become more solid).

Normally, the body temperature is a balance between heat produced by metabolism and heat loss by various means. Processes that increase body metabolism increase body heat, especially with muscle activity (e.g., shivering). Regulation of body temperature is centered in the hypothalamus (in the brain).

Pyrogens released during bacterial infections, among other causes, can affect the hypothalamus in a way that allows the body temperature to elevate higher than normal, and fever results.

The mechanisms of heat conservation include those that are always present and those elicited in emergencies (* = most important):

1. Mechanisms always present:
   - Subcutaneous fat as insulation*
   - Presence of hair or fur (lower animals)
2. Mechanisms called upon as needed:
   - Shivering—contractions of muscles produce heat*
   - Constriction of vessels to skin—prevents heat loss from surface*
   - Piloerection of hair on skin—traps air against skin; serves as an insulation
   - Increased metabolic rate

The mechanisms of heat loss include those that are always present and those elicited in emergencies (* = most important):

1. Mechanisms always present:
   - Loss of heat by radiational cooling
   - Low level of evaporation of moisture from skin—for a liquid to evaporate, heat must be supplied; this heat comes from the skin, which is cooled
2. Mechanisms called upon as needed:
   - Sweating and consequent evaporation of water—the sweat itself removes heat from the body and more is lost when this evaporates*
   - Dilation of vessels to the skin—increases the amount of radiational cooling*

The skin helps provide physical protection to the internal body. It protects the body from the bombardment of organisms that cause disease, from the physical environment (e.g., weather), and it helps prevent excessive loss of water.

Structure

The skin is made of specialized eukaryotic cells and tissues. Layers of skin are epidermis, dermis, and subcutaneous tissue. The **epidermis** (stratified squamous epithelium and lamina propria) is a layer comprised of several types of related cells and melanocytes (Figure 8-145). The deepest layer of the epidermis, the basal layer, contains dividing cells. The broad middle layer of cells is termed the **spinous layer** and is joined together

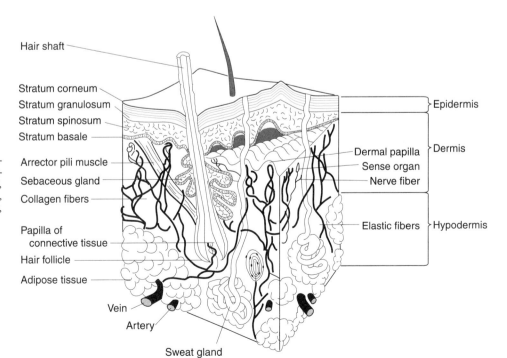

Fig. 8-145. Human skin and epidermis. (Reproduced with permission from Ville CA, Solomon EP, Davis PW: *Biology*. Philadelphia, Saunders College Publishing, 1985, p 662.)

at multiple foci by the junctional complex, the desmosome. As these cells move toward the surface, they lose their nuclei and produce a protein called **keratin** (which is stable and water insoluble). At the surface, these cells have no nuclei, are dead, are essentially keratin, and are called **stratum corneum**, which is the scaly dry surface layer of the skin. **Melanocytes**, dendritic cells found among the basal cell layer, synthesize melanin (a black to dark-brown pigment), which is responsible for the color of the skin. It also responds to ultraviolet light to produce tanning of the skin. As in all epithelia, a basal lamina attaches the epithelium to all underlying connective tissue.

The **dermis** is internal to the epidermis and contains most of the accessory structures of the skin. Blood vessels end in the dermis. Sensory endings for pain, temperature, and touch are found here and in the subcutaneous tissue. Sweat glands, hair follicles, and sebaceous glands (which secrete an oily fat substance, and, if clogged, cause acne) originate here. All of these exit at the epidermis. General connective tissue cells, fibroblasts, and macrophages, among other cells, may be found in the dermis. The **subcutaneous tissue** contains primarily fat cells.

APPLIED CONCEPTS

- Understand the biochemical structure and growth rate of fibrin; understand the biochemical structure of burns (first, second, and third degree), acne, sunburns, and skin cancer.
- Identify the biological mechanics of healing (where the edges of cut skin wounds are drawn together) and basic skin grafting techniques.
- Distinguish terminology that sounds alike and is related to the same medical term: pleura (visceral and parietal), pleural cavity, pleural fluid (composition, density, pH), intrapleural pressure, and pleurisy.
- Understand mechanisms responsible for volume changes in the thoracic cavity. Identify changes in physical and chemical properties of gases (O_2, CO_2) in liquids (volumes, partial pressures, temperature, and arterial pH related to binding with hemoglobin). Review the transport and diffusion processes of gas molecules in liquids.
- Understand basic cardiopulmonary resuscitation (CPR) techniques with emphasis on A, B, C (airway, breathing, and circulation).
- Understand what a spirogram is used for and how to read it (Figure 8-146).

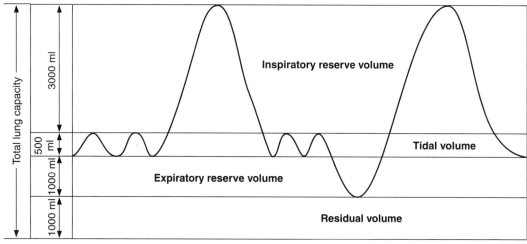

Fig. 8-146. Typical spirogram.

- Recognize the Bohr effect on hemoglobin structure, the Haldane effect, and diphosphoglycerate concentration in hemoglobin.
- Recognize respiratory disorders such as hypoxia, carbon monoxide poisoning, cyanosis, bronchial asthma, bronchitis, tuberculosis, pneumonia, emphysema, common cold, hyperventilation, hypercapnia, hypoventilation, and hypocapnia.

RESPIRATORY AND SKIN SYSTEMS: REVIEW QUESTIONS

1. The path of air into the lungs of humans is:

    A. alveoli, trachea, bronchi, bronchioles
    B. trachea, bronchi, bronchioles, alveoli
    C. bronchi, bronchioles, trachea, alveoli
    D. trachea, bronchioles, bronchi, alveoli

2. Expiration of air from the lungs:

   A. is a passive process.
   B. causes negative pressure in the chest cavity.
   C. requires contraction of the diaphragm.
   D. is an active process.

3. During inspiration of air into the lungs:

   A. the chest cavity has a positive pressure.
   B. the diaphragm moves upward.
   C. the diaphragm contracts.
   D. the rib cage moves down.

4. Which of the following structures is used to prevent the bronchi from collapsing?

   A. Cartilage rings
   B. Bony rings
   C. Fibrous tissue
   D. None of the above

5. Surfactant:

   A. is dipalmitoyllecithin.
   B. decreases surface tension.
   C. deficiency may result in respiratory distress syndrome.
   D. is all of the above.

6. Which reflex moves secretions out of the tracheobronchial tree?

   A. Cough
   B. Sneeze
   C. Baroceptor
   D. pH

7. The control center of respiration is in the:

   A. cerebrum.
   B. cerebellum.
   C. medulla.
   D. thalamus.

8. All of the following may cause an increase in respiratory rate except:

   A. increased hydrogen ion concentration.
   B. increased CO_2 tension.
   C. increased O_2 tension.
   D. anxiety.

9. CO_2 may be present in all of the following forms except:

   A. dissolved in the blood.
   B. bound to hemoglobin.
   C. as dimers.
   D. as bicarbonate.

10. The type of epithelium found lining the trachea is:

    A. pseudostratified ciliated columnar.
    B. stratified squamous.
    C. simple cuboidal.
    D. simple squamous.

11. Layers of the skin include all the following except:

    A. epidermis.
    B. dermis.
    C. lamina propria.
    D. subcutaneous tissue.

12. Dead cells are found in the:

    A. subcutaneous tissue.
    B. dermis.

C. epidermis.
D. carbuncle.

13. Melanocytes are found in the:

    A. dermis.
    B. epidermis.
    C. subcutaneous tissue.
    D. endoderm.

14. The dermis usually contains all of the following except:

    A. hair follicles.
    B. sweat glands.
    C. fat cells.
    D. fibroblasts.

15. All are functions of the skin except:

    A. exchange of gases.
    B. thermoregulation.
    C. activation site of vitamin D.
    D. protection from bacteria.

16. The main effect of extremes of temperature is on the functions of:

    A. carbohydrates.
    B. phospholipids.
    C. proteins.
    D. nucleic acids.

17. Control of body temperature is localized in the:

    A. skin.
    B. heart.
    C. cerebrum.
    D. hypothalamus.

18. Select the mechanism that is not used to conserve heat.

    A. Shivering
    B. Dilation of blood vessels
    C. Piloerection
    D. Subcutaneous fat

19. Select the mechanism that is not used to lose heat.

    A. Sweating
    B. Increase in metabolic rate
    C. Radiational cooling
    D. Dilation of blood vessels

ANSWERS AND EXPLANATIONS

1–19. 1-B, 2-A, 3-C, 4-A, 5-D, 6-A, 7-C, 8-C, 9-C, 10-A, 11-C, 12-C, 13-B, 14-C, 15-A, 16-C, 17-D, 18-B, 19-B. See text for explanation.

Hydrocarbons

SATURATED (ALKANES)

The basic ideas of nomenclature for **alkanes** are also applicable to more complex molecules. Alkanes are simple because they contain only carbon and hydrogen (they are also called hydrocarbons) and contain no aromatic rings. The longest straight carbon chain is determined and is named, depending on the number of carbons:

C_1-methane, C_2-ethane, C_3-propane, C_4-butane, C_5-pentane, C_6-hexane, C_7-heptane, C_8-octane, C_9-nonane, C_{10}-decane.

In naming hydrocarbon side chains, the suffix *-yl* is added: CH_3- = methyl, CH_3CH_2- = ethyl, $CH_3CH_2CH_2-$ = propyl, and so on.

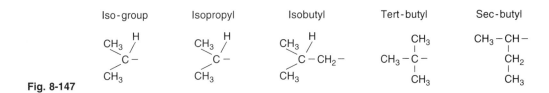

Fig. 8-147

There are special names for some branched chain alkanes as shown in Figure 8-147. Once the longest carbon chain is determined, the groups attached to it are numbered so that the lowest set of numbers is obtained. The side groups are placed in the molecule name in alphabetic order or in order of increasing size. The prefixes *di-* (two), *tri-* (three), *tetra-* (four), and so on, are used when a particular group is present more than once. The suffix indicating alkanes is *-ane* (Figure 8-148).

Fig. 8-148. 2,5,5,6-Tetramethyl-4-ethyl-6-isopropyl octane, or 2,5,5,6,7-pentamethyl-4,6-diethyl octane.

$$CH_3-CH_2-C \overset{\displaystyle CH_3}{\underset{\displaystyle \underset{CH_3\ \ CH_3}{C-H}}{|}} \ \ C \overset{\displaystyle CH_3}{\underset{\displaystyle CH_3}{|}} \ \ C \overset{\displaystyle \overset{CH_3}{|}}{\underset{\displaystyle \underset{H}{|}}{CH_2-CH-CH_3}} -CH_2-CH_3$$

Alkanes may be open chains or rings. (If there are no rings, the group is C_nH_{2n+2}; two hydrogens are lost for each ring.) The rings are named for the number of carbons that make them up (Figure 8-149).

Cyclopropane   Ethylcyclopropane   *cis*-1-Methyl-2-ethyl cyclopropane

Cyclobutane   Cyclopentane   Cyclohexane

Fig. 8-149

The main chemical features are the lack of functional groupings (e.g., ^-OH, Br) and full saturation (no double or triple bonds). These factors cause alkanes to be generally less reactive than most organic compounds with functional groups. The presence of branching and of strained ring structures leads to increased reactivity.

Physical properties of alkanes are fairly straightforward. Because they are nonpolar and have weak intermolecular forces, they have low boiling points and are not soluble in water. Branching leads to a lowering of both boiling points and melting points. This is true for other classes of compounds as well. With increasing molecular weights, the intermolecular forces increase and the boiling point increases. Melting points increase as molecular weights increase. Solubility is in nonpolar solvents and not in aqueous solvents. **Cyclopropane** is an anesthetic used in surgical procedures. Because of its low solubility in blood and its rapid elimination from the body, patients recover quickly.

Important Reactions

The main reactions of alkanes are combustion and substitution (radical) reactions:

1. **Combustion** reaction is as follows:

$$C_nH_{2n+2} + O_2 \text{ (excess)} \xrightarrow{\text{Flame}} nCO_2 + (n+1)H_2O$$

Problem Solving in the Biological Sciences 545

2. **Free radical substitution** reaction is as follows:

$$CH_3CH_3 + X_2 \xrightarrow{\text{hv or } \Delta} CH_3CH_2\,X + HX$$

$$X_2 = Cl_2 \text{ or } Br_2$$

They also get multiple substitutions.

$$CH_4 + Cl_2 \rightarrow CH_3Cl + HCl\uparrow \rightarrow CH_2Cl_2 + HCl\uparrow$$

$$\rightarrow CHCl_3 + HCl\uparrow \rightarrow CCl_4 + HCl\uparrow$$

In **initiation**, radicals are produced by homolytic bond cleavage of the halogen by the action of heat or light. Fluorine is too reactive and iodine is too unreactive to be of practical value in the laboratory without special conditions.

$$X_2 \longrightarrow 2X\cdot$$

Propagation is the generation of radicals by radicals. The following process constitutes a chain reaction that results when one intermediate reacts with a molecule to produce a new radical that can react further, allowing the process to repeat itself.

$$X\cdot + CH_3CH_3 \rightarrow HX + CH_3CH_2\cdot$$

$$CH_3CH_2\cdot + X2 \rightarrow CH_3CH_2X + X\cdot$$

Termination is the reaction of a radical with a radical to produce a stable molecule, as follows.

$$X\cdot + X\cdot \rightarrow X2$$

$$CH_3CH_2\cdot + X\cdot \rightarrow CH_3CH_2X$$

$$2CH_3CH_2\cdot \rightarrow CH_3CH_2CH_2CH_3$$

General Principles

The stability of free radicals depends on the presence of substituents that can delocalize the free electron. Alkyl groups act to stabilize a radical. Benzene rings and allylic double bonds readily delocalize electrons and are thus very effective (Figure 8-150).

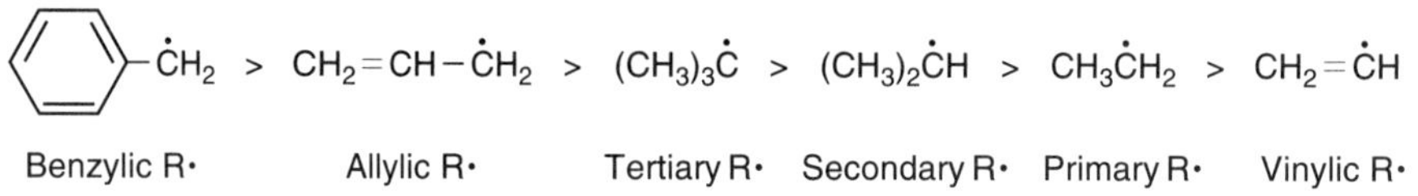

Fig. 8-150   Benzylic R·   Allylic R·   Tertiary R·   Secondary R·   Primary R·   Vinylic R·

Free radical-induced polymerizations of olefins are chain reactions. A source of radicals initiates the process in which one radical adds to the double bond of a molecule, producing a new radical that can add again, resulting in long chain polymeric molecules (Figure 8-151).

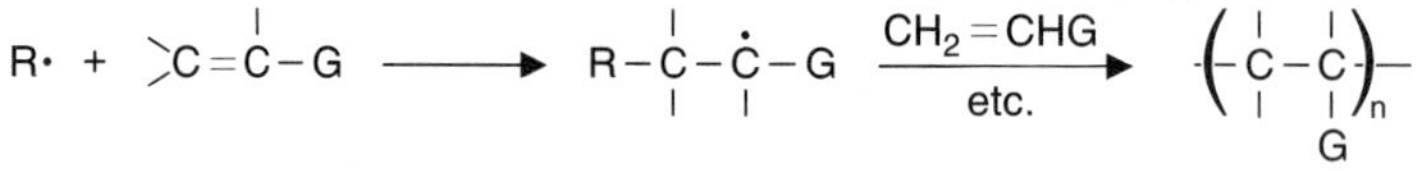

Fig. 8-151

Radicals result from homolytic cleavage of chemical bonds: $X - Y \rightarrow X\cdot + Y\cdot$

Each species is neutral (if begun neutral), and each has a free unpaired electron. Because of the free unpaired electron, radicals are paramagnetic. Most radicals are unstable and react rapidly.

The smaller the number of carbons in a ring, the less stable the ring is because of the ring strain of the bonding orbitals. The usual angle between bonds is 109.5° in the sp3 hybridized carbon. Expected bond angles in ring compounds are shown in Figure 8-152.

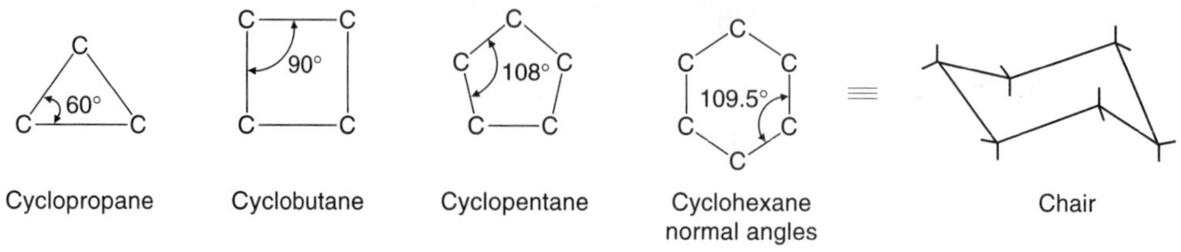

Fig. 8-152. Bond angles in ring compounds.

Cyclopropane   Cyclobutane   Cyclopentane   Cyclohexane normal angles   Chair

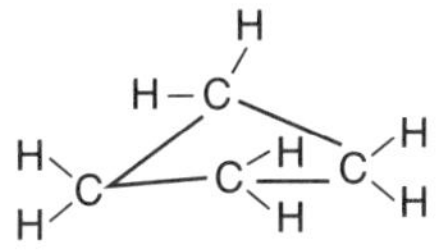

Fig. 8-153. Cyclobutane.

The ring strain is very high in cyclopropane. This makes cyclopropane as reactive with H2, Br2 as alkenes are. Cyclobutane relieves some of the ring strain by assuming a bent conformation (Figure 8-153).

Cyclopentane is puckered to relieve the strain (Figure 8-154). Cyclohexane has no strain in the chair form. Cyclobutane is fairly reactive, but cyclopentane and cyclohexane are not.

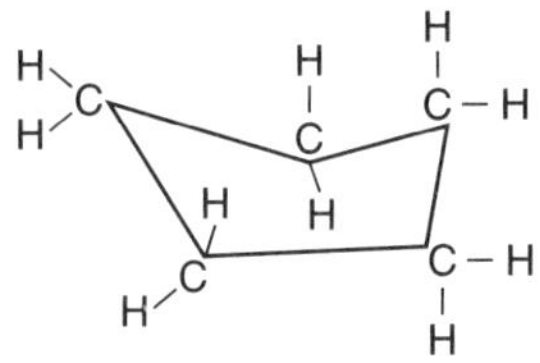

Fig. 8-154. Cyclopentane.

Planar and Nonplanar Conformations

Molecules may exist in different spatial arrangements called **conformations**, which result from rotation about a carbon–carbon single bond. The various conformations of molecules may be represented by projection drawings known as **Newman projections**, or wedge-and-dash drawings. In a Newman projection, a person sights down a carbon–carbon bond and a point represents the front carbon and an open circle represents the back carbon. In the wedge and dash projection, a wedge indicates a bond coming from the plane toward the viewer. A normal line represents a bond in the plane and a dash represents a bond away from the viewer.

The staggered conformation of ethane is approximately 3.0 kcal/mol more stable than the eclipsed conformation in which the torsional angle between adjacent substituents is 0°. The barrier to rotation in ethane (due to electron pair repulsions when the bonds are eclipsed) is called torsional strain (Figure 8-155).

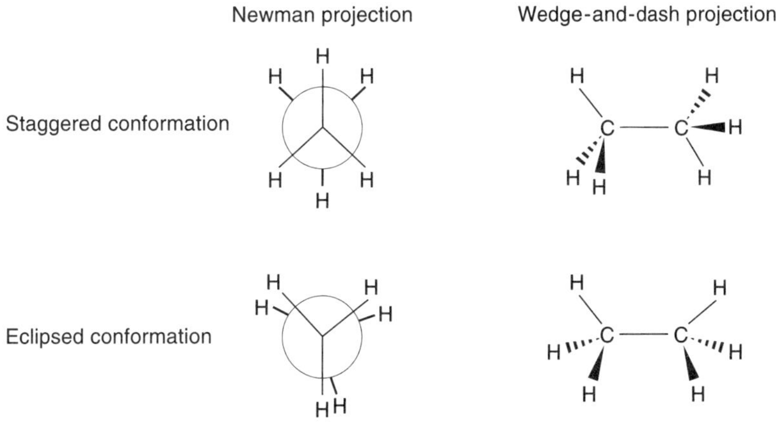

Fig. 8-155

Rotation about the C_2—C_3 bond in butane produces a number of conformations varying in energy. Rotation about a carbon–carbon bond is not completely free, but the energy barrier is low and internal rotation at room temperature is rapid. Various conformations of butane are shown in Figure 8-156.

The anti and gauche forms of butane are free of torsional strain. In the gauche form, the methyl groups are closer together than the sums of their van der Waals radii, resulting in van der Waals strain, or steric strain, due to repulsion between the methyl groups. Van der Waals strain and torsional strain are at a maximum when the methyl groups are eclipsed.

Two nonplanar conformations of cyclohexane are known as the chair and boat forms. Both forms are free of bond angle strain and the chair form is additionally free of torsional strain. The boat form has significant torsional strain because four of its carbon atoms

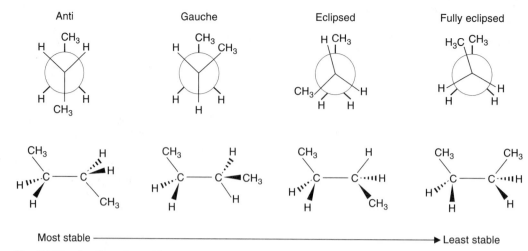

Fig. 8-156. Conformations of butane.

are eclipsed. The boat form is destabilized because of the van der Waals repulsion between the hydrogens at positions 1 and 4 of the ring.

Six of the carbon-hydrogen bonds of the chair form lie perpendicular to the plane of the ring and are called **axial bonds**. The remaining six hydrogens are located around the circumference (equator) of the ring and are designated **equatorial** (Figure 8-157).

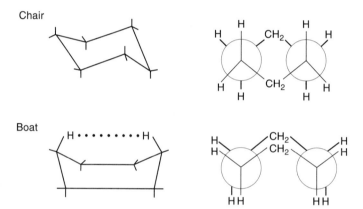

Fig. 8-157

A cyclohexane ring may have substituents in the axial or equatorial positions. Cyclohexane rings are conformationally mobile and undergo ring inversion or "ring flipping." A cyclohexane ring having an axial substituent may undergo inversion to a new chair conformation in which the substituent is equatorial by passing through the boat conformation. The chair formation with the substituent group in the equatorial position generally is the more stable. The larger the substituent, the greater the tendency for the group to be equatorial. Therefore, methylcyclohexane exists almost entirely in the chair conformation with the methyl group equatorial (Figure 8-158).

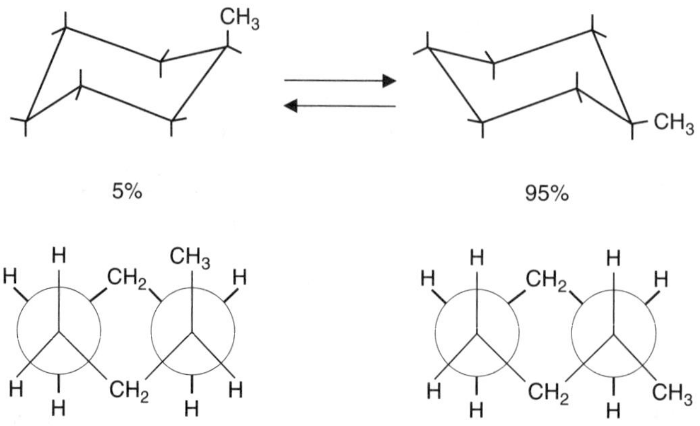

Fig. 8-158

Stability of the Intermediate Carbocations

Stability of the **intermediate carbocations** depends on the groups attached, which can stabilize or destabilize it. In general, groups that can share electrons by π orbital overlap (resonance) stabilize the carbocation, and groups that place a positive (partial or total) charge adjacent to the carbocation withdraw electrons inductively (by sigma bonds) to destabilize it (Figure 8-159).

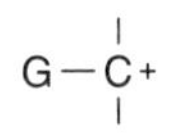

$$G-\overset{|}{\underset{|}{C}}+$$

When G is O, N, benzyl, allyl, or alkyls, the carbocation is stabilized.
The stability decreases in the following order: benzyl ~ allyl > 3°> 2°> 1°

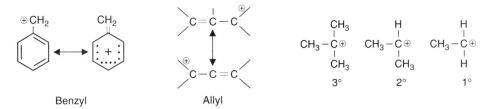

Fig. 8-159. Stability of carbocations. G = groups.

Benzyl   Allyl

G = destabilizes = carbonyl, alkyl halide

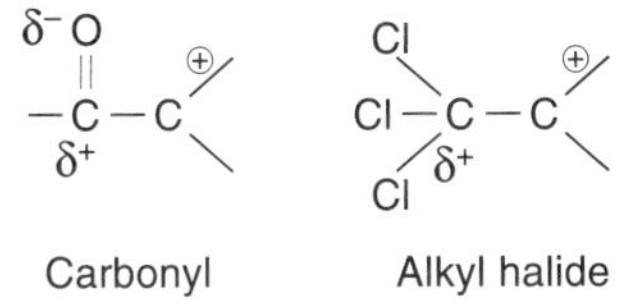

Carbonyl   Alkyl halide

These points are useful in predicting which carbon will become the carbocation and which one the electrophile and nucleophile will bond to. The intermediate carbocation formed must be the most stable. Markovnikov's rule is a sequel to this: the nucleophile (a molecule with a free pair of electrons and sometimes a negative charge that seeks out partially or completely positive charge species) will be bonded to the most substituted carbon (fewest hydrogens attached) in the product, or equivalently, the electrophile will be bonded to the least substituted (most hydrogens attached) carbon in the product (Figure 8-160).

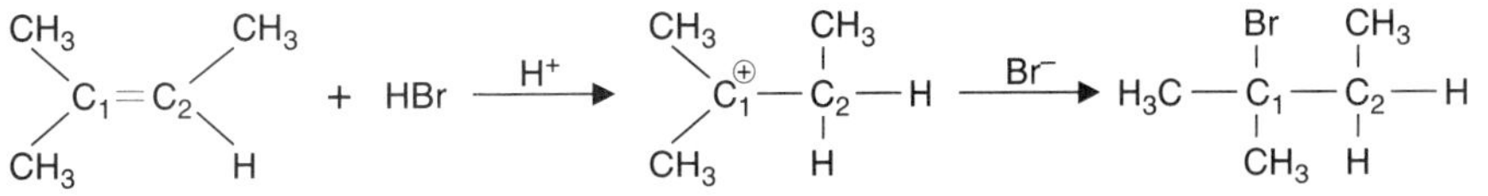

Fig. 8-160

Dienes

There are three types of **dienes** depending on the arrangement of the two double bonds. Dienes having double bonds separated by more than one single bond behave as if each double bond is isolated and they act independently of the other. Dienes in which the two double bonds share a common carbon atom are called **allenes**. Dienes having double bonds alternate with a single bond are said to be **conjugated**.

$\quad$ $RCH{=}CHCH_2CH_2CH{=}CH_2$ is a 1,5-diene (double bonds are isolated)

$\quad$ $RCH{=}C{=}CH_2$ is a 1,2-diene (an allene)

$\quad$ $RCH{=}CH{-}CH{=}CHR$ is a 1,3-diene (a conjugated diene)

Conjugated dienes are $2-4$ kcal/mol more stable than the corresponding isolated dienes due to their conjugation (overlap of π orbitals of the diene) and form preferentially during elimination reactions (Figure 8-161). Conjugated dienes form both 1,2- and 1,4- addition products (Figure 8-162).

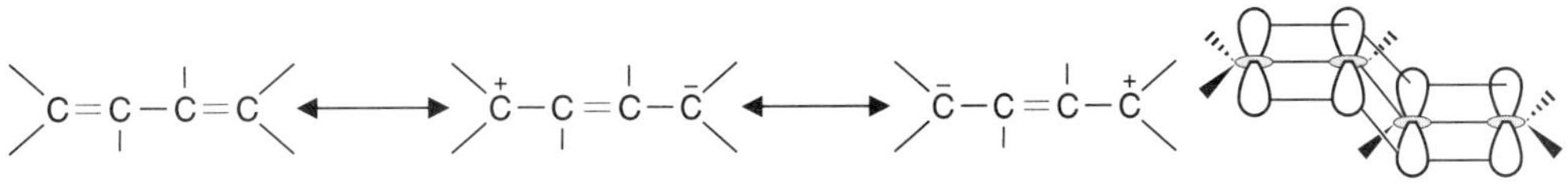

Fig. 8-161

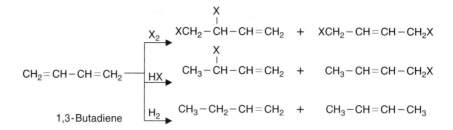

Fig. 8-162   1,3-Butadiene

Electrophilic addition to conjugated dienes involves the formation of an allylic carbocation. At low temperatures, the 1,2-product forms faster than the 1,4-product and is referred to as the **kinetic product**. At higher temperatures, the proportion of 1,4-product increases, indicating that it is the more stable or thermodynamic product (Figure 8-163).

$$CH_2=CH-CH=CH_2 \ + \ HCl \longrightarrow CH_3\overset{+}{C}H-CH=CH_2 \longleftrightarrow CH_3CH=CH-CH_2{+}$$

$$\Big\downarrow Cl^-$$

Cl
|
$$CH_3CH-CH=CH_2 \ + \ CH_3CH=CH-CH_2Cl$$

Fig. 8-163   1,2-Addition   1,4-Addition

Isoprene Rule

The carbon skeleton of isoprene, 2-methyl-1,3-butadiene, occurs in many compounds called **terpenes**, which are found in plants. The basic isoprene structure occurs as a repeat unit (**isoprene rule**). Natural rubber also may be considered a 1,4-addition polymer of isoprene (Figure 8-164).

1,4-addition polymer of isoprene

$$\underset{\displaystyle Isoprene}{CH_2=\overset{\displaystyle \overset{CH_3}{|}}{C}-CH=CH_2}$$

Menthol

Vitamin A

Fig. 8-164

Alkynes

Hydrocarbon compounds containing a carbon-carbon triple bond are called **alkynes.** They are named in a similar fashion as alkenes by replacing the *-ane* suffix with *-yne.* The simplest member of the series is also known by its common name, acetylene (Figure 8-165).

$$HC \equiv CH \qquad HC \equiv C-CH_2-CH_2-\overset{\overset{\displaystyle CH_3}{|}}{\underset{\underset{\displaystyle CH_3}{|}}{C}}-CH_2-CH_2-CH_3$$

Ethyne
(acetylene)
Fig. 8-165   5,5-Dimethyl-1-octyne

In molecules that contain both a double and triple bond, the longest continuous chain containing both bonds is numbered to give the lowest prefix numbers, with the double bond receiving the lower number if there is a choice. The *-en* suffix precedes the *-yne* suffix in the name as shown in Figure 8-166.

$$CH_3-C \equiv C-CH_2-CH=CH_2 \qquad CH_3-\overset{\overset{\displaystyle }{|}}{\underset{\underset{\displaystyle CH_3}{|}}{C}}=CH-CH_2-C \equiv CH$$

Fig. 8-166   1-Hexene-4-yne   2-Methyl-2-hexene-5-yne

Alkynes are hydrocarbons of low polarity whose physical properties are essentially the same as those of alkanes and alkenes. They are insoluble in water, soluble in low polarity organic solvents, and their boiling points are nearly the same as the corresponding alkane or alkene.

UNSATURATED (ALKENES)

Alkenes (if no ring, C_nH_{2n}) are hydrocarbons having a double bond as the functional group. For each double bond, the molecule loses two hydrogens from the alkane formula (C_nH_{2n+2}). The IUPAC name of alkenes is obtained by replacing the *-ane* ending of the corresponding alkane name with *-ene*. The longest carbon chain contained in the double bond is used to name the alkene, and the first carbon of the double bond is numbered as the lowest possible locant. Substituents are named as usual. The numbering of the double bond takes precedence over alkyl groups and halogens but not the hydroxyl group. Some of the simpler alkenes are frequently known by common names ending in *-ylene*, which are not acceptable IUPAC names (Figure 8-167).

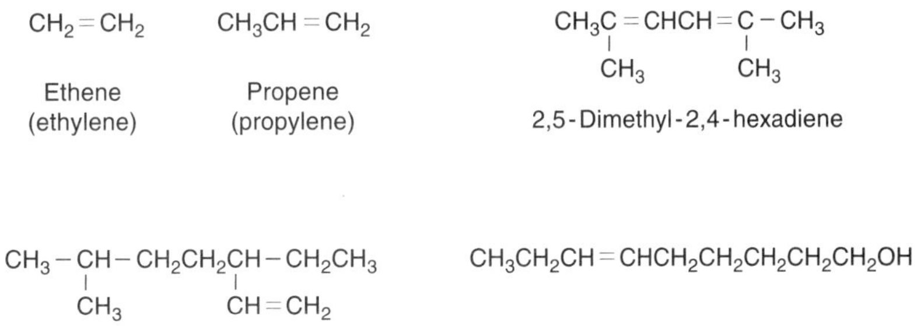

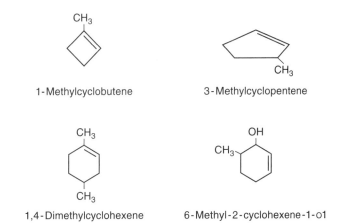

Fig. 8-167

$$CH_2=CH_2$$

Ethene
(ethylene)

$$CH_3CH=CH_2$$

Propene
(propylene)

2,5-Dimethyl-2,4-hexadiene

3-Ethyl-6-methyl-1-heptene

6-Nonen-1-ol

Cycloalkenes are named in a manner similar to alkenes, with the carbons of the double bond being carbon-1 and carbon-2 (Figure 8-168).

Fig. 8-168

1-Methylcyclobutene

3-Methylcyclopentene

1,4-Dimethylcyclohexene

6-Methyl-2-cyclohexene-1-o1

Because of the lack of rotation about the carbon double bond, alkenes may exist as stereoisomers known as **geometrical isomers**. When an alkene has two like groups or atoms on a single carbon of a double bond, this type of isomerism is not possible. Those isomers with like groups on the same side of the double bond are designated **cis** *isomers*, whereas those with the groups on opposite sides of the double bond are designated **trans** *isomers* (Figure 8-169).

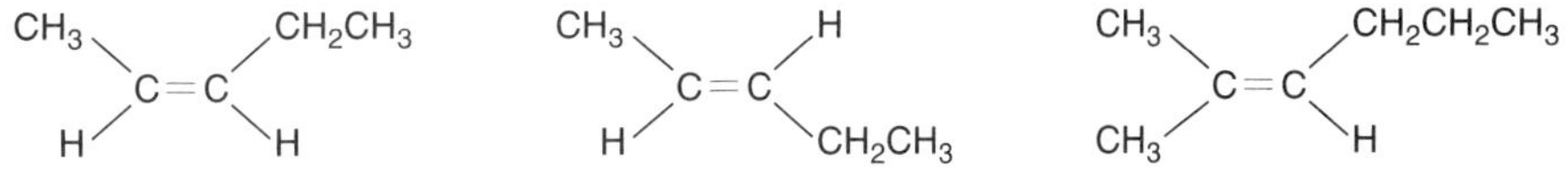

Fig. 8-169

cis-2-Pentene

trans-2-Pentene

2-Methyl-2-hexene
(no geometric isomers)

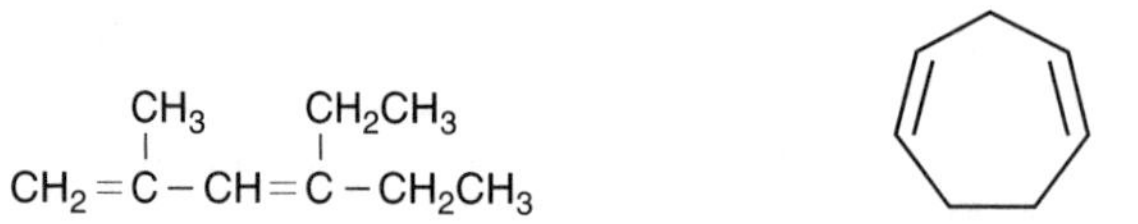

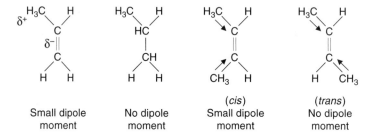

Fig. 8-170 4-Ethyl-2-methyl-1,3-hexadiene 1,4-Cycloheptadiene

A hydrocarbon having two double bonds is called a diene, one with three double bonds is called a triene, and so forth (Figure 8-170).

The physical but not chemical properties of the alkenes are much like those of the alkanes in that those with corresponding carbon skeletons have similar boiling points. The boiling point of a homologous series of alkenes increases approximately 20° to 30°C for each methylene group ($-CH_2^-$) and chain branching slightly lowers the boiling point. Alkenes are very weakly polar and are insoluble in water but soluble in nonpolar solvents such as hexane, cyclohexane, ethyl ether, dichloromethane, and benzene. One difference is that alkenes may be polar due to *cis–trans* isomers and to the nature of the double bond itself (an electron withdrawer) [Figure 8-171].

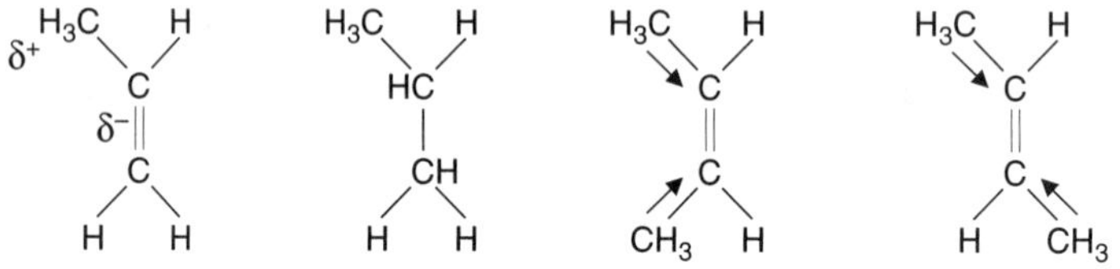

Fig. 8-171 Small dipole moment | No dipole moment | (*cis*) Small dipole moment | (*trans*) No dipole moment

Also, *trans* compounds tend to have higher melting points (due to higher symmetry) but lower boiling points (due to less polarity) than the corresponding *cis* compounds.

Nearly all the chemistry of alkenes involves addition reactions to the double bond. The pi (π) electrons of the double bond are available for reaction with reagents capable of reacting with a pair of electrons. Protons and carbocations (carbenium ions) are Lewis acids, which are electron acceptors. Carbon anions are called **carbanions**. Carbocations are electron-seeking reagents. They are also called **electrophilic reagents** or electrophiles. Alkenes, which are electron donating, are Lewis bases and are nucleophilic reagents or nucleophiles. The most important reaction of alkenes is electrophilic addition to the double bond. A general reaction is shown in Figure 8-172.

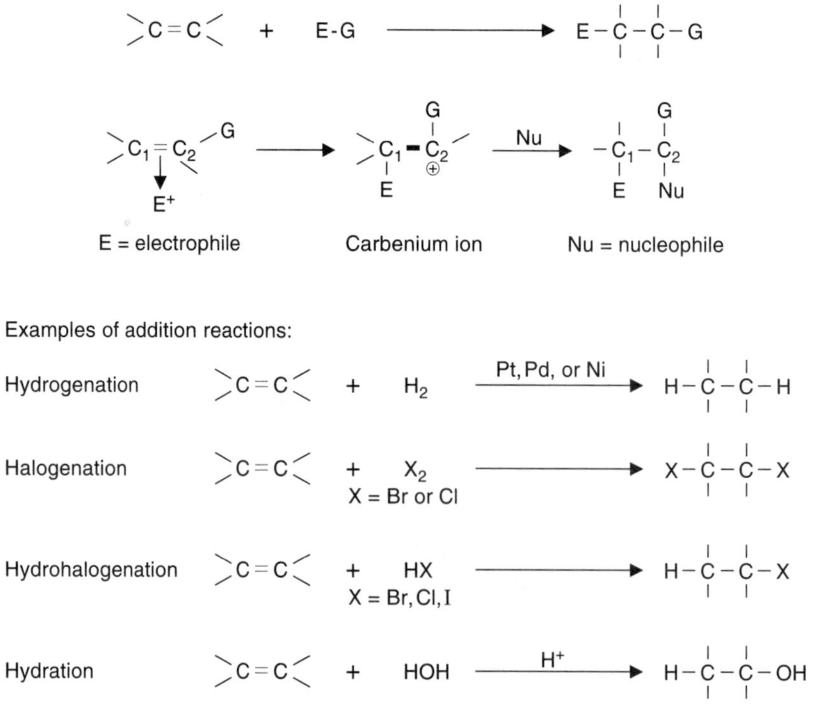
E = electrophile
Carbenium ion
Nu = nucleophile
Examples of addition reactions:
Hydrogenation
Pt, Pd, or Ni
Halogenation
X = Br or Cl
Hydrohalogenation
X = Br, Cl, I
Hydration

Fig. 8-172

Electrophilic Addition

Halogenation, hydrohalogenation, and hydration of alkenes are examples of **electrophilic addition reactions**. The electrophilic addition reactions of HX and HOH to unsymmetrical alkenes are regioselective (i.e., they give a predominance of one of the two possible addition compounds) and follow Markovnikov's rule. This rule states that, in the addition of HX and HOH reagents to unsymmetrical alkenes, the hydrogen adds to the carbon of the double bond which has the greater number of hydrogens (Figure 8-173).

Mechanism (general)

$$R-CH=CH_2 \ + \ H-X \longrightarrow R-\overset{+}{C}H-CH_3 \ + \ X^-$$

$$R-\overset{+}{C}H-CH_3 \ + \ X^- \longrightarrow R-\underset{\underset{X}{|}}{C}H-CH_3$$

Hydration

$$H_2SO_4 \ + \ HOH \longrightarrow H_3O^+ \ + \ HSO_4^-$$

$$R-CH=CH_2 \ + \ H_3O^+ \longrightarrow R-\overset{+}{C}H-CH_3 \ + \ HOH$$

$$R-\overset{+}{C}H-CH_3 \ + \ HOH \longrightarrow R-\underset{\underset{OH_2^+}{|}}{C}H-CH_3$$

$$R-\underset{\underset{OH_2^+}{|}}{C}H-CH_3 \ + \ HOH \longrightarrow R-\underset{\underset{OH}{|}}{C}H-CH_3 \ + \ H_3O^+$$

Fig. 8-173

Markovnikov's rule holds because the addition of the proton to the carbon having the greater number of hydrogens yields the more stable carbocation, which is formed via a lower energy transition state. In the example, a secondary carbocation (carbenium ion) is formed, whereas the alternate mode of addition would yield the less stable primary carbocation (Figure 8-174).

$$R-CH=CH_2 \ + \ H^+ \longrightarrow R-\overset{+}{C}H-CH_3 \quad (\text{rather than } RCH_2CH_2^+)$$

Fig. 8-174

$$R_2C=CH-R \ + \ H^+ \longrightarrow R_2\overset{+}{C}-CH_2R \quad (\text{rather than } R_2CHCHR^+)$$

The carbon skeleton of an alkene may undergo rearrangement during electrophilic addition if the initially formed carbocation can rearrange to a more stable carbocation. Rearrangement may occur by methyl or hydride shift to an adjacent carbon to form a more stable carbocation. The rearranged structure is often the major product of the reaction (Figure 8-175).

In some additions to a double bond, both atoms or groups of the reagent add to the same side of the double bond, resulting in syn addition. When the two atoms or groups add on opposite sides, anti addition occurs (Figure 8-176).

The other key feature of the double bond is its ability to stabilize carbocations, carbanions, or radicals that are on adjacent carbons (Figure 8-177). All are resonance stabilized.

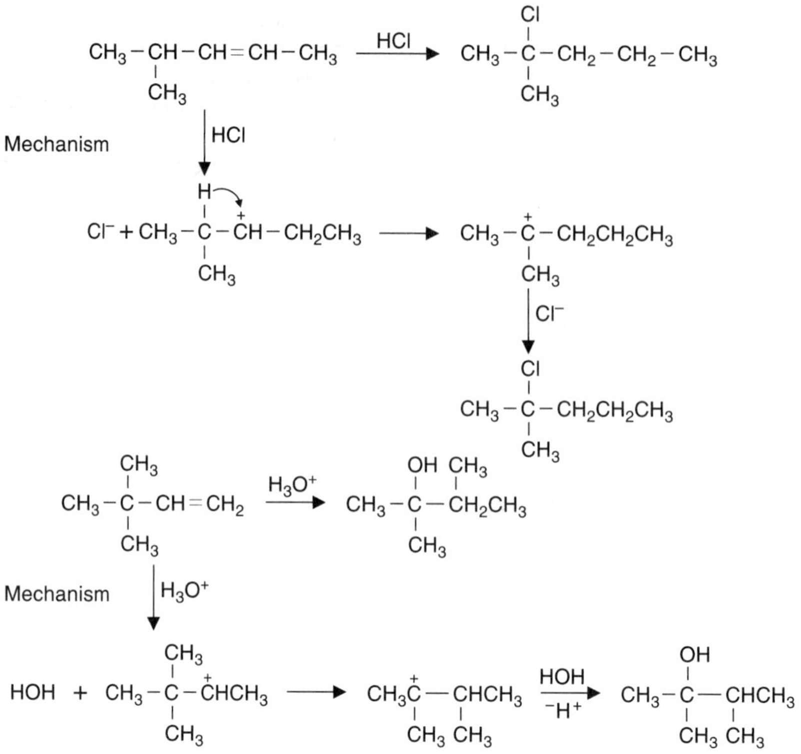

Fig. 8-175

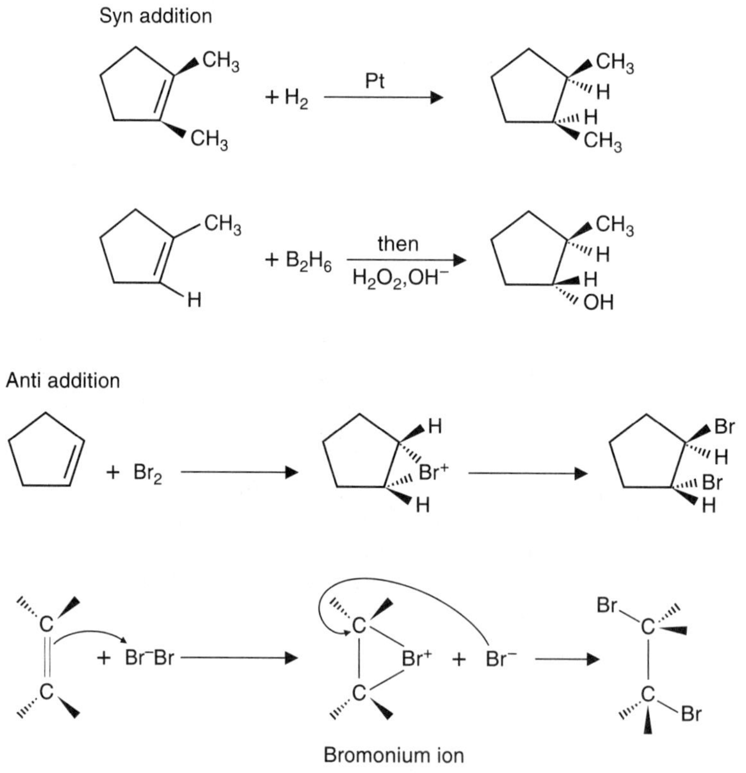

Syn addition

Fig. 8-176. Syn and anti addition.

Anti addition

Bromonium ion

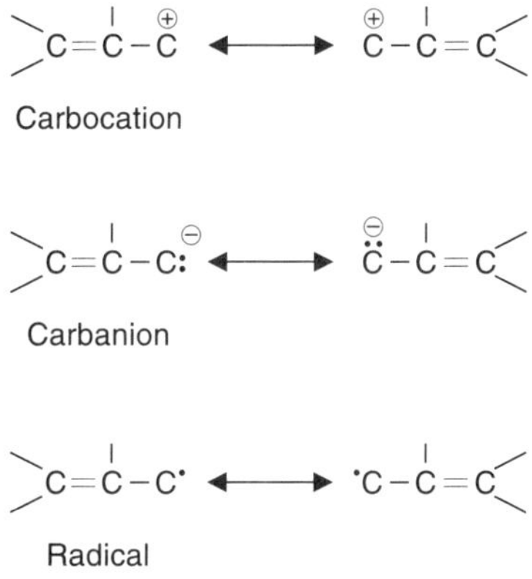

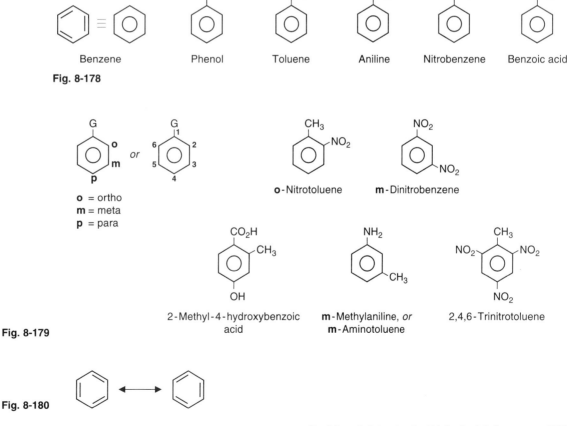

$$\underset{\text{Carbocation}}{\overset{\displaystyle>}{C}=\overset{|}{C}-\overset{\oplus}{C}< \longleftrightarrow \overset{\oplus}{C}-\overset{|}{C}=C<}$$

Carbocation

$$\underset{\text{Carbanion}}{>C=\overset{|}{C}-\overset{\ominus}{C}: \longleftrightarrow \overset{\ominus}{C}-\overset{|}{C}=C<}$$

Carbanion

$$>C=\overset{|}{C}-\overset{\centerdot}{C} \longleftrightarrow \overset{\centerdot}{C}-\overset{|}{C}=C<$$

Fig. 8-177   Radical

AROMATIC HYDROCARBONS (BENZENE)

Many **monosubstituted benzenes** have special names or they can be named by the substituent attached (Figure 8-178).

Disubstituted benzenes can be named as a derivative of the primary substituent with either numbers or the ortho (o), para (a), meta (m) system (Figure 8-179).

Trisubstituted and higher substituted benzenes require the numbering system. Benzene (C_6H_6) is a planar molecule in which the carbons are sp^2 hybridized. It often is represented by two resonance forms having alternate double and single bonds called Kekulé structures (Figure 8-180).

All of the carbon–carbon bonds are of equal length and the bond angles of benzene equal 120°. Because benzene is planar and has six sp^2 hybridized carbons, each carbon has a p orbital perpendicular to the plane of the ring. The six p orbitals, each containing one electron, lie close enough to overlap effectively in the lowest energy-bonding molecular orbital. Because of the equal overlap of the six p orbitals, benzene is often drawn as a hexagon with a circle to represent the six delocalized pi electrons (Figure 8-181).

Benzene is reduced by three molar equivalents of hydrogen to cyclohexane and has a heat of hydrogenation of 49.8 Kcal/mol. Based on the heat of hydrogenation, which would be expected for a compound with three double bonds, benzene is 36 Kcal/mol

Benzene   Phenol   Toluene   Aniline   Nitrobenzene   Benzoic acid

Fig. 8-178

o = ortho
m = meta
p = para

o-Nitrotoluene   m-Dinitrobenzene

2-Methyl-4-hydroxybenzoic acid   m-Methylaniline, or m-Aminotoluene   2,4,6-Trinitrotoluene

Fig. 8-179

Fig. 8-180

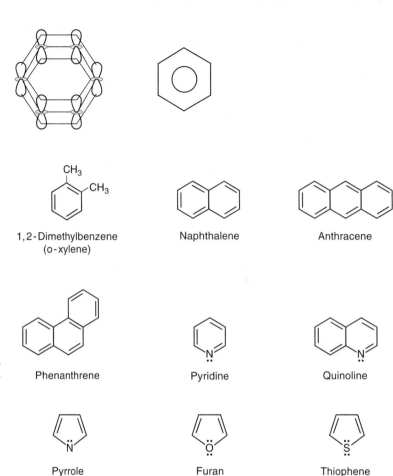

Fig. 8-181

Fig. 8-182. Examples of benzenoid, polycyclic, and heterocyclic aromatic compounds.

1,2-Dimethylbenzene
(o-xylene)

Naphthalene

Anthracene

Phenanthrene

Pyridine

Quinoline

Pyrrole

Furan

Thiophene

Indole

Purine

Pyrimidine

more stable than anticipated. That is, hydrogenation of benzene releases 36 Kcal/mol less energy than is expected for a 1,3,5-cyclohexatriene with noninteracting double bonds. This difference in energy is referred to as the **resonance energy, stabilization energy**, or **delocalization energy** of benzene. Benzene and its derivatives are the simplest and most important representatives of a large class of aromatic compounds. Aromatic compounds are those compounds that are substantially stabilized by resonance. Some examples of benzenoid, polycyclic, and heterocyclic aromatic compounds are shown in Figure 8-182. A number of heterocyclic aromatic compounds are present in biochemical systems.

The term **annulene** is used for monocyclic polyenes having alternating single and double bonds (fully conjugated). The ring size of an annulene is described by a number in a bracket. Cyclobutadiene is a [4] annulene, benzene is a [6] annulene, and cyclooctatetraene is an [8] annulene. Huckel's rule states that only planar, fully conjugated monocyclic polyenes having $4n + 2$ pi electrons, where n is an integer, that is, $n = 0, 1, 2, 3, 4$, etc., should possess aromatic stability. Therefore, Huckel's rule predicts that annulenes having 6, 10, 14, or 18 pi electrons should possess aromatic character as long as the ring is planar (Figure 8-183).

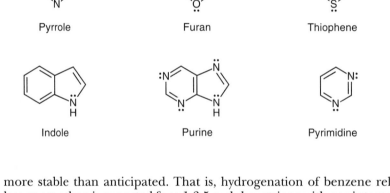

Benzene (aromatic) $4n + 2 = 6$ when $n = 1$

Fig. 8-183

Cyclobutadiene (planar) and cyclooctatetraene (nonplanar) do not meet Huckel's criteria and do not possess aromatic character. A number of [10] and [12] annulenes have been prepared and none are aromatic. The [12] annulenes have 12 pi electrons

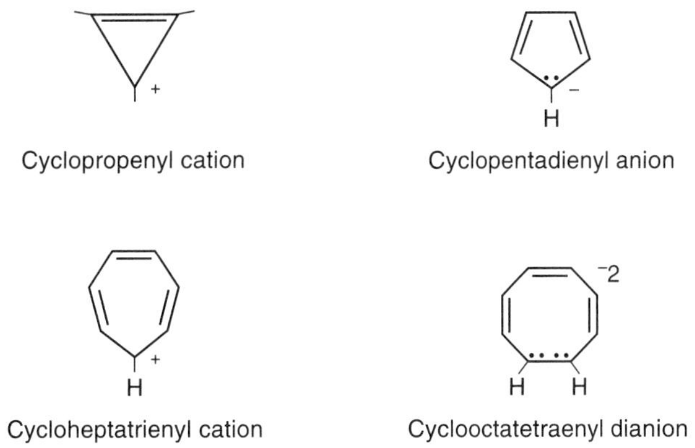

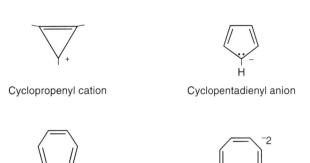

Cyclopropenyl cation

Cyclopentadienyl anion

Fig. 8-184   Cycloheptatrienyl cation

Cyclooctatetraenyl dianion

and do not obey Huckel's rule. The [10] annulenes have the correct number of pi electrons but their rings are nonplanar.

Pyrrole, furan, and pyridine are aromatic. Pyrrole has an unshared pair of electrons on the nitrogen along with four pi electrons in the diene portion, resulting in a total of six pi electrons. Furan also has six pi electrons to constitute an aromatic system. The second unshared electron pair on oxygen are in an orbital perpendicular to the pi system of the ring and do not apply to Huckel's rule. The lone electron pair on the pyridine nitrogen also lies in the plane perpendicular to the pi system of the ring and does not apply.

Certain monocyclic anions and cations exhibit enhanced stability and are considered aromatic. Some examples are shown in Figure 8-184.

RESONANCE STABILITY AND DELOCALIZATION OF ELECTRONS

The characteristic reaction of the benzene ring is electrophilic aromatic substitution in which an electrophile (E^+) is substituted for a ring hydrogen. The intermediate cation form is stabilized by charged delocalization, which is especially strong at ring carbon atoms ortho and para to the entering group (Figure 8-185).

Substituents attached to the benzene ring affect the reactivity of the ring and determine the orientation of substitution. The type of substituent greatly affects the stability of the charged intermediate formed during electrophilic substitution. Groups that donate electrons make the ring more reactive than benzene to electrophilic substitution and direct the entering electrophile to the ortho and para positions. These groups are called **ortho-para** directors. Groups that make the ring less reactive than benzene to electrophilic substitution direct the electrophile to the meta position. These groups are called **meta** directors. The halogens are unique in that they deactivate the benzene ring to substitution but are ortho-para directing.

The following are ortho-para directors (activating): $-H_2$, $-NHR$, $-NR_2$, $-OH$, $-OR$, $-NHCOR$, C_6H_5-, and $-R$. Meta directors (deactivating) are $-O_2$, $-NR_3+$, $-CF3$, $-CN$, $-COOH$, $-COOR$, $-CHO$, and $-COR$. Ortho-para directors (deactivating) are $-F$, $-Cl$, $-Br$, and $-I$.

Groups tend to withdraw or release electrons by resonance effects or inductive effects. **Resonance effects** involve delocalization of electrons to stabilize a charged species. An example of this effect is the stabilization of the charged intermediate in electrophilic substitution by an electron-releasing group such as the hydroxyl group ($-OH$). Inductive effects depend on the property of a substituent to release or withdraw electrons. The **inductive effect** of a group depends on its electronegativity and may act through the sigma bonds of a molecule or through space. Because most elements or groups are more electronegative than hydrogen is, they exert an electron-withdrawing effect. Groups such as $-CHO$, $-COR$, $-COOR$, $-COOH$, $-NO_2$, $-CF_3$, and $-NR_3+$ can only exert an electron-withdrawing effect. Groups such as $-OH$, $-OR$, $-NH_2$, $-NHR$, $-NR_2$, and the halogens may be electron releasing by resonance due to their unshared electron

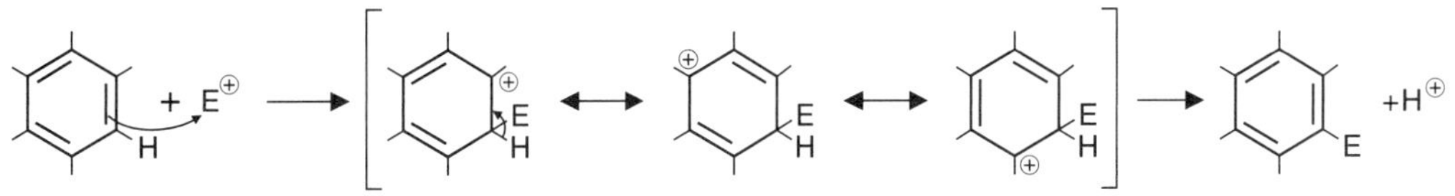

Fig. 8-185

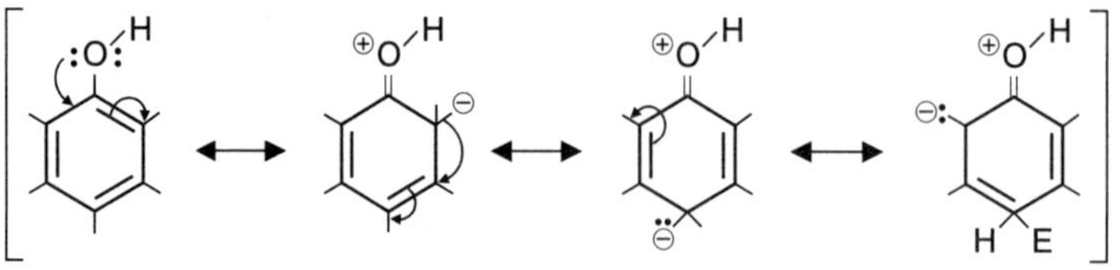

Fig. 8-186

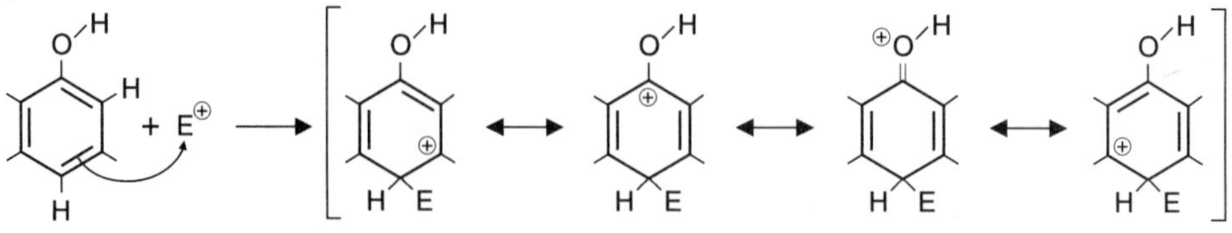

Fig. 8-187

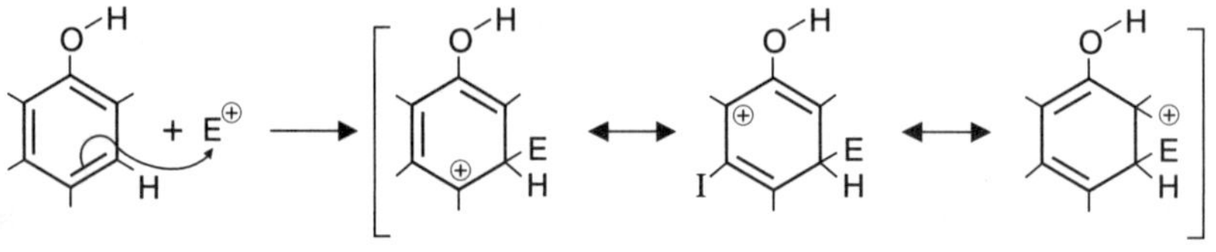

Fig. 8-188

pairs, but electron withdrawing by inductive effects due to their electronegativity. The halogens are ortho-para directing but are deactivating groups because their electron-withdrawing inductive effect reduces the electron density of the aromatic ring and thus destabilizes the cation form. The halogens direct ortho-para because they have an un-shared pair of electrons that can be donated to stabilize the intermediate cation formed by ortho or para attack. For electrophilic aromatic substitution reactions, the resonance effect is usually more important than the inductive effect of a group.

Ortho-para directors (e.g., −OH, −NH2, −OR, −NR₂, and alkyls) are shown in Figure 8-186. Note that the electron density is at the ortho-para positions so the E^+ favors attack at ortho-para positions. Figure 8-187 shows a substituent (E^+) at ortho or para to obtain good stabilization.

Figure 8-188 shows a substituent at meta. The −-OH can no longer help delocalize the positive charge, so the ortho-para is favored over the meta. Meta directors (e.g., −NO₂, −SO₂⁻, −CN) are shown without a substituent in Figure 8-189. Note that the positive charge is put at the ortho-para positions so that the E^+ favors attack at the meta position. Figure 8-190 shows a substituent at meta positions. Figure 8-191 shows a substituent at the ortho-para position.

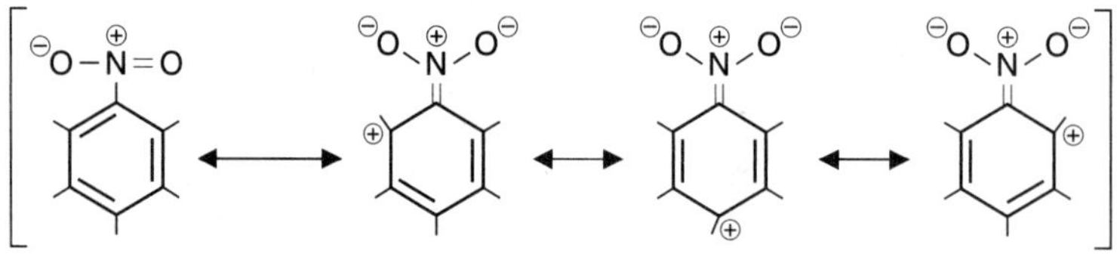

Fig. 8-189

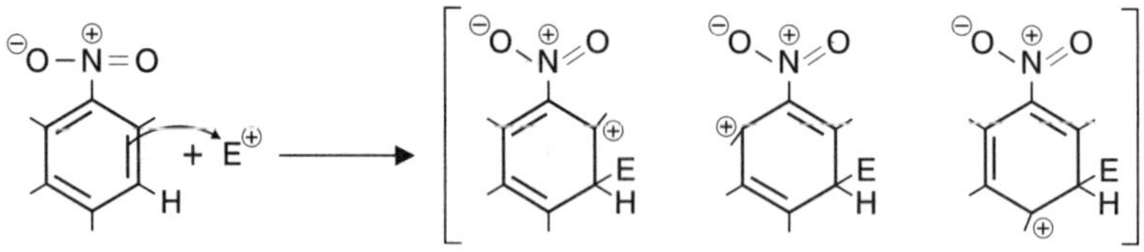

Fig. 8-190

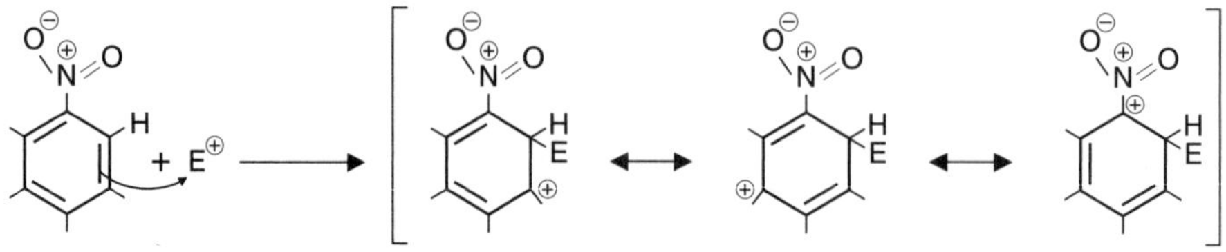

Fig. 8-191   I   II   III

Resonance form III is a noncontributor because of the adjacent positive charge; analogous situations exist with the other meta directors, so meta substitution is favored. The problem of orientation of the entering group is more complicated when there are two substituents present on a benzene ring. In some cases, the groups may be located so that the directive effect of one group reinforces that of the other. When the effects of the groups are in opposition, however, it is difficult to predict the major product, and a mixture of products may result. As a general rule, activating ortho-para directing groups are dominant over deactivating meta directing groups or groups that are less activating. For steric reasons, substitution generally does not occur between two groups, which are located meta to one another (Figure 8-192).

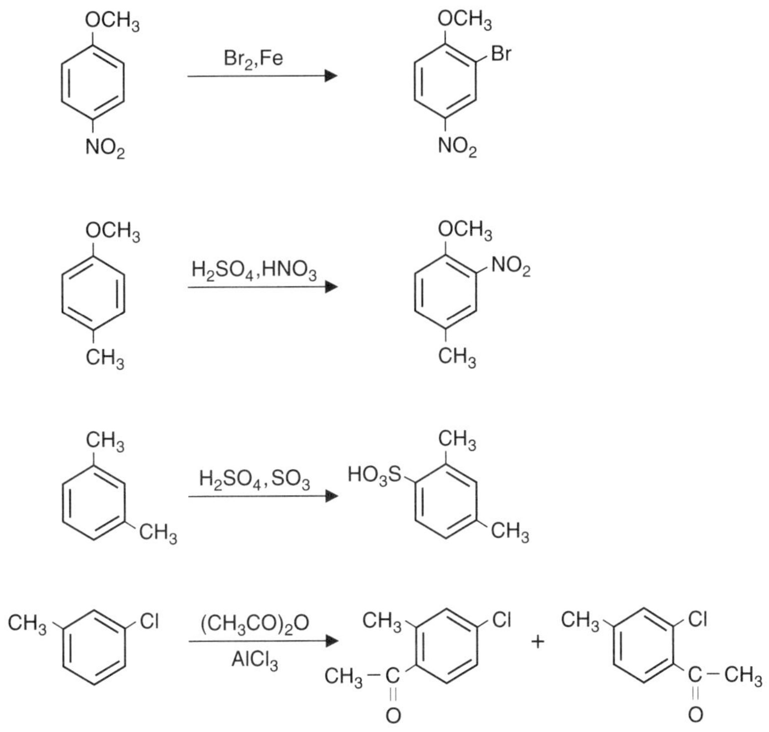

Fig. 8-192

APPLIED CONCEPTS

- Understand three types of polymers (isotactic, syndiotactic, atactic).
- Review a few laboratory procedures and experimental devices, such as a magnetic stirrer procedure and reflux condenser for two-phase mixture and the Diels-Alder reaction for dienes.
- If you are unfamiliar with Woodward-Hoffman rules, which determine molecular orbital structures, review symmetry-allowed and symmetry-forbidden concepts as they tie to the HOMO (highest occupied molecular orbital) and LUMO (lowest unoccupied molecular orbital) rules.

HYDROCARBONS: REVIEW QUESTIONS

1. Alkanes tend to have _____ boiling points because they are _____ and, hence, have _____ intermolecular forces.

   A. low; nonpolar; weak
   B. high; polar; strong
   C. low; polar; weak
   D. high; nonpolar; strong

2. Alkanes are _____ in water because they are _____.

   A. soluble; polar
   B. insoluble; polar
   C. soluble; nonpolar
   D. insoluble; nonpolar

3. Branching tends to make an alkane more _____ and this _____ the boiling point.

   A. symmetric; lowers
   B. symmetric; raises

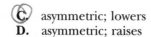

    C. asymmetric; lowers
    D. asymmetric; raises

4.   The step in which radicals react with radicals is:

    A. termination.
    B. propagation.
    C. initiation.
    D. none of these.

5.   Of the following radicals, in general, the most stable is:

    A. allylic.
    B. primary.
    C. secondary.
    D. tertiary.

6.   Which ring has the greatest ring strain?

    A. cyclohexane
    B. cyclopentane
    C. cyclobutane
    D. cyclopropane

7.   Which of the following rings has no ring strain?

    A. Cyclohexane
    B. Cyclobutane
    C. Cyclopropane
    D. None of the above

8.   The name of the compound in the following figure is:

$$CH_3-CH-CH-CH_2-CH_3$$

with CH_3 above the second carbon and CH_3 below the third carbon

    A. 2-isopropyl pentane.
    B. 2,3-dimethylpentane.
    C. 3,4-dimethyl pentane.
    D. none of the above.

9.   The name of the compound in the following figure is:

    A. 2,4,8-trimethyl-2-ethyl-5-isopropylnonane.
    B. diisoprene.
    C. 2,6,8,8-tetramethyl-5-isopropyldecane.
    D. none of the above.

10. Give the structure of 2,6-dimethyl-4-ethyloctane.

A.

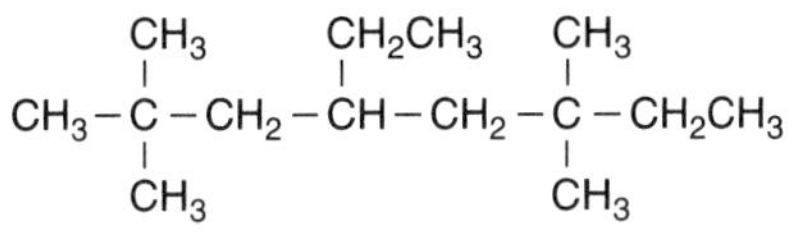

$$CH_3-\underset{\underset{CH_3}{|}}{\overset{\overset{CH_3}{|}}{C}}-CH_2-\underset{\underset{}{|}}{\overset{\overset{CH_2CH_3}{|}}{CH}}-CH_2-\underset{\underset{CH_3}{|}}{\overset{\overset{CH_3}{|}}{C}}-CH_2CH_3$$

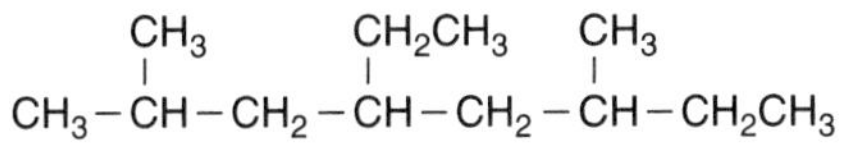

B.

$$CH_3-\overset{\overset{CH_3}{|}}{CH}-CH_2-\overset{\overset{CH_2CH_3}{|}}{CH}-CH_2-\overset{\overset{CH_3}{|}}{CH}-CH_2CH_3$$

C.

$$CH_3-\overset{\overset{CH_2CH_3}{|}}{CH}-CH_2-\overset{\overset{CH_3}{|}}{CH}-CH_2-\overset{\overset{CH_2CH_3}{|}}{CH}-CH_2CH_3$$

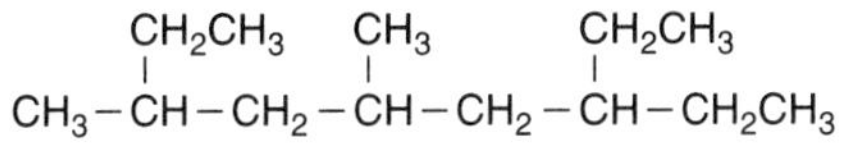

D. None of the above

11. The name of the compound in the following figure is:

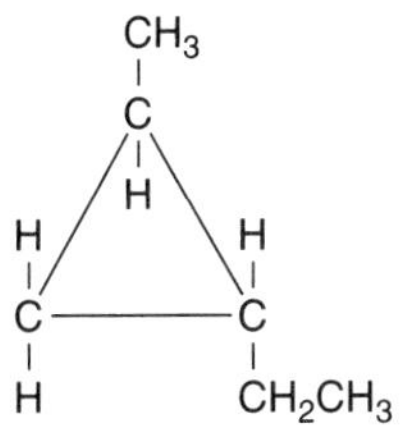

A. *cis*-1-Methyl-2-ethylcyclopropane.
B. 2,3-Methylpentane.
C. *trans*-Dimethylcylopropane.
D. none of the above.

12. What is the structure of *trans*-1-ethyl-4-t-butylcyclohexane?

A.

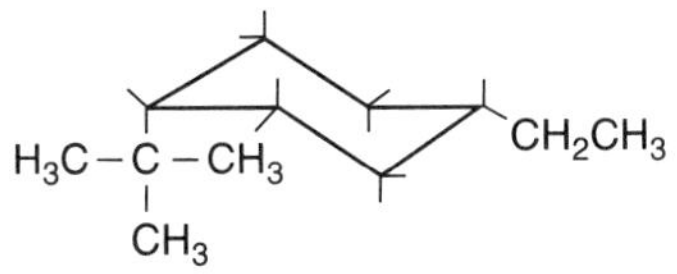

B.

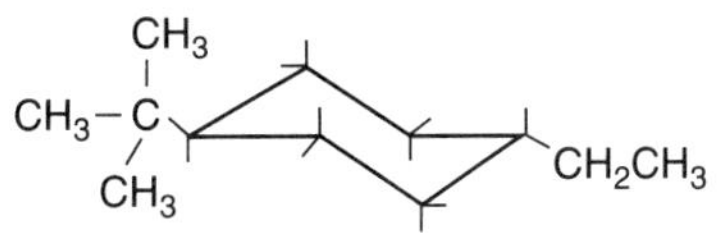

C.

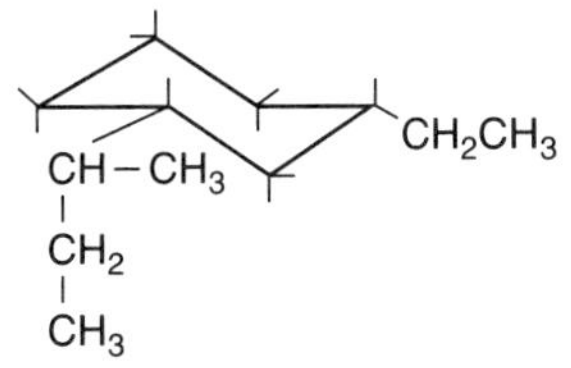

D. None of the above

13. Which of the following compounds probably has the higher boiling point?

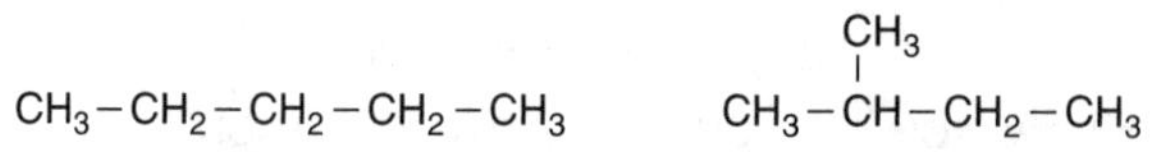

$$CH_3-CH_2-CH_2-CH_2-CH_3 \qquad \overset{\overset{\displaystyle CH_3}{|}}{CH_3-CH-CH_2-CH_3}$$

I II

A. I
B. II
C. Both have the same boiling point.
D. I and II do not boil at any temperature.

14. Which of the following compounds probably has the higher boiling point?

$$CH_3-CH_2-CH_3 \qquad CH_3-CH_2-CH_2-CH_2-CH_3$$

I II

A. I
B. II
C. Both have the same boiling point.
D. I and II do not boil at any temperature.

15. How many CO_2 molecules are produced by the complete combustion of 3,3-Diethylhexane?

A. 10
B. 8
C. 6
D. 4

16. Which of the following radicals is the most stable?

A.

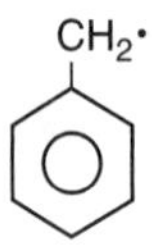

$$\overset{\displaystyle CH_2\cdot}{\bigcirc}$$

B. 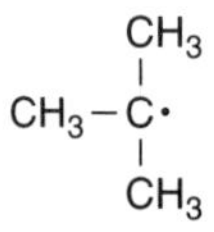 $\overset{\overset{\displaystyle CH_3}{|}}{\underset{\underset{\displaystyle CH_3}{|}}{CH_3-C\cdot}}$

C. $\overset{\overset{\displaystyle CH_3}{|}}{CH_3-\underset{\cdot}{C}H}$

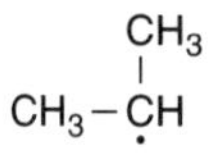

D. $CH_3\cdot$

17. In the following compound, removal of which H will result in the most stable radical?

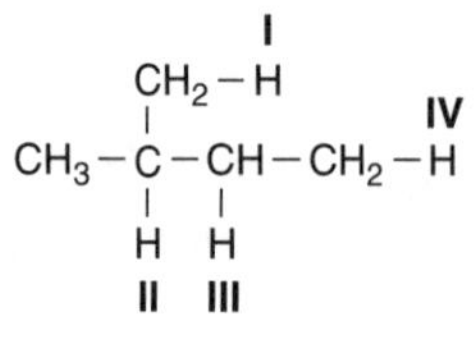

$$\overset{\overset{\displaystyle I}{|}}{\underset{\underset{\displaystyle II \quad III}{\underset{|\quad|}{H\ \ H}}}{CH_3-\underset{|}{C}-\underset{|}{CH}-CH_2-H}} \quad \overset{\displaystyle IV}{}$$
$$\overset{\displaystyle CH_2-H}{}$$

A. I
B. II
C. III
D. IV

18. The formula for an alkane is C_4H_8. This compound:

    A. is a straight chain.
    B. is branched.
    C. contains a ring.
    D. is none of these.

19. The general formula for an alkene with one double bond and no rings is:

    A. C_nH_{2n-2}
    B. C_nH_{2n+2}
    C. C_nH_n
    D. C_nH_{2n}

20. Which of the following is the most stable carbocation?

    A. 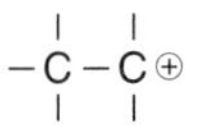 $-\overset{|}{\underset{|}{C}}-\overset{|}{\underset{|}{C}}\oplus$

    B. $-\overset{|}{\underset{|}{C}}-\overset{|}{\underset{|}{C}}\oplus$ with $-\overset{|}{\underset{|}{C}}-$

    C. $-\overset{|}{\underset{|}{C}}-\overset{|}{\underset{|}{C}}\oplus$ with $-\overset{|}{\underset{|}{C}}-$ above and $-\overset{|}{\underset{|}{C}}-$ below

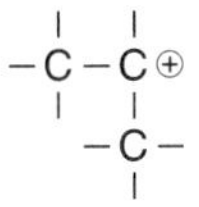

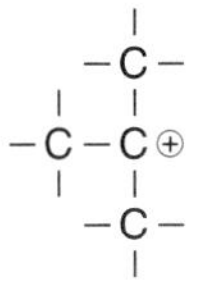

    D. 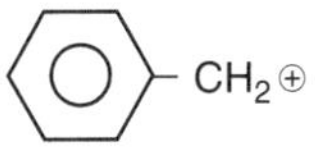 ⬡$- CH_2\oplus$

21. Which of the following is the most unstable carbocation?

    A. 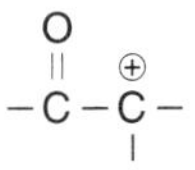 $-C-\overset{\oplus}{\underset{|}{C}}-$ with $\overset{O}{\overset{||}{}}$ on the first C

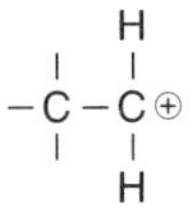

    B. $-\overset{|}{\underset{|}{C}}-\overset{H}{\underset{H}{C}}\oplus$

    C. $H-\overset{H}{\underset{H}{C}}\oplus$

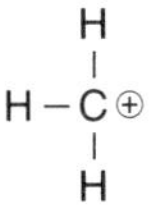

    D. 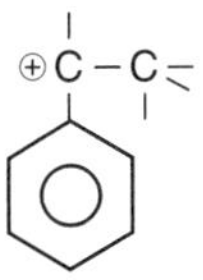 $\oplus\overset{}{C}-\overset{|}{\underset{|}{C}}$ ⬡

22. Although alkanes and alkenes are both composed of carbon and hydrogen, alkenes may show _____ due to _____.

    A. hydrogen bonding; the double bond
    B. less reactivity; the double bond
    C. polarity; *cis-trans* isomerism
    D. nonreactivity; high solubility

23. Name the compound shown in the following figure.

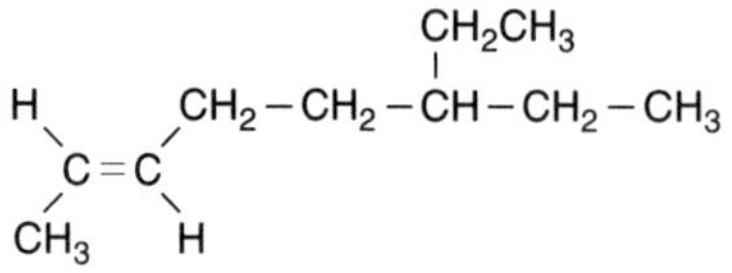

$$
\begin{array}{c}
\text{CH}_2\text{CH}_3 \\
| \\
\text{CH}_2-\text{CH}_2-\text{CH}-\text{CH}_2-\text{CH}_3
\end{array}
$$

H   CH₂–CH₂–CH–CH₂–CH₃
C=C
CH₃   H

A. 2-Ethyl-*trans*-6-octene
B. 6-Ethyl-*trans*-2-octene
C. 2-Ethyl-*cis*-6-octene
D. 6-Ethyl-*cis*-2-octene

24. Select the structure for 3,4-Dimethyl-cis-2-trans-4-heptadiene.

A. 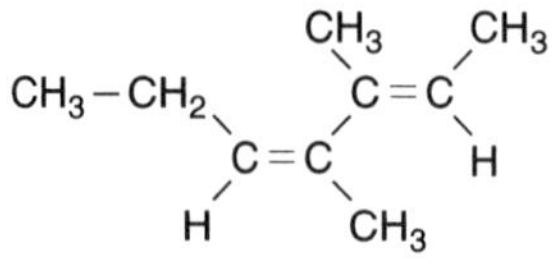
$$
\begin{array}{ccc}
 & \text{CH}_3 & \text{CH}_3 \\
\text{CH}_3-\text{CH}_2 & \diagdown \quad / & \\
 & \text{C}=\text{C} & \\
 & \diagup \qquad \diagdown & \\
 & \text{C}=\text{C} & \\
 & \diagup \qquad \diagdown & \\
 & \text{H} \qquad \text{CH}_3 & \text{H}
\end{array}
$$

B.
$$
\begin{array}{cc}
 & \text{CH}_3 \quad \text{H} \\
\text{H} & \diagdown \;\; / \\
 \diagdown & \text{C}=\text{C} \\
\text{C}=\text{C} & \diagdown \\
 / & \text{CH}_3 \\
\text{CH}_3-\text{CH}_2 \quad \text{CH}_3 &
\end{array}
$$

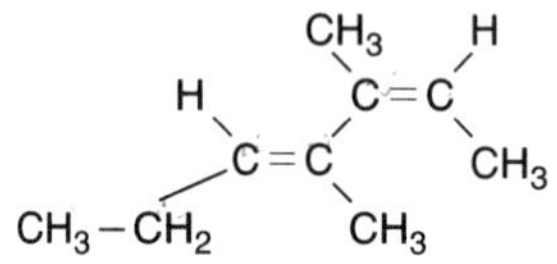

C.
$$
\begin{array}{c}
\text{CH}_3 \\
| \\
\text{CH}_3-\text{CH}_2-\text{CH} \qquad \text{CH}_2\text{CH}_3 \\
\diagdown \qquad / \\
\text{C}=\text{C} \\
/ \qquad \diagdown \\
\text{H} \qquad \text{CH}_3
\end{array}
$$

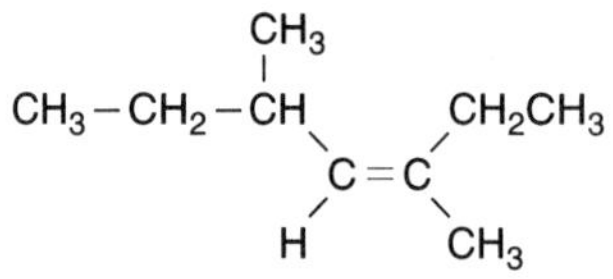

D. None of the above

25. A double bond can stabilize an adjacent carbocation by _____ (of) the positive charge with its _____-bond.

A. neutralizing; p
B. neutralizing; s
C. delocalization; p
D. delocalization; s

26. The reaction of H⁺ with the following compound will form which carbocation shown in the figure.,s(99%)

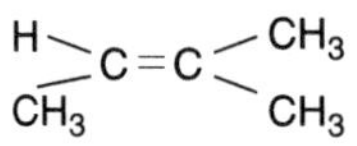

$$
\begin{array}{cc}
\text{H} & \diagup \text{CH}_3 \\
\diagdown \text{C}=\text{C} & \\
\text{CH}_3 & \diagdown \text{CH}_3
\end{array}
$$

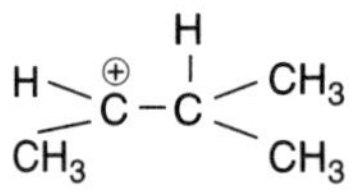

A.
$$
\begin{array}{cc}
 & \text{H} \\
 & | \\
\text{H} \diagdown \overset{\oplus}{\text{C}}-\text{C} & \diagup \text{CH}_3 \\
\text{CH}_3 & \diagdown \text{CH}_3
\end{array}
$$

B.
$$
\begin{array}{cc}
 & \text{H} \\
 & | \\
\text{H} \diagdown \text{C}-\overset{\oplus}{\text{C}} & \diagup \text{CH}_3 \\
\text{CH}_3 & \diagdown \text{CH}_3
\end{array}
$$

C.
$$
\begin{array}{cc}
 & \text{H} \\
 & | \\
\overset{\oplus}{} \diagup \text{C}-\text{C} & \diagup \text{CH}_3 \\
\text{CH}_2 \quad \text{H} \;\; \text{H} & \diagdown \text{CH}_3
\end{array}
$$

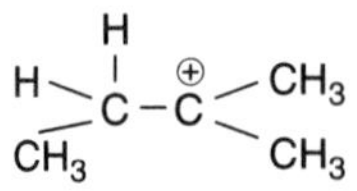

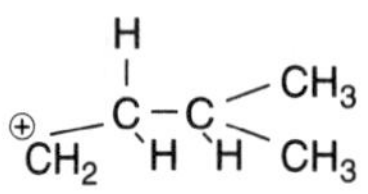

D. None of the above

27. The product of the reaction shown in the following figure is:

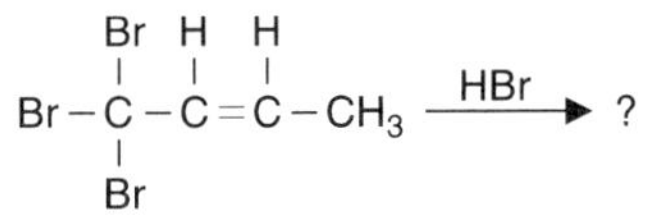

$$\text{Br}-\underset{\underset{\displaystyle \text{Br}}{|}}{\overset{\overset{\displaystyle \text{Br}}{|}}{\text{C}}}-\overset{\overset{\displaystyle \text{H}}{|}}{\text{C}}=\overset{\overset{\displaystyle \text{H}}{|}}{\text{C}}-\text{CH}_3 \xrightarrow{\text{HBr}} \text{?}$$

A. $\text{Br}-\underset{\underset{\displaystyle \text{Br}}{|}}{\overset{\overset{\displaystyle \text{Br}}{|}}{\text{C}}}-\underset{\underset{\displaystyle \text{H}}{|}}{\overset{\overset{\displaystyle \text{H}}{|}}{\text{C}}}-\underset{\underset{\displaystyle \text{H}}{|}}{\overset{\overset{\displaystyle \text{H}}{|}}{\text{C}}}-\text{CH}_3$

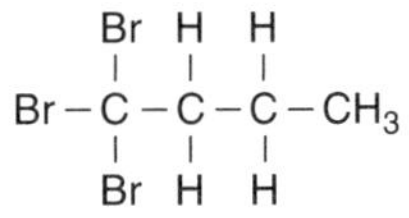

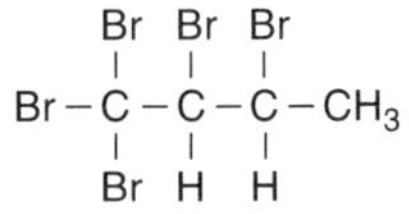

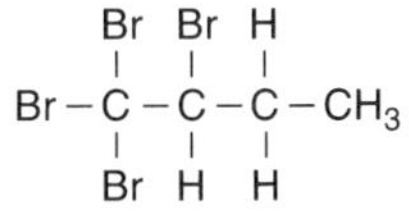

B. $\text{Br}-\underset{\underset{\displaystyle \text{Br}}{|}}{\overset{\overset{\displaystyle \text{Br}}{|}}{\text{C}}}-\underset{\underset{\displaystyle \text{H}}{|}}{\overset{\overset{\displaystyle \text{Br}}{|}}{\text{C}}}-\underset{\underset{\displaystyle \text{H}}{|}}{\overset{\overset{\displaystyle \text{Br}}{|}}{\text{C}}}-\text{CH}_3$

C. $\text{Br}-\underset{\underset{\displaystyle \text{Br}}{|}}{\overset{\overset{\displaystyle \text{Br}}{|}}{\text{C}}}-\underset{\underset{\displaystyle \text{H}}{|}}{\overset{\overset{\displaystyle \text{Br}}{|}}{\text{C}}}-\underset{\underset{\displaystyle \text{H}}{|}}{\overset{\overset{\displaystyle \text{H}}{|}}{\text{C}}}-\text{CH}_3$

(D.) $\text{Br}-\underset{\underset{\displaystyle \text{Br}}{|}}{\overset{\overset{\displaystyle \text{Br}}{|}}{\text{C}}}-\underset{\underset{\displaystyle \text{H}}{|}}{\overset{\overset{\displaystyle \text{H}}{|}}{\text{C}}}-\underset{\underset{\displaystyle \text{H}}{|}}{\overset{\overset{\displaystyle \text{Br}}{|}}{\text{C}}}-\text{CH}_3$

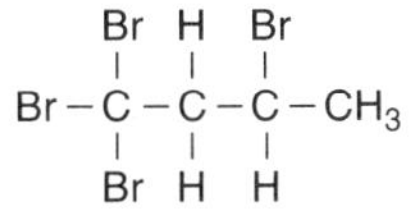

28. Which of the following compounds has the higher boiling point?

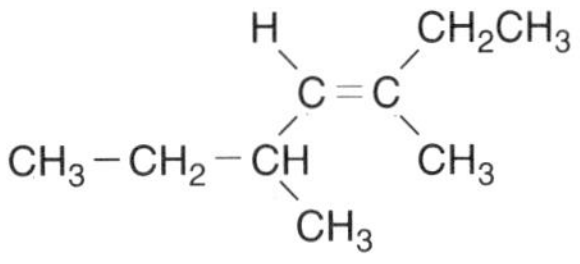

I: CH_3–CH_2–CH(CH_3) with H/CH_2CH_3 and C=C/CH_3

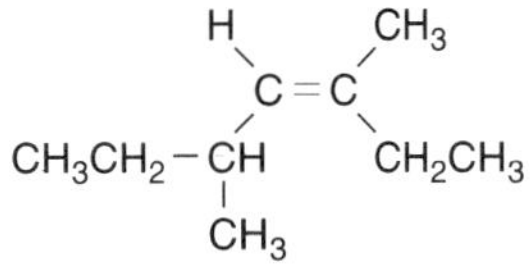

II: CH_3CH_2–CH(CH_3) with H/CH_3 and C=C/CH_2CH_3

A. I
(B.) II   *cis*
C. Both have the same boiling point.
D. I and II do not boil at any temperature.

29. Which of the following compounds has the higher dipole moment?

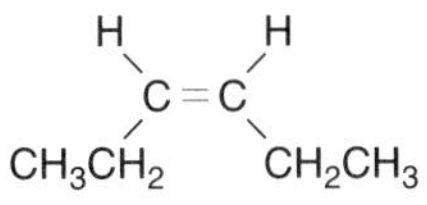

I: C=C with H/H top, CH_3CH_2/CH_2CH_3 bottom

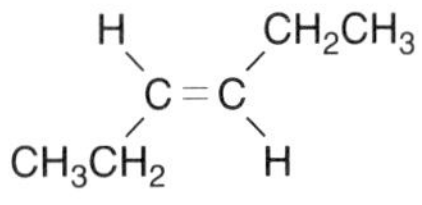

II: C=C with H/CH_2CH_3 top, CH_3CH_2/H bottom

(A.) I
B. II
C. Both have equal dipole moments.
D. I and II have no dipole moment.

30. Hydrocarbons having two double bonds are called:

A. ethenes.
(B.) dienes.
C. ethynes.
D. hexenes.

31. Which of the following hydrocarbons contains a triple bond between adjacent carbon atoms?

   A. Alkanes
   B. Alkenes
   C. Dienes
   D. Alkynes

32. Name the compound shown in the following figure.

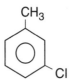

   A. o-Chlorotoluene
   B. p-Chloromethylbenzene
   C. 1-Methyl-2-chlorobenzene
   D. None of the above

33. Name the compound shown in the following figure.

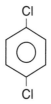

   A. p-Dichlorobenzene
   B. m-Dichlorobenzene
   C. 1,3-Dichlorobenzene
   D. None of the above

34. Select the structure of 2-chloro-4-iodonitrobenzene.

   A.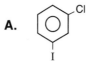

   B.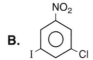

   C.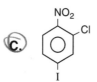

   D. None of the above

35. In the following figure, select the positions that will have the most electron density because of delocalization.

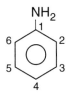

A. 1,3,5
B. 3,4,5
C. 2,5
D. None of the above

36. In the following figure, select the positions that will have the most electron density due to delocalization.

NO$_2$

A. 3,5
B. 2,4,6
C. 3,4,5
D. None of the above

37. If Br$^+$ is an electrophile (e.g., from Br$_2$ + AlCl$_3$), the most likely product of its reaction with the following compound is:

O—CH$_3$

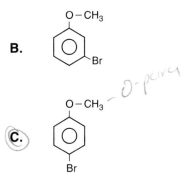

A.

B.

C.

D. None of the above

38. Assume the Br$^+$ from question 37 reacts with the following compound. The most likely product is:

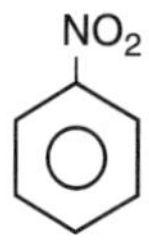

NO$_2$

A. 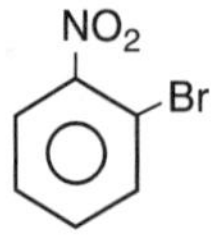 NO$_2$ Br

B. 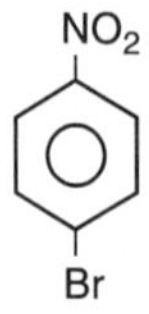 NO$_2$ Br

C. 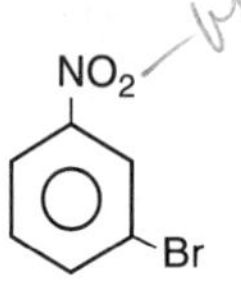 NO$_2$ —*mety* Br

D. None of the above

1–7. **1-A, 2-D, 3-C, 4-A, 5-A, 6-D, 7-A.** See text for explanation.

8. B The numbering is as shown in the following figure.

$$C$$
$$|$$
$$\underset{1}{C} - \underset{2}{C} - \underset{|3}{C} - \underset{4}{C} - \underset{5}{C}$$
$$C$$

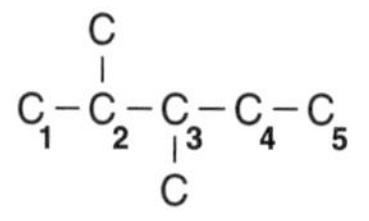

9. C The numbering is as shown in the following figure.

$$C_9 - C_{10}\ C \qquad C_4 - C_3 - \overset{C_1}{C_2}$$
$$C - C_8 - C_7 - C_6 - C_5 \qquad\qquad C$$
$$|\qquad\qquad\qquad\quad C - C$$
$$C\qquad\qquad\qquad\qquad |$$
$$\qquad\qquad\qquad\qquad\quad C$$

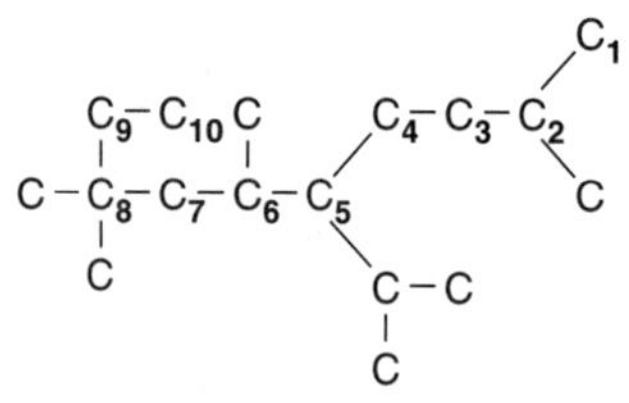

10–12. **10-B, 11-D, 12-B.** See text for explanation.
13. A Compound II is more branched than I and has a lower predicted boiling point.
14. B Compound II has the higher molecular weight and the higher predicted boiling point.
15. A The structure is as shown in the figure.

The formula is $C_{10}H_{22}$. The equation is $C_{10}H_{22} + {}^{31}\!/_2\ O_2 \rightarrow 10CO_2 + 11H_2O$.

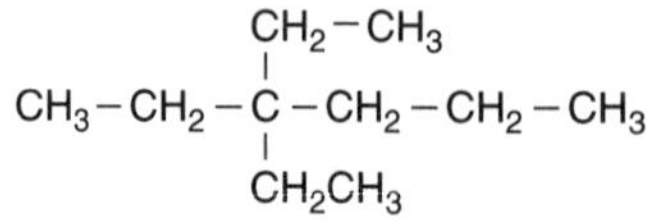

$$CH_2 - CH_3$$
$$|$$
$$CH_3 - CH_2 - C - CH_2 - CH_2 - CH_3$$
$$|$$
$$CH_2CH_3$$

16. A See text for explanation.

17. B The resulting radicals would be as shown in the figure. Then the 3° radical (II) is the most stable.

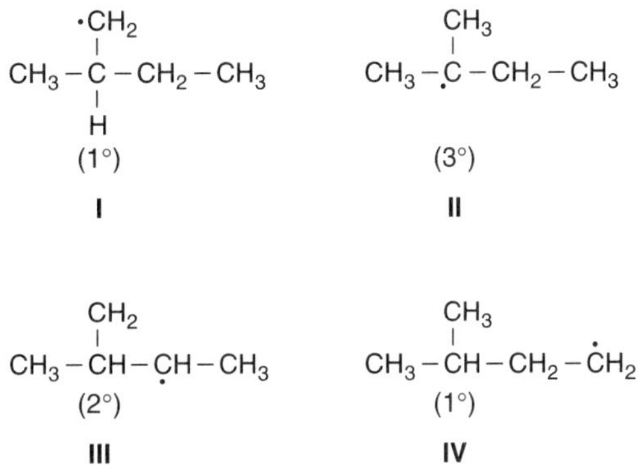

$$\underset{\text{I}}{\underset{(1°)}{\overset{\cdot CH_2}{\overset{|}{CH_3-\overset{|}{\underset{|}{C}}-CH_2-CH_3}}}} \qquad \underset{\text{II}}{\underset{(3°)}{\overset{CH_3}{\overset{|}{CH_3-\overset{|}{\underset{|}{\cdot C}}-CH_2-CH_3}}}}$$

$$\underset{\text{III}}{\underset{(2°)}{\overset{CH_2}{\overset{|}{CH_3-CH-\overset{|}{\underset{\cdot}{C}H}-CH_3}}}} \qquad \underset{\text{IV}}{\underset{(1°)}{\overset{CH_3}{\overset{|}{CH_3-CH-CH_2-\overset{\cdot}{C}H_2}}}}$$

18. C Because the compound is an alkane, there are no double or triple bonds. One would expect C_4H_{10} to be a fully saturated alkane without rings. The two missing H's (C_4H_8) suggest the presence of one ring.

19–22. 19-D, 20-C, 21-A, 22-C. See text for explanation.

23. B The numbering is as shown on the figure.

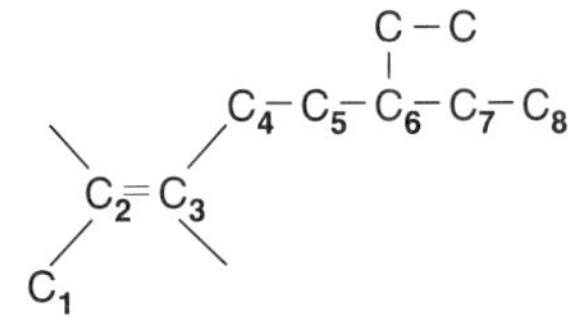

$$\overset{\displaystyle \overset{C-C}{\overset{|}{}}}{C_4^- C_5^- C_6^- C_7^- C_8}$$
$$C_2 = C_3$$
$$C_1$$

24–25. 24-B, 25-C. See text for explanation.

26. B The only possible cations from this double bond are **A**, which is 2°, and **B**, which is 3°. Tertiary (3°) is more stable than secondary (2°).

27. D The mechanism is as shown in the first figure. This carbocation is more stable than the alternate because of the adjacent brominated carbons as shown in the second figure.

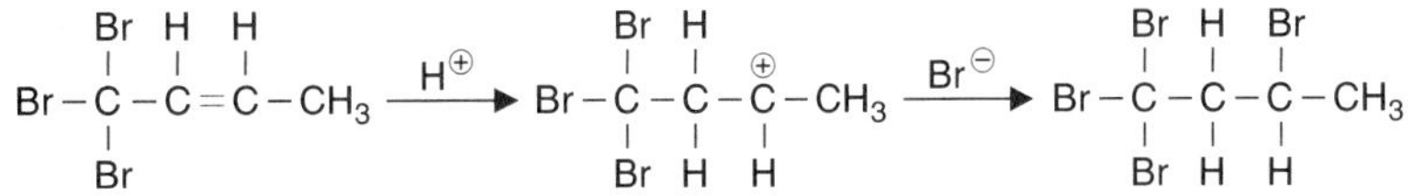

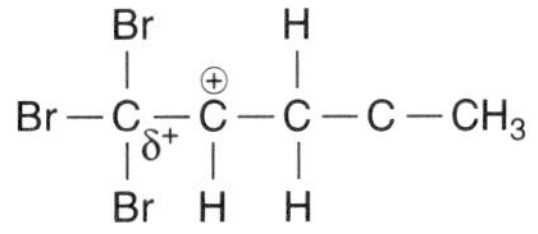

$$\underset{Br}{\overset{Br\; H\; H}{Br-C-C=C-CH_3}} \xrightarrow{H^\oplus} \underset{Br\;H\;H}{\overset{Br\;H}{Br-C-C-\overset{\oplus}{C}-CH_3}} \xrightarrow{Br^\ominus} \underset{Br\;H\;H}{\overset{Br\;H\;Br}{Br-C-C-C-CH_3}}$$

$$\underset{Br\;H\;H}{\overset{Br\qquad H}{Br-C_{\underset{\delta^+}{-}}\overset{\oplus}{C}-C-C-CH_3}} \quad \text{(alternate; less stable)}$$

28. B *Cis* compounds tend to have higher boiling points because of higher polarity than the corresponding *trans* compound.

29. A See question 10. See text for explanation.

30–31. 30-B, 31-D, 36-A. See text for explanation.

32. D The correct name is m-chlorotoluene (others are also possible).

33–36. 33-A, 34-C, 35-D, 36-A. See text for explanation.

37. C The —O—CH_3 is an ortho-para director. Of the products shown, **C** is the most likely. This para-product is also favored over the ortho-product because of steric (bulk) considerations.

38. C —NO_2 is a meta director.

Oxygen-Containing Compounds— Alcohols, Aldehydes, and Ketones

Self-Managed Learning Questions

Focus on the following experimental issues:

1. Is there any research study or hypotheses testing on the use of oxygen-containing compounds?
2. Are there any clinical laboratory tests or applications of oxygen-containing compounds related to specimen collection, specimen classification and types, collection time for specimens, specimen handling, and any experimental errors?
3. Are there any theories or laws related to oxygen-containing compounds that need clarification or synthesis with bioclinical applications? Explore at least two or three viewpoints and give a technical critique of such issues.
4. Are there any graphs, diagrams, reaction mechanisms, or sketches that require quantitative analysis? Which mathematical concepts will help in interpreting graphical data?

GENERAL PRINCIPLES

Oxygen-containing organic compounds are classified as alcohols, aldehydes, ketones, carboxylic acids and their derivatives, ethers, and phenols. See also Carboxylic Acids and Derivatives, Ethers, and Phenols. General principles of oxygen-containing compounds are broadly classified into five types: hydrogen bonds and solubility, steric effects of substituents, electronic effects of substituents, acidity and basicity, and other miscellaneous principles.

1. **Hydrogen bonding and solubility**: The carbon atom in alcohols bonded to the OH group is called carbinol carbon. Primary and secondary alcohols have at least one H on the carbinol carbon. They oxidize to carbonyl compounds in the presence of copper at approximately 300°C. Hydrogen atom in alcohols is weakly acidic. Thiols or mercaptans, which are sulfur analogs of alcohols, are represented by RSH (compared with ROH for alcohols). Hydrocarbon molecules are not associated with each other through hydrogen bonds. As the length of the alkane molecular chain gets longer, the solubility of alcohols in water decreases (e.g., ethyl alcohol is more soluble than decyl alcohol). Most alcohol reactions have O—H bond cleavage (this cleavage forms carboxylic acid esters) and C—O bond cleavage (this cleavage forms alkyl halides). The carbonyl oxygen atom in aldehydes and ketones helps form stronger hydrogen bonds with water. Carboxylic acids, which have polar molecules, can form strong hydrogen bonds with each other as well as with water. Solubility of carboxylic acids in water decreases as the length of the carbon chain increases. Carboxylic acids and alcohols are similar in solubility characteristics. Ether molecules cannot associate with each other through hydrogen bonds but can form hydrogen bonds with water. Phenols form strong hydrogen bonds like alcohols.
2. **Steric effects of substituents**: Nucleophilic reactions are affected by steric effects, especially steric hindrance. **Steric hindrance** is caused by arrangements of atomic or functional groups, causing hindrance at the reaction site and hindering rates of S_N2 reactions. Steric hindrance occurs in certain nucleophilic addition reactions (aldehydes and ketones) and in nucleophilic substitution reactions (carboxylic acid derivatives). The carbonyl carbon atom provides the reaction site or the reacting part of the molecule. Ketones with steric hindrance at the carbonyl group cannot form cyanohydrins. Aldehyde-ketone substitutions differ from carboxylic acid derivatives substitutions in that nucleophilic reactions use the addition-elimination mechanism to overcome steric hindrance.
3. **Electronic effects of substituents**: Effects of activating and deactivating substituents occur in all oxygen-containing compounds. The electronic effects include reactivity, acidity, stereoarrangements and inductive effect in carboxylic acids. Activating substituents usually increase the reaction rate, whereas deactivating substituents decrease the reaction rate. The inductive effects are more pronounced in carboxylic acids. The acidity of phenol is due to the fact that the phenoxide ion has greater resonance stabilization.
4. **Acidity and basicity**: The α-hydrogen in carbonyl compounds (aldehydes and ketones) makes them acidic. The α-hydrogen is attached to a carbon atom called α-carbon. The pK_a values for α-hydrogen are approximately 20 (for aldehydes and ketones). Resonance stability of the anion causes this higher acidity. Tautomers, which are in reversible equilibrium, are keto and enol forms of isomers, which

are interconvertible. The α, β unsaturated carbonyls react with nucleophilic reagents by simple or conjugate addition, such as with Michael additions, which are special conjugate additions. Delocalized carbanions are formed by the nucleophilic aromatic substitution mechanism (S_NAr).

5. **Miscellaneous principles**: Alcohols can typically be synthesized by hydration of alkenes under acidic conditions. A mixture of two liquids with a boiling point either higher or lower than that of the ingredients is called an **azeotrope**. In studying permeability of biological cell membranes, the role of crown ethers and host (crown) and guest (cation) relationship should be covered. An excessively acidic medium (e.g., HBr) causes dialkyl ethers to cleave and form alkyl halides. Dialkyl ethers lack reactivity with bases. Ethers have weak basicity due to their O group. Carboxylate ions or anions (negatively charged) are not reactive toward nucleophilic substitution. Proton migration from α-carbon to oxygen in aldehydes and ketones with α-hydrogen forms a special isomer called enol.

ALCOHOLS

Nomenclature and Physical Properties

See Hydrocarbons for the basics of nomenclature. Alcohols are named by replacing the -e of the corresponding alkane with -ol for simple alcohols. For example, methane (CH_4) becomes methanol, or methyl alcohol (CH_4OH) and propane ($CH_3CH_2CH_3$) becomes propanol, or propyl alcohol ($CH_3CH_2CH_3OH$).

For more complex alcohols, the numbering system is used and the carbon with the —OH should, in general, have the lowest number (if the compound is named as an alcohol) [Figure 8-193]. The use of sec-, iso-, and tert- are appropriate for common names only (Figure 8-194).

Alcohols are acidic because of the —OH group (Figure 8-195). They are very weakly acidic, being less strong than water. As the number of carbon groups attached to the C increases, the acidity decreases:

$$CH_3OH > CH_3CH_2OH \text{ in acidity (Figure 8-196).}$$

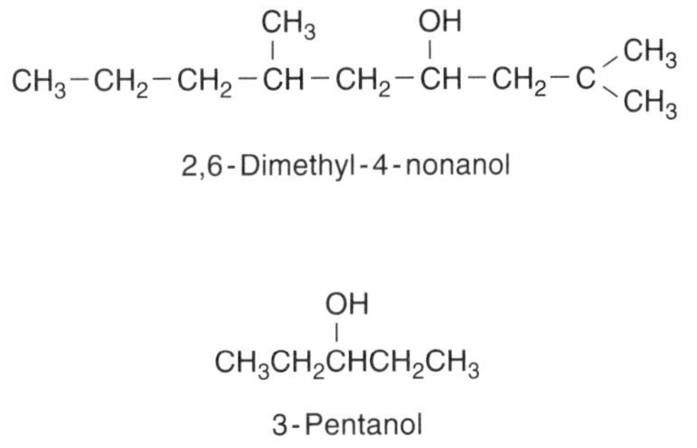

2,6-Dimethyl-4-nonanol

3-Pentanol

Fig. 8-193

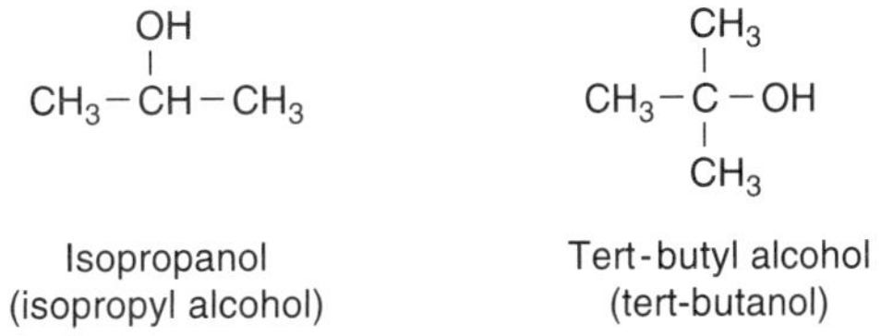

Isopropanol
(isopropyl alcohol)

Tert-butyl alcohol
(tert-butanol)

Fig. 8-194

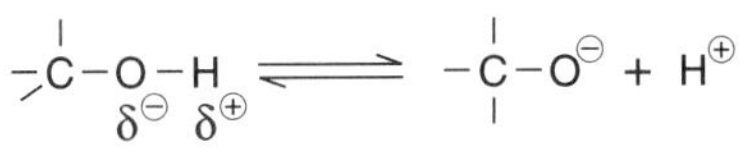

Fig. 8-195

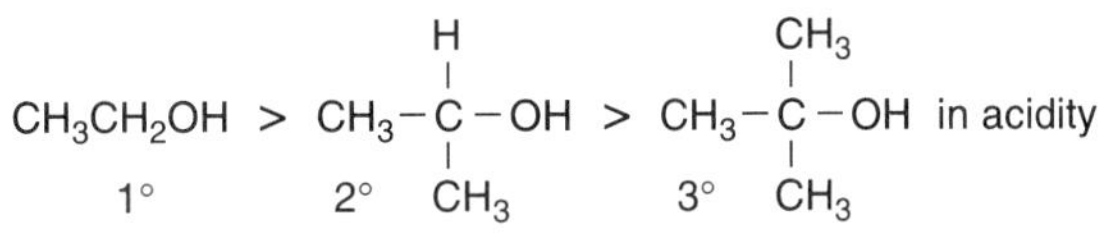

Fig. 8-196

See Hydrocarbons for general comments on physical properties of organic compounds. The greater polarity (dipole moment) and, especially, hydrogen bonding account for the greater solubility of alcohols in water and for their higher boiling points than comparable alkanes, alkenes, aldehydes, ketones, and alkyl halides. As the carbon chain gets longer, this nonpolar hydrocarbon chain overshadows the —OH group and alcohols become less soluble in water.

Chemical Reactions

The four major types of reactions of alcohols are dehydration, substitution, elimination, and oxidation.

Dehydration

The **dehydration** of alcohols is catalyzed by acids, and the relative ease of dehydration decreases in the order from tertiary to secondary to primary alcohols. In dehydration of tertiary and secondary alcohols, an intermediate carbocation is formed and the faster reaction occurs with molecules that form the more stable carbocation. Rearrangements occur if a more stable carbocation can be formed by a methyl or hydride shift. The mechanism for dehydration is shown in Figure 8-197. In general, dehydration reactions occur to yield the most substituted alkene as the major product in accordance with Zaitsev's rule. Thus, the alkene formed is the most stable. Note that a phenyl group ($C_6H_5^-$) takes preference over one or two alkyl groups (Figure 8-198).

The substitution reactions of alcohols usually involve the replacement of the —OH by a halide (usually Cl or Br) using a variety of reagents (HCl, HBr, HI, PCl_3, $SOCl_2$). The rate of reaction between an alcohol and a hydrogen halide depends on the structure of the alcohol and the nature of the halide. The mechanism for the reaction of secondary, tertiary, allylic, and benzylic alcohols involves the formation of a carbocation via an S_N1-type process, with the protonated alcohol as substrate. Methanol and primary alcohols react by an S_N2 mechanism and require more rigorous conditions or the addition of acidic reagents such as $ZnCl_2$ or H_2SO_4 to promote reaction. The reactivity of the various hydrogen halides is, in order of their decreasing acidity and reactivity, HI > HBr > HCl $\gg$ HF (in order of decreasing acidity and reactivity).

The general mechanism for reaction is

$$ROH + HX \rightarrow ROH_2^+ + X^- \rightarrow R^+ + HOH \xrightarrow{X^-} R - X$$

The mechanism for primary alcohol is

$$RCH_2OH + HX \rightarrow \overset{\delta-}{X} -- \underset{\underset{R}{|}}{CH_2} -- \overset{\delta+}{OH_2} \longrightarrow RCH_2X + HOH$$

Examples are shown in Figure 8-199. Rearrangements may occur via carbocation intermediate (Figure 8-200).

Primary, secondary, allylic, and benzyl alcohols react readily with $SOCl_2$, PCl_3, and PBr_3 to yield the corresponding halide:

$$ROH + SOCl_2 \rightarrow RCl + SO_2 + HCl$$

$$3ROH + PBr_3 \rightarrow 3RBr + H_3PO_3$$

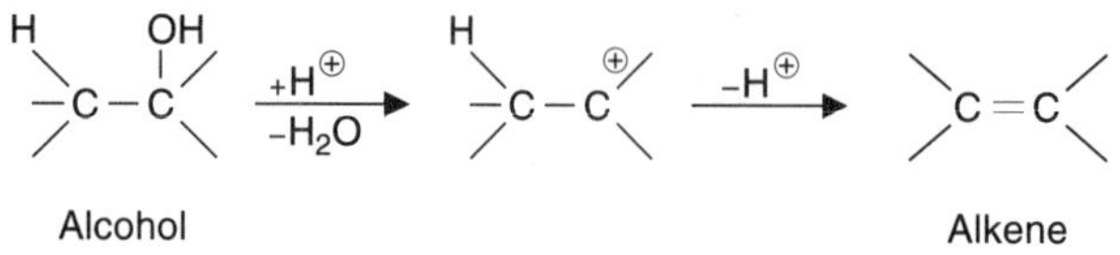

Fig. 8-197. Mechanism for dehydration.

Alcohol   Alkene

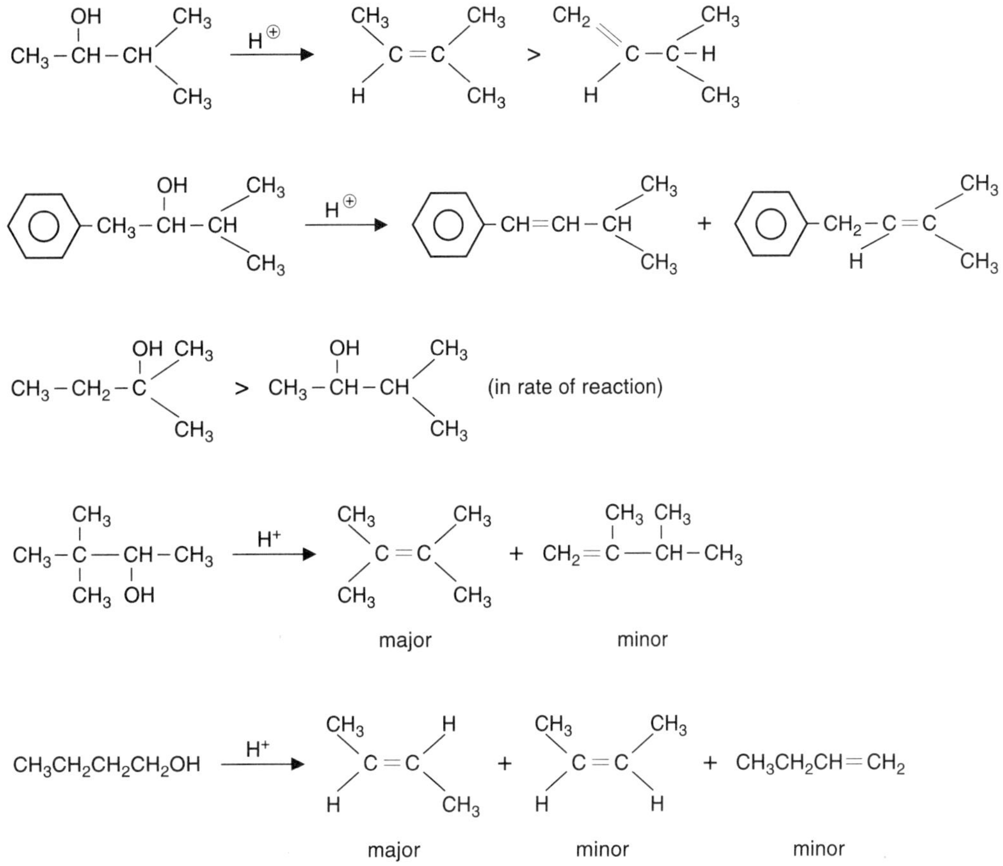

Fig. 8-198

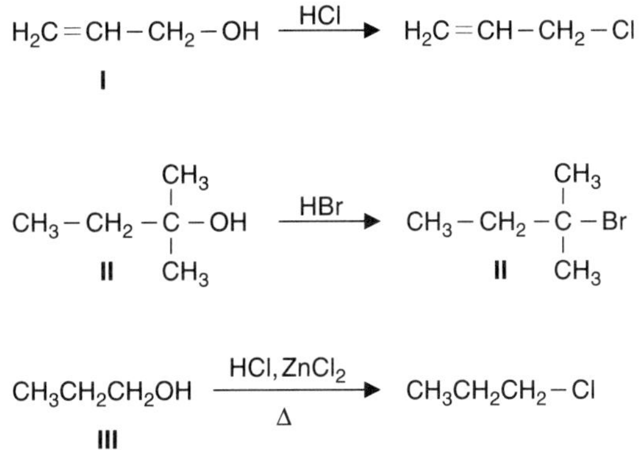

Fig. 8-199

I > II > III in rate of reaction

Fig. 8-200

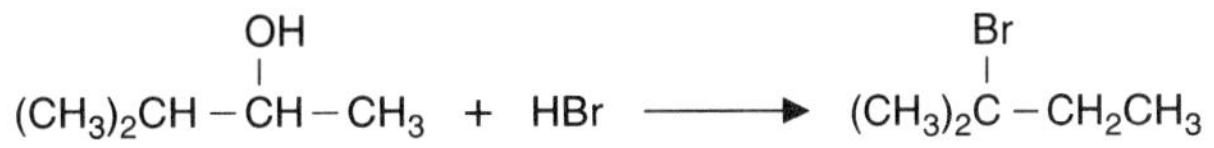

$$(CH_3)_2CH-\overset{\overset{\displaystyle OH}{|}}{CH}-CH_3 \ + \ HBr \ \longrightarrow \ (CH_3)_2\overset{\overset{\displaystyle Br}{|}}{C}-CH_2CH_3$$

Substitution Reactions of Alkyl Halides

Alkyl halides undergo a number of synthetically useful substitution reactions in which the halogen (the leaving group) is replaced by a nucleophile. The overall reaction is $R - L + Nu^- \rightarrow R - Nu + L^-$. Typical nucleophiles ($Nu^-$) include F^-, Cl^-, Br^-, I^-, CN^-, RO^-, HO^-, RS^-, HS^-, and N_3^-. Nucleophilic substitution reactions can be described by two mechanisms (1) S_N2—substitution nucleophilic bimolecular and (2) S_N1—substitution nucleophilic unimolecular.

The S_N2 mechanism involves a concerted attack by the nucleophile on the substrate in the rate-determining step. The rate follows second-order kinetics and is dependent on the concentration of the substrate and the nucleophile. Doubling the concentration of either the substrate or the nucleophile causes the rate to double. If both concentrations are doubled, the reaction proceeds four times faster: Rate = $k_2[RL][Nu^-]$. The process involves attack of the nucleophile from the side opposite the leaving group and results in inversion of configuration. The opposite enantiomer is formed if the alkyl halide is chiral to begin with (Figure 8-201).

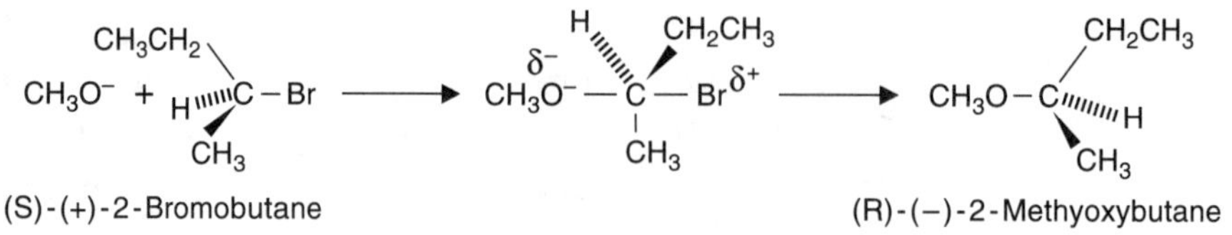

Fig. 8-201. (S)-(+)-2-Bromobutane, (R)-(−)-2-methyoxybutane.

(S)-(+)-2-Bromobutane

(R)-(−)-2-Methyoxybutane

Steric factors are important in S_N2 reactions. The less crowded the transition state, the more rapid the reaction. The order of reaction is $CH_3X > 1°RX > 2°RX > 3°RX$. Methyl halides and primary halides undergo substitution by the S_N2 process. Secondary halides may react by either mechanism, depending on the nucleophile and the solvent. In the presence of a strong nucleophile, secondary halides react by the S_N2 process, whereas, in the presence of a weak nucleophile in a polar solvent, they may react by an S_N1 process. Tertiary halides generally do not react by an S_N2 process.

The order of reactivity of leaving groups is $I^- > Br^- > Cl^- \gg F^-$. A negatively charged nucleophile is more reactive than a neutral one: $RO^- > ROH$, $RS^- > RSH$, $OH^- > ROH$. Ordinarily, if the nucleophilic atom is the same, the more basic nucleophile is the more reactive, that is, $RO^- > RCOO^-$.

The SN_1 mechanism is a two-step process involving formation of a carbocation. The rate is dependent only on the concentration of the substrate: Rate = $k_1[RL]$. Step 1 is $RL \rightarrow R^+ + L^-$ (rate-determining step). Step 2 is $R^+ + Nu^- \rightarrow RNu$.

The S_N1 process is also favored by the use of polar solvents that stabilize the transition state leading to the carbocation. If the substrate is chiral, the S_N1 reaction results in **racemization**. In most cases, racemization is not complete and more of the enantiomer having the inverted configuration is formed. In many S_N1 reactions, the solvent, such as an alcohol or water, serves as the nucleophile and the reaction is termed **solvolysis** (Figure 8-202).

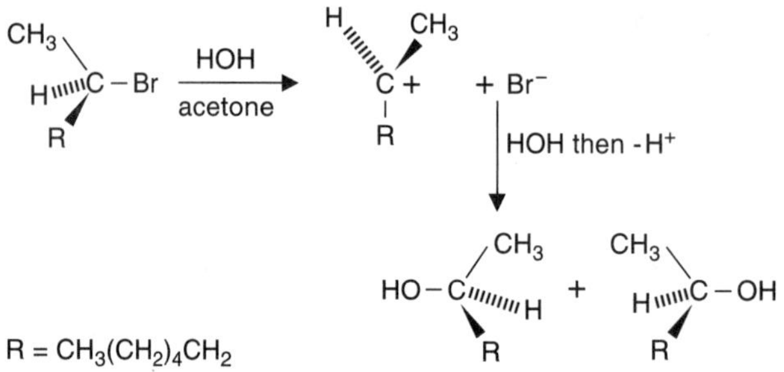

Fig. 8-202   R = $CH_3(CH_2)_4CH_2$

The rate of the reaction depends on the stability of the carbocation formed; therefore, $3°RX > 2°RX > 1°RX > CH_3X$. Generally, only tertiary and secondary halides react by an S_N1 mechanism. Because the S_N1 process involves the formation of a carbocation, rearrangements may occur as shown in Figure 8-203.

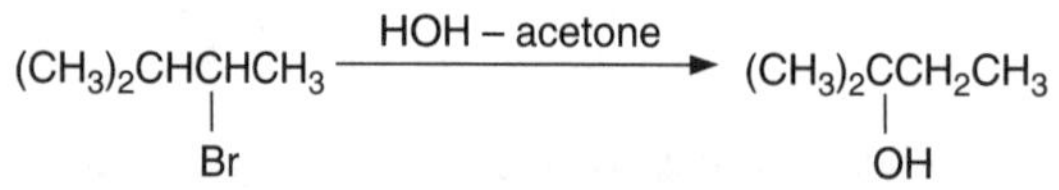

Fig. 8-203

The S_N1 process also is accompanied by alkene formation, resulting from the loss of a proton from the common intermediate, the carbocation. This elimination process is referred to as an **E_1 reaction.** E_1 reactions occur under the same conditions and simultaneously with S_N1 reactions. In solvolysis reactions at lower temperatures, the S_N1 reaction is favored over the E_1 reaction. Substitution reactions of tertiary halides are not very useful as synthetic reactions, because elimination occurs readily, especially if the nucleophile is a moderately strong base. In the presence of strong bases, tertiary halides tend to react by the E_2 process. Vinyl halides (Figure 8-204) and aryl halides (C_6H_5X) are unreactive by either S_N1 or S_N2 processes.

Fig. 8-204 Vinyl halides.

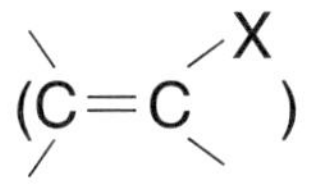

$$\left(\begin{array}{c} \diagdown \\ C = C \diagup \end{array} \begin{array}{c} X \\ \diagdown \end{array} \right)$$

The conversion of alcohols to alkyl halides may be considered as S_N1 or S_N2 processes depending on the type of alcohol.

S_N1 $ROH + HX \rightarrow ROH_2^+ + X^-$

3° and 2° ROH $ROH_2^+ \rightarrow R^+ + HOH$

                     $R^+ + X^- \rightarrow RX$

S_N2 $ROH + HX \rightarrow ROH_2^+ + X^-$

Most 1° ROH $X^- + ROH_2^+ \rightarrow X^{\delta^-} \text{--} R \text{--} {}^{\delta^+}OH_2 \rightarrow RX + HOH$

Elimination Reactions (Dehydrohalogenation Reactions of Alkyl Halides)

The treatment of an alkyl halide with a strong base such as potassium hydroxide or potassium ethoxide in ethanol on heating results in the formation of alkenes. **Dehydrohalogenation reactions**, also called β or 1,2-eliminations, generally occur by an E_2 mechanism. The E2 process is a concerted second-order reaction in which the rate is dependent on the concentration of the alkyl halide and the base: Rate = k[RX][base]. The reaction rate also depends on the nature and type of alkyl halide. The order of reactivity is as follows:

3°RX > 2°RX > 1°RX

RI > RBr > RCl > RF

E_2 reactions occur most rapidly when the hydrogen and the halogen are in an antiperiplanar relationship as shown in Figure 8-205. The reaction occurs to give the more stable

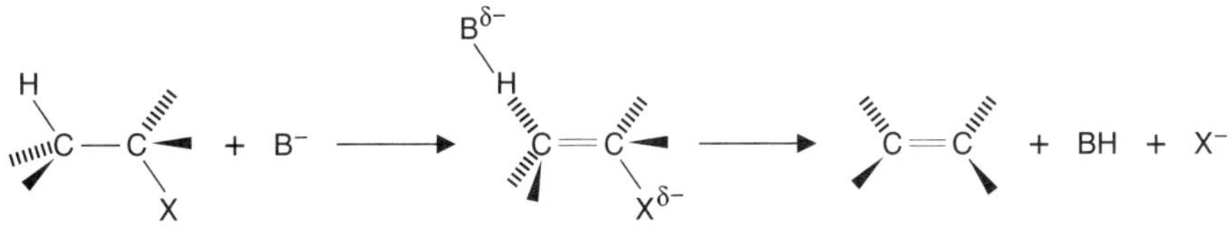

Fig. 8-205

alkene according to Zaitsev's rule and the trans isomer is favored over the cis isomer. Rearrangements do not occur. The use of a bulky base, such as potassium t-butoxide in t-butyl alcohol, favors elimination over substitution. This is especially important in the case of primary halides in which S_N2 substitution competes with E_2 elimination. Tertiary halides tend to undergo elimination reactions readily and, in the presence of a strong base, elimination is favored over substitution. Increased reaction temperature also favors elimination (Figure 8-206).

Oxidation Reactions

Oxidation can convert alcohols to aldehydes, carboxylic acids, or ketones, depending on the structure of the alcohol, the oxidizing agent, and the reaction conditions. Primary alcohols can be oxidized to aldehydes, then to carboxylic acids with potassium permanganate or acidic potassium dichromate (Figure 8-207).

Primary alcohols may be oxidized to aldehydes using chromium trioxide-pyridine complex (Collins' reagent) in an anhydrous medium such as dichloromethane or by copper oxide (Figure 8-208).

Secondary alcohols are readily oxidized to ketones by the same reagents, especially chromium compounds, that are used to oxidize primary alcohols. These oxidations usually stop at the ketone stage because further oxidation would require the breaking of a carbon–carbon bond (Figure 8-209). Tertiary (3°) alcohols are not oxidized under basic conditions but may be oxidized under acidic conditions by being dehydrated first and then oxidation of the double bond.

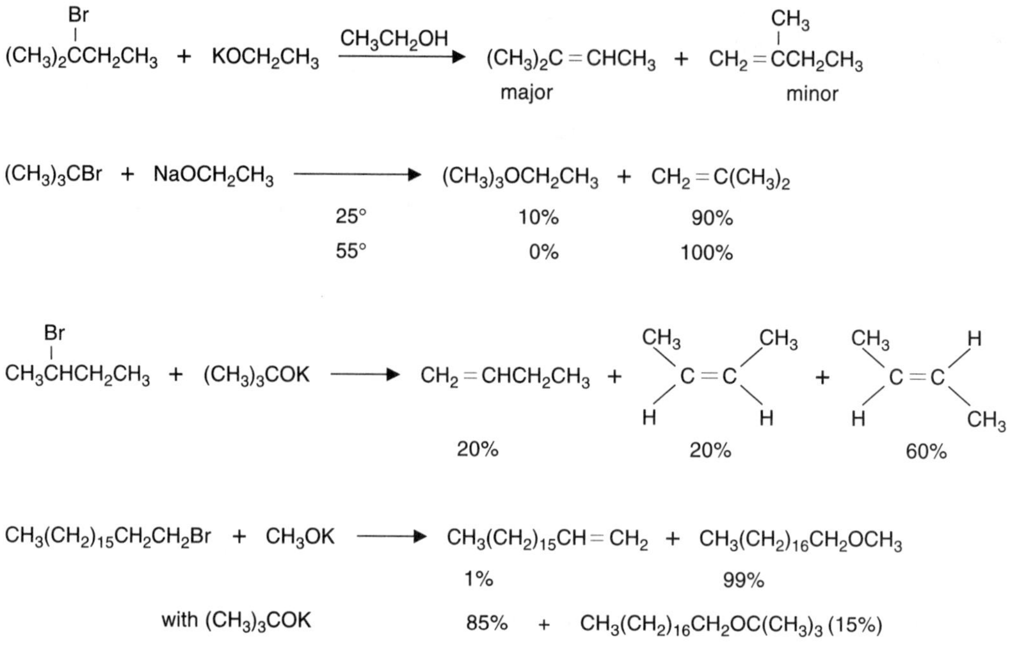

$$(CH_3)_2\overset{\displaystyle Br}{\overset{|}{C}}CH_2CH_3 \ +\ KOCH_2CH_3 \ \xrightarrow{CH_3CH_2OH}\ (CH_3)_2C{=}CHCH_3 \ +\ CH_2{=}\overset{\displaystyle CH_3}{\overset{|}{C}}CH_2CH_3$$

major   minor

$$(CH_3)_3CBr \ +\ NaOCH_2CH_3 \ \longrightarrow\ (CH_3)_3OCH_2CH_3 \ +\ CH_2{=}C(CH_3)_2$$

25°   10%   90%

55°   0%   100%

$$CH_3\overset{\displaystyle Br}{\overset{|}{C}}HCH_2CH_3 \ +\ (CH_3)_3COK \ \longrightarrow\ CH_2{=}CHCH_2CH_3 \ +\ \genfrac{}{}{0pt}{}{CH_3\quad CH_3}{\underset{H\qquad H}{C{=}C}} \ +\ \genfrac{}{}{0pt}{}{CH_3\qquad H}{\underset{H\qquad CH_3}{C{=}C}}$$

20%   20%   60%

$$CH_3(CH_2)_{15}CH_2CH_2Br \ +\ CH_3OK \ \longrightarrow\ CH_3(CH_2)_{15}CH{=}CH_2 \ +\ CH_3(CH_2)_{16}CH_2OCH_3$$

1%   99%

with (CH_3)_3COK   85% + $CH_3(CH_2)_{16}CH_2OC(CH_3)_3$ (15%)

Fig. 8-206

$$RCH_2OH \ \longrightarrow\ RCH{=}O \ \longrightarrow\ RCOOH$$

Fig. 8-207
$$RCH_2OH \ \xrightarrow{KMnO_4 \text{ or } K_2Cr_2O_7,\ H^+}\ RCOOH$$

$$RCH_2OH \ \xrightarrow{CuO,\ \Delta}\ RCH{=}O$$

Fig. 8-208
$$RCH_2OH \ \xrightarrow{(C_5H_5N)_2CrO_3}\ RCH{=}O$$

Fig. 8-209
$$R\overset{\displaystyle}{\underset{\displaystyle R^1}{\overset{|}{C}}}HOH \ \xrightarrow{K_2Cr_2O_7,\ H^+}\ R{-}\underset{\displaystyle R^1}{\overset{|}{C}}{=}O$$

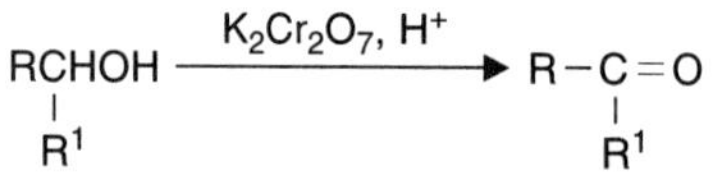

Fig. 8-210
$$R{-}\overset{\displaystyle O}{\overset{\|}{C}}{-}H$$

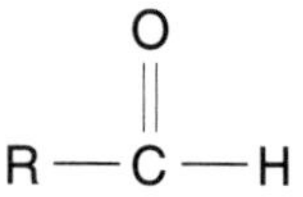

ALDEHYDES AND KETONES

See Hydrocarbons for the basics of nomenclature. Aldehydes are generally symbolized as shown in Figure 8-210.

The suffix -al replaces the -e of alkanes (Figure 8-211). Ketones are generally symbolized as shown in Figure 8-212, and the suffix -one replaces the -e of alkanes (Figure 8-213).

IMPORTANCE OF CARBONYL GROUP

The **carbonyl group** (Figure 8-214) is the basis for the chemistry of aldehydes and ketones. The key features are

1. **Polarity of C=O bond.** The oxygen is attacked by electrophiles (E⊕) and the carbon by nucleophiles (N:⊖). Both of these disrupt the double bond (Figure 8-215). Figure 8-216 shows a large dipole moment.
2. The α-hydrogen is acidic and can be abstracted by bases. It is even more acidic if it is between two carbonyls as shown in Figure 8-217.

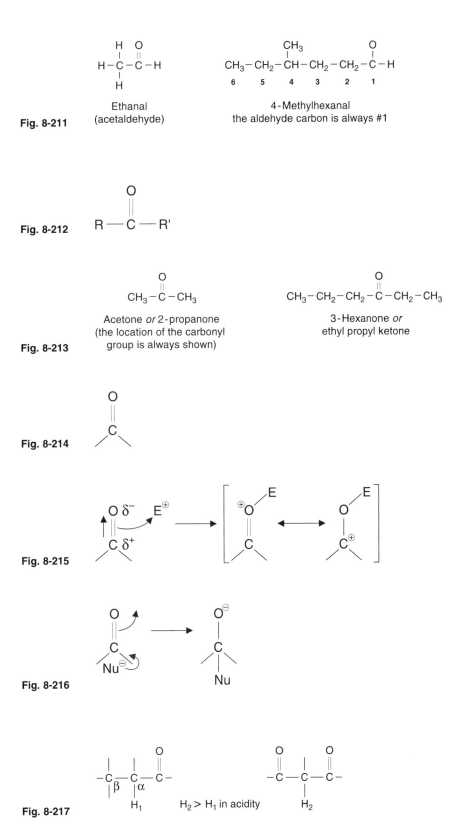

Fig. 8-211 Ethanal (acetaldehyde)

4-Methylhexanal
the aldehyde carbon is always #1

Fig. 8-212

Fig. 8-213 Acetone *or* 2-propanone
(the location of the carbonyl
group is always shown)

3-Hexanone *or*
ethyl propyl ketone

Fig. 8-214

Fig. 8-215

Fig. 8-216

Fig. 8-217 H₂ > H₁ in acidity

Important Reactions

Most of the reactions and properties of carbonyls may be understood on the basis of the following features. In general, aldehydes oxidize easier and undergo nucleophilic addition easier than ketones.

1. When adding nitrogen bases to carbonyls, the N needs two H's (Figure 8-218).

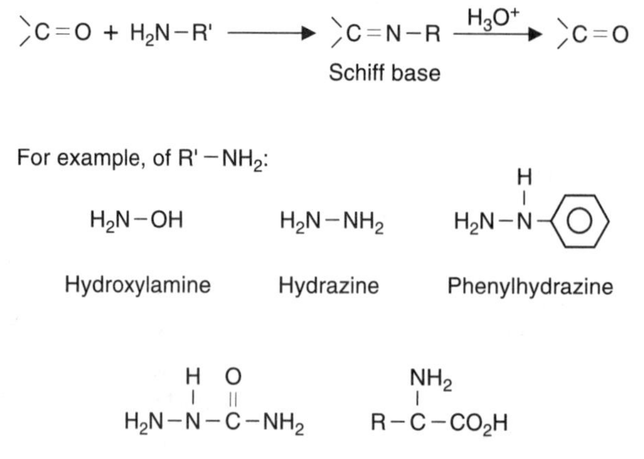

$$\underset{}{\text{>C=O}} + H_2N-R' \longrightarrow \underset{\text{Schiff base}}{\text{>C=N-R}} \xrightarrow{H_3O^+} \text{>C=O}$$

For example, of $R'-NH_2$:

$$H_2N-OH \qquad H_2N-NH_2 \qquad H_2N-N\overset{H}{|}\!\!-\!\!\bigcirc$$

Hydroxylamine   Hydrazine   Phenylhydrazine

$$\overset{H\ \ O}{\underset{|\ \ ||}{H_2N-N-C-NH_2}} \qquad \overset{NH_2}{\underset{|}{R-C-CO_2H}}$$

Fig. 8-218   Semicarbazine   Amino acids

2. Acetal (ketal) and hemiacetal (hemiketal) formations are shown in Figure 8-219.

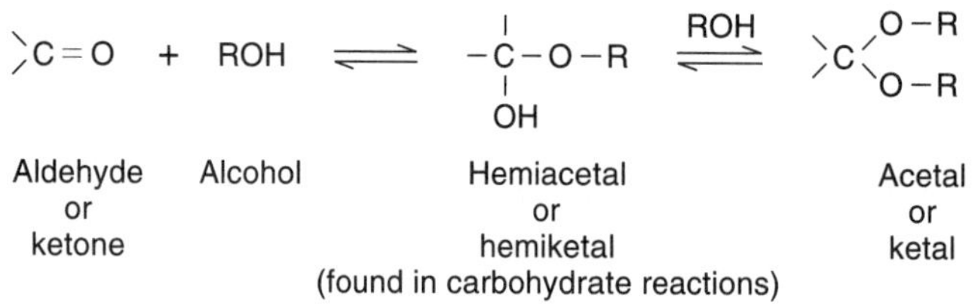

$$\text{>C=O} + ROH \rightleftharpoons \underset{\underset{OH}{|}}{-C-O-R} \xrightarrow[\rightleftharpoons]{ROH} \underset{}{\text{>C}}\overset{O-R}{\underset{O-R}{\diagdown}}$$

Aldehyde   Alcohol   Hemiacetal   Acetal
or   or   or
ketone   hemiketal   ketal

Fig. 8-219   (found in carbohydrate reactions)

3. Ammonia is a nucleophile that can react with an aldehyde or ketone. The product is called an **imine**, containing C=N groups. Schiff base is an imine (Figure 8-220). Imines are important intermediates in the biosynthesis of α-amino acids. Secondary amines (R^2NH) react with aldehydes and ketones, yielding iminium ions that convert to enamines with further reactions (Figure 8-221).

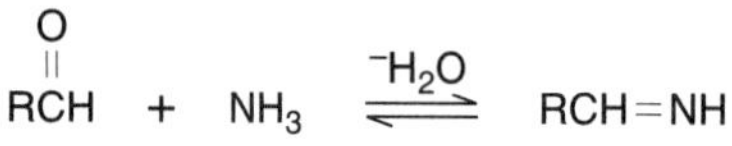

$$\overset{O}{\underset{||}{RCH}} + NH_3 \underset{\rightleftharpoons}{\overset{-H_2O}{\rightleftharpoons}} RCH=NH$$

Fig. 8-220

$$CH_3CHO + (CH_3)_2NH \rightleftharpoons CH_2=CH\overset{..}{N}(CH_3)_2$$

Aldehyde   Dimethyl   Enamine
               amine

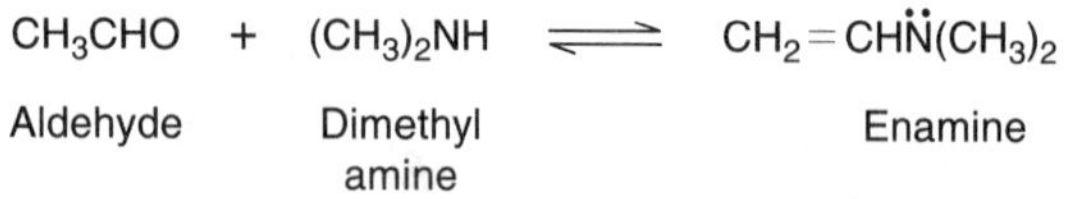

Fig. 8-221

4. In the aldol condensation of carbonyls, the α-H is important as shown in Figure 8-222.

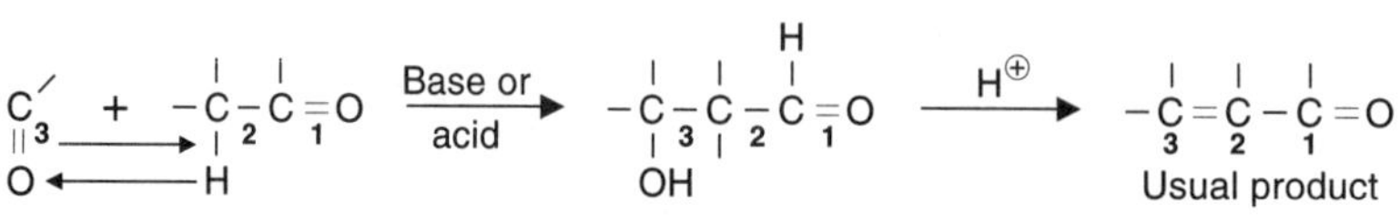

$$\underset{\underset{O}{||}}{\overset{C'}{\underset{3}{}}} + \underset{\underset{H}{|}}{-\overset{|}{\underset{2}{C}}-\overset{|}{\underset{1}{C}}=O} \xrightarrow[\text{acid}]{\text{Base or}} \underset{OH}{-\overset{|}{\underset{3}{C}}-\overset{|}{\underset{2}{C}}-\overset{\overset{H}{|}}{\underset{1}{C}}=O} \xrightarrow{H^{\oplus}} -\overset{|}{\underset{3}{C}}=\overset{|}{\underset{2}{C}}-\overset{|}{\underset{1}{C}}=O$$

Fig. 8-222   Usual product

5. A nucleophilic addition to α, β-unsaturated carbonyls is shown in Figure 8-223.

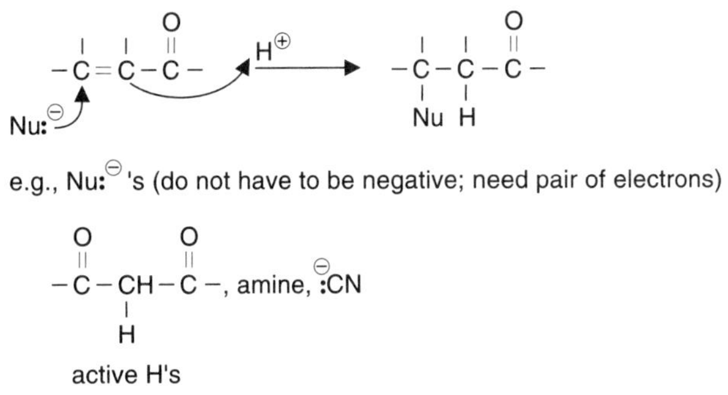

e.g., Nu:$^{\ominus}$'s (do not have to be negative; need pair of electrons)

active H's

Fig. 8-223

6. The carbonyl form of an aldehyde or ketone exists in equilibrium with the enol form. The enol form is a structure having a hydroxyl group attached to a double-bonded carbon. This equilibrium is referred to as keto-enol tautomerism. Tautomers are compounds whose structures differ in the location of an atom, normally a proton, but which exist in equilibrium. Usually, the equilibrium greatly favors

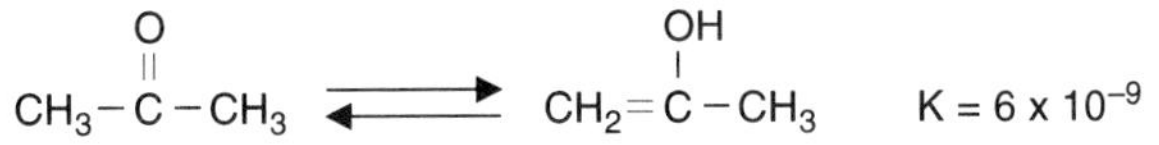

$K = 6 \times 10^{-9}$

Fig. 8-224

the keto forms (Figure 8-224). For 1,3-dicarbonyl compounds, the enol form is often the major tautomer due to the stabilization provided by intramolecular hydrogen bonding and conjugation of the carbonyl group with the double bond (Figure 8-225).

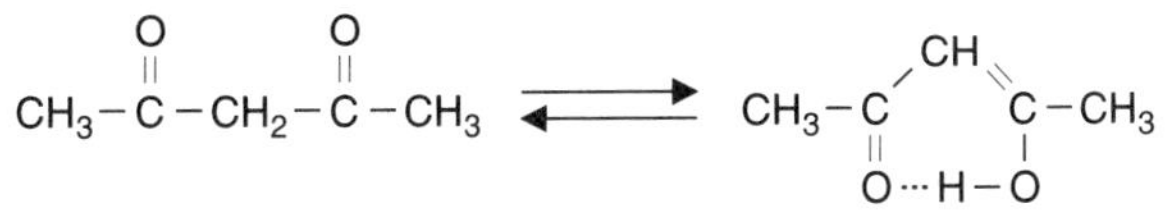

Fig. 8-225

7. The O of the carbonyl forms hydrogen bonds with H's attached to other O's or N's (Figure 8-226).

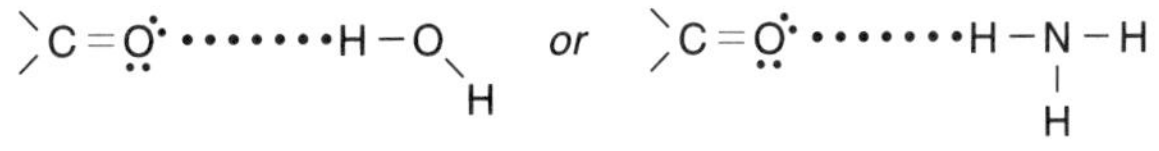

Fig. 8-226

The **boiling point** of aldehydes and ketones is higher than that of most other polar organic molecules but less than that of alcohols and acids (each can hydrogen bond to molecules of itself). The low molecular weight of aldehydes and ketones makes them soluble in water because they can form hydrogen bonds with the water—as the molecular weights increase, the hydrocarbon part dominates and solubility decreases. **Reduction reactions** of carbonyls are shown in Figure 8-227.

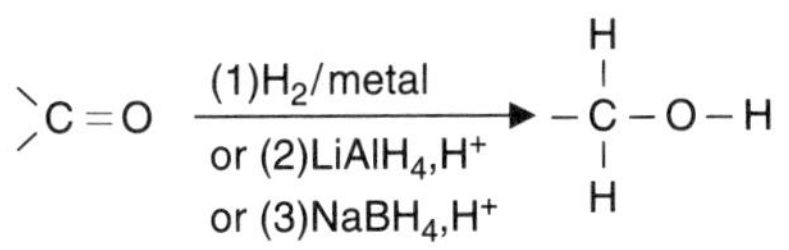

Fig. 8-227

Oxidation Reactions of Aldehydes and Ketones

Ketones are rarely oxidized. **Oxidation reactions** of aldehydes are as follows:

1. $\text{RCHO} \xrightarrow[\text{(Tollen's reagent)}]{\text{Ag(NH}_3)_2 + \text{H}_2\text{O}} \text{R—CO}_2\text{H} + \text{Ag(mirror)}$

    (Ar)   (Ar)

    Ar = Aromatic; Benedict's reagent is also used.

2. $RCHO \xrightarrow[\text{or}]{(1)KMnO_4}$ RCO_2H

$(Ar)(2)K_2Cr_2O_7$ (Ar)

The main reason for the acidity of the α-H is that the resulting α-carbanion is stabilized by resonance. This stabilization also allows for nucleophilic addition at the β-carbon in α-β unsaturated carbonyls as shown in Figure 8-228.

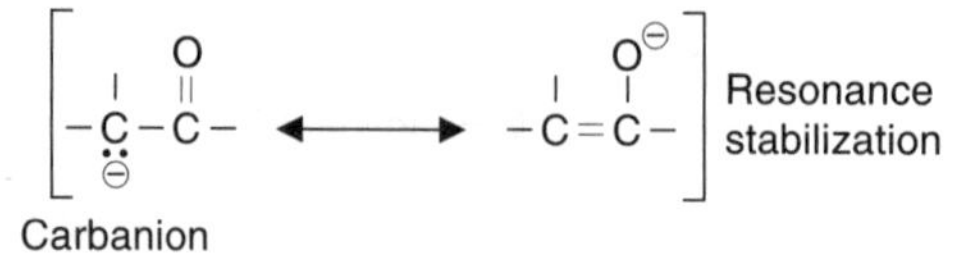

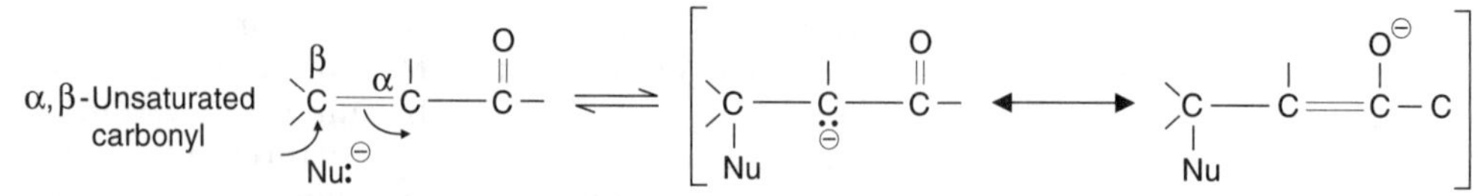

Carbanion

Resonance stabilization

α,β-Unsaturated carbonyl

Fig. 8-228

A carbanion is a species in which there is a carbon atom with a pair of nonbonding electrons and a negative charge. Most carbanions are strong bases.

APPLIED CONCEPTS

The following is a list of tools to analyze and understand alcohols, aldehydes, and ketones.

- Understand how reactions are related to basic mechanisms, how reaction rates are affected, and what bonding arrangements, resonance stability structures, and stereoarrangements are possible. Elucidate each mechanism in a visual format.
- Ponder how organic chemistry of medical compounds (alcohols, aldehydes, and ketones) can be investigated, identified, and linked to the biological side effects (both microscopic and physiologic).
- What biological disorders (e.g., protein deficiency, enzyme deficiency) result from deficiency or abundance of medical compounds (aldehydes, alcohols, and ketones), especially bioorganic molecules?
- Determine how organic reaction mechanisms translate into biochemical reaction mechanisms, such as metabolism.
- Look for hidden assumptions behind each experimental technique or procedure, theoretic explanation, and practical explanation of each mechanism.
- Alcoholism: Methanol is a highly toxic alcohol whose ingestion may lead to blindness and death. In the body, methanol is oxidized to formaldehyde and then to formic acid. It is not certain whether the formaldehyde or the formic acid attacks the cells of the retina and causes blindness. It is known, however, that the formation of formic acid can cause acidosis in the blood, leading to death. Ethanol is first oxidized to acetaldehyde by an enzyme, alcohol dehydrogenase, and then to other products. One treatment of alcohol addiction involves the use of the drug disulfiram (Antabuse), which prevents further oxidation of acetaldehyde, leading to its buildup in the body, causing nausea, vomiting, and sweating. Taking disulfiram may cause aversion to drinking alcohol.

ALCOHOLS, ALDEHYDES, AND KETONES: REVIEW QUESTIONS

1. Alcohols have _____ boiling points and _____ solubility in water than corresponding alkanes and alkenes, which is due to _____.

   A. lower; lesser; hydrogen bonding
   B. higher; greater; hydrogen bonding
   C. lower; lesser; polarity
   D. higher; lesser; polarity

2. In the dehydration reaction of alcohols, the _____ stable double bond is formed.

   A. most
   B. least
   C. complete
   D. incomplete

3. Which of the following alcohols undergoes a substitution reaction the fastest?

   A. Primary
   B. Secondary
   C. Tertiary
   D. Benzyl

4. Which of the following types of alcohols is not normally oxidizable?

   A. Primary
   B. Secondary
   C. Tertiary
   D. All are oxidizable

5. Which type of alcohol probably undergoes substitution by an S_N2 mechanism?

   A. Primary
   B. Tertiary
   C. Allyl
   D. None of the above

6. Name the alcohol shown in the following figure.

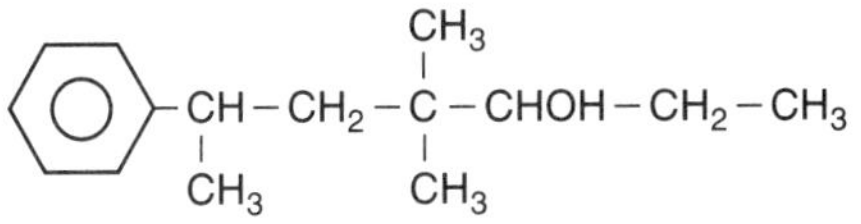

   A. 2-Phenyl-4,4-dimethyl heptanol
   B. 4,4-Dimethyl-6-phenyl-3-heptanol
   C. Phenyl-2-heptanol
   D. None of the above

7. Select the strongest acid shown.

   A. $CH_3-CH-OH$ with CH_3

   B. $CH_3-CH_2-CH-OH$ with CH_3

   C. CH_3-CH_2-C-OH with CH_3 and CH_3

   D. $CH_3-CH_2-CH_2-OH$

8. Which of the following alcohols is least soluble in water?

   A. $CH_3-CH-CH_2-OH$ with CH_3

   B. $CH_3-CH_2-CH_2-CH_2-CH_2-CH_2-OH$

   C. CH_3-CH_2-OH

   D. CH_3OH

9. What is the most likely (or greatest) product of the following reaction?

$$CH_3-CH-\underset{\underset{OH}{|}}{\overset{\overset{CH_3}{|}\quad\overset{CH_2-CH_3}{|}}{C}}-CH_3 \xrightarrow{\ H^{\oplus}\ } ?$$

A.
$$\underset{H_3C}{\overset{H_3C}{>}}C=C\underset{CH_3}{\overset{CH_2-CH_3}{<}}$$

B.
$$\underset{CH_3}{\overset{H_3C}{>}}CH-C\underset{CH_3}{\overset{CH-CH_3}{<}}$$

C.
$$\underset{H_3C}{\overset{H_3C}{>}}CH-C\underset{CH_2}{\overset{CH_2-CH_3}{<}}$$

D. All are equal

10. Which of the following alcohols undergoes the fastest reaction with HBr?

A.

B. CH_3CH_2OH

C. $CH_3-\underset{\underset{OH}{|}}{\overset{\overset{CH_3}{/}}{CH}}$

D. 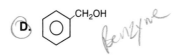 benzyne

11. The carbonyl group is _____ with the carbon being slightly _____ and the oxygen being slightly _____.

   A. polarized; negative; positive
   B. polarized; positive; negative
   C. polarized; positive; positive
   D. polarized; negative; negative

12. Which hydrogen is the most acidic?

$$H-\underset{\underset{H}{|}}{\overset{\overset{H_3}{|}}{C}}-\underset{\underset{H}{|}}{\overset{\overset{H_2}{|}}{C}}-\underset{\underset{H}{|}}{\overset{\overset{H_1}{|}}{C}}-\overset{\overset{O}{||}}{C}-H_4$$

   A. H_1
   B. H_2
   C. H_3
   D. H_4

13. Which of the following will undergo nucleophilic addition more easily?
    A. Aldehydes
    B. Alkenes
    C. Aldehydes and alkenes equally
    D. Neither aldehydes nor alkenes

14. Aldehydes and ketones have higher boiling points than corresponding compounds (similar carbon structures) of all the following except:
    A. alkanes.
    B. alkenes.
    C. ethers.
    D. alcohols.

15. Which of the following groups are rarely oxidized?
    A. Aldehydes
    B. Ketones
    C. Neither A nor B
    D. Both A and B

16. Name the compound shown.

$$CH_3-\underset{\underset{Cl}{|}}{\overset{\overset{CH_3}{|}}{C}}-CH_2CHO$$

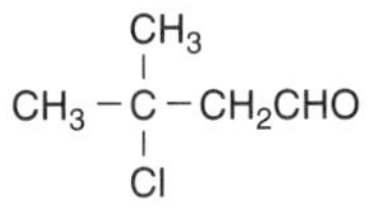

    A. tert-Chlorobutanol
    B. tert-Chlorobutyl ketone
    C. Hydrogen chloro-tert-butyl ketone
    D. 3-Chloro-3-methyl-butanal

17. Name the compound shown.

$$\underset{CH_3}{\overset{CH_3}{>}}CH-\overset{\overset{O}{\|}}{C}-CH_2CH_3$$

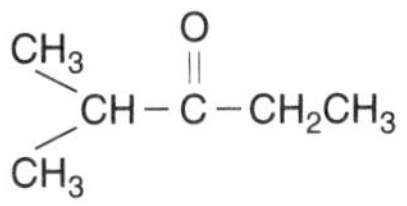

    A. 2-Methyl-3-pentanone
    B. Diethyl methyl ketone
    C. 2-Methyl-3-butanal
    D. Isobutyl ethyl ketone

18. Select the product of the following reaction.

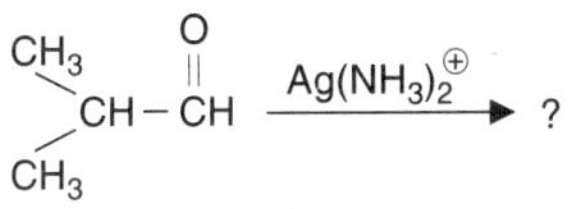

$$\underset{CH_3}{\overset{CH_3}{>}}CH-\overset{\overset{O}{\|}}{C}H \xrightarrow{Ag(NH_3)_2^{\oplus}} ?$$

    A. $$\underset{CH_3}{\overset{CH_3}{>}}CH-\underset{\underset{}{|}}{\overset{\overset{OH}{|}}{C}}H-\underset{\underset{}{|}}{\overset{\overset{OH}{|}}{C}}H-CH\overset{CH_3}{\underset{CH_3}{<}}$$

    B. $$\underset{CH_3}{\overset{CH_3}{>}}CH-\underset{\underset{H}{|}}{\overset{\overset{O-H}{|}}{C}}-H$$

    C. $$\underset{CH_3}{\overset{CH_3}{>}}C=CH_2$$

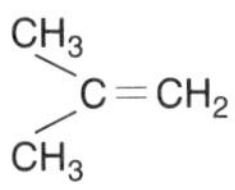

    D. 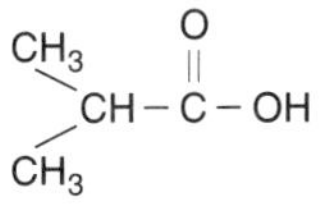 $$\underset{CH_3}{\overset{CH_3}{>}}CH-\overset{\overset{O}{\|}}{C}-OH$$

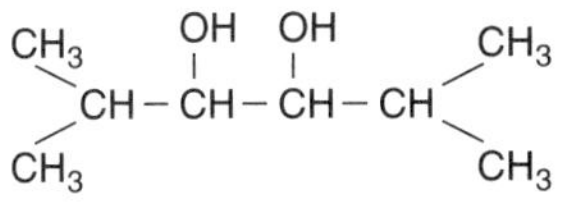

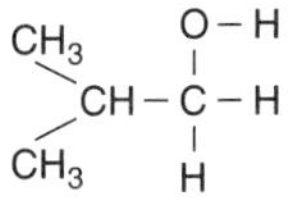

1–5. **1-B, 2-A, 3-C, 4-C, 5-A.** See text for explanation.
6. **B** The numbering is as shown.

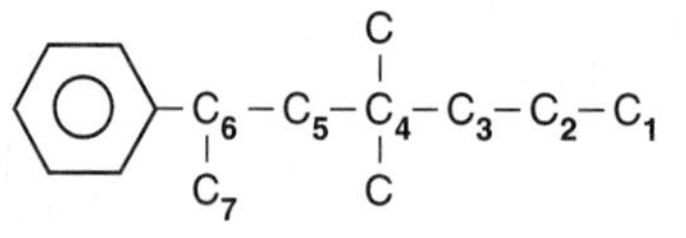

7. **D** Primary alcohols are stronger than similar 2° or 3° alcohols.
8. **B** The longer the carbon chain, the lower the solubility in water.
9. **A** The most substituted double bond will be the one that is formed.
10. **D** Substitution reactions are faster for benzyl (shown) or allyl type alcohols.
11–15. **11-B, 12-A, 13-A, 14-D, 15-B.** See text for explanation.
16. **D** This aldehyde is numbered as shown.

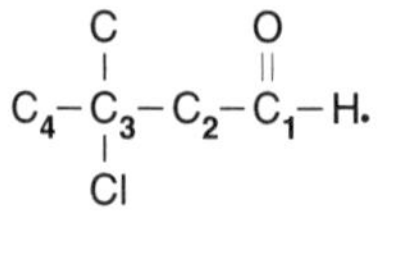

17. **A** The numbering of this ketone is as shown.

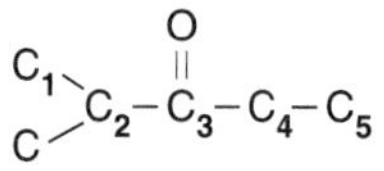

An alternate name is ethyl isopropyl ketone.
18. **D** This is an oxidation reaction as discussed in the text.

Carboxylic Acids and Derivatives, Ethers, and Phenols

Self-Managed Learning Questions
Focus on the following experimental issues:

1. Are there any clinical laboratory tests or applications of carboxylic acids, ethers, and phenols related to specimen collection, specimen classification and types, collection time for specimens, specimen handling, and any experimental errors?
2. Are there any theories or laws related to carboxylic acids, ethers, and phenols that need clarification or synthesis with bioclinical applications? Explore at least two or three viewpoints and technically critique such issues.
3. Are there any graphs, diagrams, reaction mechanisms, or sketches that require quantitative analysis? Which mathematical concepts help in interpreting graphical data?

See Bioorganic Molecules and Hydrocarbons to review general nomenclature. The *-e* of alkanes is replaced by *-oic acid* for carboxylic acids:

$$CH_3—CH_2—CH_2—CH_3 \qquad CH_3—CH_2—CH_2—CO_2H$$

Butane   (4)   (3)   (2)   (1)

Butanoic acid

The $-CO_2H$ carbon is always numbered as 1. Figure 8-229 is an example.

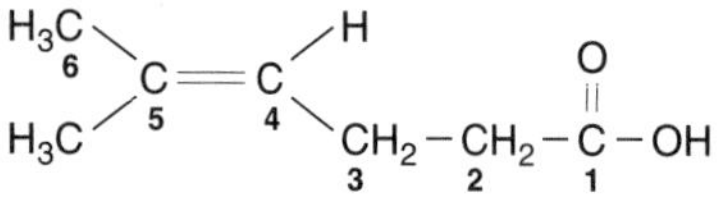

Fig. 8-229   5-Methyl-4-hexenoic acid

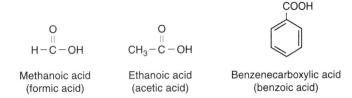

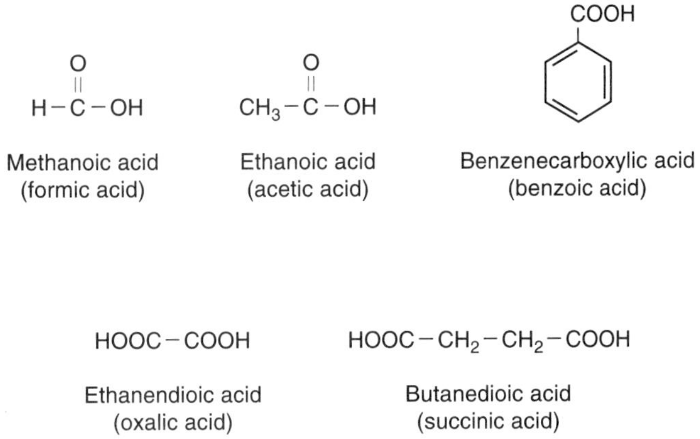

Methanoic acid
(formic acid)

Ethanoic acid
(acetic acid)

Benzenecarboxylic acid
(benzoic acid)

HOOC − COOH

HOOC − CH₂ − CH₂ − COOH

Ethanendioic acid
(oxalic acid)

Butanedioic acid
(succinic acid)

Fig. 8-230

Figure 8-230 shows some common carboxylic acids and their IUPAC names. The common names are stated in parentheses. Many acids are better known by their common names and the IUPAC nomenclature rules are prone to accept such common names as benzoic acid as permissible alternatives to the systematic ones. Note that, in naming dicarboxylic acid, the *e* of the alkane name is not dropped.

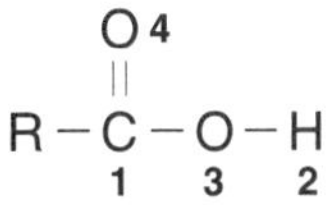

$$R - \underset{1 \quad 3 \quad 2}{\overset{\overset{\text{O} \, 4}{\|}}{C} - O - H}$$

Fig. 8-231

The key functional group of these compounds is the carboxyl (Figure 8-231).

CARBOXYLIC ACIDS

Carboxylic acids are the acids of organic chemistry. The only other compounds that approach their acid strength are substituted phenols. Organic classes of molecules by decreasing acid strength are $RCO_2H > ArOH > HOH > ROH > HC = CH > NH_3 > RH$ (substituted phenols may be stronger acids than H_2O).

The relative base strength is just the reverse. In decreasing base strength, the order is $R^- > NH_2^- > HC = CH^- > RO^- > HO^- > ArO^- > RCO_2^-$.

The relative acid strength of carboxylic acids depends primarily on the groups attached and the distance of these groups from the carboxyl (Figure 8-232).

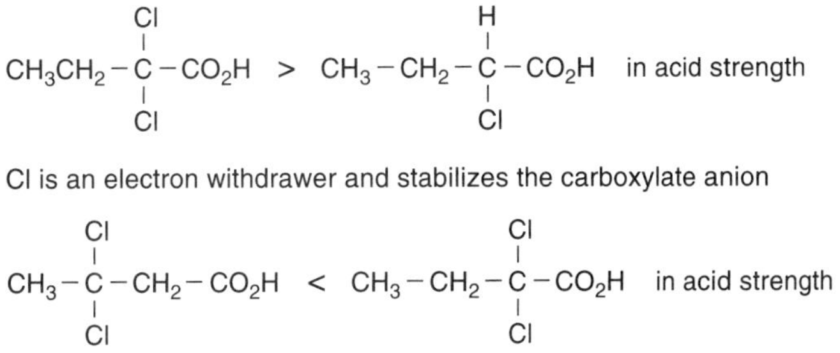

$$CH_3CH_2 - \underset{Cl}{\overset{Cl}{\underset{|}{\overset{|}{C}}}} - CO_2H \quad > \quad CH_3 - CH_2 - \underset{Cl}{\overset{H}{\underset{|}{\overset{|}{C}}}} - CO_2H \quad \text{in acid strength}$$

Cl is an electron withdrawer and stabilizes the carboxylate anion

$$CH_3 - \underset{Cl}{\overset{Cl}{\underset{|}{\overset{|}{C}}}} - CH_2 - CO_2H \quad < \quad CH_3 - CH_2 - \underset{Cl}{\overset{Cl}{\underset{|}{\overset{|}{C}}}} - CO_2H \quad \text{in acid strength}$$

Fig. 8-232

Dicarboxylic acids have two ionization constants (K_1 and K_2). The first ionization constant is larger than that for a comparable monocarboxylic acid because there are two sites for ionization and because one carboxyl group is electron withdrawing, aiding the ionization of the other. The ionization constant of the second carboxyl group is lower because it is more difficult to remove a proton from an anion than from a neutral molecule.

CH_3—CH_2—COOH $K = 1.3 \times 10^{-5}$ HOOC—CH_2—COOH $K_1 = 1.4 \times 10^{-3}$
Propanoic acid   Propanedicarboxylic acid $K_2 = 2 \times 10^{-6}$
(propionic acid)   (malonic acid)

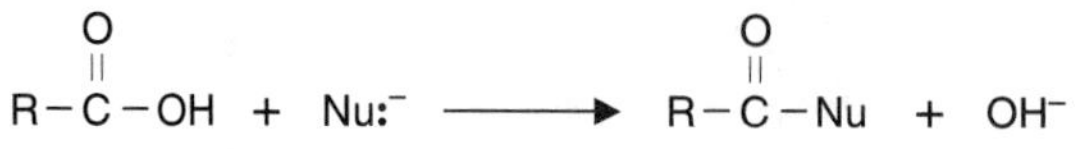

Fig. 8-233

$$R-\overset{\overset{\displaystyle O}{\|}}{C}-OH \ + \ Nu{:}^- \ \longrightarrow \ R-\overset{\overset{\displaystyle O}{\|}}{C}-Nu \ + \ OH^-$$

Important Carboxyl Group Reactions

Nucleophilic substitution reactions can involve a variety of nucleophiles (Nu) reacting under a variety of conditions (Figure 8-233):

Nu: = $-OR'$ in which R' is an alkyl ($1° > 2° > 3°$), ester results
= $-NH_2$, amides result
= $-Cl_2$ from $SOCl_2$ or PCl_3 or PCl_5, acid chlorides result

Figure 8-234 shows the ester reaction. **Esterification reactions** occur when alcohols react with carboxylic acids and carboxylic acid derivatives to yield esters of carboxylic acids. Esterification is acid catalyzed and reversible. The rate of esterification of a carboxyl acid depends on the steric hindrance in the alcohol and the carboxylic acid. The strength of the acid plays only a small role in the rate of ester formation.

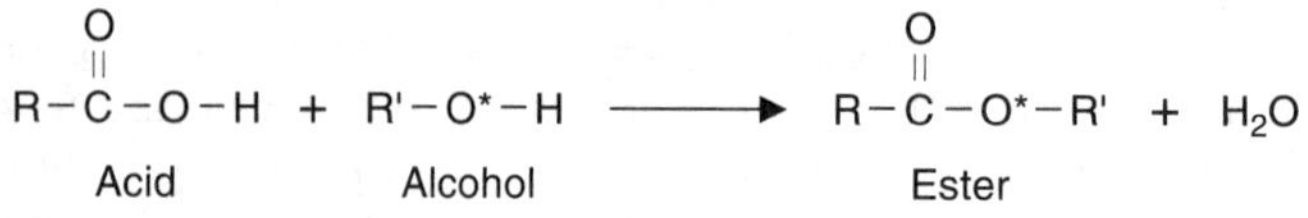

$$\underset{\text{Acid}}{R-\overset{\overset{\displaystyle O}{\|}}{C}-O-H} \ + \ \underset{\text{Alcohol}}{R'-O^*-H} \ \longrightarrow \ \underset{\text{Ester}}{R-\overset{\overset{\displaystyle O}{\|}}{C}-O^*-R'} \ + \ H_2O$$

Fig. 8-234   (Note the origin of the O*)

The major **reduction reaction** is with $LiAlH_4$ (Figure 8-235). Acids can be converted to esters or amides and then reduced also.

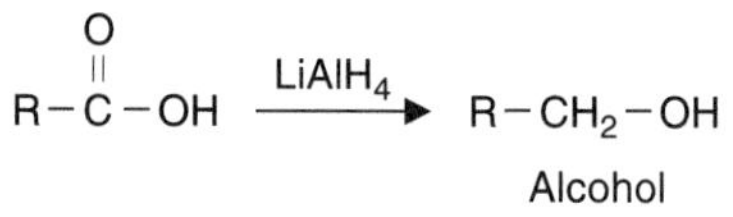

$$R-\overset{\overset{\displaystyle O}{\|}}{C}-OH \ \xrightarrow{\ LiAlH_4\ } \ \underset{\text{Alcohol}}{R-CH_2-OH}$$

Fig. 8-235

Decarboxylation reaction involves β-diacids or β-ketoacids as shown in Figure 8-236.

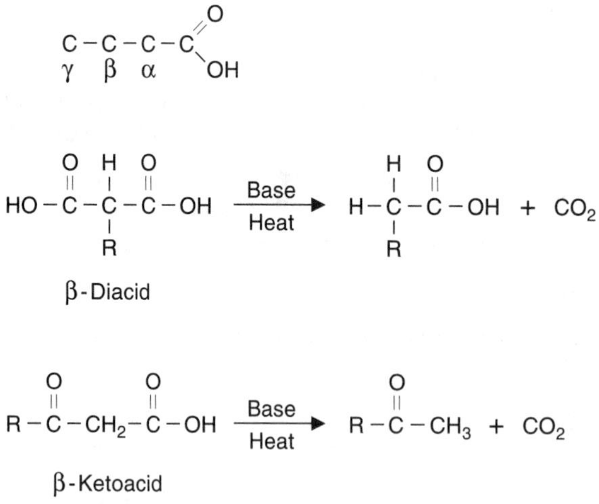

$$\underset{\gamma \quad \beta \quad \alpha}{C-C-C-C}\diagup^{O}_{\diagdown OH}$$

$$\underset{\beta\text{-Diacid}}{HO-\overset{\overset{\displaystyle O}{\|}}{C}-\overset{\overset{\displaystyle H}{|}}{\underset{\underset{\displaystyle R}{|}}{C}}-\overset{\overset{\displaystyle O}{\|}}{C}-OH} \ \xrightarrow[\text{Heat}]{\text{Base}} \ H-\overset{\overset{\displaystyle H}{|}}{\underset{\underset{\displaystyle R}{|}}{C}}-\overset{\overset{\displaystyle O}{\|}}{C}-OH \ + \ CO_2$$

$$\underset{\beta\text{-Ketoacid}}{R-\overset{\overset{\displaystyle O}{\|}}{C}-CH_2-\overset{\overset{\displaystyle O}{\|}}{C}-OH} \ \xrightarrow[\text{Heat}]{\text{Base}} \ R-\overset{\overset{\displaystyle O}{\|}}{C}-CH_3 \ + \ CO_2$$

Fig. 8-236

General Principles

Low-molecular-weight aliphatic carboxylic acids tend to be soluble in water due to hydrogen bonding with water; aromatic acids generally are not soluble. The acids are also soluble in dilute bases, NaOH or $NaHCO_3$, for example, because of their acid properties. The boiling points are high because of the hydrogen bonding possible between molecules.

Reactions of the carboxylic acids center around the four central features of the carboxyl group:

1. The H is acidic because it is weakly attached to the O and because the resulting carboxylate anion is stabilized by resonance (Figure 8-237).

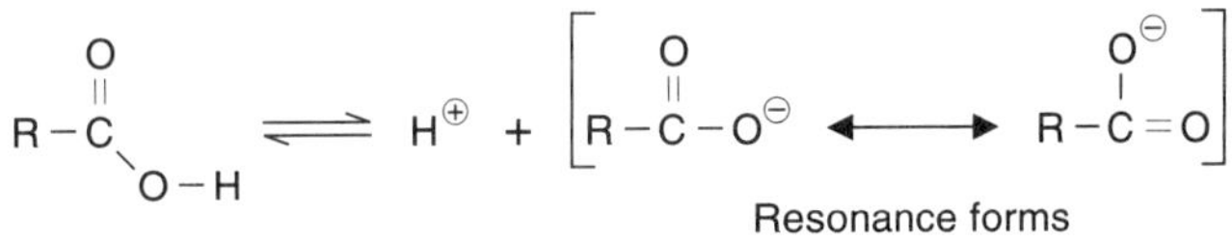

Fig. 8-237

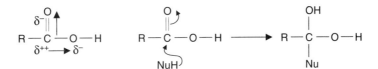

Resonance forms

2. The carboxyl carbon is susceptible to attack by nucleophilic agents (Nu) because it has attached electronegative oxygens and the carbonyl oxygen as shown in Figure 8-238.

Fig. 8-238

3. The hydroxyl can become a good leaving group by appropriate solvent conditions (e.g., if basic) or by protonating if the solution is acidic; this also promotes nucleophilic substitution (Figure 8-239).

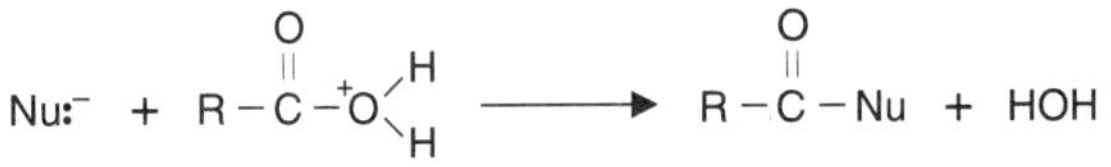

Fig. 8-239

4. Hydrogen bonding is possible between molecules (intermolecular) or within the same molecule (intramolecular) because of the carbonyl and hydroxyl moieties (Figure 8-240).

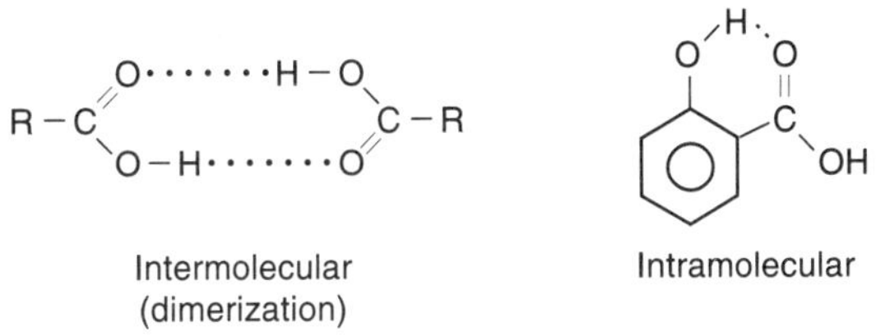

Intermolecular
(dimerization)

Intramolecular

Fig. 8-240

Inductive effects help illuminate why carboxylic acids are more acidic than alcohols. **Inductive effect** is an intrinsic electron-attracting ability that is transmitted through space and through the bonds of the molecule. Inductive effects weaken as the distance from the substituent increases. Transmission of the effect through bonds results from the polarization of one bond, which causes the polarization of an adjacent bond. Transmission of the effect through space is considered to be the more important mode of transmission; it results from simple electrostatic effects.

Electrons of 2s orbitals have a lower energy than 2p orbitals because the electrons in the 2s orbitals usually are closer to the nucleus than the electrons in 2p orbitals. With hybrid orbitals, having more s character means that the electrons of the anion usually have lower energy, making the anion more stable.

COMMON ACID DERIVATIVES

A derivative of a carboxylic acid is a compound that yields a carboxylic acid when it reacts with water. Carboxylic acids and some of their derivatives are found in nature. In the nomenclature of carboxylic acids, the *-oic acid* (or *-ic acid*) is changed to *-amide* as shown in Figure 8-241. If the N is substituted, this feature is added as shown in Figure 8-242.

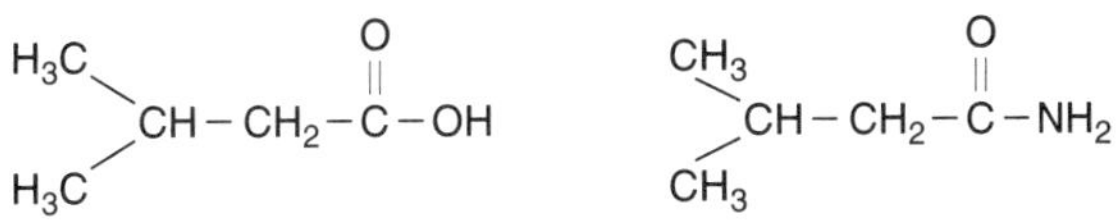

Fig. 8-241

3-Methyl butanoic acid

3-Methyl butanamide

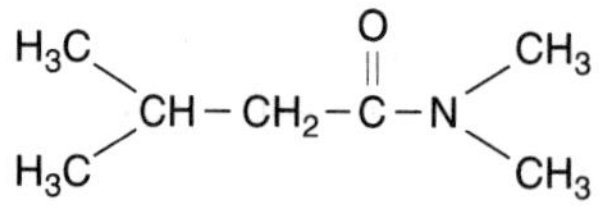

Fig. 8-242   N,N-Dimethyl-3-methyl butanamide

The boiling points of unsubstituted and monosubstituted amides are very high due to strong intermolecular hydrogen bonds. Disubstituted amides have boiling points like ketones or aldehydes (due to the carbonyl moiety). Amides have essentially no acidity (as compared with carboxylic acids) and no basicity (as compared with amines).

Amides are formed from carboxylic acids (or its derivatives) by the mechanism shown in Figure 8-243. Amides are susceptible to nucleophilic substitution at the carbonyl carbon (Figure 8-244). Amides undergo hydrolysis back to the original acid and amine under basic or acidic conditions (Figure 8-245).

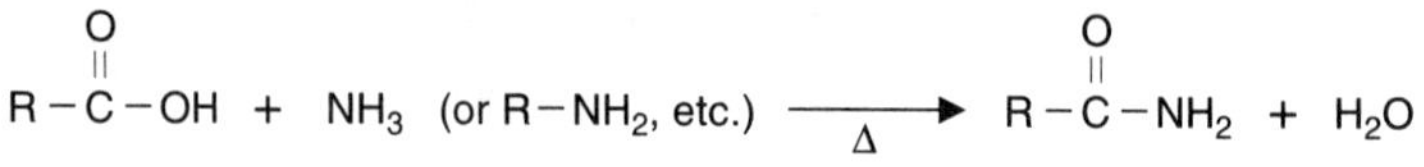

Fig. 8-243

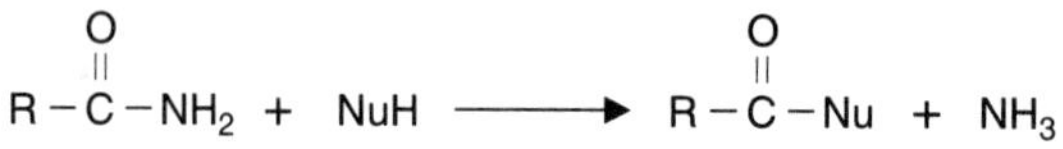

Fig. 8-244

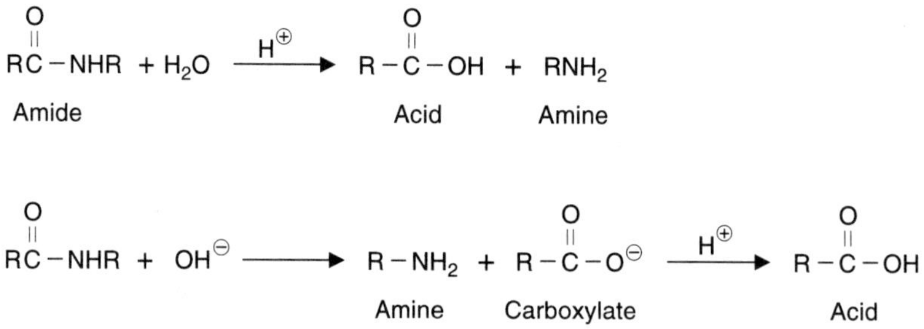

Fig. 8-245

ESTERS

The *-oic acid* of carboxylic acids is replaced by *-oate* and the carbon fragment of the ester precedes the base name as shown in Figure 8-246. Esters have no acidity (because they have no —OH) and have boiling points comparable to ketones and aldehydes because they have carbonyl groups but not hydrogen bonding.

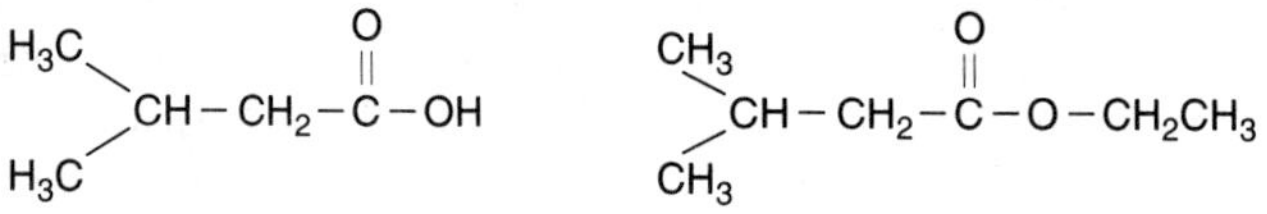

Fig. 8-246   3-Methyl butanoic acid   Ethyl-3-methyl butanoate

Esters are formed from carboxylic acids (or derivatives), usually under acidic conditions (Figure 8-247).

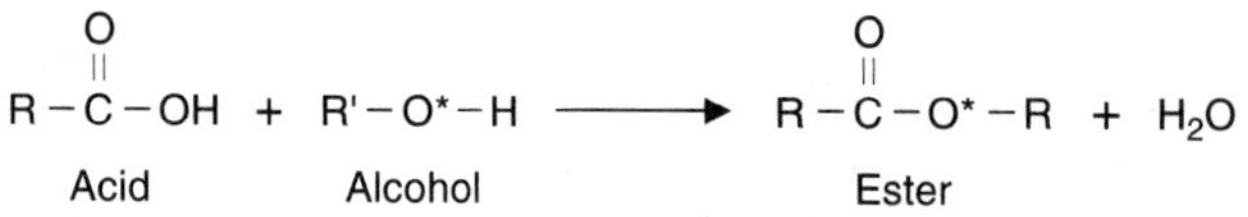

Fig. 8-247   Acid   Alcohol   Ester

Esters undergo nucleophilic substitution at the carbonyl carbon (Figure 8-248). Esters

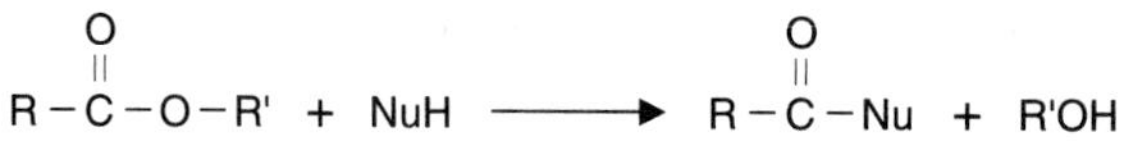

Fig. 8-248   Nu = Nucleophile

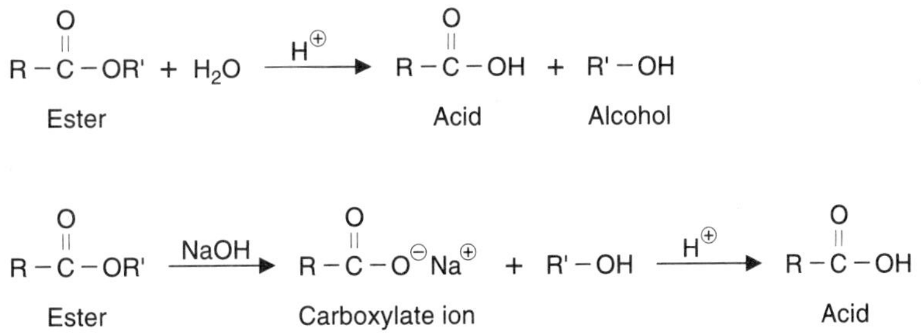

O
||
R − C − OR' + H₂O $\xrightarrow{H^\oplus}$ R − C − OH + R' − OH

Ester   Acid   Alcohol

O   O   O
|| || ||
R − C − OR' $\xrightarrow{NaOH}$ R − C − O⊖Na⊕ + R' − OH $\xrightarrow{H^\oplus}$ R − C − OH

Fig. 8-249   Ester   Carboxylate ion   Acid

are hydrolyzed by acid or base back to the original acid and alcohol as shown in Figure 8-249.

Fats are a special class of esters of biologic importance. They are formed as shown in Figure 8-250.

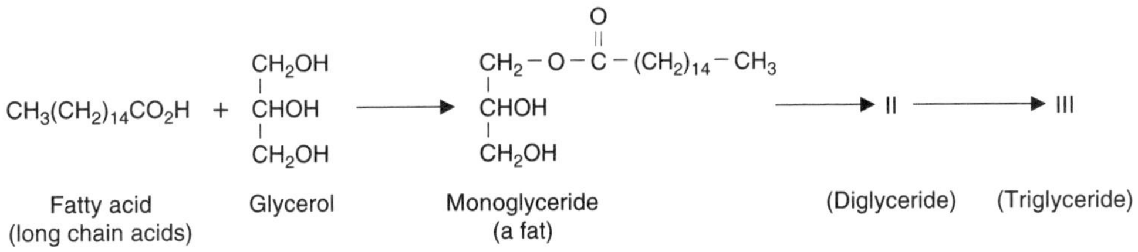

O
||
CH₂ − O − C − (CH₂)₁₄ − CH₃

CH₂OH |
| CH₂OH
CH₃(CH₂)₁₄CO₂H + CHOH $\longrightarrow$ CHOH $\longrightarrow$ II $\longrightarrow$ III
| |
CH₂OH   CH₂OH

Fig. 8-250 Fatty acid   Glycerol   Monoglyceride   (Diglyceride) (Triglyceride)
                (long chain acids)   (a fat)

More fatty acids (FAs) can be added to the glycerol to form diglycerides (II) and triglycerides (III). Fats may be hydrolyzed back to FAs and glycerol by base, a process called saponification (Figure 8-251).

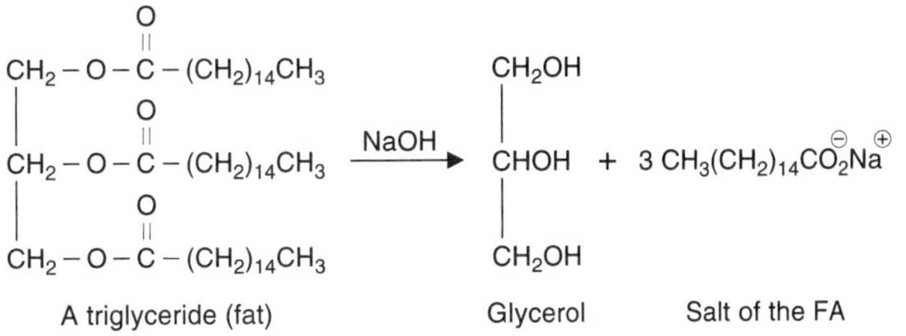

O
||
CH₂ − O − C − (CH₂)₁₄CH₃   CH₂OH
| O |
              ||
CH₂ − O − C − (CH₂)₁₄CH₃ $\xrightarrow{NaOH}$ CHOH + 3 CH₃(CH₂)₁₄CO₂⊖Na⊕
| O |
              ||
CH₂ − O − C − (CH₂)₁₄CH₃   CH₂OH

Fig. 8-251   A triglyceride (fat)   Glycerol   Salt of the FA

Amides undergo **hydrolysis** when they are heated with an aqueous acid or aqueous base. Whichever method is used, amide hydrolysis takes place more slowly than the comparable hydrolysis of an ester. Thus, amide hydrolyses usually require more forcing conditions. In an acidic hydrolysis, water acts as a nucleophile and attacks the protonated amide. The leaving group is ammonia (or an amine). In a basic hydrolysis, there is evidence that hydroxide ions act both as nucleophiles and as bases. A hydroxide ion attacks the acyl carbon, then removes a proton to give to a dianion. The dianion loses a molecule of ammonia. This process is synchronized with a proton transfer from water.

General Principles

Carboxylic acid derivatives contain leaving groups that are bonded to the acyl carbons. Reagents substitute for the leaving groups of acid derivatives. With good leaving groups, acid chlorides and acid anhydrides are readily attacked by water. Because of this, these compounds are not found in animal or plant cells. These acid derivatives are invaluable in the synthesis of other organic compounds because of their high reactivity. A relatively nonreactive carboxylic acid may be converted to one of these more reactive derivatives and then converted to a ketone, ester, or amide.

ETHERS

Ethers have the general structure R—O—R'. R, R' are aliphatic or aromatic groups. Ethers are named by naming the R and R' and following these by *ether* as shown in Figure 8-252.

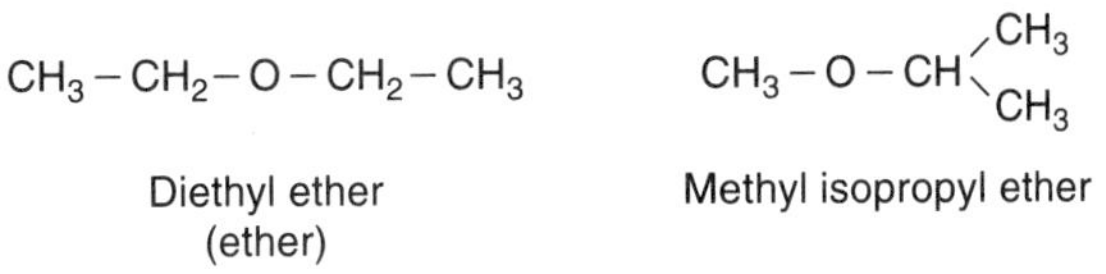

CH₃−CH₂−O−CH₂−CH₃   CH₃−O−CH⟨CH₃/CH₃

Diethyl ether   Methyl isopropyl ether
(ether)

Fig. 8-252

The physical properties of ethers reflect the polar oxygen and the nonpolar hydrocarbon component. There is some solubility in water due to the O hydrogen bonding with H_2O. The boiling points are less than those of alcohols and about the same as those of alkanes because there is no hydrogen bonding between the molecules of ether.

Ethers may exist in a cyclic form in which the oxygen is part of the ring. Three important cyclic ethers are shown in Figure 8-253. The preparation and the physical and chemical properties of cyclic ethers are generally similar to those of their open-chain counterparts.

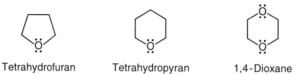

Fig. 8-253   Tetrahydrofuran   Tetrahydropyran   1,4-Dioxane

Three-member ring ethers are called **epoxides**, or oxiranes. They are frequently known by their common names as oxides of alkenes (Figure 8-254).

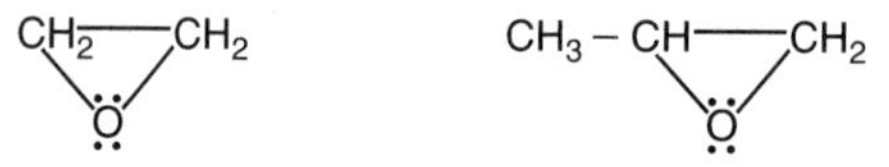

Fig. 8-254

Epoxyethane
(ethylene oxide)

Epoxypropane
(propylene oxide)

Because of bond angle strain, epoxides are much more reactive than are other ethers. They readily undergo acid catalyzed hydrolysis to produce diols. Epoxides also react readily with HX, hydroxide ion, alkoxide ions, and Grignard reagents (Figure 8-255).

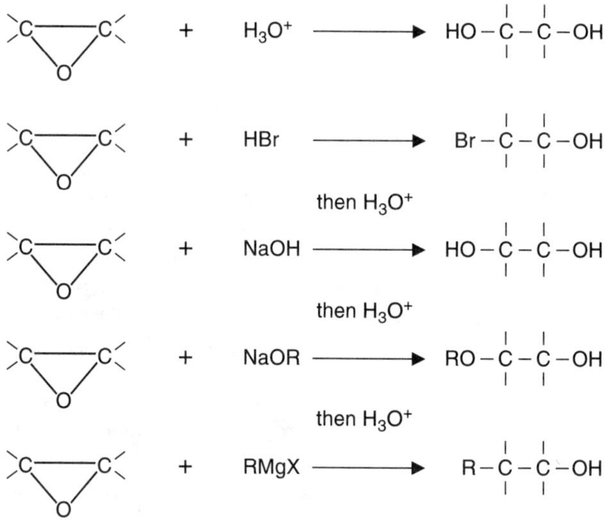

Fig. 8-255

Cleavage by Acid

Ether cleavage with HI or HBr follows almost the same path as the reaction of an alcohol with HX, in which the first step is the protonation of the oxygen.

Weak Basicity of Ethers

Basicity is a measure of the ability of the reagent to accept a proton in an acid-base reaction. This means that the relative base strength of reagents is determined by comparing the relative positions of their equilibria in an acid-base reaction (e.g., measuring the degree of ionization in water).

PHENOLS

A phenol consists of a hydroxyl group attached to an aromatic ring. For nomenclature, refer to Hydrocarbons. Some phenols that have counterparts in biochemistry and medicine are shown in Figure 8-256. Phenols also are powerful o-p directors.

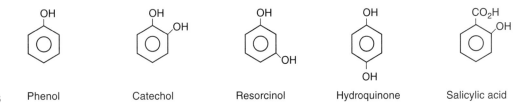

Fig. 8-256

| Phenol | Catechol | Resorcinol | Hydroquinone | Salicylic acid |

General Principles

Phenols are acidic due to the dissociable hydrogen on the oxygen. Phenols are more acidic than alcohols because of the electron-withdrawing and resonance stabilization effects of the aromatic ring (Figure 8-257).

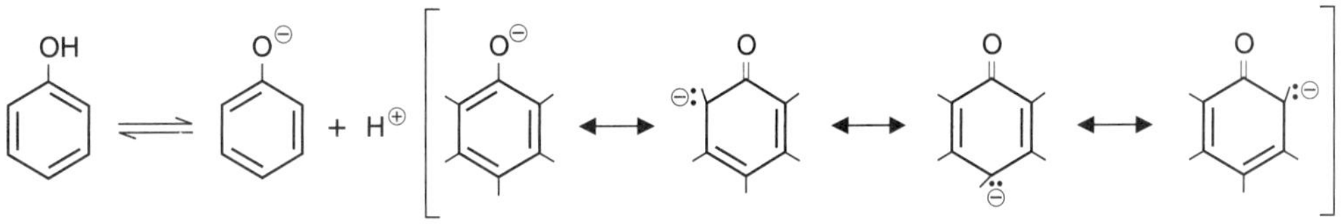

Fig. 8-257

Phenols are less acidic than carboxylic acids but more acidic than alcohols. The ionization constant, or acidity constant (K_a), for most phenols is approximately 10^{-10} ($pK_a = 10$), whereas most carboxylic acids have a K_a of approximately 10^{-5} ($pK_a = 5$). The K_a of alcohols is in the 10^{-16} to 10^{-20} range (pK_a 16-20). Note that $pK_a = -\log K_a$. These differences in acidity are of practical importance and useful in separating phenols from alcohols or carboxylic acids. Phenols react with dilute sodium hydroxide to form the water-soluble sodium phenoxide salt, but phenols do not react with dilute sodium bicarbonate. Carboxylic acids react with dilute sodium bicarbonate or sodium hydroxide to form sodium carboxylate salts, whereas alcohols do not react with either sodium hydroxide or sodium bicarbonate.

The resonance forms discussed show that electron-withdrawing meta-directing groups such as $-NO_2$, $-CN$, $-COR$, and $-COOH$, when placed at the ortho-para positions, should make the phenol more acidic. These groups can delocalize the negative charge and stabilize the phenoxide ion. Groups that can destabilize (and make less acidic) the phenoxide ion are the electron-donating ortho-para directors.

Phenols form **intramolecular** and **intermolecular** hydrogen bonds. Physical properties are understood by considering the hydrogen bond-forming capacity and the hydrophobic nature of aromatic rings. Even phenol itself is only slightly soluble in water (due to its hydrogen bonding), but most other phenols are insoluble due to their aromatic ring. Most phenols have high boiling points, primarily because of the hydrogen bonding between molecules. Within the disubstituted phenols, the ortho compounds tend to have lower boiling points because they have the potential for intramolecular hydrogen bonding, whereas meta and para have intermolecular hydrogen bonding (and higher boiling points) [Figure 8-258].

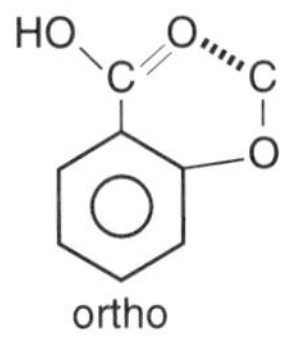

ortho

Intramolecular hydrogen bonding

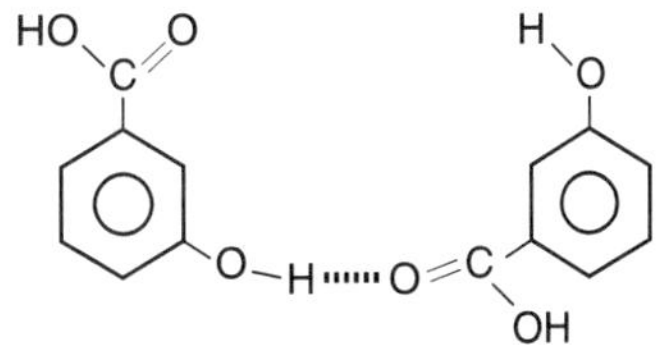

Meta (or para) intermolecular hydrogen bonding

Fig. 8-258

APPLIED CONCEPTS

The following is a list of tools to analyze and understand carboxylic acids, esters, amides, anhydrides, ethers, and phenols.

- Understand how reactions are related to basic mechanisms, how reaction rates are affected, and what bonding arrangements, resonance stability structures, and stereoarrangements are possible. Elucidate each mechanism in a visual format.
- Ponder how organic chemistry of medical compounds (carboxylic acids and derivatives) can be investigated, identified, and linked to the biological side effects (both microscopic and physiologic).
- What biological disorders (e.g., protein deficiency, enzyme deficiency) result from deficiency or abundance of medical compounds (carboxylic acids and derivatives), especially bioorganic molecules?
- Determine how organic reaction mechanisms translate into biochemical reaction mechanisms (e.g., metabolism).

CARBOXYLIC ACIDS AND DERIVATIVES, ETHERS, AND PHENOLS: REVIEW QUESTIONS

1. Which atom shown is susceptible to nucleophilic attack?

- A. I
- B. II
- C. III
- D. IV

2. A high – molecular-weight carboxylic acid may be soluble in _____ but probably not in _____.

- A. dilute acid; dilute base
- B. water; dilute acid
- C. water; dilute base
- D. dilute base; water

3. For comparable compounds, which of the following would be most acidic?

- A. Water
- B. Alcohol
- C. Alkene
- D. Carboxylic acid

4. Name the compound shown in the following figure.

$$CH_3-\underset{\underset{CH_3}{|}}{\overset{\overset{CH_3}{|}}{C}}-CH=\underset{\overset{|}{Cl}}{C}-CH_2-CO_2H$$

- A. 3-Chloro-5,5-dimethylhexenoic acid
- B. 3-Chloro-5,5-dimethyl-3-hexenoic acid
- C. 2,2-Dimethyl-4-chloro-3-hexenoic acid
- D. None of the above

5. Select the compound shown that is most acidic.

A.
$$Cl-\underset{\underset{Cl}{|}}{\overset{\overset{Cl}{|}}{C}}-CH_2-CO_2H$$

B. $CH_3-CH_2-CO_2H$

C. 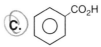 a benzene ring with a CO_2H substituent

D. All are equal

6. What is the product of the reaction shown in the following figure?

$$\text{(benzene ring)}-CH_2-CH_2-\overset{\overset{O}{\|}}{C}-OH \ + \ CH_3-NH_2 \ \xrightarrow{\Delta} \ ?$$

A. $H_3C-\underset{\overset{|}{}}{\overset{\overset{H}{|}}{N}}-\text{(benzene ring)}-CH_2-CH_2-\overset{\overset{O}{\|}}{C}-OH$

B. $\text{(benzene ring)}-CH_2-CH_2-CH_2-OH$

C. $\text{(benzene ring)}-CH_2-CH_2-CH_2-NH-CH_3$

D. None of the above

7. Which of the following compounds has the potential for decarboxylation?

A. benzene ring with $\overset{\overset{O}{\|}}{C}-CH_2CO_2H$ substituent

B. benzene ring with $\overset{\overset{O}{\|}}{C}-CH_2-CO_2H$ substituent

C. $CH_3-CH_2-\underset{\underset{CH_2-CO_2H}{\diagdown}}{\overset{\diagup CO_2H}{CH}}$

D. None of the above

8. Amides have essentially no:

   A. acidity.
   B. basicity.
   C. hydrogen bonding.
   D. acidity or basicity.

9. Fats are _____ and are made of _____ and _____.

   A. esters; glycerol; fatty acids
   B. amides; an amine; fatty acids
   C. ethers; glycerol; fatty acids
   D. none of the above

10. Saponification is the _____ of _____.

    A. alkaline hydrolysis; fats
    B. acidic hydrolysis; fats
    C. neutral hydrolysis; amides
    D. osmosis; amides

11. Name the compound shown in the following figure.

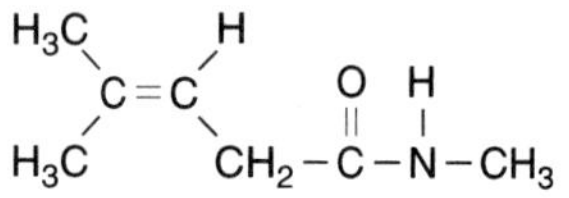

    A. N-Methyl-4-methyl-3-pentenamide
    B. 2-Methyl-2-pentenamide
    C. Dimethyl pentenamide
    D. None of the above

12. Which of the compounds shown probably has a boiling point similar to comparable molecular weight ketones or aldehydes?

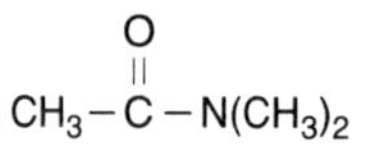

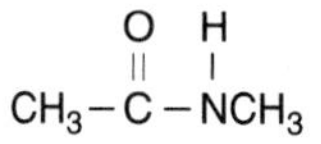

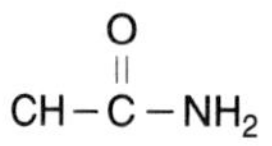

    D. None of the above

13. Name the compound shown in the following figure.

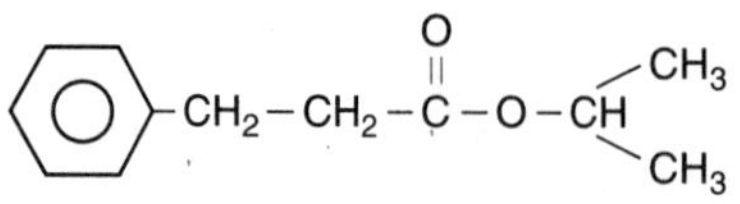

    A. Isopropyl benzoate
    B. Isopropyl 3-phenyl propanoate
    C. Phenyl isopropyl ester
    D. None of the above

14. Give the product of the reaction shown in the following figure.

$$\underset{\underset{CH_3}{|}}{\overset{\overset{CH_3}{|}}{CH}}-\overset{\overset{O}{||}}{C}-O-CH_3 \xrightarrow{\text{NaOH}} ?$$

A. $\underset{\underset{CH_3}{|}}{\overset{\overset{CH_3}{|}}{C}}=CH_2$

B. $\underset{\underset{CH_3}{|}}{\overset{\overset{CH_3}{|}}{CH}}-CH_2OH$

C. $\underset{\underset{H_3C}{|}}{\overset{\overset{CH_3}{|}}{CH}}-\overset{\overset{O}{||}}{C}-O^{\ominus}Na^{\oplus}$

D. None of the above

15. The compound shown in the following figure is a:

$$\begin{array}{l} CH_2-O-\overset{\overset{O}{||}}{C}-(CH_2)_8CH_3 \\ | \qquad\qquad \overset{O}{||} \\ CH_2-O-\overset{}{C}-(CH_2)_{10}CH_3 \\ | \qquad\qquad \overset{O}{||} \\ CH_2-O-\overset{}{C}-(CH_2)_{12}CH_3 \end{array}$$

A. nucleotide.
B. monosaccharide.
C. amino acid.
D. triglyceride.

16. Name the compound shown in the following figure.

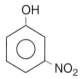

A. o,m-Hydroxynitrobenzene
B. 2-Nitrophenol
C. o-Nitrophenol
D. m-Nitrophenol

17. Which of the following compounds probably has the highest boiling point?

A. $CH_3(CH_2)_2-CH=CH_2$

B. CH_3-O-CH_3

C.

D. CH_3-CH_3

18. Rank the following compounds in order of decreasing acid strength (most acidic to least acidic):

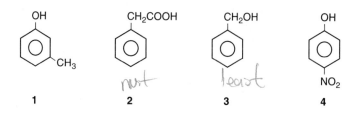

1   2   3   4

    A. $1 > 2 > 3 > 4$
    B. $2 > 3 > 4 > 1$
    C. $3 > 1 > 2 > 4$
    D. $2 > 4 > 1 > 3$

ANSWERS AND EXPLANATIONS

1–3. 1-B, 2-D, 3-D.
  4. B   The numbering is as shown in the figure. Note how the double bond is handled.

$$C-\underset{|\atop C}{\overset{C\atop |}{\underset{6}{C}}}-\overset{\ }{\underset{5}{C}}=\overset{Cl\atop |}{\underset{4}{C}}-\underset{3}{C}-\underset{2}{C}-\underset{1}{CO_2H}$$

  5. C   The benzene ring withdraws electrons, and, therefore, increases the acidity. The Cl's on option **A** are one carbon from the $-CO_2H$, and they are much less effective than a benzene ring attached to the carboxyl group.
  6. D   The correct product is shown.

$$\text{⟨O⟩}-CH_2-CH_2-\overset{O\atop ||}{C}-NHCH_3$$

  7. B   Option B is the only β-ketoacid (no β-diacids) given.
8–10. 8-D, 9-A, 10-A.
 11. A   The numbering is as shown.

$$\underset{C}{\overset{C}{\underset{5}{\diagdown}}}C=\underset{3}{\overset{4}{C}}\diagdown\underset{2}{C}-\overset{O\atop ||}{\underset{1}{C}}-\overset{|}{N}-C$$

 12. A   Disubstituted amides have boiling points similar to carbonyls because there is no intermolecular hydrogen bonding.
 13. B   The numbering is as shown.

$$\text{⟨O⟩}-\underset{3}{C}-\underset{2}{C}-\overset{O\atop ||}{\underset{1}{C}}-O-C\diagup^{C}\diagdown_{C}$$

 14. C   This is the alkaline hydrolysis of an ester, so a carboxylate anion results.
 15. D
 16. D   The compound is named as a phenol with ortho-meta-para as shown.

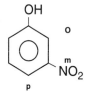

17. C The phenol can hydrogen bond to itself, which increases the boiling point; the others cannot.

18. D Number 2 is a carboxylic acid and the most acidic. Number 3 is an alcohol and the least acidic. Numbers 1 and 4 are phenols, and number 4 is the more acidic of the two phenols due to the p-NO$_2$.

Nitrogen-Containing Compounds—Amines

Self-Managed Learning Questions

Focus on the following experimental issues:

1. Is there any research study or hypotheses testing on the use of amines?
2. Are there any clinical laboratory tests or clinical applications of amines related to specimen collection, specimen classification and types, collection time for specimens, specimen handling, and any experimental errors?
3. Are there any theories or laws related to amines that need clarification or synthesis with bioclinical applications? Explore at least two or three viewpoints and technically critique such issues.
4. Are there any graphs, diagrams, reaction mechanisms, or sketches that require quantitative analysis? Which mathematical concepts help in interpreting graphical data?
5. Review special properties related to basicity and electronic effects of substituents (e.g., stabilization of carbocations). Review the structure of choline and acetylcholine (quaternary ammonium salt) as neurotransmitters. Understand the structure of the pyridine ring and derivatives such as NAD$^+$ and NADP$^+$ used in cellular metabolism. Identify the structural and mechanistic differences between histamines and antihistamines.

DESCRIPTIONS

Stereochemistry and Physical Properties

Amines are symbolized generally as shown in Figure 8-259. All the R's (R$_1$, R$_2$, R$_3$) or any combination can be carbon groups or hydrogens. If R's are carbon groups, as shown in Figure 8-260, amines may be named by locating the −NR$_2$ in a compound by numbers (Figure 8-261) or by naming each group attached to the N (Figure 8-262).

Nearly all the chemistry of amines depends on the free pair of electrons on nitrogen (Figure 8-263). Groups that withdraw electron density (e.g., aromatics, halides) from

Fig. 8-259

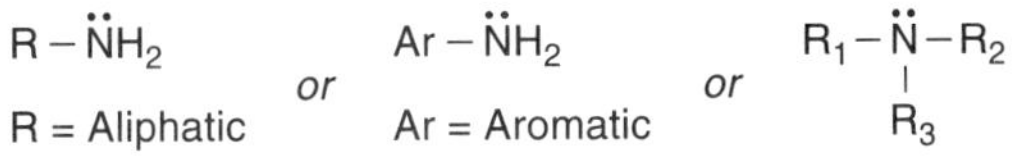

Fig. 8-260

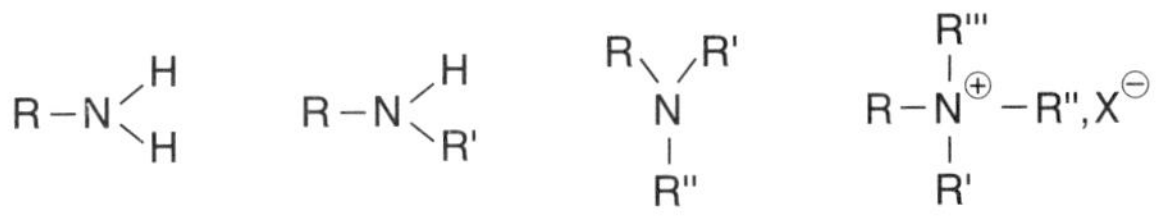

Fig. 8-261

Fig. 8-262

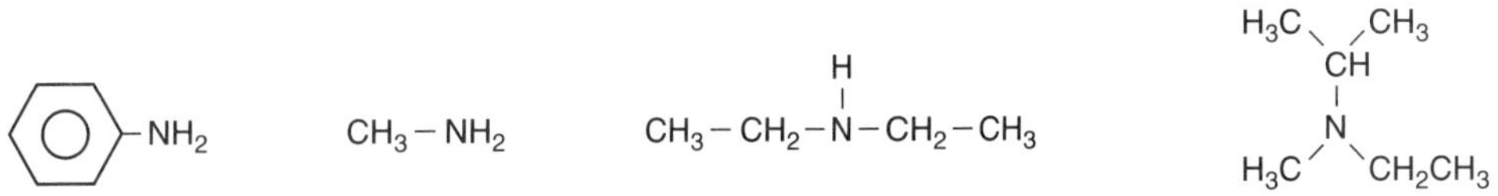

Fig. 8-263

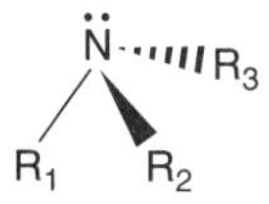

nitrogen decrease the availability of this electron pair. Groups that donate electron density (especially alkyls) increase the availability. The exception to this rule is the secondary amine, which is the most basic because the combination of the alkyls and the single hydrogen (provides hydrogen bonding, e.g., with water) stabilizes the ion and makes the electrons more available. The availability of the electrons is reflected in the sequence of decreasing **base strengths** shown in Figure 8-264.

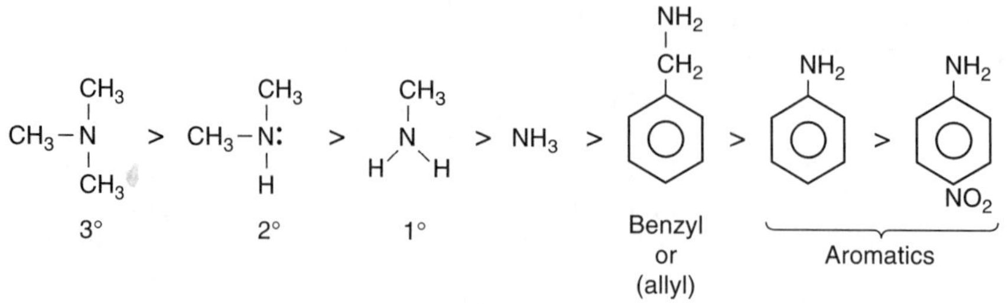

Fig. 8-264

The available electron pair classifies amines as **Lewis bases**. Amines are also nucleophiles.

The N can form hydrogen bonding via its electron pair with hydrogens attached to other nitrogen or oxygen atoms, and it can form hydrogen bonds from hydrogens at-

Fig. 8-265

tached to it with electron pairs of N, O, F, or Cl (Figure 8-265). Note that 1° or 2° amines can hydrogen bond with each other (intermolecularly) but 3° amines cannot (no H's are attached to the N). For this reason 1° or 2° amines have higher than expected boiling points for compounds of similar molecular weight (but lower than for similar alcohols or carboxylic acids). Low-molecular-weight amines are also soluble in water (due to their H-bonding).

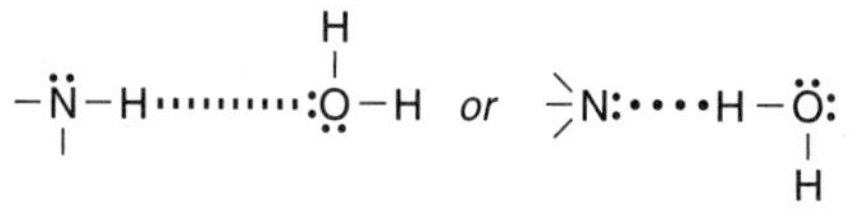

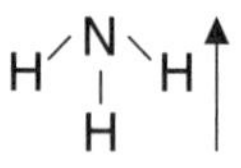

Fig. 8-266

A dipole moment is possible (Figure 8-266). Amines are also ortho-para directors.

MAJOR REACTIONS

The key reaction of amines is the nucleophilic attack by it upon an electron-deficient carbon.

Amide Formation

A very important reaction of 1° and 2° amines is with carboxylic acids (or usually their derivatives) to form amides (Figure 8-267). This is the reaction important in protein synthesis.

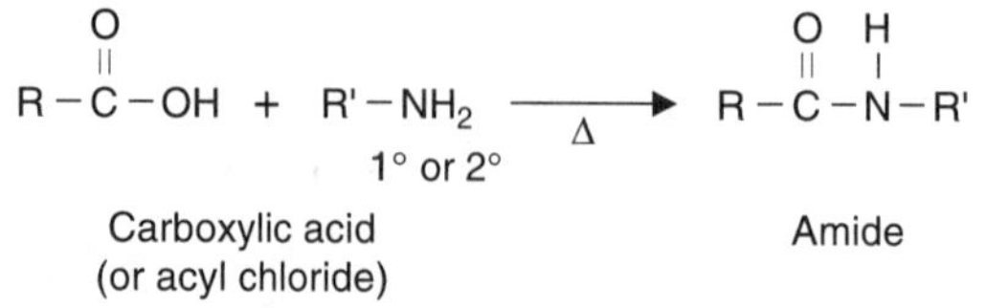

Fig. 8-267

Alkylation

Another common reaction of amines is alkylation of amines by alkyl halides (Figure 8-268). Both amide formation and alkylation make use of the nucleophilic character of the electrons on nitrogen.

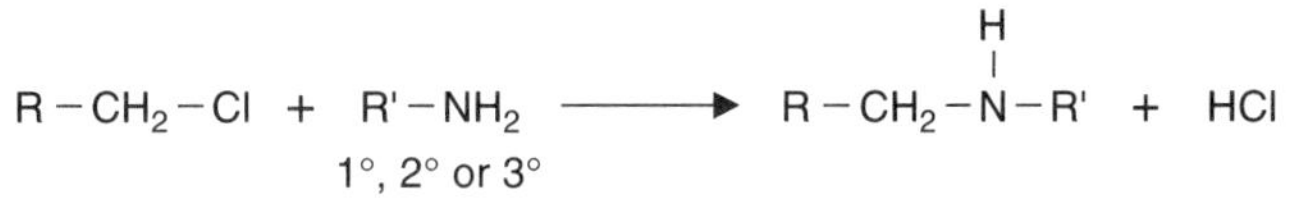

Fig. 8-268

$$R-CH_2-Cl \ + \ R'-NH_2 \longrightarrow R-CH_2-\overset{\overset{\displaystyle H}{|}}{N}-R' \ + \ HCl$$

1°, 2° or 3°

GENERAL PRINCIPLES

Basicity

Basicity measures the ability of a reagent to accept a proton in an acid-base reaction. The base strengths of a series of reagents can be determined by comparing the relative positions of their equilibria in an acid-base reaction (e.g., the degree of ionization in water). In contrast to basicity, nucleophilicity is a measure of the ability of a reagent to cause a substitution reaction. The basicity equilibrium constant is K_b. This results from the reversible reaction of a weak base with water, which results in a small and constant concentration of ions at equilibrium. When the strength of the base increases, the K_b value increases and the pK_b value decreases. The smaller the pK_b value, the stronger the base.

Stabilization of Adjacent Carbonium Ions (Carbocations)

Carbocations are electron deficient, having only six electrons. They are electron-seeking reagents called electrophiles; they seek the extra electron or electrons that will give them a stable octet. Carbocations usually exist as short-term intermediates in organic reactions. A few of them are stable enough to be isolated but only when special groups are attached to the carbon atoms that allows the positive charge to be stabilized.

NITROGEN-CONTAINING COMPOUNDS—AMINES: REVIEW QUESTIONS

1. Name the following compound.

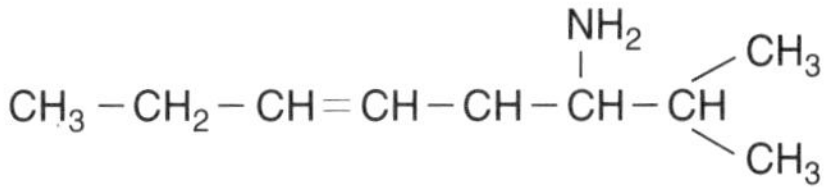

$$CH_3-CH_2-CH=CH-CH-\overset{\overset{\displaystyle NH_2}{|}}{CH}-CH\overset{\nearrow CH_3}{\searrow_{CH_3}}$$

  A. 6-Amino-7-methyl-3-octene
  B. Isononenyl amine
  C. 2-Methyl-3-aminooctene
  D. None of the above

2. Select the structure of isopropyl diethyl amine.

A. 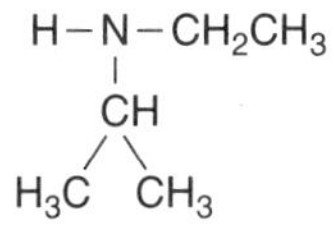
$$\underset{H_3C \quad CH_3}{\overset{H-N-CH_2CH_3}{\underset{\diagup \diagdown}{|}}} CH$$

B. 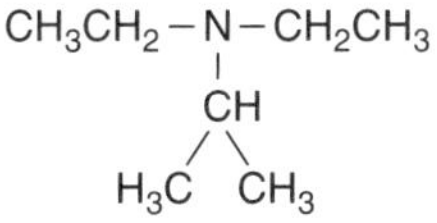
$$\underset{H_3C \quad CH_3}{\overset{CH_3CH_2-N-CH_2CH_3}{\underset{\diagup \diagdown}{|}}} CH$$

C. 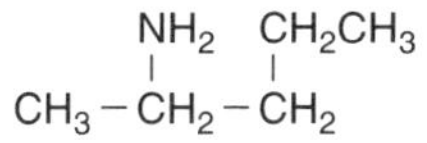 $CH_3-CH_2-\overset{\overset{\displaystyle NH_2}{|}}{\underset{}{CH_2}}\;\overset{\overset{\displaystyle CH_2CH_3}{|}}{}$

D. None of the above

3. Which compound shown has the greatest base strength?

A. CH_3-NH_2

B. 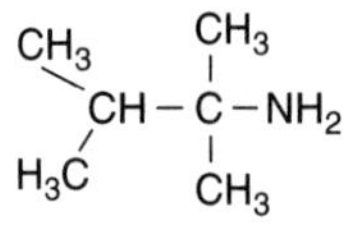
$$\begin{array}{cc} CH_3 & CH_3 \\ \diagdown & | \\ CH-C-NH_2 \\ \diagup & | \\ H_3C & CH_3 \end{array}$$

C.
$$\begin{array}{c} CH_2-CH_2-CH_3 \\ | \\ N-CH_3 \quad \text{tertiary} \\ | \\ CH_3 \end{array}$$

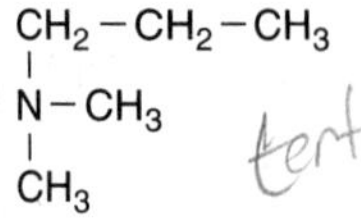

D. All are equal

4. Which compound shown has the greatest base strength?

A. 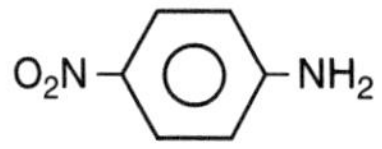 $O_2N-\langle \bigcirc \rangle-NH_2$

B. 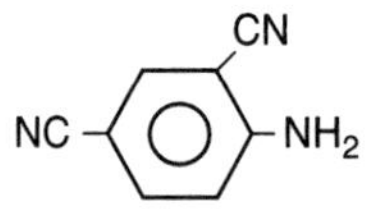
$$NC-\langle \bigcirc \rangle \overset{CN}{-}NH_2$$

C. 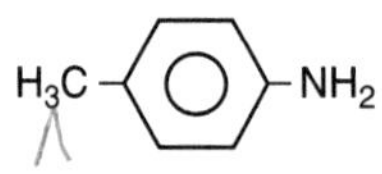 $H_3C-\langle \bigcirc \rangle-NH_2$

D. None of the above

5. Which of the compounds shown probably has the lowest boiling point?

A. 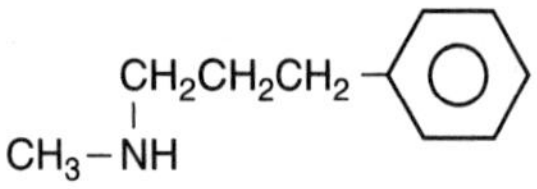
$$\begin{array}{c} CH_2CH_2CH_2-\langle \bigcirc \rangle \\ | \\ CH_3-NH \end{array}$$

B. $\langle \bigcirc \rangle-(CH_2)_3-NH_2$

C.
$$\langle \bigcirc \rangle-CH_2-\overset{\overset{\displaystyle |}{N}}{\underset{\displaystyle |}{}}-CH_3 \quad \text{tertiary} \\ CH_2CH_3$$

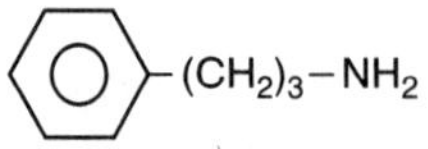

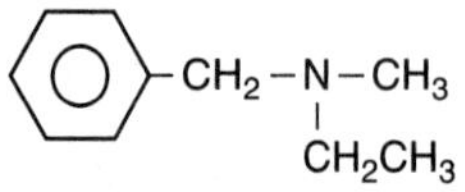

D. All are equal

6. Give the product of the reaction shown in the figure.

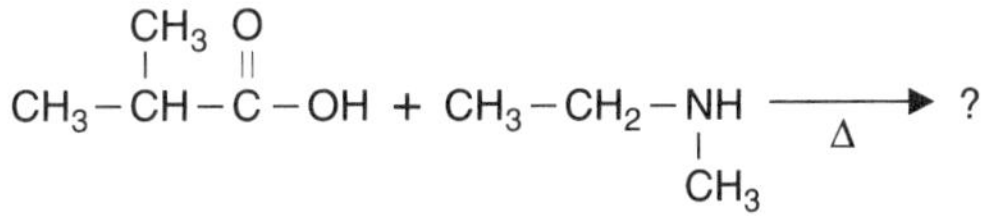

$$CH_3-\underset{\underset{CH_3}{|}}{CH}-\underset{\overset{O}{\|}}{C}-OH \ + \ CH_3-CH_2-\underset{\underset{CH_3}{|}}{NH} \xrightarrow{\Delta} \ ?$$

A. $CH_3-\underset{\underset{CH_3}{|}}{CH}-\underset{\overset{H}{|}}{C}=N-CH_2CH_3$

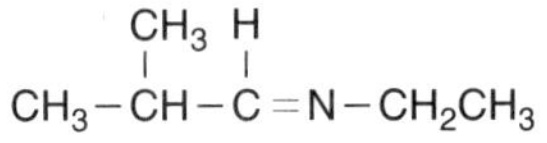

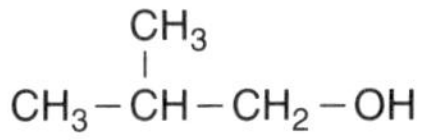

B. $CH_3-\underset{\underset{CH_3}{|}}{CH}-CH_2-OH$

C. $CH_3-\underset{\underset{CH_3}{|}}{CH}-\underset{\underset{CH_3}{|}}{\overset{\overset{\displaystyle CH_3}{|}}{CH}-N-CH_2CH_3}}$ ... $CH_3-\underset{\underset{CH_3}{|}}{CH}-\underset{\underset{CH_3}{|}}{CH}-\underset{}{\overset{\overset{CH_3\ \ N-CH_2CH_3}{}}{N}}-CH_2CH_3$

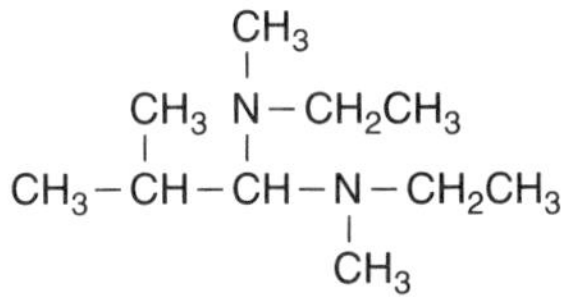

D. 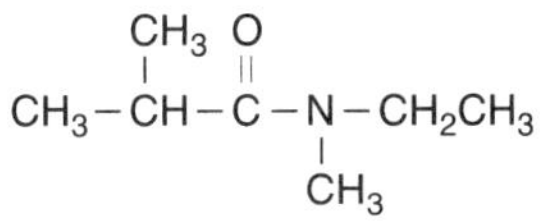 $CH_3-\underset{\underset{CH_3}{|}}{CH}-\underset{\underset{CH_3}{|}}{\overset{\overset{O}{\|}}{C}}-N-CH_2CH_3$

7. Give the product of the reaction shown in the figure.

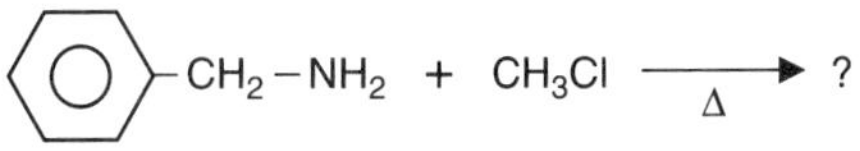

$-CH_2-NH_2 \ + \ CH_3Cl \xrightarrow{\Delta} \ ?$

A. 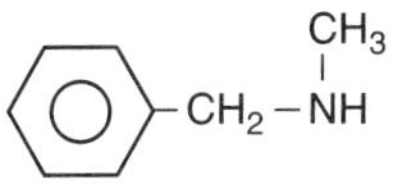 $-CH_2-\underset{\underset{}{}}{\overset{\overset{CH_3}{|}}{NH}}$

B. 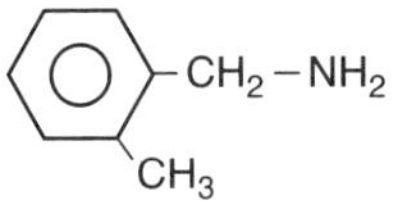 $-CH_2-NH_2$

C. 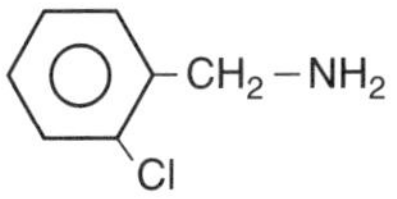 $-CH_2-NH_2$

D.   None of the above

1. **A** The compound is named as an alkene and the amino group is considered to be a substituent (it could have been named as an amine also). The numbering is as shown.

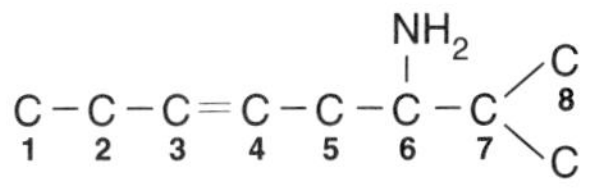

$$\underset{1}{C}-\underset{2}{C}-\underset{3}{C}=\underset{4}{C}-\underset{5}{C}-\underset{6}{\underset{\underset{NH_2}{|}}{C}}-\underset{7}{C}\overset{\diagup C \ _8}{\diagdown C}$$

2. **B** Review the structure of methyl-ethylisopropylamine.
3. **C** Tertiary amines have greater base strength than primary or secondary amines.
4. **C** Aromatic amines have low base strength in general, but electron-withdrawing groups ($-CN$, $-NO_2$) placed ortho-para decrease it even more. Electron-donating groups ($-CH_3$) placed ortho-para can increase base strength.
5. **C** Tertiary amines have lower boiling points than 1° and 2° because there is no intermolecular hydrogen bonding.
6. **D** This is the amide-forming reaction.
7. **A** This is the alkylation reaction.

Separations and Purifications

EXTRACTION

Solvent extraction is a means of purifying a compound by partitioning it between two immiscible liquids in such a fashion that the compound of interest is held strongly in one solvent, preferentially over other solutes. Quantitatively, the preference of a solute for a given solvent A over another solvent B may be expressed as its **partition coefficient**: $K_{A/B}$ = [solute]$_A$/[solute]$_B$ = (grams solute/volume of A)/(grams solute/volume of B). For example, if 1.20 g of a substance is partitioned between 50.0 ml CH_2Cl_2 and 50.0 ml of H_2O and it is determined that 0.95 g are in CH_2Cl_2 and 0.25 g are in H_2O, then the partition coefficient is calculated as: KCH_2Cl_2/H_2O = (0.95 g/50.0 ml)/(0.25 g/50.0 ml).

The higher the value of the partition coefficient, the more soluble the compound is in one solvent compared with the other.

It is often useful to take advantage of differences in the acid-base properties of solutes and to separate them on that basis. Chemical reactions ionize functional groups in organic molecules and render them soluble in water. Compounds containing very acidic protons (i.e., carboxylic acids) are extracted readily from organic solvents, such as dichloromethane, into aqueous solutions of a weak base, such as $NaHCO_3$. Compounds containing less acidic protons (i.e., phenols) are extracted from dichloromethane by stronger aqueous bases such as NaOH. Compounds that are moderately basic (i.e., amines) are extracted from dichloromethane by aqueous hydrochloric acid. Once the compound of interest has been obtained in the aqueous medium to the virtual exclusion of other compounds, the aqueous solution can be brought to neutral pH and back extracted into an organic solvent. The separation and purification of a mixture of toluene, benzoic acid, phenol, and aniline illustrate the concept (Figure 8-269).

CHROMATOGRAPHY

Chromatography, as a technique for separation and purification, is similar to solvent extraction. Chromatographic separations may be viewed as continuous partitions between a mobile phase and a stationary phase. Compounds with different partition coefficients between the mobile and stationary phase are separated because they move at different rates. The greater a compound favors the mobile phase, the faster it moves. The greater the difference in partition coefficients between compounds, the greater the difference in their respective velocities, and the easier their separation. The generalization that "like dissolves like" is applicable to chromatographic separations too.

Gas-Liquid Chromatography

Gas-liquid chromatography, or as it is more commonly called, gas chromatography, permits the quantitative separation of mixtures of compounds that can be vaporized. The *gas* frequently refers to either helium or nitrogen gas as the mobile phase in this separation technique. The *liquid* refers to a high–molecular-weight liquid, such as octadecane, coated on an inert solid support, such as finely ground firebrick, as the stationary phase. The stationary phase is packed into glass or metal tubing called a column. A typical gas chromatograph is shown in Figure 8-270.

Gas chromatography is frequently used to establish the purity of a sample, identify components in the sample, and quantitatively measure the amount of each component present in the sample. It is also possible to use gas chromatography for preparative separation of milligram quantities of reaction mixtures. A solution containing the sample to be separated and analyzed is introduced via a microliter syringe into an injector port that instantaneously vaporizes the entire sample. The vapor produced is partitioned between the high–molecular-weight liquid stationary phase and the helium or nitrogen mobile phase. The greater affinity a component has for the stationary phase, the longer it is retained in the stationary phase. Components of a mixture that have a larger difference in affinity for the stationary phase have an easier separation. Identification of compounds is based on the **retention time** of authentic compounds, or the length of time it takes from injection until a component exits the column and is detected. In addition to

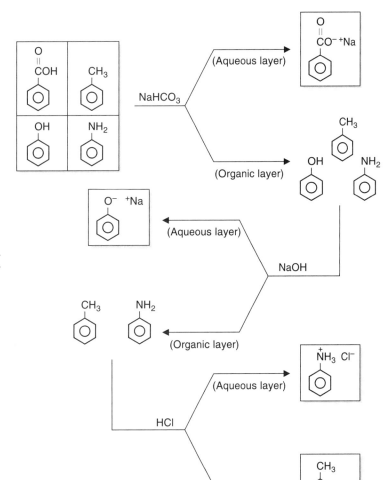

Fig. 8-269. Separation of benzoic acid, toluene, phenol, and aniline by solvent extraction.

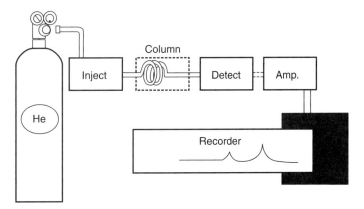

Fig. 8-270. A typical gas chromatograph.

the affinity considerations, the higher the boiling point of a compound, the longer its retention time. The detector drives a strip-chart recorder that produces peaks whose area is proportional to the amount of material passing the detector. Quantitative data can be obtained from calibration curves based on known amounts of authentic material. The free radical chlorination of cyclohexane produces a combination of unreacted cyclohexane, chlorocyclohexane, and some isomeric dichlorocyclohexanes. The presence of each compound can be detected and its concentration determined if authentic samples of each compound are available for comparison and calibration.

Problem Solving in the Biological Sciences   603

Thin-Layer Chromatography

Thin layer chromatography (TLC) is useful for the rapid separation of small quantities of materials. Such separations are valuable for determining purity of a sample, identifying the components of a mixture, and establishing conditions for the separation and purification of larger quantities of material using a buret packed with silica gel or alumina. It is possible to use TLC for preparative separations of milligram quantities of compounds. TLC is not generally used for quantitative analyses. The most common stationary phase is a plastic sheet coated with silica gel or alumina cut into small strips called plates. Both silica gel and alumina are polar because they contain —O—H groups. A nonpolar solvent, such as hexane, is used as the mobile phase or is mixed with a polar solvent, such as dichloromethane or diethyl ether, to adjust the polarity of the mobile phase for the best separation. A nonpolar mobile phase has minimal electrostatic interaction with the stationary phase, so compounds separate according to their polarity—the most polar compound moves slowest in the mobile phase whereas the least polar compound travels fastest. A more polar mobile phase interacts with the polar stationary phase and hastens the movement of all compounds, because the stationary phase interacts with the solvent to a greater extent than the sample due to the greater abundance of the solvent. A few microliters of a solution of the mixture to be separated is spotted near the bottom of a TLC plate. The plate is placed in a covered beaker or jar containing the mobile phase. The mobile phase rises on the plate by capillary action, carrying with it components of the mixture to be separated. Figure 8-271 shows schematically the separation of a three-component mixture on a silica gel plate. Compound *a* is the most polar component, *c* is the least polar component, and *b* is of intermediate polarity. Identification of the components is based on the ratio (R_f) of the distance moved by a given spot to the distance traveled by the solvent (mobile phase).

Such R_f values are, by definition, equal to or less than unity. It is often convenient to spot authentic samples on the same plate as an unknown to measure their R_f values under identical conditions. The basis for the separation of fluorene from fluorenone on silica gel is shown in Figure 8-272. Fluorene, a nonpolar compound, has an R_f value close to 1.00, whereas the polar fluorenone has an R_f of nearly half that using silica gel as a stationary phase and hexane as the mobile phase. For the separation of large quantities of fluorene from fluorenone, a solvent or solvent mixture is selected by TLC. For the separation of fluorene and fluorenone, hexane provides two readily distinguishable, separated spots. A buret is filled with a suspension of silica gel in hexane, excess hexane is drained off, and the stopcock of the buret is closed. The mixture to be separated is introduced as a concentrated solution at the top of the buret and the stopcock is opened. Additional hexane must be added to the buret to replace the mobile phase that flows out. As the hexane moves down the buret, it carries with it the fluorene, leaving the fluorenone near the top of the silica gel. Once the nonpolar fluorene has eluted, dichloromethane is used as the mobile phase to chase out the polar fluorenone (Figure 8-273).

$$R_f = \frac{\text{Distance spot "A" moves from the origin}}{\text{Distance solvent "S" moves from origin}} = A/S$$

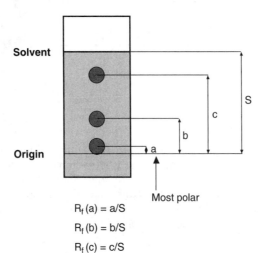

Fig. 8-271. Thin layer chromatography separation of a three-component mixture.

$R_f (a) = a/S$

$R_f (b) = b/S$

$R_f (c) = c/S$

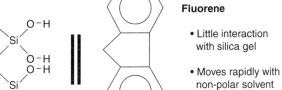

Fluorene

• Little interaction
with silica gel

• Moves rapidly with
non-polar solvent

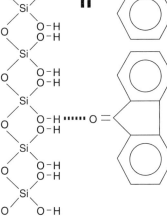

Fig. 8-272. Silica gel interaction with fluorene and fluorenone.

Fluorenone

• Hydrogen bonding
to silica gel

• Little movement with
non-polar solvent

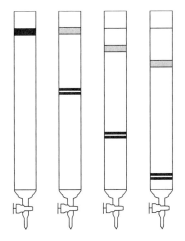

Fig. 8-273. Column chromatographic separation of fluorene and fluorenone.

▬ Fluorenone – fluorene mixture

▦ Fluorenone

≡ Fluorene

DISTILLATION

Distillation is a means of purifying a liquid by vaporizing it, separating its vapor from that of impurities or other compounds, and condensing the purified vapor back to a liquid and collecting it in a separate container.

Every volatile liquid compound has molecules above it in the vapor phase. Heating the liquid increases the kinetic energy of the molecules in the liquid state to the point where they are no longer attracted to other molecules of the liquid and therefore pass into the gas or vapor phase. This, in turn, increases the partial pressure of vapor above the liquid. When the temperature at which the partial pressure of vapor above the liquid equals ambient pressure, the liquid boils. The actual temperature required to boil a liquid depends on the presence or absence of factors that hold molecules of liquid near each other. Such factors include van der Waals forces, dipolar electrostatic attractions, and hydrogen bonding.

The distillation process can be viewed as a series of vaporizations and condensations that enrich the vapor in the more volatile compound. In an equimolar mixture of two liquids (A and B), if A is the more volatile substance, the vapor above the A/B mixture is richer in A than in B. That vapor is condensed back to a liquid, now enriched in A. The vapor above this enriched liquid is even richer in A, the more volatile compound.

Each vaporization-condensation cycle is termed a "theoretical plate." In research and academic laboratories, this theoretical plate has no physical being (i.e., it really is theoretical). In industrial distillations, each theoretical plate corresponds to a distinctly different heating-condensing apparatus. Liquids with widely different boiling points require few theoretical plates to achieve a vapor that is practically pure in the low boiling, more volatile compound. Similarly, two liquids whose boiling points are close together require several vaporization-condensation cycles to obtain a vapor that contains only one compound because the enrichment of each step is smaller.

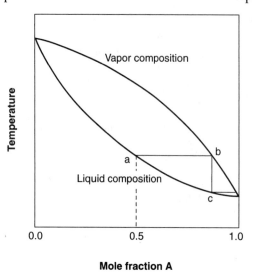

Fig. 8-274. Liquid and vapor composition of an ideal two-component mixture as a function of temperature.

Figure 8-274 shows an idealized graph of the vapor and liquid compositions for mixtures of A and B, where A is the more volatile liquid. Point *a* represents the starting point of 0.5 mole fraction A in the liquid phase. Point *b* represents the composition of the vapor in equilibrium with the liquid in A at the same temperature. Note that the vapor has a greater mole fraction of A than does the liquid (approximately 0.85 mole fraction A in the vapor phase). Point *c* represents the vapor from point *b* condensed to a liquid with the same 0.85 mole fraction A. The path from point *a* to *b* to *c* represents one theoretical plate. The figure shows that two theoretical plates are needed to produce a vapor of nearly pure A. A third plate would lead to a further increase in the concentration of A in the liquid phase. From a practical standpoint, the number of theoretical plates in a research or academic laboratory distillation may be increased by increasing the surface area available for condensations and the length of the distillation column. Experimentally, this is accomplished by packing the fractionating column with glass beads, ceramic "saddles," or stainless steel wool.

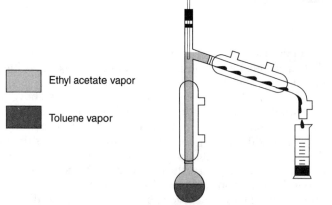

Fig. 8-275. Distillation of ethyl acetate and toluene.

Ethyl acetate vapor

Toluene vapor

Figure 8-275 shows the apparatus for the distillation of a mixture of ethyl acetate (boiling point is 78°C) and toluene (boiling point is 111°C). Note that the vapor about to distill is virtually free of toluene, whereas the vapor closer to the distilling flask contains increasingly higher amounts of that compound.

As each pure material is distilled, the temperature remains constant at the boiling

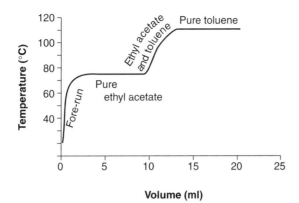

Fig. 8-276. Variation of temperature with volume during the distillation of ethyl acetate and toluene.

point for the compound distilling. An idealized graph of temperature as a function of volume for the fractional distillation of a mixture of ethyl acetate and toluene is shown in Figure 8-276. Four regions or fractions on the graph may be discerned. There is an initial fraction for which the temperature increases from room temperature (25°C) to the boiling point of ethyl acetate. The liquid collected during that region is termed "fore-run." Although the liquid collected in this fore-run is largely ethyl acetate, it is not pure and should not be combined with the fraction that will contain the pure material. Experimentally, the fore-run is usually small in volume. The second fraction that is observed is where the temperature remains constant at 78°C, the boiling point of pure ethyl acetate. This is collected in a separate container as a pure liquid. The third fraction is observed as the temperature increases from 78°C to 111°C, the boiling point of toluene. This fraction contains both ethyl acetate and toluene. Accordingly, it should be collected in a different container. The fourth fraction boils at a constant 111°C and is pure toluene.

RECRYSTALLIZATION

Recrystallization is a technique for the purification of a solid by breaking down the crystal lattice structure of the solid by dissolving it in a suitable solvent and then allowing the crystal lattice to form again. A saturated solution of an impure solid is prepared at an elevated temperature. When the solution cools, it becomes supersaturated with respect to the compound of interest and crystals of that compound form. The more slowly the solution cools, the larger are the resulting crystals. The original impurities are excluded from the crystals that form for two reasons: (1) the solution is not supersaturated with respect to the impurities (i.e., they remain dissolved), and (2) the impurities do not easily fit into the growing crystal lattice structure. Once the solution has deposited all the crystals that it will yield, the crystals are filtered from the solution, washed with cold solvent, and dried. If the recrystallization has indeed improved the purity of the solid sample, its melting point should increase over that recorded for the initial material and it should melt over a narrower temperature range.

A good choice of solvent is crucial to the success of a recrystallization. The following criteria should be met: (1) the solvent must not react chemically with the sample, (2) the solubility of the sample in the solvent should increase greatly by increasing the temperature, (3) the impurities should remain largely in solution at the crystallization temperature of the desired compound, and (4) the solvent should be reasonably easy to evaporate from the purified sample.

Water, methanol, ethyl acetate, dichloromethane, hexane, and toluene were tested as potential solvents for the recrystallization of a solid with the following results, where S = soluble, S_h = soluble in hot solution, and I = insoluble:

water—I, methanol—S_h, ethyl acetate—S, dichloromethane—S, hexane—S, and toluene—S.

Based on the second criterion, methanol would be the solvent of choice to purify the solid by recrystallization, assuming that the other criteria are also met by methanol. Ethyl acetate, dichloromethane, hexane, and toluene dissolved the sample at room temperature. To induce crystallization, the volume of solution would have to be substantially reduced to obtain any crystals on cooling. Water failed to dissolve the sample in the first place, so it is an unacceptable recrystallizing solvent for this solute.

Fractional crystallization can be used to separate a mixture of two solids if a solvent can be found that dissolves one compound readily even cold and dissolves the other only when it is hot. A typical example is the separation of trans-cinnamic acid from urea. Both

TABLE 8-7. Typical Observations in Solubility

Compound	Water	Methanol	Ethyl Acetate	Dichloromethane	Hexane	Toluene
Cinnamic acid	S_h	S	S	S	S	S
Urea	S	S	I	I	I	I

I = insoluble; *S* = soluble; S_h = soluble in hot solution.

melt at nominally 132°C, but the mixture has a melting point that is considerably less than that.

Table 8-7 lists typical observations on solubility. From these data, it can be seen that a mixture of cinnamic acid and urea dissolved in hot water would yield crystals of cinnamic acid on cooling. Urea remains dissolved in the cold water. The crystals thus obtained should melt at close to 132°C. Proof of the identity of the crystal as *trans*-cinnamic acid can be obtained by a mixed melting point with authentic *trans*-cinnamic acid.

SEPARATIONS AND PURIFICATIONS: REVIEW QUESTIONS

1. For two compounds to be separated by NaHCO₃ extraction, they must have:

    A. different dipole moments.
    B. different acid-base properties.
    C. different boiling points.
    D. different molecular weights.

2. Which pair of compounds could be separated most readily by solvent extraction?

    A. Aminocyclohexane and chlorocyclohexane
    B. Cyclohexanol and cyclohexanone
    C. Phenol and p-cresol
    D. Butanoic acid and 2-methylpropanoic acid

3. Carboxylic acids are generally separated as their methyl esters in gas chromatography. Why are the carboxylic acids themselves difficult to separate by this technique?

    A. Carboxylic acids all have the same nominal polarity.
    B. Carboxylic acids are insoluble in most organic solvents, whereas their methyl esters are soluble.
    C. Carboxylic acids decompose readily in a gas chromatographic column.
    D. Carboxylic acids do not vaporize readily but their methyl esters do so easily.

4. Which pair of compounds shown would be separated most readily on silica gel by thin layer chromatography?

    A.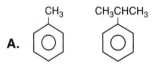

    B. CH₃CH₂CH₂CH₂CH₂Cl
       CH₃CH₂CH₂CH₂CH₂Br

    C. $$CH_3CH_2CH_2CH_2\overset{\overset{\displaystyle O}{\|}}{C}CH_3$$
       $$CH_3CH_2CH_2\overset{\overset{\displaystyle O}{\|}}{C}CH_2CH_3$$

    D.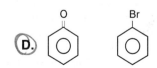

5. Fractionating columns in distillations are frequently packed with glass beads, ceramic saddles, or stainless steel wool to:

   A. increase the condensation of the vapor in the fractionating column.
   B. decrease the rate at which pure liquid distills.
   C. maintain a constant temperature in the fractionating column.
   D. provide a surface on which impurities may be absorbed and removed.

6. According to the temperature vs. volume graph of the distillation, how many compounds were present in the initial mixture?

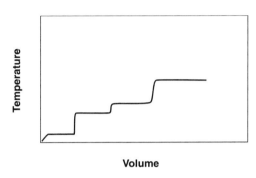

Volume

   A. One
   B. Two
   C. Three
   D. Four

7. An impure solid gives the following solubility test results, where I = insoluble; S = soluble; S_h = soluble when the solvent is hot: water—I, methanol—I; hexane—S_h, dichloromethane—S. Which solvent would be most appropriate to attempt the recrystallization of this impure solid?

   A. Water
   B. Methanol
   C. Hexane
   D. Dichloromethane

8. Impurities are removed in the recrystallization process because of the following factors:

   I. Impurities do not "fit" into a growing crystal lattice.
   II. Impurities lower the melting point of the compound.
   III. Impurities remain dissolved in the solvent used.
   A. I only
   B. I and II
   C. I and III
   D. I, II, and III

ANSWERS AND EXPLANATIONS

1. B Separation by solvent extraction requires different acidity-basicity. Sodium bicarbonate is a weak base. For it to serve as the basis of a separation, one compound must be capable of reacting with $NaHCO_3$ while the other does not.

2. A Separation by solvent extraction requires different acidity-basicity. This is an application of the same principle as in question 1 using HCl. An amine can be protonated and therefore water solubilized, leaving behind the alkyl halide. The remaining pairs of compounds are not readily distinguishable by their acid-base properties.

3. D By definition, compounds to be separated by gas chromatography must be capable of being vaporized. Carboxylic acids form hydrogen bonded dimers that keep their vapor pressure low. Hydrogen-bonded dimers do not form from the methyl esters.

4. D Thin layer chromatography separates compounds on the basis of polarity. A ketone and an alkyl halide have different polarities, whereas the other compounds are similar in theirs.

5. A Distillation is a series of vaporizations and condensations. The efficiency of the distillation is improved by increasing the surface area in the fractionating column on which liquid–vapor exchange can take place and by increasing the length of the column.

6. **D** A pure compound distills at constant temperature. There are four regions at which temperature remains constant, so four compounds were initially present.

7. **C** The best solvent for recrystallization on the basis of solubility tests is the one that needs to be heated for the solute to dissolve. In that manner, obtaining pure crystals is obtained by cooling the solution below room temperature.

8. **C** Crystals grow in highly ordered patterns into which impurities do not fit unless the impurities look very much like the compound of interest. With a properly chosen solvent, the impurities should remain in solution as the pure crystals form.

Use of Spectroscopy in Structural Identification

Self-Managed Learning Questions
Focus on the following experimental issues:

1. Is there any research study or hypotheses testing on the use of spectroscopy?
2. Are there any clinical laboratory tests or applications of spectroscopy related to specimen collection, specimen classification and types, collection time for specimens, specimen handling, and any experimental errors?
3. Are there any theories or laws related to spectroscopy that need clarification or synthesis with bioclinical applications? Explore at least two or three viewpoints and technically critique such issues.
4. Are there any graphs, diagrams, reaction mechanisms, or sketches that require quantitative analysis? Which mathematical concepts help in interpreting graphical data?
5. Review laboratory and commercial spectroscopic techniques and identify differences. Understand the mechanical and electric design, working, and accuracy of various types of spectrometers.

INFRARED SPECTROSCOPY

Intramolecular Vibrations and Rotations

Infrared spectroscopy, sometimes called "vibrational spectroscopy," is useful for identification of functional groups present in a molecule. Bonds that vibrate in a manner that changes the net dipole moment of the molecule absorb infrared radiation according to Hooke's law for the vibration of a spring. In the case of carbon dioxide, there are four possible vibrational modes: symmetric stretching, asymmetric stretching, in-plane bending, and out-of-plane bending. These are shown schematically in Figure 8-277. The symmetric stretching vibration does not alter the net dipole moment of the compound because the vector sum of the dipoles is still zero. Accordingly, this vibrational mode of carbon dioxide is not "infrared active."

Frequencies are given in wave numbers (cm^{-1}), which is the reciprocal of wavelength, or in microns (μm), which is also a unit of wavelength. The two frequency units may be interconverted by the following formulae; $v = 1/\lambda$ (λ in cm) $= 10,000/\lambda$ (λ in μm). Texts and laboratory manuals give extensive correlation tables of frequencies and functional groups. A concise summary of important functional groups and their characteristic

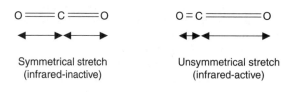

Symmetrical stretch
(infrared-inactive)

Unsymmetrical stretch
(infrared-active)

Fig. 8-277. Vibrational modes of carbon dioxide.

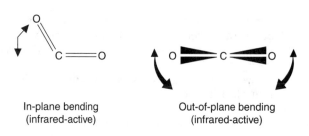

In-plane bending
(infrared-active)

Out-of-plane bending
(infrared-active)

TABLE 8-8. Common Characteristic Group Absorptions

Frequency (cm^{-1})	Functionality	Comments
3500 (broad)	OH, NH	Hydrogen bonding causes broadness of the peak
3000	CH	Virtually every organic compound has this
2200	alkyne, nitrile	
1715	C=O	Exact frequency varies with the type of C=O
1600	C=C	
1500–600		Fingerprint region—each compound has a unique pattern
1100	C—O	Useful to identify esters and ethers
600–800	Aromatic C—H	One peak = ortho or para disubstituted; two peaks = mono substituted or meta disubstituted

frequencies is given in Table 8-8. The frequencies listed are not absolute; structural features of different compounds shift the vibrational frequencies of the functionality.

NUCLEAR MAGNETIC RESONANCE SPECTROSCOPY

Protons in a Magnetic Field, Equivalent Protons

Proton magnetic resonance spectroscopy measures the number and types of different protons in a compound. Certain nuclei rotate on an axis and precess about that axis in much the same manner that the earth rotates and precesses on its axis. This rotation and precession sets up a magnetic moment of the nucleus—it can be aligned with or against an externally applied magnetic field. Alignment in the same direction as the external field is easier, just as it is easier to swim downstream than upstream. The difference in energy required for each magnetic orientation is measured by radio frequency radiation according to the equation $\Delta E = h\nu$. A plot of radiation absorbed as a function of frequency provides information about the local magnetic environment of the nuclei examined. Protons are one of a number of such nuclei that rotate. In proton magnetic resonance spectroscopy (PMR), only protons are observed. The presence of carbon can only be inferred. Equally important is the fact that substitution of deuterium (D) = H_1^2 for a type of proton H_1^1 will render that type of proton invisible.

Diasterotopic and Enantiotopic Protons

The number of different signals depends on the number of magnetically different protons that are present in a molecule. Figure 8-278 shows different compounds and an indication of the number of magnetically different protons on each. There are two means by which protons can be considered identical—by **symmetry** or by being **geminal** (twins on the same carbon atom). The four protons of methane are all geminal; therefore, only one signal is observed. Similarly, all six protons of ethane are identical by symmetry, but the two methyl groups of methyl ethanoate (methyl acetate) are not identical. One methyl

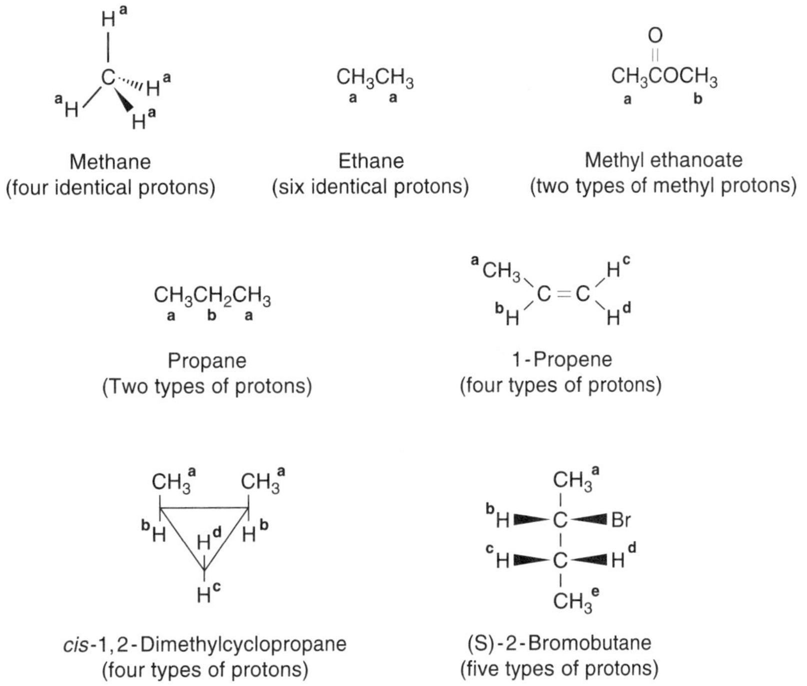

Fig. 8-278. Magnetically different protons.

group is attached to a carbonyl carbon and the other is attached to an oxygen. Each methyl group is then in a different magnetic environment. Propane is symmetric about carbon-2 and so has two magnetically different types of protons. Propene offers the chance to make a careless error in selecting the number of magnetically different protons present. There are four. Protons (c) and (d) are not identical. Proton (c) is *cis* to a methyl group, whereas proton (d) is *trans* to the methyl group. Again, this gives a different magnetic environment to these protons. In an analogous fashion, protons (c) and (d) of 1,2-dimethylcyclopropane are not identical. Here, (d) is *cis* to two methyl groups and (c) is *cis* to two protons. (S)-2-bromobutane is a more difficult case. Protons (c) and (d) here are again superficially the same, but in fact they are not. They are called diastereotopic protons. Replacing each of these protons with some other group results in diastereomers, which are easily distinguished by chemical and physical properties. Proton (d) is affected by the effects of the bromine atom of carbon-2 more so than is proton (c) in the configuration shown. Each is in a magnetically different environment. If replacement of each of two suspected identical protons with another group yields enantiomers, the protons are called "enantiotopic" and are magnetically indistinguishable.

Chemical Shifts for Protons

The **chemical shift** of a proton resonance is the difference in frequency between a signal absorbed by a sample and the frequency at which **tetramethylsilane** (TMS), a common reference material, absorbs radiation in the same instrument. This difference is expressed in a δ scale in units of parts per million (ppm). TMS is a good reference standard because its resonance frequency is different from most other types of protons, it is chemically inert, it has 12 identical protons so it gives a very strong signal, and it is easy to remove from the sample after the spectrum is recorded (boiling point = 26°C–28°C). Protons that absorb at lower frequencies than TMS are said to be "shielded" from the external magnetic field because less energy is required to meet the resonance condition $\Delta E = h\nu$. Some instruments maintain a constant radio frequency and use an electromagnet to vary the strength of the magnetic field applied. The same shielded protons resonate upfield of TMS, that is, at higher magnetic field strength than TMS. Such shielding stems from a local magnetic flux that opposes the external field. Protons may also be "deshielded" or shifted downfield of TMS by local magnetic flux that reinforces the applied field. [18]-Annulene provides a compound with examples of both phenomena. Protons on the inside of the ring are shielded by a magnetic field that opposes the applied external field while the outside protons are deshielded by the same field. This field that shields and deshields is induced by the ring current that flows in the aromatic [18]-annulene ring. Its flux opposes the external applied field for the inside protons and it reinforces the external applied field for the outside protons (Figure 8-279).

Protons along the perimeter of an aromatic ring are then deshielded (shifted to higher δ). Protons attached to carbons bearing an electronegative element, such as O or Cl are also deshielded from their customary resonance frequency in the absence of the electronegative element. The electron density near such electronegative elements is greater, so that higher magnetic field strength is required to achieve the resonance condition. The chemical shift of a proton gives information about its magnetic environment.

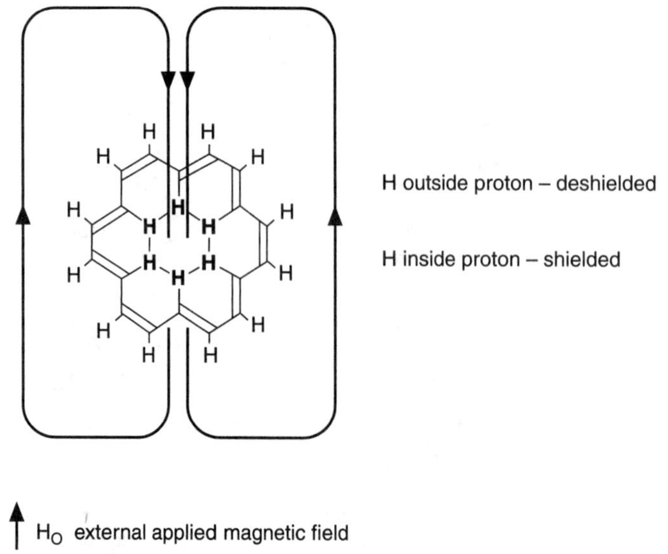

Fig. 8-279. [18]-Annulene showing shielding and deshielding.

H outside proton – deshielded

H inside proton – shielded

H₀ external applied magnetic field

Textbooks and laboratory manuals provide detailed tables of chemical shifts for a variety of different types of protons. Although such tables may be helpful in predicting the chemical shift of a given type of proton, they are not as crucial to structure determination. For that purpose, there are only three chemical shift values that need to be memorized:

Chemical shift (δ ppm)	Proton type
7	Aromatic C—H
9	Aldehyde RCHO
11	Carboxylic acid RCO_2H

Spin-Spin Splitting

It is sometimes useful to note that methyl protons (CH_3) give a typical resonance near δ 1 ppm and methylene protons (CH_2) generally give a resonance in the range d 2–3 ppm. The fine structure or multiplicity of the signal **(splitting pattern)** provides a great deal of information about the protons in the vicinity of the one at resonance. This is because protons "couple" with protons that are one carbon atom away. The magnetic environment of a proton is slightly altered by the magnetic orientation of those nearby protons. The fine structure or multiplicity is defined as follows: Multiplicity of PMR signal = 1 + (total number of protons on adjacent carbon atoms).

The fine structure of PMR signals is symmetric and in relative ratios that are defined by Pascal's triangle (the coefficients for the binomial expansion of [a + b]n) as follows:

Singlet (1 let)	1
Doublet (2 let)	1 1
Triplet (3 let)	1 2 1
Quartet (4 tet)	1 3 3 1
Quintet (5 tet)	1 4 6 4 1

Thus, a triplet consists of three peaks of relative intensity 1:2:1 and is indicative of a proton with a total of two protons on the adjacent carbon atoms. The term **multiplet** (m let) is used when the relative intensity of the first peak is too small to detect and accurately count. Aromatic protons are described as a singlet, broad singlet, or multiplet depending on the specific compound. The chemical shift is more useful than multiplicity in the identification of the presence of aromatic rings.

If there are other spinning nuclei, for example F-19, protons also couple with that nucleus so that multiplicity then becomes: Multiplicity of PMR signal = 1 + (total number of protons on adjacent carbon atoms) + number of F-19 atoms on the same carbon.

The proton spectrum of cumene shown in Figure 8-280 illustrates the splitting of

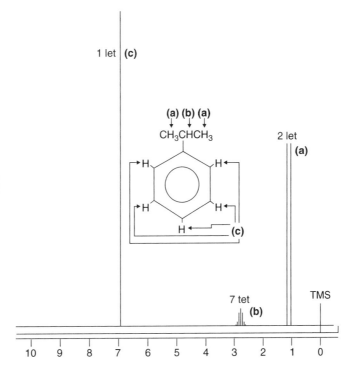

Fig. 8-280. Proton magnetic resonance spectroscopy spectrum of ethylbenzene.

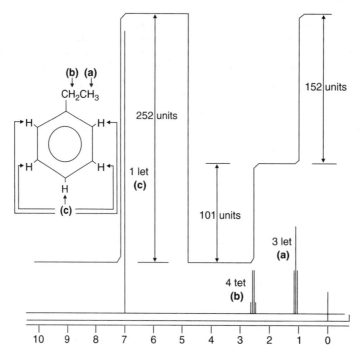

Fig. 8-281. Potential structures for sample spectroscopy problem.

adjacent protons. (The multiplicity of the two identical methyl groups is 1 plus the number of protons on the adjacent carbon atoms.) There is only one proton on that "adjacent" carbon, so the methyl protons appear as a doublet. In the same manner, the methine proton (CH) appears as a septet because there are six protons on the adjacent carbons. The benzene ring appears as a singlet because, in this case, the ortho-meta-para protons are nearly alike.

There are two splitting patterns that are especially important: (1) 3 let and 4 tet ethyl group and (2) 2 let and 7 tet iso-propyl group.

To count the protons that give a signal, the area under each peak is electronically determined by charging a capacitor and plotting the charge on that capacitor as a function of the frequency scanned. The change in capacitor charge plotted on the y-axis is proportional to the number of protons at a given resonance position. A ratio is established between the total integration distance and the total number of protons in the structure, and that ratio is used to determine the number of protons on signal. The spectrum in Figure 8-281 for a compound of formula C_8H_{10} (ethyl benzene) illustrates the use of this methodology.

The total integral distance is 505 units. A proportion is then set up as follows: total integral distance/total protons in molecule = integral distance of one signal/protons giving rise to the signal. That translates into the following for the triplet: 505 units/10H = 152 units/xH. Solving for x gives 3.01 protons, which is close enough to 3 to be correctly identified with a set of methyl protons.

APPLIED CONCEPTS

The following is a list of tools to analyze and understand use of spectroscopy in structural identification.

- Improve review of observations linked with types and quantities of reactants and products. Identify all possible experiments to be performed. Propose any experimental modifications or new procedures to be used.
- Understand how reactions are related to basic mechanisms, how reaction rates are affected, and what bonding arrangements, resonance stability structures, and stereoarrangements are possible. Elucidate each mechanism in a visual format.
- Learn how to judge the influence of new experimental evidence on each conclusion, including experimental conditions, experimental errors, and practical limitations on experiment.
- Look for hidden assumptions behind each experimental technique or procedure, theoretical explanation, and practical explanation of each mechanism.
- Look for scientific reasons behind each observation (laboratory observations, untaught observations from experimental data, and completely new observations).

- Determine deductive conclusions from observations to approve or nullify your hypotheses.

USE OF SPECTROSCOPY IN STRUCTURAL IDENTIFICATION: REVIEW QUESTIONS

1. In the structure shown, how many magnetically different protons are present?

$$CH_3CH_2CHCH_2CH_3$$
$$|$$
$$CH_2CH_3$$

   A. Three
   B. Four
   C. Five
   D. Seven

2. Which pair of compounds cannot be readily distinguished by infrared spectroscopy?

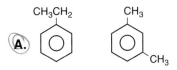

   A.

$$O$$
$$||$$
$$CH_3CH_2CH_2CH_2CCH_3$$
   B. $CH_3CH_2CH_2CH_2CH_2CH_2OH$

$$O$$
$$||$$
$$CH_3CH_2CH_2CH_2COH$$
   C. $CH_3CH_2CH_2CH=CHCH_2CH_3$

$$CH_3CH_2CH_2CH_2CH_2CH_2Cl$$
   D. $CH_3CH_2CH_2CH_2CH_2CH_2OH$

3. In the molecule shown, in the proton magnetic resonance spectrum, the indicated protons should appear as a:

$$CH_3CH_2CHCH_3$$

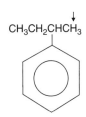

   A. singlet
   B. doublet
   C. triplet
   D. quartet

4. A compound of formula C_5H_{12} is studied by proton magnetic resonance spectroscopy. The total integral distance was measured as 144 mm. One signal gave an integral distance of 72 mm. How many protons give that signal?

   A. Two
   B. Three
   C. Six
   D. Nine

$$\frac{144}{12} = \frac{12 \cdot 6}{x}$$

$$12 = \frac{72}{x}$$

$$12 \times c = 72$$
$$x = \frac{72}{12} = 6$$

Problem Solving in the Biological Sciences   615

5. The signals shown represent magnetic resonance signals. Which one is a quartet?

A

B

C

(D) 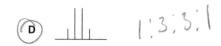 1:3:3:1

6. A broad peak in the 3500–3000 cm^{-1} region of the infrared spectrum is due to:

A. O—H vibrations damped by hydrogen bonding.
B. C=C vibrations damped by hydrogen bonding.
C. C=O vibrations damped by hydrogen bonding.
D. aromatic ring vibrations.

7. In the compound shown, which of the indicated protons will give their resonance signal farthest downfield (highest δ)?

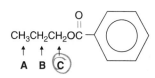

D. All protons will have the same nominal chemical shift.

8. In the proton magnetic resonance spectrum, a singlet that corresponds to one proton disappears on addition of D_2O. This disappearance is due to the fact that:

A. deuterium exchanges with all protons.
B. deuterium exchanges with acidic protons.
C. deuterium causes instrument malfunctions.
D. the deuterium signal is much stronger than the proton signal.

9. How many magnetically different protons are present in the molecule shown?

$$CH_3CH_2\diagdown \qquad \diagup CH_3$$
$$C = C$$
$$\diagup \qquad \diagdown$$
$$H \qquad \qquad CH_2CH_3$$

A. Three
B. Four
C. Five
D. Six

10. An unknown compound has been determined to be either *cis*-1,2-dimethylcyclopropane or its *trans* isomer. The magnetic resonance spectrum of the compound revealed four magnetically different types of protons. Which isomer is the unknown?

A. *trans* — 3
B. *cis* — 4
C. Mixture of both
D. Cannot tell

11. An unknown molecule has been found to contain oxygen. From the infrared spectrum shown, it is clear that the oxygen is present as which functional group?

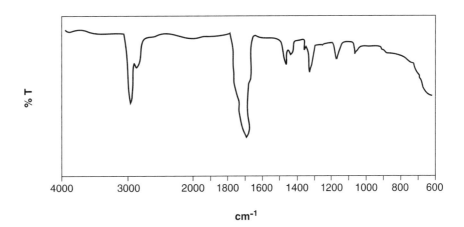

cm⁻¹

A. Alcohol
B. Carboxylic acid
C. Ether
D. Ketone

12. Which structure is consistent with the spectral data listed for $C_4H_8O_3$?
3 let δ 1.27 (3H)
4 tet δ 3.66 (2H) ir: 2500–3000 cm⁻¹ broad
1 let δ 4.13 (2H) 1715 cm⁻¹
1 let δ 10.95 (1H)

A. $CH_3\overset{\overset{O}{\|}}{C}CH_2OCH_2OH$

B. $CH_3\underset{\underset{CH_3}{|}}{CH}\overset{\overset{O}{\|}}{C}OOH$

C. $CH_3CH_2OCH_2\overset{\overset{O}{\|}}{C}OH$

D. $CH_3OCH\underset{}{}OCH_3$, $\overset{CH_2OH}{|}$ (CH₃OCHOCH₃)

ANSWERS AND EXPLANATIONS

1. A There are three identical ethyl groups (two types of protons) and one methine (CH) proton. Thus, there are three different types of protons present.

2. A Monosubstituted benzenes and meta disubstituted benzenes both give two major peaks in the 600–800 cm⁻¹ region of the infrared spectrum.

3. B The multiplicity of a proton magnetic resonance signal is 1 plus the number of protons on adjacent carbons. In this case, there is one carbon adjacent to the terminal methyl group and it has but one proton. The multiplicity is (1 + 1) = 2 = doublet.

4. C A ratio of total integration distance:total protons = signal distance:signal protons is set up as 144 mm/12 H = 72 mm/x. Solving for x gives six protons.

5. D Magnetic resonance signals are symmetric and follow Pascal's triangle for their relative intensity. The correct ratio for a quartet is 1:3:3:1.

6. A Peak broadening in the ir spectrum is due to hydrogen bonding. Of the choices listed, alcohols are the only functionality capable of hydrogen bonding to other like molecules.

7. **C** Protons on carbons bonded to electronegative elements or electron withdrawing groups have their resonance condition shed to higher δ (downfield).

8. **B** Deuterium exchange for protons causes a PMR signal to disappear. For such an exchange to take place, the proton must first be removed and then replaced. That can only happen with D_2O when the protein is acidic (e.g., in alcohols, carboxylic acids).

9. **D** The two ethyl groups are not identical. One is *cis* to a methyl group, whereas the other is *cis* to a proton. Each has a slightly different magnetic environment.

10. **B** The *trans* isomer has three magnetically different types of protons, whereas the *cis* isomer has four.

11. **D** The peak near 1700 cm^{-1} is characteristic of C$=$O.

12. **C** The triplet and quartet are characteristic of an ethyl group. The singlet of two protons corresponds to a CH_2 with no protons on atoms on either side of it. A singlet at δ 10.95 is due to a carboxylic acid, a functionality confirmed in the infrared spectrum.

Bibliography

Davis W, Soloman EP. *The World of Biology*, 4th ed. Philadelphia, Saunders College Publishing, 1990.

Durst HD, Gokel GW. *Experimental Organic Chemistry*, 2nd ed. New York, McGraw-Hill, 1986.

Friefelder D. *Molecular Biology*, 2nd ed. Boston, Jones and Bartlett, 1983.

Keeton WT, Gould JL. *Biological Science*, 5th ed. New York, WW Norton, 1993.

Loudon GM. *Organic Chemistry*, 2nd ed. Redwood City, CA, Benjamin-Cummings, 1988.

Morrison RT, Boyd RN. *Organic Chemistry*, 6th ed. Englewood Cliffs, NJ, Prentice-Hall, 1992.

Purves WK, Orians GH, Heller HC. *Life: The Science of Biology*, 4th ed. Sunderland, MA, Sinauer Associates, 1995.

Solomons TWG. *Organic Chemistry*, 5th ed. New York, John Wiley & Sons, 1992.

Williamson KL. *Microscale and Macroscale Organic Experiments*, Lexington, MA, DC Heath, 1989.

Zubrick JW. *The Organic Chem Lab Survival Manual: A Student's Guide to Techniques*, 3rd ed. New York, John Wiley & Sons, 1992.

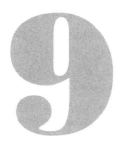

Full-Length Practice MCAT

Verbal Reasoning

Directions: You are provided with nine passages in the Verbal Reasoning test. Each passage is followed by several questions. After reading a passage, select the one best answer to each question. If you are not certain of an answer, eliminate the alternatives that you know to be incorrect and then select an answer from the remaining alternatives.

Passage I (Questions 1–7)

Computerized transactions of all kinds are becoming ever more pervasive. More than half a dozen countries have developed or are testing chip cards that would replace cash. In Denmark, a consortium of banking, utility, and transport companies has announced a card that would replace coins and small bills. In France, the telecommunications authorities have proposed general use of the smart cards now used at pay telephones. The government of Singapore has requested bids for a system that would communicate with cars and charge their smart cards as they pass various points on a road (as opposed to the simple vehicle identification systems already in use in the U.S. and elsewhere). And cable and satellite broadcasters are experimenting with smart cards for delivering pay-per-view television. All these systems, however, are based on cards that identify themselves during every transaction.

If the trend toward identifier-based smart cards continues, personal privacy will increasingly be eroded. But in this conflict between organizational security and individual liberty, neither side emerges as a clear winner. Each round of improved identification techniques, sophisticated data analysis or extended linking can be frustrated by widespread noncompliance or even legislated limits, which in turn may engender attempts at further control.

Meanwhile, in a system based on representatives and observers, organizations stand to gain competitive and political advantages from increased public confidence (in addition to the lower costs of pseudonymous record-keeping). And individuals, by maintaining their own cryptographically guaranteed records and making only necessary disclosures, will be able to protect their privacy without infringing on the legitimate needs of those with whom they do business.

From David Chaum, "*Achieving Electronic Privacy*" (Scientific American, August, 1992), p. 101.

1. The passage suggests that chip cards are being developed because:

    A. they are easier to handle than cash.
    B. they provide greater privacy.
    C. they generate sophisticated data to analyze.
    D. the technology exists and should be used.

2. How does the author characterize the trend toward identifier-based smart cards?

    A. Representing a technologic advance
    B. Posing a potential threat to personal privacy
    C. Providing a competitive edge for innovative corporations
    D. Offering greater choices to consumers

3. It can be inferred from the passage that the key technologic innovation that made the use of smart cards possible was:

    A. sophisticated data analysis.
    B. miniaturization of computer components.

C. sophisticated security systems.
D. advances in telecommunications.

4. According to the passage, all of the following are advantages of a system based on representatives EXCEPT:

    A. competitive advantages for organizations.
    B. protection of individual privacy.
    C. increased public confidence.
    D. improved identification systems.

5. All of the following groups could gather data generated by identifier-based smart cards EXCEPT:

    A. businesses.
    B. governments.
    C. individuals.
    D. organizations.

6. In the context of the passage, what is the meaning of cryptographically?

    A. Simple
    B. Complex
    C. Coded
    D. Anonymous

7. What does the author suggest is the difference between identifier-based systems and systems based on representatives and observers?

    A. Identifier-based systems are more economical.
    B. Systems based on representatives and observers threaten organizational security.
    C. Systems based on representatives and observers can better protect individuals.
    D. Identifier-based systems can deliver a larger range of services.

Passage II (Questions 8–15)

Tropical, shallow-water ecosystems, coral reefs are found around the world in the latitudes that generally fall between the southern tip of Florida and mid-Australia. They rank among the most biologically productive of all marine ecosystems. Because they harbor a vast array of animals and plants, coral reefs are often compared to tropical rain forests. Reefs also support life on land in several ways. They form and maintain the physical foundation for thousands of islands. By building a wall along the coast, they serve as a barrier against oceanic waves. And they also sustain the fisheries and tourist diving industries that help to maintain the economies of many countries in the Caribbean and Pacific.

Although corals seem almost architectural in structure—some weigh many tons and stand between 5 and 10 meters high—they are composed of animals. Thousands of tiny creatures form enormous colonies; indeed, nearly 60% of the 220 living genera of corals do so. Each colony is made up of many individual coral animals, called polyps. Each polyp is essentially a hollow cylinder, closed at the base and interconnected to its neighbors by the gut cavity. The polyps have one or more rings of tentacles surrounding a central mouth. In this way, corals resemble sea anemones with skeletons. The soft external tissues of the polyps overlie a hard structure of calcium carbonate.

Many of the splendid colors of corals come from their symbionts, creatures that live in a mutually dependent relation with the coral. Symbiotic algae called zooxanthellae reside in the often transparent cells of the polyps. There are between one and two million algae cells per square centimeter of coral tissue. Through photosynthesis, the algae produce carbon compounds, which help to nourish the coral—some species receive 60% of their food from their algae. Algal photosynthesis also accelerates the growth of the coral skeleton by causing more calcium carbonate to be produced. The corals provide algae with nutrients, such as nitrogen and phosphorus, [which are] essential for growth, as well as housing. The association enables algae to obtain compounds that are scarce in the nutrient-poor waters of the tropics (where warm surface waters overlie and lock in cold, nutrient-rich waters—except in restricted areas of up welling).

When corals bleach, the delicate balance among symbionts is destroyed. The corals lose algae, leaving their tissues so colorless that only the white, calcium carbonate skeleton is apparent. Other organisms, such as anemones, sea whips, and sponges, all of which harbor algae in their tissue, can also whiten in this fashion. Some of this loss is routine. A healthy coral or anemone continuously releases algae, but in very low numbers. Under natural conditions, less than 0.1% of the algae in a coral is lost during processes of regulation and replacement. When subject to adverse changes, such as temperature increases, however, the corals release increased number of algae. For example, transferring coral from a reef to a laboratory can cause a fivefold elevation in the number of algae expelled.

The mechanism of algae release is not fully understood. Even defining bleaching is tricky. The current definition has its basis in laboratory measurements of the loss of algae and the reduction in algal pigments. The laboratory approach, however, is rarely, if ever, applied in the field. There, judgment must rely on the naked eye's ability to detect loss of coloration. Although such methods may be reliable for instances of severe bleaching, a determination that pale colonies are bleached can be extremely arbitrary, given the natural variability of pigmentation.

From Barbara E. Brown and John C. Ogden, "*Coral Bleaching*" (Scientific American, January, 1993), pp. 65–66.

8. What is the effect of algal photosynthesis on coral?

   A. It produces carbon compounds.
   B. It provides nourishment.
   C. It provides nitrogen nutrients.
   D. It accelerates bleaching.

9. The definition of coral bleaching is:

   A. destruction of more than 0.1% of coral algae.
   B. a fivefold increase above normal algae replacement.
   C. judgment of the naked eye.
   D. not provided in the passage.

10. What provides the colors of many corals?

    A. Zooxanthellae
    B. Phosphorus
    C. Carbon compounds
    D. Warm surface waters

11. Corals do NOT provide algae with:

    A. nitrogen.
    B. phosphorus.
    C. housing.
    D. carbon compounds.

12. According to the passage, coral reefs are analogous to:

    A. barriers against oceanic waves.
    B. marine ecosystems.
    C. tropical rain forests.
    D. elaborate architectural structures.

13. What happens when corals bleach?

    A. Polyps die.
    B. Algal photosynthesis accelerates.
    C. 0.1% of algae are lost.
    D. Balance among symbionts is destroyed.

14. Coral reefs provide all of the following EXCEPT:

    A. warming of surface waters.
    B. barriers against waves.
    C. physical foundations for islands.
    D. fisheries.

15. According to the passage, corals most closely resemble:

    A. coastal walls.
    B. sea anemones with skeletons.
    C. a rich marine ecosystem.
    D. hollow cylinders.

Passage III (Questions 16–22)

To search for clues about the earth's youthful nature, geophysicists make use of an assortment of radioactive dating methods. These methods vary in their strengths and weaknesses, but they all rely on determining the relative abundance of a radioactive isotope and the subsequent isotope, or daughter nucleus, into which it decays. Every radioactive isotope eventually produces a final, stable decay product. Knowing the rate at which the nuclear transformation occurs (which can be measured to high precision in the laboratory) allows one to infer how long the decay products have been collecting in a rock. That information, taken with other evidence, reveals much about geologic history.

In the ongoing search for the oldest continental remnants, researchers primarily examine isotopes of uranium. Uranium ultimately decays into lead, so the relevant dating technique is called the uranium-lead method. That approach greatly benefits from the fact that samples of uranium and lead large enough to analyze can usually be extracted from zircon crystals. Such crystals are very commonly found in granite and metamorphic rocks, and in some volcanic rocks and sedimentary material derived from any of these rocks. Zircons also resist heat and weathering strongly, so they may survive intact in rocks that have experienced one or more metamorphic episodes.

From Derek York, *"The Earliest History of the Earth"* (Scientific American, January, 1993), p. 90.

16. What is the main idea of the passage?

    A. The nature of geologic dating techniques
    B. The search for tools to measure radioactive decay in rocks
    C. The search for geologic clues to the early earth
    D. The relative value of different dating techniques

17. What is the primary virtue of the uranium-lead method?

    A. Lead is a stable element.
    B. Sufficient samples can be found.
    C. Uranium decays very slowly.
    D. Scientists can precisely measure the decay rate of uranium.

18. All of the following statements describe benefits of zircons EXCEPT:

    A. they resist heat well.
    B. they resist weathering strongly.
    C. they are abundant.
    D. they always survive metamorphic episodes.

19. What do decay products allow scientist to infer?

    A. Geologic age
    B. Abundance of minerals
    C. Location and place of origin of rocks
    D. Relative abundance of a radioactive isotope

20. What is the daughter nucleus of uranium isotopes?

    A. Zircon
    B. Lead
    C. Granite
    D. Volcanic rock

21. What is the importance of zircon crystals to the uranium-lead method?

    A. They are easily analyzed.
    B. They are very old.
    C. They contain large samples of uranium and lead.
    D. They are often found in metamorphic rocks.

22. Geophysicists use an assortment of radioactive dating techniques because:

    A. every radioactive isotope produces a decay product.
    B. the uranium-lead method is not always reliable.
    C. the methods vary in strengths and weaknesses.
    D. rocks experience one or more metamorphic episodes.

Passage IV (Questions 23–29)

There are many paradoxes about the nuclear age in which we live. Recognizing them is an important first step on the road to resolving them. The Neanderthal had little patience with paradoxes, puzzles, and games. If he recognized them at all, he either bulled his way through or promptly forgot. Homo sapiens, on the other hand, had always been intrigued by such logical problems; in fact, paradoxes have often been the steppingstones to his highest achievements in philosophy and science. Here are a few of the paradoxes of the world today.

Paradox I. The greater the destructive capacity of the weapons in our hands, the less most people seem to worry about it. I have heard it estimated by a physicist friend of mine that if all the destructive energy in nuclear weapons now stockpiled were to be transformed into 10 million tons of TNT and so forth—and if then it were to be spread evenly over the surface of our country, we would all be wading around nearly up to our ankles in dynamite! Be that as it may, it is certainly true that never before in human history have so few been able to destroy so many and so much in so little time. Yet how many people are as worried about this as they are about the next raise or about what the fellow next door thinks of them? How many intellectuals have fully committed themselves to working on this problem, which surely by all odds is the most significant of all times? How much effort have our mass media given to the search for fresh alternatives to war? Let one madman loose on the streets of our town, and we form citizens' posses; but let hundreds of millions of tons of destruction hang over our heads, and we couldn't be less concerned, apparently.

Paradox II. While feverishly engaged in a nuclear arms race, both sides express peaceful intentions and fervently hope that these weapons will never be used. I believe that these hopes and intentions are sincere, on both sides. Nobody wants a nuclear war. Yet roughly half the national budgets of the two polar powers go into military preparations—that is, into producing things no one expects ever to use. The Russians resume testing, and we condemn them for polluting the air with radioactive fallout. And then, with almost the same breath, we claim we must also resume testing in the atmosphere, to keep ahead in the arms race and thereby defend ourselves. Surely future generations will look back upon these grim years as the Age of Unreason.

Paradox III. The more nations spend for what they call "Defense," the less real security their people have. Who will deny that over the past ten years we have been steadily increasing our expenditures for weapons? And who will deny that now we are really less safe, less secure, less defended than ever before in our national history? The reason for this is to be found in a basic fact about military technology in a nuclear age. This is the fact that offensive capability has completely outstripped defensive capability. Policy-makers are fond of talking about great defensive "shields" or "umbrellas," but these defenses are more in men's minds than their weapons. Defense in this nuclear age adds up to more than mutual fear.

Paradox IV. The greater a nation's military power, the less seems to be its freedom of initiative in foreign policy. Witness the squashing of the Suez situation, the attempts on all sides to neutralize Laos, the Soviet back down in

the Congo, or the ambivalence of the mighty American elephant in dealing with the little Cuban mouse. Quite apart from fears of retaliation, the mere possession of nuclear weapons has a sobering, restraining effect. For rational men, at least, possession of power brings along with it a sense of responsibility. And so we find this nuclear age characterized by a Great Freeze on initiative in foreign policy.

From Charles E. Osgood and Oliver C.S., eds., *"Language, Meaning, and Culture: The Selected Papers of Charles E. Osgood"* (Westport CT, Praeger Publishers, an imprint of Greenwood Publishing Group, Inc. Copyright 1990 by Charles E. Osgood). Reprinted by permission.

23. The author's primary contention is that:

    A. there are many paradoxes in the nuclear age.
    B. the spending on defensive weapons is equal to the spending on offensive weapons.
    C. Neanderthal man had little understanding of puzzles.
    D. spending on national defense provides security.

24. The author states that with greater military power comes:

    A. greater ability to defend one's self from aggression.
    B. greater need to develop more sophisticated weaponry.
    C. less flexibility in the area of foreign policy.
    D. less flexibility in the area of foreign aid.

25. The author believes that in the nuclear arms race:

    A. nations respond only to perceived threat.
    B. the Russians break arms agreements more than the United States.
    C. more than half of the national budgets for the polar powers has been used for military preparation.
    D. the polar power countries have not acted in a reasonable manner.

26. According to the passage, which of the following statements is true?

    I. Nations in the nuclear age often act in an irrational manner.
    II. The behaviors of nations can be compared to the behaviors of individuals.
    III. Nuclear science has brought about the age of missiles and bombs.

    A. I, II, and III
    B. I and II
    C. I only
    D. II and III

27. Enactment of an arms accord agreement between the United States and Russia to reduce nuclear and chemical weapons while permitting underground nuclear testing would:

    A. strengthen the author's position.
    B. weaken the author's position.

    C. neither strengthen nor weaken the author's position.

    D. eliminate paradoxes II and IV.

28. In the statement, "Defense in this nuclear age adds up to more than mutual fear," the author implies:

    A. countries have a mutual distrust for each other.

    B. defense is costly to the countries involved.

    C. defense is not based on nuclear fear.

    D. defense is more complex than economic or political realities.

29. Regarding the increase of weapons, the author criticizes today's society by stating that:

    A. the Neanderthal man had little time or patience to worry about paradoxes, puzzles, and games.

    B. in spite of the increase of the number of nuclear weapons, people are more worried about their neighbors' opinions and their next raise.

    C. we are falling behind other countries in the nuclear arms race.

    D. policy makers are fond of talking about defensive shields or umbrellas.

Passage V (Questions 30–37)

Much of the stellar archaeologic information on which astronomers decipher the evolution of the galaxy resides in two regions of the Milky Way: the halo and the disk. The halo is a slowly rotating, spherical region that surrounds all the other parts of the galaxy. The stars and star cluster in it are old. The rapidly rotating, equatorial region constitutes the disk, which consists of young stars and stars of intermediate age, as well as interstellar gas and dust. Embedded in the disk are the sweepingly curved arms that are characteristic of spiral galaxies, such as the Milky Way. Among the middle-aged stars is our sun, which is located about 25,000 light-years from the galactic center. (When you view the night sky, the galactic center lies in the direction of Sagittarius.) The sun completes an orbit around the center in approximately 200 million years.

Less than 70 years ago, astronomers discovered that the sun is part of the Milky Way galaxy. At the time, Bertil Lindblad of Sweden and Jan H. Oort of the Netherlands hypothesized that the Milky Way system is a flattened, differentially rotating galaxy. A few years later, John S. Plaskett and Joseph A. Pearce of Dominion Astrophysical Observatory accumulated three decades' worth of data on stellar motions that confirmed the Lindblad-Oort picture.

In addition to a disk and halo, the Milky Way contains two other subsystems: a central bulge, consisting primarily of old stars, and, within the bulge, a nucleus. Little is known about the nucleus because it is obscured by dense gas clouds in the central bulge. The nuclei of some spiral galaxies, including the Milky Way, may contain a large black hole. A black hole in the nucleus of our galaxy, however, would not be as massive as those that seem to act as the powerful cores of quasars.

30. Which region of the Milky Way surrounds the galaxy?

   A. Star clusters
   B. A black hole
   C. The halo
   D. The disk

31. Which of the following statements best expresses the main idea of the passage?

   A. The sun was only recently discovered to be part of the Milky Way.
   B. The Milky Way is a spiral galaxy.
   C. Structures within the Milky Way allow astronomers to study its evolution.
   D. The halo and the disk are the two most important regions of the Milky Way.

32. The authors mention all of the following astronomic elements as confirmed components of the Milky Way EXCEPT for the

   A. nucleus.
   B. disk.
   C. black hole.
   D. halo.

33. Approximately how long does it take the sun to complete an orbit around the center of the galaxy?

   A. 200 million years
   B. 70 million years
   C. 70 years
   D. 25,000 light years

34. What is the significance of the work of Plaskett and Pearce?

   A. They hypothesized that the Milky Way is a flattened differentially rotating galaxy.
   B. They confirmed through observation that the sun is a middle-aged star.
   C. They confirmed through observation the Linblad-Oort hypothesis.
   D. They hypothesized that the Milky Way contains a large black hole.

35. What kind of stars make up the central bulge?

   A. Large
   B. Undetermined
   C. Old
   D. Rapidly rotating

36. According to the passage, what is the most likely location of the sun in the Milky Way?

   A. The spherical region surrounding the galaxy
   B. The equatorial region
   C. The halo
   D. The gaseous central bulge

37. What evidence does the passage offer to support the claim that the Milky Way is a differentially rotating galaxy?

   A. The disk contains rotating curved arms.
   B. The nucleus is obscured by dense gas clouds.
   C. The halo rotates slowly and the disk rotates rapidly.
   D. The sun orbits the center of the galaxy.

Among intelligence, police, and military agencies, there exists no agreement on the definition of terrorism. Some parameters need to be delineated and it obviously would be highly desirable if these parameters could be universally accepted. Clearly, this is unrealistic, given the attachment of those doing the defining to their particular views on this emotionally charged and highly political issue.

However, while a definitive description of terrorism might be politically useful, it would not change the nature or gravity of the threat, nor should it affect the way in which our government responds to terrorism.

Over 30 different government agencies are involved in the war against terrorism. Each one perceives and interprets the phenomenon differently. "Think tanks" and the new flock of private terrorist experts exacerbate the problem by adding different biases.

U.S. government definitions have only one commonality. They dismiss the root cause theory, which has been expressed by Yassir Arafat: "Nobody is a terrorist who stands for a just cause." The government does not accept that terrorism—the commission of terrorist acts—is justifiable if used to remedy political or social injustices or for any other reason. Therefore, terrorism cannot subsist as part of a "just" war.

The 1986 Public Report of the Vice President's Task Force on Combating Terrorism was supposed to be the definitive document regarding international terrorism and the U.S. role in combating it. The high-level panel of experts who prepared the report defined terrorism as the unlawful use or threat of violence against persons or property to further political or social objectives. Terrorism is generally intended to intimidate or coerce a government, individuals, or groups to modify their behavior or politics.

Already the report's definition is outdated, if ever it was valid. (Whose law applies—American, Soviet, Iranian, etc.?) Violence, the focal point of this definition, excludes nonviolent acts or passive resistance as well as many actions that are logically considered self-defense. Many actions of terrorists have been destructive and fearsome without being violent. Witness the recent "computer viruses" injected into the Defense Department computer system as one example of the devastating effect a terrorist could have on our nation's infrastructure and ability to defend itself. Rather than taking people hostage, such terrorists hold integral and vulnerable systems hostage. Other nonviolent actions could terrorize populations by disrupting communication or transportation systems. For example, residents of New York could consider stoppage of rush hour traffic to be a terrorist act. Trucks or other barriers placed on all streets leading out of New York City would disrupt and terrorize the lives of millions without physically harming anyone. The spectrum of nonviolent acts is limited only by the imagination of the perpetrators.

The third aspect of the report's definition, that terrorism is to "further political or social objectives," is also too limiting. There are many categories of terrorism that are not motivated by political or social objectives. Narcoterrorism, perpetrated by narcotics traffickers, may be aimed at reducing the threat of competition or capture. Many left-wing European terrorists of the late 1960s were driven by their personal inadequacies and the need to increase the level of fear and anarchy in their victims, believing that they would have no impact on the society at large.

As further evidence that terrorism cannot be defined only by motive, much of contemporary American terrorism, such as narcoterrorism and extortion rings, is devoted to personal economic gain. Terrorist objectives range from divine orders to retribution to no logical reason at all. Some "looney tunes" and "mad-men," as President Reagan labeled them, perpetrate terrorist activities for reasons alien to the rational mind. Jerrold Post writes that some people commit these acts solely for the inner catharsis they feel—terror for terror's sake. Just as the rapist's act may be motivated by the desire for some gratification other than sexual, the terrorist may act out of inner motivations not related to any stated political or social objective, although he generally asserts one.

From James Prince, "*Is There a Role for Intelligence in Combating Terrorism?*" (Conflict 9:3, 1989), pp 302–303. Reprinted by permission from Taylor & Francis, Inc., publisher and copyright holder.

38. Without a definition of terrorism, the author states that:

    A. combating it should be held in check until nations agree.
    B. a task force should be convened to expand the existing definition.
    C. legal prosecution is not valid against terrorists.
    D. governments should go forward based on existing policies.

39. When the author states that the United States dismisses the root cause, he means terrorism:

    A. has no viable reason for existence.
    B. can exist for a just cause.
    C. is outdated.
    D. is agreed on by other countries.

40. According to the author's point of view, the definition of the Vice President's Task Force on Combating Terrorism:

    I. became valid in 1986.
    II. may never have been valid.
    III. was politically motivated.
    A. I only
    B. I and II
    C. II only
    D. II and III

41. According to the Task Force definition, which of the following actions would NOT be considered an act of terrorism?

    I. A deliberate black-out of a major metropolitan area
    II. The downing of a military aircraft
    III. Scrambling of the air controllers' interactions with pilots
    A. I only
    B. I and II

C. II only

D. I and III

42. If the United States sent troops to assist Cambodia in combating a drug cartel, how might the author define such action?

   A. State terrorism
   B. A justifiable act
   C. Furthering a social objective
   D. An irrational act

43. J. Post believes that terrorists are motivated by:

   A. a desire to hold society responsible for its actions.
   B. a need to free themselves from sin or guilt.
   C. the desire to stimulate competition.
   D. acts of desperation.

44. According to the author, all of the many U.S. definitions of terrorism:

   A. accept that terrorism subsists as part of a just war.
   B. agree that terrorism uses unlawful use or threat of violence against people.
   C. accept that Yassir Arafat is a terrorist.
   D. dismiss the root cause theory.

45. The author states that the Task Force's definition of terrorism is too limiting because:

   A. stopping traffic from leaving New York City during rush hour has terrorized millions without harming anyone.
   B. terrorists can be motivated by things other than political or social injustices.
   C. narcoterrorists aim to reduce the threat of competition or capture.
   D. President Reagan has defined some terrorists as "looney tunes" or "mad-men."

Passage VII (Questions 46–52)

The first studies of the mental effects of the adrenocorticotropic hormones (ACTH) showed that a learned response was maintained longer in rats treated with ACTH than in those rats that did not receive ACTH. Later results demonstrated that rats that had their pituitaries removed (hypophysectomized) proved less capable of learning responses than intact animals. In addition, when hypophysectomized animals received ACTH, their learning disturbance was partially eliminated. Thus, the pituitary seemed to be involved in brain function.

In subsequent investigations, scientists studied the influence of ACTH and hypophysectomy on the learning of conditioned avoidance behavior in rats and confirmed that ACTH was indeed involved in learning. The 39 amino acids that make up the ACTH molecule were broken down into fragments. They determined that the behavioral effect of ACTH was attributable to only four amino acids, those numbering 4 to 7 in the ACTH sequence. These simple sequences of amino acids are known collectively as short-chain polypeptides.

The ACTH 4 to 7 fragment, or the more common fragment, 4 to 10, and a similar sequence of amino acids from another hormone, called alpha-MSH, have been studied in human volunteers. Alpha-MSH mediates the control of skin color in frogs, but in humans, its effect seems to be on behavior. These simple peptides, when administered to humans, produce decreased anxiety and generally influence the occipital electroencephalogram (EEG) toward a pattern consistent with increased attention.

Although just how these peptides influence the brain is still largely a mystery, scientists have noted a clear decrease in the levels of ribonucleic acid (RNA) and of protein synthesis in the brains of hypophysectomized rats. This disturbance in protein synthesis was limited to a small fraction of rapidly turning over protein, and when these animals received ACTH, the rate of protein synthesis was restored to close to that of normal animals. This finding suggests that the rapidly turning over proteins are involved in learning behaviors, and peptides exert an influence on these proteins.

46. Mental changes can be induced by ACTH and adrenocortical hormones when they are:

    A. excessive.
    B. deficient.
    C. both A and B.
    D. neither A nor B.

47. Treating hypophysectomized rats with ACTH resulted in:

    A. increasing their intelligence quotients (IQ).
    B. deficient intelligence quotients (IQ).
    C. both A and B.
    D. neither A nor B.

48. Removal of the pituitary gland causes rats to exhibit:

    A. aggressive behavior.
    B. impaired muscular control.
    C. both A and B.
    D. neither A nor B.

49. Studies of the 4–10 ACTH fragment in human subjects have shown that it can affect:

    A. learning.
    B. behavior.
    C. both A and B.
    D. neither A nor B.

50. In humans, alpha-MSH has been shown to:

    A. decrease anxiety.
    B. control skin color.
    C. both A and B.
    D. neither A nor B.

51. Human subjects have been used in studies of the effect of:

    A. ACTH 4–10.
    B. alpha-MSH.
    C. both A and B.
    D. neither A nor B.

52. Studies have shown that ACTH is related to protein synthesis in:

    A. rats.
    B. humans.
    C. both A and B.
    D. neither A nor B.

Passage VIII (Questions 53–58)

Paul was diagnosed as having cystic fibrosis at 5 years of age. During his childhood, he was watched over and guarded by adults who were oriented to the possibility of imminent death. He was usually avoided by peers and potential friends who would "take a step back" once they learned that he had a serious illness. Teachers from grade school through college were reluctant to make demands or encourage long-range tasks that might prove stressful or would be abruptly terminated by death.

Paul had difficulty dealing with the attitudes of others toward illness and death. Rather than confront people and ask for clarification of their ideas about his situation, he would withdraw to avoid exposing his feelings regarding the implications of his grave medical problems.

Paul considered seeking psychiatric help to learn to cope with his everyday problems of living, but he did not pursue this idea because he was uncertain whether his vague depression and anxieties were appropriate to take to a psychiatrist. Even when seen by a counselor in college, he found it difficult to describe his needs and guide the therapist toward his areas of discomfort. The therapist, in turn, tended to be more concerned about his illness, following the pattern of seeing him primarily as a sick person.

A doctor friend helped Paul change his self-image from a seriously ill person to a man with a serious illness, a shift of attitude that proved successful in all areas of his life. He was able to broaden his horizons and persevere in his search for a job. He had graduated from college with a business degree, but interviewers routinely refused his application on hearing that he had a chronic illness. With support from his doctor friend, he finally was hired in a managerial capacity with a major distribution and retail firm. His drive to success carried him rapidly into additional areas of responsibility. Having given up a death orientation, Paul decided to marry. Although at present he denies neither the threat of death nor the reality of being alive, his newfound confidence and strength in dealing with himself and others has led to a more productive, rewarding life.

53. Which of the following phrases best describes the central idea of the passage?

   A. Changing one's lifestyle
   B. Coping with mental illness
   C. Adjusting to life's demands
   D. Learning to live with serious illness

54. The college counselor's primary concern for Paul was:

   A. his future career.
   B. his imminent death.
   C. his physical illness.
   D. his emotional health.

55. Which adjective best describes people's attitude toward Paul during his childhood?

   A. Authoritarian
   B. Compassionate
   C. Hostile
   D. Protective

56. Why did Paul not seek psychiatric help?

   A. He considered his illness only a physical disorder.
   B. He refused to talk with others about his emotional distress.
   C. He doubted the suitability of psychiatric help for solving his coping problems.
   D. He felt inhibited when talking with medically trained people about his inner feelings.

57. Paul's success in dealing with his illness was due to:

   A. his desire to get well.
   B. his change in mental attitude.
   C. his having completed a college degree.
   D. his strict adherence to medical treatments.

58. From information in the passage, one can infer that:

   A. cystic fibrosis cannot be cured.
   B. cystic fibrosis can be inherited.
   C. cystic fibrosis is difficult to diagnose.
   D. cystic fibrosis is an emotionally disabling disease.

For two centuries, federal, state, and local governments have worked together in constantly changing patterns . . . The challenge is to assure that each level of government retains the freedom and authority it needs to carry out its own responsibilities well, without unnecessary limits and constraints.

The Supreme Court's recent decisions have made it clear that little protection is provided for the states under the 10th Amendment. The Court has suggested that the states must seek to limit federal power through the political process, rather than relying on the limitation included in the initial delegation of powers to the federal government . . .

While the simplest answer is the model established 200 years ago—for the states to convene a constitutional convention to renew the commitment to power shared between states and the federal government—current fear of a runaway convention has forced the states to rely on the Congress to voluntarily give up powers it has centralized on the national level. History makes it clear, however, that power is rarely given up voluntarily.

The impact of this problem is now more acute as a result of South Carolina vs Baker. In that case, the Court repealed the last vestiges of intergovernmental tax immunity and reinforced its intent to remove itself from defining clear lines between state and federal authority.

For this reason, the governors are convinced that a measured, practical constitutional solution to the federalism issue is needed—a solution that restores the state's ability to initiate constitutional change without being stymied by the threat of the perceived problem associated with a convention, a solution that assures the people of a continued say in the decisions about the basic structure of the nation and the appropriate roles of each level of government.

Such a solution is clearly possible within the current intergovernmental structure. As the Governors' Task Force on Federalism noted, "The Constitution envisioned that amendments could be initiated by both federal government and the states. However, the fear of a 'runaway' convention has effectively closed the door to state-initiated amendments. Until recently, the 10th Amendment was thought to protect the states and localities from an uncontrolled expansion of federal power through legislation and regulatory action." Now, however, the Supreme Court has effectively removed that protection, and the Congress is free to act without constitutional constraints. Furthermore, the concern over a constitutional convention has blunted the balancing capacity originally provided in the Constitution.

Therefore, the governors have called on the Congress to restore the intended states' ability to initiate amendments. Congress can do this by referring to the states a constitutional amendment that would create a more practical route under Article V for states to initiate amendments to the Constitution.

Under this approach, two-thirds of the states could pass memorials that seek the addition of a specific constitutional amendment. Unlike the petitions for a constitutional convention that must be served on the Congress, these memorials would be filed with every state. When the necessary 34 states are reached, the proposing states would appoint representatives to a Committee on Style to reconcile the details of the language of the various memorials. When a majority of the states represented on the Committee of Style approve the proposed amendment, it would be submitted to the Congress. A two-thirds vote by both houses within the next congressional session would be necessary to stop the amendment from going back to the states for ratification. If the Congress did not vote by two-thirds to stop the amendment, it would be submitted to the states for ratification by the required three-fourths. This reasonable, measured approach can restore the balance of power without any radical alteration of the structure, process or specific responsibilities exercised today.

From John Sununu, "*The Spirit of Federalism: Restoring the Balance.*" (The Journal of State Government, 62:1, January/February, 1989; copyright 1989, The Council of State Governments), pp 26–27. Reprinted by permission.

59. The passage indicates that the Supreme Court has suggested to the states that an appropriate way to limit federal power is to:

A. wait for the federal government to voluntarily transfer power.
B. use the political process.
C. stand on the limitation in the initial delegation of powers.
D. sue the federal government for breach of contract.

60. The importance of the South Carolina vs Baker decision is that it:

A. emphasized states' rights.
B. emphasized the federal government's supremacy over states.
C. decreased the role of the Supreme Court as a mediator between the states and the federal government on issues of authority.
D. mandated tax immunity for the state of South Carolina.

61. The author implies that neither the states nor the government want to risk a constitutional convention. The most likely reason is:

A. too many issues will be addressed that do not deal with the limitation of the federal government's role.
B. the states think the Supreme Court will take a stand against them.
C. the 10th Amendment will be enforced to limit states' powers.
D. the states fear that if they use the convention to confront the issue, the federal government might find a way to block future uses.

62. The most fundamental right that the states wish to protect is the authority to:

A. initiate amendments to the constitution.
B. ratify decisions made by the congress by three-fourths majority.
C. repeal the 10th Amendment.
D. have representatives on the Committee of Style.

63. What would be the effect on the states' rights issue if the President chose new members for the Supreme Court who had been recorded as promoting the powers of central government?

A. No effect, because the Supreme Court has limited power over state governments.

B. No effect, because previous views of Supreme Court justices have no effect on future cases.

C. Possible effect, in that the Supreme Court justices may have preconceived opinions limiting the role of the states.

D. Possible effect, in that the Supreme Court justices may wish to initiate an arbitration system between the states and the federal government.

64. The author states that within the current intergovernmental structure, it is possible to:

A. solve the federalism issue by restoring a state's ability to initiate a constitutional convention.

B. solve the federalism issue by allowing states to initiate constitutional change and assuring the public's voice in the structure and function of government.

C. assure that states have a vote in the basic structure of the Congress without being stymied by the perceived problems associated with a convention.

D. force the federal government to come up with a measured, practical constitutional solution to the federalism issue.

65. What is the central theme of the passage?

A. The states and the federal government must battle each other to gain control over the basic function and structure of the government.

B. The states must convene a constitutional convention to renew the commitment to power shared between states and the federal government.

C. The state and federal governments must each retain the authority needed to effectively carry out its respective responsibilities.

D. The Supreme Court has encouraged states to seek to limit federal power through the political process.

Physical Sciences

Directions: Most questions in the Physical Sciences test are organized into groups, each of which is preceded by a descriptive passage. After studying the passage, select the one best answer to each question. Some questions are not based on a descriptive passage and are also independent of each other. Select the one best answer to these independent questions. A periodic table is provided for your reference.

PERIODIC TABLE OF THE ELEMENTS

IA																	VIIIA
1 H 1.0	IIA											IIIA	IVA	VA	VIA	VIIA	2 He 4.0
3 Li 6.9	4 Be 9.0											5 B 10.8	6 C 12.0	7 N 14.0	8 O 16.0	9 F 19.0	10 Ne 20.2
11 Na 23.0	12 Mg 24.3											13 Al 27.0	14 Si 28.1	15 P 31.0	16 S 32.1	17 Cl 35.5	18 Ar 39.9
19 K 39.1	20 Ca 40.1	21 Sc 45.0	22 Ti 47.9	23 V 50.9	24 Cr 52.0	25 Mn 54.9	26 Fe 55.8	27 Co 58.9	28 Ni 58.7	29 Cu 63.5	30 Zn 65.4	31 Ga 69.7	32 Ge 72.6	33 As 74.9	34 Se 79.0	35 Br 79.9	36 Kr 83.8
37 Rb 85.5	38 Sr 87.6	39 Y 88.9	40 Zr 91.2	41 Nb 92.9	42 Mo 95.9	43 Tc 98.0	44 Ru 101	45 Rh 102	46 Pd 106	47 Ag 108	48 Cd 112	49 In 115	50 Sn 119	51 Sb 122	52 Te 128	53 I 127	54 Xe 131
55 Cs 133	56 Ba 137	57 La 139	72 Hf 179	73 Ta 181	74 W 184	75 Re 186	76 Os 190	77 Ir 192	78 Pt 195	79 Au 197	80 Hg 201	81 Tl 204	82 Pb 207	83 Bi 208	84 Po 209	85 At 210	86 Rn 222
87 Fr 223	88 Ra 226	89 Ac 227															

58 Ce 140	59 Pr 141	60 Nd 144	61 Pm 145	62 Sm 150	63 Eu 152	64 Gd 157	65 Tb 159	66 Dy 163	67 Ho 165	68 Er 167	69 Tm 169	70 Yb 173	71 Lu 175
90 Th 232	91 Pa 231	92 U 238	93 Np 237	94 Pu 244	95 Am 243	96 Cm 247	97 Bk 247	98 Cf 251	99 Es 252	100 Fm 257	101 Md 258	102 No 259	103 Lr 260

Passage I (Questions 66–73)

Frictional forces are forces in nature that are not always contrary. For example, the force of friction between the tires of a car and the road is the reason why the tires can grip without slipping. The frictional force between two surfaces depends on the nature of the materials with which the surfaces are made. Such dependence is exhibited through the use of a dimensionless quantity known as the coefficient of friction. The force of friction itself is proportional to the magnitude of the normal force that acts on the body, with the constant of proportionality being the coefficient of friction. If the two surfaces in contact are not moving with respect to each other, the maximum force of friction acting between the surfaces is proportional to the normal force, with the constant of proportionality being a coefficient of friction, μ_s. When there is some relative motion of the surfaces, a coefficient of kinetic friction, μ_k, is used to determine the actual magnitude of the force of friction.

In Figure 1, boxes A, B, C, and D have coefficients of friction equal to 0.2, 0.5, 2, and 5, respectively.

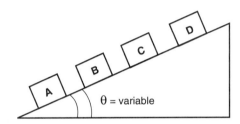

66. A person has to push four boxes of equal mass made of four different materials. What is the most efficient way to arrange the boxes to minimize the force required to push?

    A. Pile the boxes up with box A at the bottom.
    B. Pile the boxes up with box D at the bottom.
    C. Align the boxes with box B in front.
    D. Align the boxes with box C in front.

67. Box A has a weight of 500 N. A force of 200 N is applied to the box horizontally. What is its acceleration? Take $g = 10$ m/sec^2.

    A. 1 m/sec^2
    B. 2 m/sec^2
    C. 4 m/sec^2
    D. 8 m/sec^2

68. Box B is not placed on top of box A. What total force is needed to push the boxes together horizontally with an acceleration of 2 m/sec^2?

    A. 700 N
    B. 200 N
    C. 300 N
    D. 550 N

69. Suppose you reverse the order of boxes A and B. What would happen to the force required to keep the boxes moving with an acceleration of 2 m/sec^2?

    A. It would double.
    B. It would increase, but not necessarily by a factor of two.
    C. It would decrease.
    D. It would remain the same.

70. Assume that box B is back on top of box A. Using the given friction coefficients for A, B, C, and D, determine the maximum angle of incline possible before boxes A and B start sliding down the incline. Assume that the boxes do not slide relative to one another.

    A. $\theta = \tan^{-1}(0.2)$
    B. $\theta = \tan^{-1}(0.5)$
    C. $\theta = \tan^{-1}(2)$
    D. $\theta = \tan^{-1}(0.1)$

71. If box A is glued to the top of box B, what is the effect on the maximum angle that the incline can have before the two boxes slide down?

    A. It would remain the same.
    B. It would always decrease by a factor of 1.2.
    C. It would increase.
    D. It would decrease by a factor other than 1.2.

72. At what angle will box B slide on top of box A if the coefficient of static friction between A and B is 0.1?

    A. $\theta = [1/\tan^{-1}(0.1)]$
    B. $\theta = \cos^{-1}(0.1)$
    C. $\theta = \tan^{-1}(0.4)$
    D. $\theta = \tan^{-1}(0.1)$

73. Which of the boxes would not slide on a 45° incline?

    A. A and B
    B. C and D
    C. A and D
    D. B and C

Passage II (Questions 74–77)

The percentage content of an element A in a compound C is obtained by using the general rule:

$$\text{Percent element} = \frac{\text{Amount of element A}}{\text{Amount of compound C}} \times 100\%$$

Take the case in which "amount" represents a mass. The percentage of the total mass contributed by each element of a compound is determined using the following formula:

$$\frac{\text{Percent}}{\text{element}} = \frac{\text{Mass of element (g)}}{\text{Molecular mass of compound (g)}} \times 100\%$$

A balanced chemical equation allows the determination of the quantitative relationships that exist between the reactants and the products. It is important to know the amount of each reactant needed, as well as the amount of each product yielded by the reaction. For example, consider the reaction $A + 3B \rightarrow 2C + D$. In this reaction, 1 mole of A always reacts with 3 moles of B to yield 2 moles of C and 1 mole of D. The Cl_2 formed by the decomposition of 0.8 mole of PCl_3 is used to convert carbon to CCl_4.

74. How many grams of PCl_3 are involved in the reaction?

   A. 109.9
   B. 137.3
   C. 220.0
   D. 274.7

75. How many grams of Cl_2 are produced?

   A. 70.9
   B. 85.1
   C. 106.3
   D. 213.0

76. What is the quantity of C needed to react with the Cl_2 produced to form CCl_4?

   A. 4.0
   B. 6.0
   C. 7.2
   D. 12.0

77. What is the quantity of CCl_4 produced?

   A. 38.4
   B. 76.9
   C. 85.0
   D. 92.3

Passage III (Questions 78–88)

Consider a horizontal string or wire under tension. When a transverse wave is generated at one end of the string (or wire) at a certain frequency, the wave is reflected at the other end of the string. At the right frequencies, the incident wave and the reflected wave combine to produce a regular pattern of waves that appear to be stationary. One or more envelopes or loops are observed on the string. Each envelope or loop corresponds to half a wavelength. If the frequency of the incident wave is not cautiously selected, the wave pattern, if produced, may be irregular.

The first possible mode of vibrations, in which the entire string vibrates as one envelope is called the fundamental mode of vibrations. Higher modes are referred to as overtones. In the vibrations of a guitar string or other musical instrument, it is the overtones that make the music interesting. The fundamental mode should sound dull. The frequency of the nth harmonic is represented by $f_n = nf_0$, in which f_0 is the fundamental frequency.

Standing waves are established on a rope with $L = 4$ m and a total mass of $m = 4$ kg (Figure 1). The tension in the rope is 400 N.

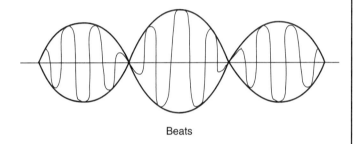

Beats

78. A string of length L resonates in n loops at a frequency f. If you used a string of the same length with a greater mass, you would expect an increase in:

A. the speed of the waves.
B. the wavelength of the waves.
C. the number of loops.
D. the wave speed and wavelength.

79. If four loops are established in the rope, what is the wavelength of the incident waves?

A. 4 m
B. 2 m
C. 1 m
D. 0.5 m

80. How is the wavelength of the reflected wave related to the wavelength of the incident wave?

A. They are equal.
B. The wavelength of the reflected wave is always less than the wavelength of the incident wave.
C. The wavelength of the reflected wave is less than the wavelength of the incident wave for frequencies that are multiples of the fundamental frequency.

D. The wavelength of the reflected wave is always greater than the wavelength of the incident wave.

81. The speed of the transverse wave is:

A. 1 m/sec.
B. 10 m/sec.
C. 20 m/sec.
D. 2 m/sec.

82. What is the frequency of the wave?

A. 10 Hz
B. 5 Hz
C. 1 Hz
D. 100 Hz

83. For the entire length of the rope to represent one full wavelength, if the frequency is 10 Hz, then the tension in the rope must be:

A. 800 N.
B. 200 N.
C. 400 N.
D. 1600 N.

84. Two blocks are pulled upward, as shown in the following figure, at a rate of 2 m/sec². The mass of the disk-shaped pulley is 50 kg, and its radius is 0.5 m. The two attached masses are $m_1 = 10$ kg and $m_2 = 20$ kg. The moment of inertia of the pulley $= \frac{1}{2}MR^2$. Tension T_2 is:

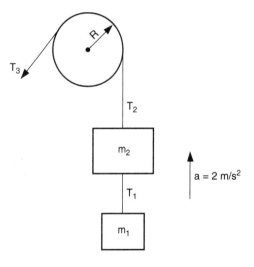

A. 50 N.
B. 100 N.
C. 200 N.
D. 340 N.

85. The blade of a fan with a moment inertia of 1.5 kg · m² is turned on at t = 0. The blade accelerates at a constant angular rate of 6 rad/sec² for the first 10 seconds. The fan continues to rotate at a constant angular speed. The fan is switched off at t = 20 seconds, at which time the blade starts decelerating uniformly. The blade comes to a complete stop at t = 30 seconds. What is the magnitude of the net torque exerted on the fan blade at t = 17?

A. 60 N · m
B. 9 N · m
C. 102 N · m
D. None of the above

86. Consider the equilibrium PCl_3 (g) + Cl_2 (g) $\rightleftharpoons$ PCl_5 (g). The addition of PCl_3 will:

    A. move the equilibrium to the left.
    B. move the equilibrium to the right.
    C. not affect the equilibrium position.
    D. move the equilibrium constant to the right only if P < 5 atm.

87. How many different states are possible for an electron with a principal quantum number of n = 2?

    A. 2
    B. 4
    C. 8
    D. 16

    $2n^2 =$

88. What is the molarity of the chloride ion (Cl^-) in a solution containing 12 g of calcium chloride ($CaCl_2$) in 645 ml of the solution?

    A. 0.169 M
    B. 0.338 M
    C. 0.507 M
    D. 0.676 M

    $\dfrac{12}{116.1} = .1033$

    $1L = 1000 mL$

    $.645 mdx \dfrac{L}{100 mL}$

    $.645 L$

    $\dfrac{12}{111.1}$

Passage IV (Questions 89–95)

Acids containing more than one atom of hydrogen that can be lost on dissociation are known as polyprotic acids. Vitamin C, or ascorbic acid $H_2C_6H_6O_6$ is a polyprotic acid and contains two ionizable hydrogens. Polyprotic acids lose their hydrogens, one at a time, in a stepwise fashion. Thus, two steps for the dissociation of vitamin C are written as:

$$H_2C_6H_6O_6 \rightleftharpoons H^+ + HC_6H_6O_6^-$$

$$K_{A1} = 7.9 \times 10^{-5}$$

$$HC_6H_6O_6^- \rightleftharpoons H^+ + C_6H_6O_6^{-2}$$

$$K_{A2} = 1.6 \times 10^{-12}$$

89. Assuming all the H^+ comes from the first dissociation, what is the equilibrium H^+ concentration in a 0.1 M aqueous solution of vitamin C?

  A. 1.6×10^{-12} M
  B. 8.0×10^{-6} M
  C. 3.0×10^{-4} M
  D. 2.8×10^{-3} M

90. What is the equilibrium concentration of $HC_6H_6O_6^-$ in a 0.1 M aqueous solution?

  A. 1.6×10^{-12} M
  B. 7.9×10^{-6} M
  C. 8.5×10^{-5} M
  D. 2.8×10^{-3} M

91. A liquid at equilibrium in a sealed container is at 300 K. All of the following statements are true EXCEPT:

  A. raising the temperature of the system will increase the number of molecules in the vapor phase.
  B. a small increase in the size of the container while keeping the temperature at 300 K will eventually cause the pressure of the vapor to decrease.
  C. opening the container will cause the temperature of the liquid to fall.
  D. a different liquid that has weaker attractive forces between its molecules will have a higher vapor pressure (under the same conditions).

92. The equilibrium $C_6H_6O_6^{-2}$ concentration at 0.1 M aqueous solution in this passage is:

  A. 1.6×10^{-12} M.
  B. 2.5×10^{-6} M.
  C. 7.9×10^{-4} M.
  D. 2.8×10^{-3} M.

93. Which of the following graphs represents the shape of the titration curve of ammonia with nitric acid?

A
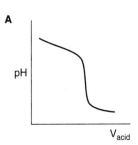

B
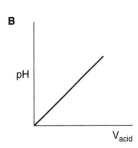

C
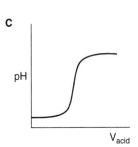

D
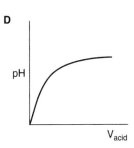

94. The equilibrium $H_2C_6H_6O_6$ concentration in 0.1 M aqueous solution in this passage is:

  A. 6.1×10^{-3} M.
  B. 9.7×10^{-2} M.
  C. 2.1×10^{-2} M.
  D. 1.2×10^{-2} M.

95. Fluids in the stomach have a pH $\cong$ 1.0. Assume all the H^+ comes from the first dissociation. If the volume of fluids in the stomach is 200 ml, the fraction of vitamin C in a 500-mg tablet that will be dissociated is:

  A. 1.6×10^{-12}.
  B. 3.6×10^{-6}.
  C. 7.9×10^{-4}.
  D. 2.8×10^{-3}.

Passage V (Questions 96–100)

Microscopes, telescopes, eye glasses, and cameras are only a few examples of the large number of optical instruments that we have become accustomed to over the last few decades. Microscopes, which are used widely in the fields of medicine and biology, consist of a pair of lenses, the eyepiece, and the objective. These lenses are separated by a distance (d). A simple system of two lenses is the closest model to a microscope that can be analyzed.

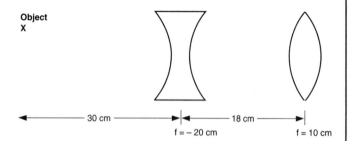

Object
X

30 cm   18 cm
f = – 20 cm   f = 10 cm

Consider the system of lenses shown in Figure 1 (this system is not a microscope). An object is placed 30 cm to the left of a diverging lens of focal length 20 cm. A converging lens of focal length 10 cm is located 18 cm to the right of the diverging lens. For a single lens, the distance s' between the image and the lens can be obtained if the distance s between the lens and the object is known, by using the lens equation:

$$\frac{1}{s} + \frac{1}{s'} = \frac{1}{f}$$

in which f is the focal length of the lens.

96. What is the location of the image formed by the first lens?

    A. 12 cm to its left
    B. 12 cm to its right
    C. 60 cm to its left
    D. 60 cm to its right

97. Objects seen through the first lens will appear:

    A. bigger and erect.
    B. bigger and inverted.
    C. smaller and inverted.
    D. smaller and erect.

98. The location of the final image is:

    A. 15 cm to the left of the converging lens.
    B. 15 cm to the right of the converging lens.
    C. 7.5 cm to the left of the converging lens.
    D. 7.5 cm to the right of the converging lens.

99. What is the magnification of the second lens?

    A. +0.25
    B. −0.25
    C. +0.50
    D. −0.50

100. Which of the following terms best describe the final image?

    A. Enlarged and erect
    B. Enlarged and inverted
    C. Reduced and erect
    D. Reduced and inverted

Passage VI (Questions 101–112)

Although it was first suggested that atoms are indivisible, it is now known that atoms are composed of three kinds of subatomic particles: electrons, protons, and neutrons. Electrons and protons have electrical charge, whereas the neutron is an uncharged particle. According to the quantum theory, one can only specify the probability that any one electron in an atom is at a certain position in that atom. The electrons in orbitals with a high probability of being close to the nucleus are held tightly by the positive charge of the nucleus. These inner-core electrons are not significantly affected by chemical reaction. On the other hand, electrons that have a high probability of being relatively far from the nucleus are bound less tightly to the nucleus than are the inner-core electrons. These valence electrons are principally involved when an atom bonds to other atoms, which explains why elements with the same number of valence electrons have similar chemical properties.

Research probes, such as the Galileo atmospheric probe, provide evidence leading scientists to believe that Io's torus is formed when SO_2 is spewed from the moon's surface, breaking into atomic sulfur and oxygen. As photons from the sun or electrons in Jupiter's magnetosphere ionize an atom of sulfur or oxygen, the magnetic field grabs and holds onto that ion. It must go with the lines of force, so it is immediately accelerated to temperatures up to 30,000 to 40,000 K, which are as hot as the solar corona. The dynamics of the jovian atmosphere are fairly complex at a subatomic level, which means more studies on new particles will continue far into the twenty-first century. Electron maps of such particles will be useful chemical tools for future scientists.

101. Which of the following statements is NOT true?

- **A.** Most of the mass of an atom is in its nucleus.
- **B.** The nucleus of an atom occupies a small fraction of the volume of the atoms.
- **C.** An atomic nucleus contains protons and electrons.
- **D.** A neutral atom has the same number of protons and electrons.

102. What is the valence shell of 16S?

- **A.** $2s^22p^2$
- **B.** $3s^23d^1$
- **C.** $3s^23p^4$
- **D.** $4s^23d^1$

103. Which of the following valence electron configurations corresponds to an excited state?

- **A.** $2s^22p^6$
- **B.** $3s^23d^1$
- **C.** $3s^23p^4$
- **D.** $4s^23d^1$

104. How many unpaired electrons are present in sulfur?

- **A.** Zero
- **B.** One
- **C.** Two
- **D.** Three

105. Which of the following elements is an exception to the rules of electronic configuration orbital diagram?

- **A.** Ca
- **B.** Cu
- **C.** Co
- **D.** Cd

106. Which of the following electron configurations is incorrect?

- **A.** $1s$
- **B.** $1s^22s^2$
- **C.** $1s^22s^22p^6$
- **D.** $1s^22s^22p^63s^3$

107. Which of the following is not an isotope of hydrogen?

- **A.** $_1^1H$
- **B.** $_1^2H$
- **C.** $_2^2H$
- **D.** $_1^3H$

108. What is the formal charge on C in CO_2?

- **A.** -2
- **B.** 0
- **C.** $+2$
- **D.** None of the above

109. A small steel ball falls in water. What is the net force on the ball after it reaches terminal velocity?

- **A.** The force of gravity only.
- **B.** The force of viscosity only.
- **C.** The force due to the water pressure.
- **D.** The net force is zero.

110. A man's upper body has a mass of 60 kg. Assuming the center of mass of his upper body rises by 25 cm when he does situps, what is the work done per situp?

- **A.** 150 J
- **B.** 300 J
- **C.** 200 J
- **D.** 450 J

111. An object accelerating at a constant rate a m/sec^2 starts from rest and travels a distance d in the first t seconds. What total distance does the object travel in twice as much time?

- **A.** Three times the distance traveled in the first t seconds.
- **B.** Twice the distance traveled in the first t seconds.
- **C.** Four times the distance traveled in the first t seconds.
- **D.** None of the above.

112. The emf of the cell for the reaction M + 2H$^+$ (1.0 M) → H^2 (1.0 atm) + M^{2+} (0.1 M) is 0.50 V. What is the standard reduction potential for the M^{2+}|M couple?

- **A.** -0.47 V
- **B.** -0.30 V
- **C.** $+0.50$ V
- **D.** $+0.95$ V

Passage VII (Questions 113–120)

When an object moves through a fluid, as when a ball falls through air or a glass sphere falls through water, the fluid exerts a viscous force F on the object. This force tends to slow the object. For a small sphere of radius r, moving slowly at a speed v, the magnitude of the viscous force is given by Stoke's law, $F_v = 6\pi\eta rv$. In this formula, η is the coefficient of viscosity of the fluid, which is the proportionality constant that determines how much tangential force is required to move a fluid layer at a constant speed v, when the layer has an area A and is located a perpendicular distance z from an immobile surface. The magnitude of the force is given by $F = \eta Av/z$. For a viscous fluid to move from location 2 to location 1 along a pipe of radius R and length L, the pressure at location 2 must exceed that at location 1. Poiseuille's law gives the volume flow rate Q that results from such a pressure difference $P_2 - P_1$. The flow rate is expressed by the formula:

$$Q = \frac{\pi R^4 (P_2 - P_1)}{8\eta L}$$

Poiseuille's law remains valid as long as the fluid flow is laminar. For a sufficiently high speed, however, the flow becomes turbulent. Flow is laminar as long as the Reynolds number is less than approximately 2000. This number is given by the formula:

$$Re = \frac{2\bar{v}\rho R}{\eta}$$

in which $\bar{v}$ is the average speed, ρ is the density, η is the coefficient of viscosity of the fluid, and R is the radius of the pipe. Take the density of water to be $\rho = 1000 \text{ kg/m}^3$.

113. Which of the following may be concluded from the information in the passage?

   A. The volume flow rate and the mass flow rate are greater for the more viscous fluids.
   B. The volume flow rate is smaller for more viscous fluids, whereas the mass flow rate is greater for more viscous fluids.
   C. The volume flow rate is greater for more viscous fluids, whereas the mass flow rate is smaller for more viscous fluids.
   D. The volume flow rate and the mass flow rate are greater for less viscous fluids.

114. The following figure is a hypodermic syringe filled with a solution of viscosity 1.5×10^{-3} Pa · s. The plunger area of the syringe is 8×10^{-5} m², and the length of the needle is 0.025 m. The internal radius of the needle is 4×10^{-4} m, and the gauge pressure in a vein is 1900 Pa. What force must be applied to the plunger, so that 1×10^{-6} m³ of solution can be injected in 3.0 seconds?

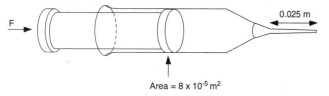

Area = 8 x 10⁻⁵ m²

A. 0.20 N
B. 0.25 N
C. 0.50 N
D. 1.00 N

115. A blood vessel is 0.10 m in length and has a radius of 1.5×10^{-3} m. Blood flows at a rate of 1×10^{-7} m³/sec through this vessel. The pressure difference that must be maintained for this flow, between the two ends of the vessel, is 20 Pa. What is the viscosity coefficient of blood?

A. 2×10^{-3} Pa · s
B. 1×10^{3} Pa · s
C. 4×10^{-3} Pa · s
D. 5×10^{4} Pa · s

116. Motor oil is more viscous than alcohol. The viscous force on a spherical object is:

A. greater in the alcohol than in the motor oil.
B. greater in the motor oil than in the alcohol before the object reaches a terminal speed.
C. greater in the motor oil than in the alcohol at all times.
D. the same in the motor oil as in the alcohol at all times.

117. A spherical object of radius R and mass m is dropped in a 2% alcohol solution. An identical object is dropped in a more viscous oil solution. Which object reaches terminal velocity over the shorter distance?

A. The object dropped in the alcohol.
B. The object dropped in the oil.
C. Both reach terminal velocity over the same distance.
D. More information about atmospheric pressure is needed.

118. Calculate the highest average speed that blood ($\rho \approx 1000 \text{ kg/m}^3$) could have and still remain in laminar flow when it flows through the aorta (R = 8×10^{-3} m). Take the coefficient of viscosity of blood to be 4×10^{-3} Pa · s.

A. 0.5 m/sec
B. 1.0 m/sec
C. 1.5 m/sec
D. 2.0 m/sec

119. What is the viscous force on a glass sphere of radius r = 1 mm falling through water ($\eta = 1 \times 10^{-3}$ Pa · s) when the sphere has a speed of 3 m/sec?

A. 2.7×10^{-2} N
B. 2.5×10^{-2} N
C. 5.7×10^{-5} N
D. 9.5×10^{-5} N

120. If the sphere in question 119 has a mass of 1×10^{-5} kg, what is its terminal velocity when falling through water? ($\eta = 1 \times 10^{-3}$ Pa · s)

A. 1.3 m/sec
B. 3.4 m/sec
C. 5.3 m/sec
D. 6.5 m/sec

Real gas behavior deviates from the ideal gas law because the assumptions made in the kinetic molecular theory are not absolutely valid. When the pressure of the gas is not ordinary, i.e., when the pressure is either too high or too low, the ideal gas law no longer reasonably approximates the behavior of gases. The van der Waals equation does a better approximation:

$$\left(P + \frac{n^2a}{V^2}\right)(V - nb) = nRT$$

in which a and b are constants for the gas. The equation takes into account both intermolecular forces of attraction and finite molecular volumes, both of which are assumed negligible in the kinetic theory. The van der Waals constants for carbon tetrachloride are a = 20.39 liter$^2 \cdot$ atm/mole^2 and b = 0.1383 liter/mole. Assume that 1 mole occupies a volume of 30 liters at 77°C.

121. The pressure of this sample according to ideal gas law is:

  A. 1.98 atm.
  B. 1.00 atm.
  C. 0.96 atm.
  D. 2.94 atm.

122. The pressure of the sample according to van der Waals equation is:

  A. .70 atm.
  B. 1.00 atm.
  C. 3.96 atm.
  D. none of the above.

123. The ideal gas law is used in the limit of small pressures. Assuming the pressure is small enough, which of the following conditions must be met in order that the van der Waals equation reduces to the ideal gas law?

  A. The constant a must be set equal to zero in the van der Waals equation.
  B. The constant b must be set equal to zero in the van der Waals equation.
  C. Both constants a and b must be set equal to zero.
  D. None of the above.

124. The percentage change with respect to P_{ideal} is:

  A. 6%.
  B. −2%.
  C. 24%.
  D. −12%.

125. If the volume of 1 mole of CCl_4 is held at 30 liters while it is cooled from 77°C to −200°C, what is the final pressure according to van der Waals equation?

  A. 0.20 atm
  B. 0.18 atm

  C. 0.25 atm
  D. 0.38 atm

126. Using the information given in question 125, what is the percentage change with respect to P_{ideal}?

  A. 4%
  B. −5%
  C. 20%
  D. −10%

127. The spring constant, k, of a spring is defined by the equation

$$\Delta F = -k\Delta L$$

where F is force and L is length. The negative sign signifies that the force exerted by the spring is opposite to the displacement. Written in a different way this becomes (See figure)

$$F_f - F_i = -k(L_f - L_i)$$

where the subscripts signify final and initial states. Suppose a spring has a spring constant of −2 N/meter and initially has length 0.1m with a mass of .5 Kg hanging from it. If a 1 Kg mass is added to the .5 Kg mass, by how much will the spring change length?

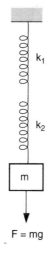

F = mg

  A. 1 m
  B. 2 m
  C. 4.9 m
  D. None of the above

128. An object that produces sound waves at a frequency of 350 Hz is dropped from a 20-m high building. Assume the speed of sound is v = 340 m/sec. One second after the object is dropped, what is the frequency heard by a person on top of the building?

  A. 330 Hz
  B. 340 Hz
  C. 350 Hz
  D. 360 Hz

129. A rectangular loop of wire carries a current of 2 A. Let the sides of the rectangle be a, b, c, and d, as shown in the following figure. Nearby, in the plane of the loop, is a long straight wire carrying a current of 1 A. Take $\mu_0 = 4\pi \times 10^{-7}$. What is the force due to the long wire on the b segment of the loop?

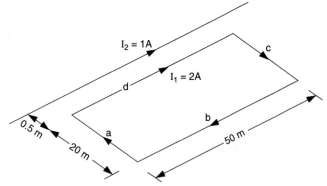

I₂ = 1A
I₁ = 2A
d
c
b
a
0.5 m
20 m
50 m

    A. 4.0×10^{-7} N and attractive
    B. 4.0×10^{-7} N and repulsive
    C. 2.4×10^{-7} N and attractive
    D. 9.8×10^{-7} N and repulsive

130. Consider the circuit shown in the following figure. The equivalent resistance of the circuit is:

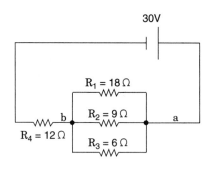

30V

$R_1 = 18\,\Omega$
$R_2 = 9\,\Omega$
$R_3 = 6\,\Omega$
$R_4 = 12\,\Omega$
b
a

    A.   3 Ω.
    B.   9 Ω.
    C.   15 Ω.
    D.   35 Ω.

131. Which of the following indicators would you choose for the titration of NH_3 with HNO_3?

    A.   Bromocresol green (pH range 3.8–5.4)
    B.   Bromothymol blue (pH range 6.0–7.6)
    C.   Phenolphthalein (pH range 8.2–10.0)
    D.   Any of the above

Passage IX (Questions 132–137)

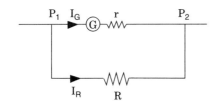

Figure 1

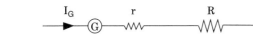

Figure 2

Measurements and interpretations of voltage and electric current signals are common in modern medicine. Occasionally, a situation arises in which a voltmeter or an ammeter is needed but it is not available. A galvanometer is an instrument that can be used to construct an ammeter (for measuring electric currents). It can also be used to construct a voltmeter (to measure voltages). In both cases, a resistor R must be connected to the galvanometer to effect the change.

To turn the galvanometer into an ammeter, the resistor R is connected in parallel, as shown in Figure 1. The resistor R is connected in series with the galvanometer in order to turn it into a voltmeter, as shown in Figure 2. The current required to produce a full scale deflection in a galvanometer is 10 mA. The internal resistance of the galvanometer is 100 Ω. Let V_r be the voltage across r and V_R the voltage across R.

132. Which of the following formulas correctly applies to the ammeter circuit?

 A. $V_r > V_R$
 B. $V_r < V_R$
 C. $V_r = V_R$
 D. More information is needed.

133. What resistance must be connected in parallel to the galvanometer to turn it into an ammeter capable of reading electric currents of up to 10.01 A?

 A. 0.1 Ω
 B. 1 Ω
 C. 10 Ω
 D. None of the above

134. What resistance R must be connected in series to the galvanometer in order to convert it to a 100 V voltmeter?

 A. 900 Ω
 B. 1000 Ω
 C. 9900 Ω
 D. 10,000 Ω

135. In the voltmeter circuit, the current in the resistor R must be:

 A. negligible, so that it only has a small effect on the voltage reading.
 B. substantial, but does not have any effect on the voltage reading.

 C. substantial, but does have some effect on the voltage reading.
 D. none of the above.

136. Which of the following formulas correctly applies to the voltmeter circuit?

 A. $V_r > V_R$
 B. $V_r < V_R$
 C. $V_r = V_R$
 D. $V_r = 2 V_R$

137. To double the full scale voltage reading of any galvanometer turned into a voltmeter, you must:

 A. double the resistance R.
 B. halve the resistance R.
 C. reduce the resistance R.
 D. do none of the above.

Passage X (Questions 138–142)

In quantum mechanics, some quantities are discrete and cannot be continuous. One of these quantities is the energy. Energy can only take certain values—E_1, E_2, E_3, E_4 ..., which are called energy levels. The energy cannot take any values between E_1 and E_2, or E_2 and E_3, or E_3 and E_4, etc. Certain transitions from one energy level to another result in the emission of a photon of radiation, whereas others can only take place if a photon is absorbed. The energy levels in a newly discovered gas are expressed as:

$$E_n = \frac{-E_1 z^2}{n^2}$$

in which $-E_1 z^2$ is the ground state energy. Take $z = 1$ for simplicity, but do not assume that the gas is hydrogen. An experiment is designed to measure the energy as a function of the level. The results obtained are as follows:

n	E_n(eV)
2	−144
3	−64
4	−36

138. The ionization energy of the gas must be:

- **A.** 244 eV.
- **B.** 576 eV.
- **C.** 144 eV.
- **D.** +13.6 eV.

139. The ground state energy is:

- **A.** −144 eV.
- **B.** +144 eV.
- **C.** −244 eV.
- **D.** none of the above.

140. Which of the following shapes is most likely to represent the graph of E_n versus $1/n^2$?

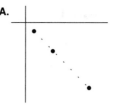

A.

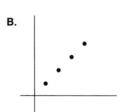

B.

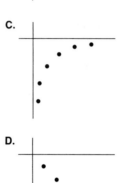

C.

D.

141. A transition from the n = 2 state to the n = 3 state results:

- **A.** in emission of a photon of energy 144 eV.
- **B.** in emission of a photon of energy 80 eV.
- **C.** in emission of an ultraviolet photon.
- **D.** only accomplished if a photon is absorbed.

142. A transition from the n = 4 state to the n = 3 state results:

- **A.** in emission of a photon of energy 28 eV.
- **B.** in emission of a photon of energy 13.6 eV.
- **C.** in emission of an infrared photon.
- **D.** only accomplished if a photon is absorbed.

Writing Sample

Directions: You have 30 minutes to complete Essay Topic 1. When time is called, you must stop working on this essay. Draw a line below the last sentence in Essay 1 to mark your stopping point. You then have 30 minutes to complete Essay Topic 2. You may not work on Essay Topic 1 during the second 30-minutes period allotted for Essay Topic 2.

Your essays will be written on the pages provided with the answer sheets, with three pages provided for each response, or a total of 6 pages. Use pages marked with "1" for the first essay and those marked with "2" for the second essay. You are not expected to use all three pages. Do not skip lines between sentences. Illegible essays will not be scored.

ESSAY TOPIC 1

Consider this statement:

What is essential is invisible to the eye.

Write a unified essay in which you perform the following tasks. Explain what you think the above statement means. Describe a specific situation in which something essential is visible to the eye. Discuss what you think determines whether essential things are perceived to be invisible or really are invisible.

1 1 1 1 1

_____

_____

_____

_____

_____

_____

_____

_____

_____

_____

_____

_____

_____

_____

_____

_____

_____

_____

_____

_____

_____

IF YOU NEED MORE SPACE, PLEASE CONTINUE ON THE NEXT PAGE.

1   1   1   1   1

IF YOU NEED MORE SPACE, PLEASE CONTINUE ON THE BACK OF THIS PAGE.

1   1   1   1   1

Consider this statement:

In business, the chairperson of the team should be someone with easy conversational access to the very top management.

Write a unified essay in which you perform the following tasks. Explain what you think the above statement means. Describe a specific situation in which a person with easy conversational access to the top management should not be the team leader. Discuss what you think is criteria for selecting an effective team leader.

_____

_____

_____

_____

_____

_____

_____

_____

_____

_____

_____

_____

_____

_____

_____

_____

_____

_____

_____

_____

_____

_____

_____

IF YOU NEED MORE SPACE, PLEASE CONTINUE ON THE NEXT PAGE.

2 2 2 2 2

_____
_____
_____
_____
_____
_____
_____
_____
_____
_____
_____
_____
_____
_____
_____
_____
_____
_____
_____
_____
_____
_____
_____

IF YOU NEED MORE SPACE, PLEASE CONTINUE ON THE BACK OF THIS PAGE.

Biological Sciences

Directions: Most questions in the Biological Sciences section are organized into groups, each of which is preceded by a descriptive passage. After studying the passage, select the one best answer to each question. Some questions are not based on a descriptive passage and are also independent of each other. Select the ONE best answer to these independent questions. A periodic table is provided for your reference.

PERIODIC TABLE OF THE ELEMENTS

IA																	VIIIA
1 H 1.0	IIA											IIIA	IVA	VA	VIA	VIIA	2 He 4.0
3 Li 6.9	4 Be 9.0											5 B 10.8	6 C 12.0	7 N 14.0	8 O 16.0	9 F 19.0	10 Ne 20.2
11 Na 23.0	12 Mg 24.3											13 Al 27.0	14 Si 28.1	15 P 31.0	16 S 32.1	17 Cl 35.5	18 Ar 39.9
19 K 39.1	20 Ca 40.1	21 Sc 45.0	22 Ti 47.9	23 V 50.9	24 Cr 52.0	25 Mn 54.9	26 Fe 55.8	27 Co 58.9	28 Ni 58.7	29 Cu 63.5	30 Zn 65.4	31 Ga 69.7	32 Ge 72.6	33 As 74.9	34 Se 79.0	35 Br 79.9	36 Kr 83.8
37 Rb 85.5	38 Sr 87.6	39 Y 88.9	40 Zr 91.2	41 Nb 92.9	42 Mo 95.9	43 Tc 98.0	44 Ru 101	45 Rh 102	46 Pd 106	47 Ag 108	48 Cd 112	49 In 115	50 Sn 119	51 Sb 122	52 Te 128	53 I 127	54 Xe 131
55 Cs 133	56 Ba 137	57 La 139	72 Hf 179	73 Ta 181	74 W 184	75 Re 186	76 Os 190	77 Ir 192	78 Pt 195	79 Au 197	80 Hg 201	81 Tl 204	82 Pb 207	83 Bi 208	84 Po 209	85 At 210	86 Rn 222
87 Fr 223	88 Ra 226	89 Ac 227															

58 Ce 140	59 Pr 141	60 Nd 144	61 Pm 145	62 Sm 150	63 Eu 152	64 Gd 157	65 Tb 159	66 Dy 163	67 Ho 165	68 Er 167	69 Tm 169	70 Yb 173	71 Lu 175
90 Th 232	91 Pa 231	92 U 238	93 Np 237	94 Pu 244	95 Am 243	96 Cm 247	97 Bk 247	98 Cf 251	99 Es 252	100 Fm 257	101 Md 258	102 No 259	103 Lr 260

Protein synthesis is carried out by ribosomes that bind to mRNA and decode the information that it carries in the form of proteins. The process of protein synthesis, known as translation, is divided into three distinct phases: initiation, elongation, and termination.

Two basic steps are involved in the making of proteins from genetic information in DNA. First, a copy is made of the information in the DNA that is needed to make a certain protein — which is called messenger RNA (mRNA). This process is similar to DNA replication in that the mRNA strand is formed by complementary base pairing with one strand of DNA.

Because the synthesis of mRNA involves the production of a copy of nucleic acid information (DNA) in the form of another nucleic acid (RNA), the process is called transcription. During the second stage of the process, the transcribed information in the mRNA is converted into the amino acid sequence of a protein. Because that process involves transformation of the "nucleic acid language" in the mRNA molecule into the "amino acid language" of the protein, it is called translation of the genetic code. The information contained within the mRNA is in the form of a three-base genetic code. A group of three bases in the mRNA that specifies an amino acid is called a codon. Each codon in the mRNA specifies one of the amino acids in the protein encoded by the gene. Translation involves the recognition and decoding of codons in the mRNA, which is accomplished by "adapter" molecules, called transfer RNA (tRNA). Each tRNA molecule has a sequence of three bases, called the anticodon, which can recognize a codon on the mRNA by complementary base pairing. The amino acid specified by the anticodon is attached to another part of the tRNA molecule.

143. During initiation of protein synthesis, the small subunit of ribosome binds to which of the following part(s) of mRNA?

  A. The 5′ end
  B. The 3′ end
  C. Both the 5′ and 3′ ends
  D. Either the 5′ or 3′ end

144. The proteins involved in the start of peptide synthesis are called:

  A. start proteins.
  B. initiation factors.
  C. elongation factors.
  D. peptide factors.

145. What is the sequence of the anticodon of initiator ammoniacal tRNA?

  A. 3′ UAB 5′
  B. 5′ UAB 3′
  C. 5′ AUG 3′
  D. 3′ AUG 5′

146. The first amino acid in a peptide is almost always:

  A. alanine.
  B. methionine.
  C. arginine.
  D. glycine.

147. During elongation of peptide chain, the formation of peptide bonds between the existing peptide and the incoming amino acid is catalyzed by:

  A. peptidyl transferase.
  B. peptide kinase.
  C. peptidase.
  D. peptide synthetase.

148. A protein called "release factor" is involved in:

  A. transcription initiation.
  B. initiation of translation.
  C. termination of translation.
  D. termination of transcription.

149. Termination of translation occurs when:

  A. the A site of ribosome reaches a termination codon.
  B. the P site of ribosome reaches a termination codon.
  C. a termination specific tRNA puts in a termination-specific amino acid.
  D. none of the above.

150. If five codons are deleted from the middle of a gene so that they are not present in the mRNA, which of the following effects may occur?

  A. A frameshift mutation
  B. Loss of a ribosome binding site
  C. Loss of five amino acids from the resulting protein
  D. No protein will be produced

Passage II (Questions 151–154)

The plasma membrane maintains homeostasis of the cell by its property of selective permeability. The cell membrane regulates the passage of materials in and out of the cell. This function allows the cell to maintain its structural and functional integrity. Water passes through the cell by bulk flow, diffusion, or osmosis. Bulk flow is the overall movement of water molecules as a group. Diffusion involves the random movement of molecules and results in a net movement down a concentration gradient.

Carbon dioxide and oxygen are two important molecules that move into and out of cells by diffusion across the membrane. Osmosis is the movement of water through a membrane that permits the passage of water but inhibits the movement of solutes. The movement of water in osmosis is from a region of lower solute concentration, and therefore of higher water potential, to one of higher solute concentration.

Controlled movement into and out of a cell may also occur by endocytosis or exocytosis, in which substances are transported in vacuoles composed of portions of the cell membrane. Endocytosis of solids is called phagocytosis. Endocytosis of dissolved molecules is called pinocytosis.

151. Which of the following passes through the plasma membrane most readily?

    A. Gases
    B. Lipid soluble molecules
    C. Nonlipid soluble molecules
    D. Both gases and nonlipid soluble molecules

152. The main difference between diffusion and osmosis is that osmosis involves:

    A. movement across a semipermeable membrane.
    B. expenditure of energy in the form of ATP.
    C. endocytosis.
    D. both A and C.

153. Which of the following statements about endocytosis is correct?

    A. It is the functional opposite of exocytosis.
    B. It may be illustrated by phagocytosis.
    C. It may be illustrated by pinocytosis.
    D. All of the above.

154. A desmosome is a:

    A. broken chromosome.
    B. connection between the cytoplasmic membrane of two adjacent cells.
    C. self-replicating DNA molecule.
    D. vacuole.

Passage III (Questions 155–165)

After a compound is isolated in the laboratory, it is necessary to determine what functional groups are present in it. Before subjecting the isolated compound to elaborate procedures for structural determination, it is often desirable to gather information about compounds of similar kind. Spectroscopy is one way of determining compound structures but it requires expensive instruments. A simple chemical test can help to identify a particular functional group. Such a test usually consists of a single reagent that, when mixed with the compound in question, indicates the presence of a particular functional group.

Consider three compounds, A, B, and C, that have the same molecular formula C_5H_8. Compound A gives a precipitate when treated with ammoniacal silver nitrate, but compounds B and C do not. Compounds A and B both yield pentane when treated with excel hydrogen in the presence of a platinum catalyst. Under the same conditions, C absorbs only 1 mole of hydrogen to yield a product with formula C_5H_{10}.

155. Choose a possible structure for compound A.

A. $CH_3—CH_2—CH_2—C≡CH$
B. $CH_3—C≡C—CH_2CH_3$

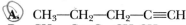

C.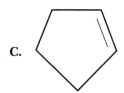

D. $CH_3—CH=CH—CH=CH_2$

156. Choose a possible structure for compound C.

A. $CH_3—CH_2—CH_2—C≡C—H$
B. $CH_3—C≡C—CH_2—CH_3$

C.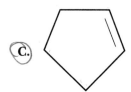

D. $CH_3—CH=CH—CH=CH_2$

157. If oxidative cleavage of B with hot basic potassium permanganate gives acetic acid and $CH_3CH_2CO_2H$ after acidification, what is the structure of B?

A. $CH_3—CH_2—C≡C—H$
B. $CH_3—C≡C—CH_2—CH_3$

C.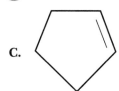

D. $CH_3—CH=CH—CH—CH_2$

158. Which of the following compounds does not dissolve when added to cold concentrated sulfuric acid?

A. $CH_3CH=CHCH_2CH_3$
B. $CH_3—C≡C—CH_2CH_3$
C. $CH_3CH_2CH_2CH_2OH$
D. $CH_3CH_2CH_2CH_2Br$

159. Which of the following would both decolorize bromine in carbon tetrachloride in the absence of light?

A. Alkanes and alkyl halides
B. Alkanes and alkenes
C. Alcohol and alkynes
D. Alkenes and alkynes

160. Which of the following reagents would be used as a first step in the conversion of cyclopentene to *cis* 1,2 cyclopentanediol?

A. Cold dilute potassium permanganate
B. Hot potassium permanganate
C. A peroxy acid
D. Ozone

161. With DNA replication, a difference between the leading and lagging strand is that the lagging strand is:

A. not synthesized until the leading strand is completely synthesized.
B. longer than the leading strand.
C. synthesized in fragments that are later joined together.
D. never used by the cell as a template for transcription.

162. Which of the following is most likely to occur in a cell infected by an actively reproducing virus?

A. Decreased synthesis of the host cell's protein
B. Breakdown of the host cell's ribosomes
C. Breakdown of the host cell's tRNA
D. Cessation of amino acid biosynthesis in the host cell

163. Energy production is the principal function of which organelle?

A. Nucleolus
B. Endoplasmic reticulum
C. Mitochondria
D. Golgi apparatus

164. In mitosis, daughter chromosomes pull apart and move toward opposite poles during:

A. telophase.
B. metaphase.
C. anaphase.
D. prophase.

165. What is the number of possible isomers for tetrapeptides containing one ala, one gly, one lys, and one val?

A. 4
B. 8
C. 16
D. 24

Passage IV (Questions 166–171)

The interaction of the human body with its external environment is based on the movement of nerve impulses from the peripheral regions of the body to the brain via sensory neurons and from the brain to the peripheral regions via motor neurons. This conduction of nerve impulses involves a complex series of changes in the ion content of the neurons that causes the generation of an action potential in a previously resting neuron. After a nerve impulse has traveled along the length of a neuron, it has to be conducted across the synapse. Several chemicals can block the conduction of nerve impulses at the synapse.

Once a receptor has been stimulated, the information must be conducted through a sequence of neurons. The transmission of a nerve impulse down the length of a neuron is an electrochemical process that depends on changes in the ion distribution. In general, the transmission from one neuron to another across a synapse is a chemical phenomenon involving the secretion of a neurotransmitter by the axon and the action of chemoreceptors in the dendrite.

An electrical, chemical, or mechanical stimulus may alter the resting potential of a neuron. The resting neuron is said to be electrically polarized. Excitory stimuli are thought to open sodium gates in the plasma membrane, allowing sodium to enter a cell and depolarize the membrane. Inhibitory stimuli hyperpolarize the membrane. When the extent of depolarization reaches a threshold level, an action potential wave may be generated, which is a wave of depolarization that spreads along the axon. As the action potential wave moves down the axon, repolarization occurs quickly. In the millisecond or so during which it is depolarized, the axon membrane is in an absolute refractory period, when it cannot transmit an action potential no matter how great the stimulus might be.

166. In what order are the following states seen during nerve stimulation starting with a resting nerve?

   I. Polarization
   II. Hyperpolarization
  III. Repolarization
  IV. Depolarization
   A. II, I, IV, III
   B. I, IV, III, II
   C. IV, III, II, I
   D. I, II, IV, III

167. Once depolarization is complete:

   A. Na$^+$ channels open.
   B. K$^+$ channels close.
   C. K$^+$ channels open.
   D. both A and B.

168. Which of the following statements about an action potential is true?

   A. It can be generated only with low level stimuli.
   B. It is an all-or-none phenomenon.
   C. It does not involve a change in permeability.
   D. All of the above.

169. As an action potential is generated, the nerves go through a period during which they do not respond to additional stimuli. This period is known as:

   A. the summation period.
   B. the refractory period.
   C. tetanus.
   D. the silence period.

170. An action potential would travel faster through:

   A. an axon with a small diameter.
   B. an axon with a large diameter.
   C. a nonmyelinated axon.
   D. a neuron lacking dendrites.

171. What is the effect of the myelin sheath on the transmission of nerve impulses?

   A. It increases the velocity.
   B. It decreases the velocity.
   C. It lowers the threshold potential.
   D. None of the above.

Passage V (Questions 172–176)

All bacteria contain DNA that is organized in the bacterial cell as a single circular chromosome. The bacterial chromosome contains all the genes necessary for its survival, metabolism, and growth. In addition, some bacteria have genes that render them pathogenic for humans and animals. Many bacteria possess an additional form of DNA molecule known as a plasmid, which is an independently replicating, closed circular double-stranded DNA molecule. Plasmids can be isolated from the bacterial cells in pure form and then introduced into other cells by a method called transformation, which involves altering the bacterial cell wall to make it permeable to the DNA molecules. Once a plasmid enters a cell, it is replicated and will be distributed to the daughter cells during cell division. A single cell can carry up to thousands of copies of a single plasmid. Many cells carry several different types of plasmid. Plasmids carry genes that are not required for the survival of a bacterium but may provide a selective growth advantage to it.

172. The fact that a plasmid replicates independently of the bacterial chromosome implies that the plasmid must have at least its own:

   A. transcription factors.
   B. ribosomes.
   C. origin of replication.
   D. DNA polymerase.

173. Plasmids can be removed from bacteria by a process known as t curing. Which of the following would be an effect of curing on the metabolism of the host bacteria?

   A. The bacteria will die.
   B. The bacteria will not be able to synthesize proteins.
   C. The bacterial chromosome will not be able to replicate.
   D. None of the above.

174. Salmonella typhimurium is a pathogenic organism. Select the experimental method or methods that prove that the ability of this organism to cause disease is primarily related to a plasmid.

   A. Curing to remove pathogenic traits.
   B. Treatment with DNase to remove pathogenic traits.
   C. Re-introduction of the plasmid in the cured bacterium to restore pathogenesis.
   D. Both A and C.

175. A plasmid is introduced experimentally into a bacterial cell. The resulting cell gains the ability to grow in the presence of ampicillin. You may conclude that:

   A. the plasmid contained the gene for resistance to ampicillin.
   B. the plasmid produces ampicillin so that the bacterial cell becomes insensitive to it.
   C. genes may play a role in resistance to antibiotics.
   D. both A and C are plausible.

176. Plasmids can transfer from one bacterium to another in nature by a process known as:

   A. transformation.
   B. transduction.
   C. conjugation.
   D. plasmid donation.

Passage VI (Questions 177–189)

The immune system is an essential component of the human body. It consists of cellular and noncellular components that interact with invading organisms and substances that are not native to the human body, clearing the body to maintain a state of health. Thus, health or disease can depend on proper functioning of the immune system.

Antibodies are highly specific proteins called immunoglobulins (Ig). They are produced in response to specific antigens. Antibodies are grouped in five classes according to their structure. At the constant end, the heavy chains of an antibody have amino acid sequences characteristic of the particular antibody class. They are: IgG, IgM, IgA, IgD, and IgE. In humans, 75% of the antibodies in the blood belong to the IgG group. IgG contributes to immunity against many blood-borne pathogens, including bacteria, viruses, and some fungi.

Transplanted tissues possess protein markers (major histocompatibility complex) that stimulate graft rejection, an immune response (launched mainly by T-cells) that destroys the transplant.

Humoral immunity is antibody-mediated immunity residing in the body fluids that is based on immunoglobulin proteins produced by B-lymphocytes. B-lymphocytes (B-cells) are a type of white blood cells responsible for antibody-mediated immunity. When stimulated, B-lymphocytes differentiate to become plasma cells that produce antibodies. T-cells are lymphocytes that are processed in the thymus. T-cells have a wide variety of immune functions but are primarily responsible for cell-mediated immunity.

177. Before an organism can cause disease, it has to deal with a number of nonspecific defenses of the body. Which of the following are nonspecific defenses?

   I. B-lymphocytes
   II. Antibodies in the blood circulation
   III. Lysozymes in the tears
   IV. Interferons
   A. I and III
   B. III and IV
   C. I and IV
   D. Only III

178. Which of the following statements about humoral immunity is incorrect?

   A. It is a result of proliferation of antibodies as a result of exposure to an antigen.
   B. It requires normal function of B-lymphocytes.
   C. After the first exposure to an antigen, a 1- to 2-week time interval is required for the humoral immunity to become evident.
   D. It requires normal function of cytotoxic T-cells.

179. Which of the following statements about T-lymphocytes are true?

   I. They mature in the bone marrow.
   II. A subpopulation of T-cells called suppressor T-cells are involved in regulation of the immune response.

   III. They secrete interleukins.
   IV. They secrete antibodies that have heavy and light chains.
   A. I and II
   B. II and IV
   C. II and III
   D. All statements are correct.

180. Some individuals with defective immune systems have antibodies in their circulation that have a defective heavy chain. Which of the following cells may be defective in these people?

   A. Macrophages
   B. Helper T-cells
   C. B-cells and memory B-cells
   D. Neutrophils

181. What are the five classes of immunoglobulins?

   A. IgM, IgA, IgD, IgG, and IgE
   B. IgA, IgD, IgB, IgG, and IgE
   C. IgG, IgB, IgE, IgM, and IgD
   D. IgM, IgG, IgD, IgL, and IgE

182. The class of an immunoglobulin is specified by:

   A. the molecular weight of its molecule.
   B. the constant region of its heavy chain.
   C. the constant region of its light chain.
   D. the variable region of its heavy chain.

183. The antigen-binding sites of an immunoglobulin molecule are at:

   A. the constant regions of the heavy chains.
   B. the constant regions of the light chains.
   C. the variable regions of both the heavy and the light chains.
   D. the constant regions of both the heavy and light chains.

184. Sometimes when a tissue is transplanted from a donor to a recipient, the body of the recipient rejects the transplant because it recognizes the transplanted tissue as foreign and mounts an immune response against it. What cells are responsible for this reaction?

   A. Neutrophils
   B. Macrophages
   C. Cytotoxic T-cells
   D. Helper T-cells

185. The metabolic activity of a neuron is controlled within the:

   A. axon.
   B. dendrites.
   C. cell body.
   D. nodes of Ranvier.

186. The enzyme phosphodiesterase (present in the cytoplasm) has which of the following activities?

   A. It stimulates cAMP activity.
   B. It inhibits cAMP activity.
   C. It recruits co-factors for cAMP.
   D. It acts as a coenzyme for cAMP.

187. The nature of the blood vessel wall is an important factor in both the maintenance of a steady flow of blood as well as rapid exchange of substances. The most elastic of the following blood vessels is the:

A.   posterior vena cava.
B.   aorta.
C.   pulmonary artery.
D.   mesenteric artery.

188. Na^+ movement in the kidney tubules:

A.   is influenced by aldosterone.
B.   requires active transport in the proximal convoluted tubule.
C.   occurs via passive diffusion in the loop of Henle.
D.   all of the above.

189. How many s and π bonds are present in the following compound?

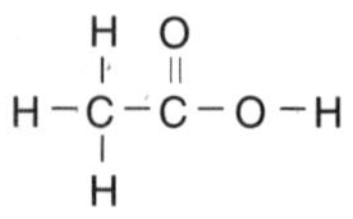

```
        H   O
        |   ||
   H — C — C — O — H
        |
        H
```

A.   Six s and two π bonds
B.   Six s and one π bond
C.   Seven s and two π bonds
D.   Seven s and one π bond

Passage VII (Questions 190–195)

The mammalian skeletal system consists of bones and cartilage. The human body comprises 206 bones that form movable and immovable joints. The movable joints are instrumental in locomotion and the immovable joints provide structural support. The human skeletal system is divided into the axial skeleton and the appendicular skeleton.

In the human body, the axial skeleton, located along the central axis, consists of the skull, vertebral column, ribs, and sternum (breast bone). The appendicular skeleton consists of the bones of the appendages, the upper and lower extremities (arms and legs), plus the bones making up the girdles that connect the appendages to the axial skeleton—the shoulder girdle and the pelvic girdle.

The human spine, or vertebral column, supports the body and bears its weight. It consists of 24 vertebrae, and two fused bones, the sacrum and coccyx. The regions of the vertebral column are as follows: cervical (neck), 7 vertebrae; thoracic (chest), 12 vertebrae; lumbar (back), 5 vertebrae; sacral (pelvic), 5 fused vertebrae; and coccygeal, also made up of fused vertebrae.

The pectoral girdle (shoulder girdle) consists of the two collarbones, or clavicles, and the two shoulder blades, or scapulas. The pelvic girdle consists of a pair of large bones, each composed of three fused hipbones. Whereas the pelvic girdle is securely fused to the vertebral column, the pectoral girdle is loosely and flexibly attached to the spine by muscles.

190. Which of the following structures is not a part of the axial skeleton?

   A. Vertebral column
   B. Skull
   C. Ribs
   D. Femur

191. An important function of the vertebral column is to:

   A. form blood cells.
   B. regulate the release of pituitary hormones.
   C. protect the spinal cord against physical damage.
   D. all the above.

192. The mandible is part of the:

   A. axial skeleton.
   B. appendicular skeleton.
   C. pectoral girdle.
   D. sacrum.

193. The ulna is a part of the:

   A. axial skeleton.
   B. upper extremities.
   C. pectoral girdle.
   D. lower extremities.

194. The humerus is an important bone of the appendicular skeleton. At its lower extremity, it ends at the elbow joint. Which of the following bones articulate with the humerus at the upper extremity?

   A. Femur
   B. Sternum
   C. Scapula
   D. Atlas

195. The sternum is found in which region of the body?

   A. Thorax
   B. Vertebral column
   C. Skull
   D. Extremities

Benzene belongs to a class of organic substances called aromatic compounds. The benzene molecule is highly unsaturated and although its formula (C_6H_6) indicates the presence of several double bonds, benzene does not show any behavior characteristic of alkenes. Benzene is a monocyclic conjugated molecule. It has a closed shell of six pi electrons that makes it unusually stable. Benzene is susceptible to electrophilic attack, but it undergoes substitution reactions rather than addition reactions. Substitution reactions allow the aromatic sextet of pi electrons to regenerate after attack by the electrophile, which retains the cyclic conjugation. Addition reactions, on the other had, tend to destroy the conjugation.

196. Which of the following choices represents the expected product for the following reaction?

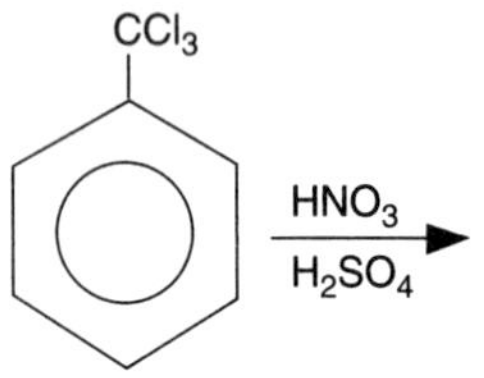

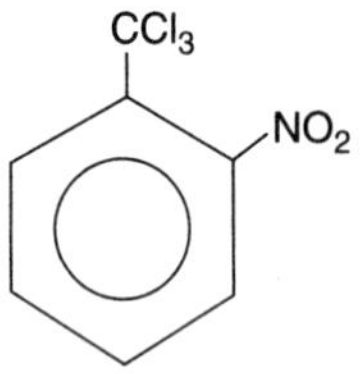

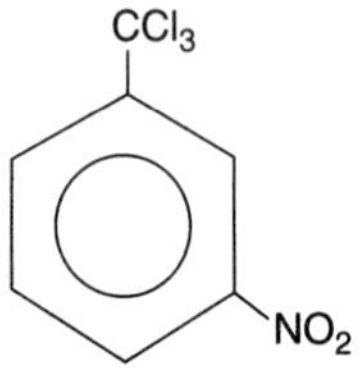

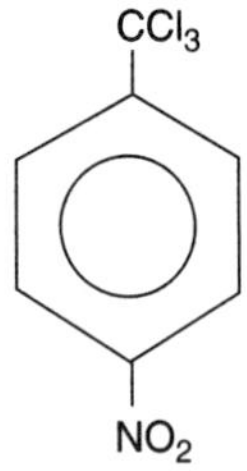

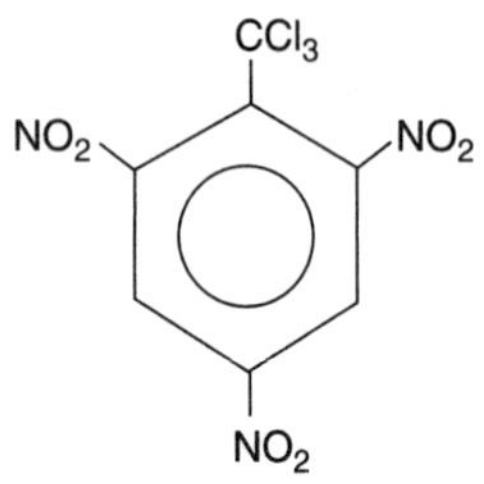

197. Which of the following choices represents the expected product for the following reaction?

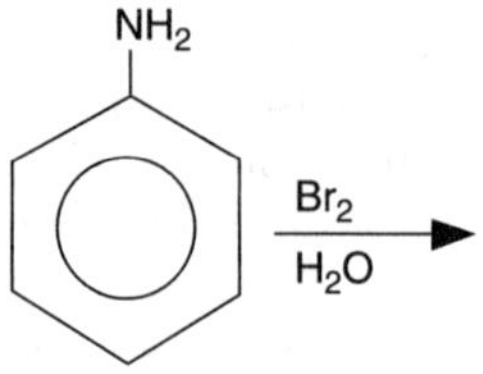

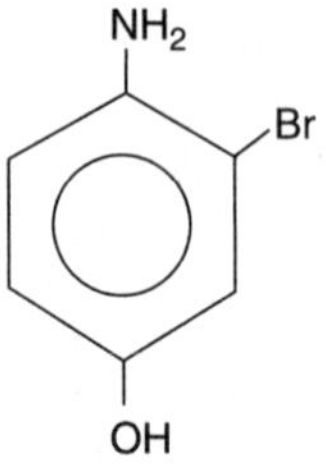

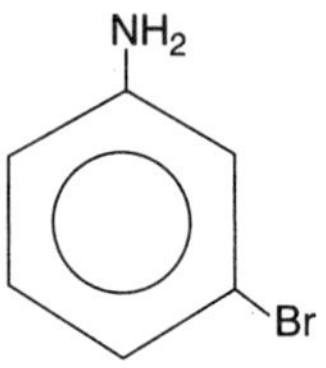

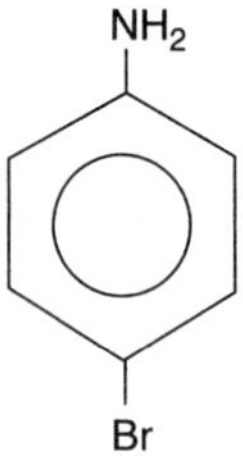

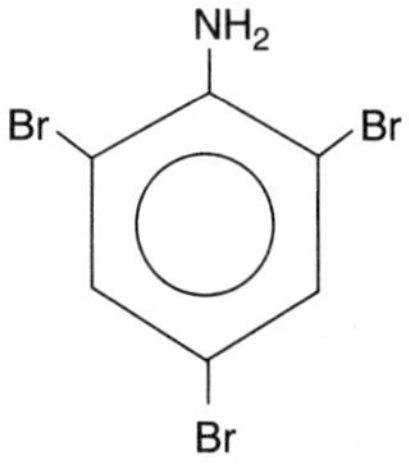

198. The most stable structure among the following resonance structures is:

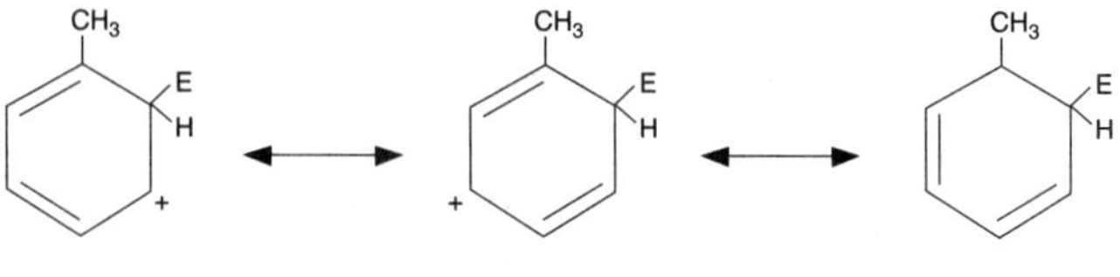

A. I.
B. II.
C. III.
D. all structures are equally stable.

199. The least stable structure among the following resonance structures is:

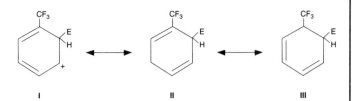

I   II   III

    A. I.
    B. II.
    C. III.
    D. all structures are equally stable.

200. Which of the following choices represents the expected product for the following reaction?

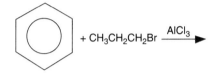

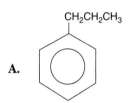

    A.

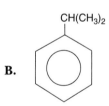

    B.

    C. A mixture of A and B, with A in greater
        amount
    D. A mixture of A and B, with B in greater amount

201. A muscle can atrophy if it is immobilized in a cast
for a long period of time. This type of atrophy is
known as:

    A. muscle fatigue.
    B. hypertrophy.
    C. denervation atrophy.
    D. disuse atrophy.

202. For the respiratory process to proceed normally, the
integrity of the alveoli must be maintained at all
times. A total collapse of the alveoli during expiration is prevented because of the presence of:

    A. surfactant.
    B. mucus.
    C. goblet cells.
    D. both mucus and goblet cells.

203. One potential mechanism leading to the various differentiation patterns is the:

    A. asymmetric distribution of cytoplasmic con-
        tents.
    B. asymmetric cleavage of the nucleolus.
    C. asymmetric replication of the mitochondrial
        DNA.
    D. none of the above.

204. A recessive sex-linked trait is usually expressed:

    A. only in females.
    B. only in males.
    C. more often in females than in males.
    D. more often in males than in females.

205. The NMR spectrum of ethyl chloride is characterized by:

    A. a triplet and a quartet.
    B. a doublet and a triplet.
    C. a quartet and a doublet.
    D. a singlet and a triplet.

Passage IX (Questions 206–211)

Reproduction is the process by which a species ensures its perpetuation. In humans, the female gametes, oocytes, are fertilized inside the female reproductive tract by the male gametes, spermatozoa. After fertilization, the zygote undergoes a complex series of developmental processes within the female reproductive tract. Because the reproductive tract of the female hosts all the events that eventually lead to the perpetuation of the species, it is important to understand its anatomy and physiology.

The female reproductive system includes the ovaries, which produce ova and the hormones estradiol and progesterone; the uterine tubes; the vagina; the vulva; and the breasts. After ovulation, the ovum enters the uterine tube, where it may be fertilized. The uterus serves as an incubator for the developing embryo. Fertilization restores the diploid chromosome number, determines the sex of the offspring, and triggers development.

Embryology (embryo development) involves a series of cell divisions, followed by the process of differentiation. A zygote formed by the union of a sperm and an oocyte gives rise to a multicellular organism with highly specialized organs that not only carry out specific functions but also coordinate with each other in an organized fashion.

206. The ovaries are the sites for the production of female gametes. Which of the following statements about ovaries are correct?

   I.   They are found in the abdominal cavity.
   II. Each human female has two ovaries.
   III. They are found in the pelvic cavity.
   IV. Their primary function is to produce ova and androgens.
   A.   I and II
   B.   II and III
   C.   I, II, and IV
   D.   II and IV

207. The thousands of structures in each ovary that give rise to ova are called the:

   A.   corpus luteum.
   B.   follicles.
   C.   ovarian cysts.
   D.   sertoli cells.

208. Which of the following statements about the ovarian follicles are true?

   I.   They are multilayered.
   II. They are single layered.
   III. They secrete estrogens.
   IV. They secrete androgens.
   A.   I and II
   B.   II and III
   C.   I and III
   D.   I and IV

209. Which of the following statements is true about the ovaries as they apply to a newborn female?

   A.   They are nonfunctional structures called ovules that develop into ovaries later on in life.

   B.   They contain primary oocytes that are arrested at prophase I of meiosis.
   C.   They produce only LH, not estrogen.
   D.   They produce testosterone for the first 10 days of life before initiating the production of other hormones.

210. The menstrual cycle marks the onset of puberty in the female. The first menstrual cycle means that:

   A.   pregnancy is possible even if ovulation does not take place.
   B.   a primary oocyte has completed meiosis I to form a secondary oocyte.
   C.   a primary oocyte has developed into tertiary oocyte and is ready for fertilization.
   D.   the corpus luteum has atrophied.

211. The rapid cell division that occurs in the early development of an embryo is called:

   A.   cleavage.
   B.   modulation.
   C.   blastulation.
   D.   meiosis.

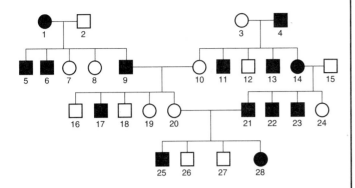

○ Healthy females

● Females with defect

□ Healthy males

■ Males with defect

The inheritance of a nonlethal genetic defect in a human family is illustrated. It is known that the defect is attributable to the inheritance of a single gene and not to spontaneous mutations in the various generations.

A birth defect is simply one that is present at birth. It may or may not be inherited. Some congenital abnormalities are inherited, and others are produced by environmental factors.

Within each chromosome are many genes, each generally different from the others, and each controlling the inheritance of one or more characteristics. Genes that govern variations of the same characteristics and that occupy corresponding loci on homologous chromosomes are called alleles. The fact that some alleles may be dominant and others recessive means that the alleles carried by an organism cannot always be determined by simply looking at the organism. The term used to specify the appearance of an individual in a given environment with respect to a certain inherited trait is known as its phenotype. The genetic constitution of that organism is called its genotype.

212. Which of the following conclusions is plausible?

   A. The defect is autosomal.
   B. The defect is sex-linked.

   C. Affected females have only one defective allele.
   D. Affected males have both defective alleles.

213. Which of the following statements is true about the genotype of individual 3?

   A. She has both normal alleles.
   B. She has both defective alleles.
   C. She has one normal and one defective allele.
   D. Insufficient information is provided.

214. Individual 5 has:

   A. both X and Y chromosomes.
   B. X chromosomes only.
   C. only one defective allele.
   D. both A and C.

215. The genotype of individual 6:

   A. has no defective allele.
   B. could have no defective allele.
   C. cannot be determined.
   D. has no defective allele and could not have a defective allele.

216. This trait is attributable to a:

   A. dominant allele.
   B. recessive allele.
   C. Y chromosome.
   D. dominant homozygous pair.

217. Why do males 17 and 26 show the trait?

   A. They have a depressed immune response.
   B. Their Y chromosome is dominant.
   C. They lack the dominant allele.
   D. They are homozygous for the allele.

218. One normal and one defective allele may be found in which individual?

   A. 13
   B. 14
   C. 20
   D. None of the above

219. The expected offspring of individual 9 with individual 4 would have:

   A. all normal males and females.
   B. all defective males and females.
   C. only defective males.
   D. only defective females.

Answers and Explanations

VERBAL REASONING

Passage I

  1. A The correct answer is found in the first paragraph, in particular with reference to Denmark.

  2. B In the first sentence of the second paragraph, the correct response is phrased in the conditional, using the term "potential," which is consistent with the author's tone.

  3. B In the first paragraph, the author writes that chip cards are increasingly replacing cash.

  4. D The second paragraph includes the fact that this system is a possible danger to personal privacy.

  5. C It is important to recognize that individuals would not have any reason to gather data and that the author is concerned about the individual maintaining privacy.

6. **C** The correct response can be either a vocabulary recognition problem or drawn from the context of "guaranteed records."

7. **C** Consider the contrasting information presented in the second and third paragraphs.

Passage II

8. **B** Although it is true that algal photosynthesis produces carbon compounds (response A), the question asks for the "effect" on coral.

9. **D** Although it is the correct response, test-takers dislike responses like D. The authors state that the definition of bleaching is tricky and then proceed to explain why by detailing the shortcomings of current incomplete definitions. These definitions all lack precision.

10. **A** The correct response is contained in the first two sentences of paragraph three.

11. **D** The relationship between corals and their algal symbionts is discussed in paragraph three. Response D is inverted; i.e., coral provide algae with carbon compounds.

12. **C** This analogy and the correct response are contained in the first paragraph.

13. **D** The correct response may seem too general, but examination of the fourth paragraph reveals that the other responses are either too specific or simply incorrect.

14. **A** The first paragraph addresses this question. The key term is "provide." Although coral reefs may exist in warm waters, they do not cause them.

15. **B** Corals are explicitly compared to sea anemones in the second paragraph.

Passage III

16. **C** The last sentence of the first paragraph offers a vital clue as to the author's purpose in presenting information on dating methods.

17. **B** The second sentence of the passage contains the necessary information.

18. **D** Use of the term "always" in response D should raise suspicions. A search through the paragraph reveals that there is no basis for assuming that zircons always survive metamorphic episodes.

19. **A** This first paragraph of the passage is essentially devoted to this topic.

20. **B** Re-read the second sentence of the second paragraph.

21. **C** The answer is provided in the third sentence of paragraph two.

22. **C** It can be presumed that the passage is an excerpt from a longer article and that while the uranium-lead method is the primary focus, the first sentence of the passage suggests that other methods have value and might be discussed later in the passage.

Passage IV

This passage discusses a series of predicaments, which the author calls paradoxes, related to the current war-making capabilities of the great powers. The core of the argument is that rational humans have created a so-called defense system that is essentially irrational.

23. **A** B is not stated in the passage, whereas D is false. C is a correct statement but is not the primary emphasis.

24. **C** Stated as paradox IV. D is not stated in the passage. A is incorrect and B refers to a "need" to develop weaponry when it is indicated that weapons are now stockpiled.

25. **D** The Age of Unreason is discussed in paradox II. Answer C is close, but the article states that it is "roughly half" instead of "more than half."

26. **C** II and III are not discussed.

27. **A** The example provides a paradox with two irreconcilable actions, which fits into the author's view.

28. **D** A and B are correct, but are not sufficiently comprehensive for the meaning of the quotation. C is incorrect. D addresses both economic and political concerns, and thus is closer to the meaning of the quote.

29. **B** In paragraph two, the author criticizes people for worrying more about raises and their neighbor's opinions than about the nuclear threat that could destroy the entire world.

Passage V

30. **C** The halo and disk are mentioned in the first sentence and the halo is specifically defined in the second sentence.